Life-span Cognitive Development

George W. Rebok

State University of New York, Geneseo

HOLT, RINEHART AND WINSTON

New York   Chicago   San Francisco   Philadelphia
Montreal   Toronto   London   Sydney
Tokyo   Mexico City   Rio de Janeiro   Madrid

To my family
and in loving memory of my grandfather,
George A. Rebok

Cover photo by John Giannicchi—Photo Researchers, Inc.

Library of Congress Cataloging-in-Publication Data

Rebok, George W.
  Life-span cognitive development.

  Bibliography: p.
  Includes index.
  1. Cognition. 2. Developmental psychology. I. Title.
BF311.R353 1987   155   86-21670

ISBN 0-03-064182-9

CBS COLLEGE PUBLISHING
Holt, Rinehart and Winston
The Dryden Press
Saunders College Publishing

Preface

I decided to write this book because of the rapid acceleration of knowledge about cognition and the growing prominence of a life-span perspective within cognitive developmental psychology. Over the past decade the number of publications on cognition and cognitive development has escalated dramatically, forcing students and instructors alike to master several theoretical viewpoints and disciplinary perspectives. However, most current textbooks offer the reader a very narrow view of cognitive development by emphasizing a single theoretical approach or age period. Even recent textbooks which claim to be comprehensive limit their topical coverage to childhood cognitive development, thereby giving students the misimpression that truly significant cognitive changes are confined to early life. It is the purpose of this textbook to provide students with a more balanced, truly comprehensive overview of the constantly changing process of cognitive development from infancy through old age.

The book is intended primarily for advanced undergraduate and beginnning-level graduate students enrolled in a single-term course in cognitive development, cognitive psychology, or the psychology of thinking. It is also appropriate as an adjunct text in courses on developmental psychology or life-span human development. Because many students will not have had background coursework in developmental psychology or cognitive psychology, the introduction summarizes the major approaches in these two areas.

Point of View

A broad life-span perspective on cognitive development seems especially appropriate at the present time in light of the increasing conceptual and methodological sophistication of developmental researchers. While the cognitive theory of Piaget dominated the field for many years and continues to wield considerable influence, information-processing theories now pose a serious challenge to structural models of cognition. Furthermore, developmental theorists increasingly recognize the need to integrate contextualistic notions into their models, regardless of their theoretical predilections. This book adopts a contextualistic perspective and stresses the need for theoretical pluralism. Although I have attempted to integrate various theoretical viewpoints when I can, much theoretical integration remains to be done. I also pay much more attention to methodological and design issues than is usually the case in childhood cognitive development textbooks. The latter emphasis reflects the sensitivity of life-span researchers to research methods that span long time periods and involve multiple sources of causation.

While I have tried to write a comprehensive life-span textbook, the knowledge explosion in the cognitive development field created a real problem in choosing appropriate material. My goal has been to cover the literature selectively and to emphasize topics in depth rather than to try to cover everything. In pursuing that goal I had to make many difficult decisions about what information to include and what information to exclude. The principal focus is on recent theoretical and empirical advances in cognitive developmental psychology, although pioneering contributions to the field are considered. The book also focuses on normal cognitive development in human beings rather than on abnormal thought or animal cognition. Because major gaps exist in our knowledge about life-span cognitive changes and continuities, I point out areas where data are lacking and where additional research is needed.

Content and Organization

A fairly general definition of cognition was used to select topics for this text. Areas of traditional emphasis, such as perceptual and attentional development, language, memory, problem solving, and intellectual development, are covered. So, however, are relatively newer and less emphasized areas such as spatial cognition, creativity, social cognitive development, and cognitive intervention. The book also relates the findings from research studies in these substantive areas of cognitive development to practical problems in everyday life contexts.

The author of a developmental text must decide whether to organize material chronologically, topically, or by age as well as topic. Each arrangement presents clear advantages and disadvantages. A chronological ordering allows the author to highlight the most salient developmental issues during particular age periods, whereas a topical ordering permits the author to present cognitive changes that characterize individual development over time or age. I have opted for the latter organization because it is most in line with my objective of presenting a coherent picture of cognitive developmental trends for each of the major content areas and age divisions across the entire life span. Moreover, in contrast to many child-oriented cognitive development texts, my book emphasizes not only age- and stage-related changes, but also cohort- and other time-related effects.

Learning Aids

Numerous learning aids are included in the book to promote student interest and understanding.

Box Inserts
Several box inserts are included in Chapters 2–10. These boxes draw attention to major issues, debates, innovations, and practical applications of cognitive developmental psychology. Each of these boxes was carefully selected to reinforce the themes discussed in the text. Some boxes deal with in-depth discussions of important research, for example Terman's longitudinal study of gifted men and women. Others focus on innovative theoretical developments, (for example Sternberg's triarchic theory of intelligence); practical models, (for example Pastalan's empathic model of perceptual changes); classroom exercises, (for example a concept learning problem); and exceptional cognition (for example skilled memory).

Chapter Overviews and Chapter Summaries
Chapter overviews introduce the major concepts and help students focus on the most important material. Each chapter ends with a numbered list of the key points in the chapter. These summaries highlight the major points to remember and help students consolidate the material from the chapter.

Definitions and Key Terms
Key terms are boldfaced in the text and concise definitions are given adjacent to each. A list of key terms is also provided at the end of each chapter.

Suggested Readings
Annotated lists of suggested readings at the end of each chapter are provided for students who wish to go into a topic in more depth. The readings enable students and instructors to keep pace with the current knowledge explosion in cognitive developmental psychology.

Comprehensive Glossary
A comprehensive glossary is included at the end of the text to assist students in defining key terms and concepts in cognitive development.

Test Bank

A comprehensive test bank has been developed by Cheryl L. Raskind. The test bank is available to all instructors who adopt *Life-span Cognitive Development*. The test item file consists of 20–30 multiple-choice questions per chapter plus several essay questions. These questions focus on conceptual knowledge as well as knowledge of factual material. They have been categorized as "basic," "moderate," or "advanced" to make them easy to use.

Acknowledgments

During the countless hours I spent preparing this book, I developed a keen appreciation for the indispensable roles played by so many individuals in making *Life-span Cognitive Development* a reality. I owe an incalculable debt to Margaret W. Matlin whose initial encouragement and enthusiastic support convinced me that I was capable of writing a textbook. Other colleagues and associates of mine also deserve special gratitude for reading initial drafts of the manuscript. I especially want to thank Kenneth Kallio, Shahin Hashtroudi, and Lynn Offermann for their constructive feedback and suggestions. Many colleagues and students shared information and articles that I used in the book. I would like to thank Jacques Chevalier, William Hoyer, Jerome Meyer, Paul Olczak, Leisa Welch, and James Van Haneghan.

Many other individuals made important contributions to this book. First, I wish to thank everyone at Holt, Rinehart and Winston for their unswerving support, hard labor, and attention to detail that made working with them a pleasure. Special thanks goes to my editors, Steve Helba and Alison Podel, for their tireless work to keep the writing and revising process moving smoothly and to Sondra Greenfield, Senior Project Editor, for her expert management of the copyediting and production. I also wish to thank the members of the production staff, Annette Mayeski and Stefania Taflinska, for their contributions to the finished product.

Vee Richardson and Linda Matthews of the Ability Group deserve special mention for expertly wordprocessing and proofing several drafts of the manuscript. Their perpetual good humor, patience, and understanding made even the most difficult times in the writing process more bearable.

I also want to thank my academic reviewers for their detailed comments and suggestions. Their insights proved invaluable as I revised various portions of the manuscript. The reviewers include Susan A. Todd, Bridgewater State College; Dean Richards, University of California, Los Angeles; John C. Cavanaugh, Bowling Green State University; Ross A. Thompson, University of Nebraska-Lincoln; Dana W. Birnbaum, University of Maine at Orono; David F. Hultsch, University of Victoria; David J. Townsend, Columbia University; Nancy L. Mergler,

University of Oklahoma; Thomas Mehle, University of Nebraska-Lincoln.

Finally, I want to thank Lynn for her love, support, and deep understanding. She patiently endured my all-too-frequent absences during the long writing process.

Contents

Life-span Cognitive Development

CHAPTER 1

Introduction

OVERVIEW

Psychologists who study cognition seek to understand how we gain knowledge and information about our physical and social world. The scientific study of cognition and cognitive development is important for many reasons: to learn more about human beings as thinkers, to understand other aspects of our lives and personalities, to improve human communication, and to develop effective educational programs.

Recently, scientific interest in the nature and development of cognitive processes has been so phenomenal that many psychologists believe we are in the so-called cognitive revolution. Even though the cognitive revolution is relatively new, scientific investigation of cognitive processes dates back over 100 years. Three factors have contributed to the cognitive revolution in psychology: (1) dissatisfaction with the behavioristic approach, (2) influence of the cognitive developmental work of Jean Piaget, and (3) advances in the fields of computer science and linguistics.

A second revolution—labeled the life-span revolution—has important implications for the study of cognition. The life-span view suggests that (1) our knowledge changes continually from infancy to old age, (2) there is a dynamic interaction between the developing person and the changing environment, and (3) development can take many forms and is determined by multiple factors. The life-span approach expands and enriches more static, age-specific views of cognition and behavior.

WHY STUDY COGNITION?

The acquisition of complex cognitive abilities is one of the crowning achievements of human development. Our abilities to organize and to remember information, to be self-conscious, to plan and be decisive, and to use symbolic communication are the skills which make us uniquely human. These cognitive skills allow us not only to gain information about our physical and social world but also to structure our experience in the form of complex rules and social organizations. Without these abilities, our present scientific and artistic achievements, technological advancements, and social-cultural systems would be unthinkable. We would lack a complex moral and legal code; a viable economic, political, and religious system; and unique family structures. We would have no education, mathematics, philosophy, or literature. In brief, we would have no humanity.

In our fast-changing modern society, sophisticated cognitive abilities have become increasingly important for leading effective, successful lives. It is not surprising, therefore, that investigators show great interest in the study of cognition and in how our cognitive skills develop and change with age. The growth in scientific interest in the nature and development of cognitive processes has been so phenomenal that one psychologist has defined the past two decades as "The Period of the Cognitive Revolution" (Sigel, 1981). Although some psychologists express concern about the extensive study of cognitive processes to the exclusion of other areas such as social and emotional growth, no psychologist can remain unaffected by the tremendous outpouring of work on cognition and closely related topics such as language.

Even if you do not plan to become a psychologist, the study of cognition and cognitive development can contribute to your knowledge and improve your life in many significant ways. For example, have you ever wondered why most people, young and old, occasionally experience lapses of memory, even though their mental apparatus remains intact? Do we forget a name or an appointment because we have failed to pay attention to the information? Is it because we are overloaded with too many things to recall? Or are we simply unmotivated to learn and remember the information in the first place?

We may also ask whether a poor memory has implications for other cognitive processes. Does memory ability play a significant role in problem solving, decision making, and other complex thinking skills? How does memory affect creativity and other higher-order thought processes such as wisdom? Is the reason young children fail to solve many logical problem-solving tasks related to basic cognitive processes such as memory and perception, or is it related to lack of experience with certain kinds of problems? Further, can anything be done to improve memory skills and enhance cognitive processing? What sorts of cognitive skills are required to become an expert memorizer?

One important reason to study cognition is to learn more about ourselves as thinkers and about how our thinking changes with development. The knowledge of one's own cognitive processes, termed **metacognition,** is currently a topic of great interest to cognitive developmental psychologists.

A second reason for studying cognition is that thinking is related to so many other aspects of our lives. For example, how we think about ourselves and our personalities is related to our cognitive state. The more complex the thinking skills we possess, the more abstract, differentiated, and internally focused our self-concepts and self-perceptions will be. Furthermore, disturbed patterns of thinking such as irrational belief systems or an inability to filter out irrelevant information may lead to abnormal personality disorders.

The study of cognitive development can also lead to better communication and improved social relations with other people. Indeed, as will be argued in Chapter 9, cognitive development is inseparable from social development. For example, the ability to understand the perspective of other people and empathize with them enables us to put ourselves in "another's shoes." It allows us to be friendly, kind, generous, and cooperative. Perspective-taking ability also can serve to stimulate a deeper level of communication with others. For example, two different perspectives can be shared "at the level of superficial information, at the level of common interests, or at the level of deeper and unverbalized feelings" (Selman & Jaquette, 1978, p. 274). Moreover, different perspectives can become generalized to form a societal perspective or a moral point of view.

Finally, the more we understand about the development of cognition, the better we will be able to develop effective training or intervention programs. For example, understanding cognitive development is important for estimating the potential effectiveness of various educational intervention programs such as Project Head Start.

In this chapter the recent surge of interest in cognition and the current major areas of concern will be examined. At the same time an emerging approach to the study of cognitive processes called life-span developmental psychology will be considered. We will examine why more and more psychologists are moving beyond the narrow confines of child psychology or adolescent psychology to answer questions about the nature of the human condition across the entire life cycle. But first we must define what psychologists mean by the concept of cognition.

THE CONCEPT OF COGNITION

Before describing the nature of the cognitive revolution that has occurred since the 1960s, we must know exactly what the term **cognition** means. In general, the term refers to "any process which allows an organism to know and be aware" (Wolman, 1973, p. 66). It encompasses processes by which we acquire, store, interpret, understand, and use information in the external environment as well as information stored internally.

Virtually every human activity involves cognition to a significant degree. In driving a car, we may be attending to road signs along the highway, trying to figure out a map, conversing with a friend, and listening to the radio. In reading this book, you are scanning the words on the page, relating the information to your knowledge, memorizing relevant material, and so on. Traditionally, everyday activities such as attending, remembering, and problem solving were described under the heading of *thinking*. However, thinking is a vague, imprecise term, and an understanding of these activities and processes is better conveyed by the term *cognition*.

As you will discover in Chapters 3–8, cognition cuts across a broad range of higher-order mental processes including perception and attention, spatial cognition and imagery, language, memory, problem solving and creativity, and intelligence; and in each of these areas there exist competing theoretical frameworks. Currently, psychologists disagree over whether cognitive processes are really different systems or are manifestations of the same underlying system explainable by the same set of principles (J. R. Anderson, 1983). Although we will present them as separate topics in this book, there is considerable overlap among different cognitive processes such as attention, memory, and problem solving. For instance, to solve a problem you must attend to the essential details, mentally represent the problem space, generate plans and strategies, remember previous solution attempts, and perform various reasoning operations.

Although it would not be desirable to exclude any of the above activities from the cognitive domain, it would not be difficult to expand the list of topics. Motor skills, learning, and social and emotional processes are just a few other topics that involve cognition to a significant degree. However, as Flavell (1985) indicates, once we start to implicate other higher mental processes in our definition, it is difficult to know where to stop. We would be hard-pressed to think of a human activity that does not implicate cognitive processes, at least to some extent.

In this introduction we will resist the temptation to limit the definition of cognition to a precise set of mental processes or mental contents. No simple definition can adequately convey the complexity of cognition and cognitive development. You can probably gain a better sense of the topic by understanding the origins of the cognitive revolution in psychology, and the guiding assumptions, principles, and methods of its researchers. Let us begin by defining what is meant by a "revolution" in scientific thinking.

SCIENTIFIC REVOLUTIONS

Many researchers in psychology and other scientific fields view the present state of knowledge about physical and psychological processes as the most advanced and most complex yet achieved. In certain respects, reaching our current level of scientific knowledge can be viewed as a process that parallels the achievement of the more sophisticated levels of cognition by the individual person (Piaget, 1978).

However, just as cognitive processes continue to change in individuals as they grow and age, so too does scientific thinking continue to develop in a society. As discussed in Chapter 2, some cognitive developmental psychologists believe that individuals undergo dramatic shifts or reorganizations in their thinking processes when their view of the world no longer conforms to reality. According to this view, thinking processes do not grow simply by adding more and more information, but they become different in their organization and structure.

In a classic essay entitled *The Structure of Scientific Revolutions*, T. Kuhn (1970) argued that science does not progress solely by accumulating more information or facts but also by undergoing **paradigmatic shifts.** These shifts occur when the information or body of data that scientists collect does not agree with prevailing ways of thinking about scientific phenomena. When this happens, scientists are sooner or later forced to abandon their old habits of thought and develop new models and theories, which give rise in turn to new paradigms. *Paradigms* are more general or global than theories and consist of the beliefs and concepts shared by scientific investigators. A famous example of a paradigmatic shift is the scientific revolution in astronomy that occurred when Copernicus successfully documented that the planets revolve around the sun, and the rotation of the earth on its axis is responsible for the rising and setting of the stars. The Copernican system replaced the Ptolemaic system, which considered the earth as the center of the universe around which the planets and stars revolved. (The Ptolemaic system remains useful for some navigational purposes.) In biology, the rise of Darwinian theory during the nineteenth century and the recent interest in molecular biology are other examples of major scientific revolutions (R. Lachman, Lachman, & Butterfield, 1979).

Although T. Kuhn's (1970) ideas have been criticized by other philosophers of science (e.g., Lakatos, 1978), they offer an excellent description of scientific activity and are appropriate to the study of psychology. According to Kuhn, scientific paradigms serve two principal functions: (1) they integrate knowledge and focus scientific attention on the most relevant problems, and (2) they provide a direction for future scientific work. It is important to note that the paradigms we will be reviewing in the next chapter cannot be objectively proven true or false. Rather, they should be seen as more or less useful to the scientist in providing a framework or context for investigation. At the same time, paradigms may blind the scientist to other ways of describing and understanding the world. A good example of this blinding process is the fact that Copernicus won few converts to his theory until almost a century after his death.

THE PERIOD OF THE COGNITIVE REVOLUTION

To help you understand the distinguishing features of the cognitive approach to psychology and what led to the cognitive revolution in psychology, we will review the history of cognitive study. A full review would be impossible because how knowledge is acquired is a centuries-old philosophical question. The discussion will be limited to scientific investigations into the nature of cognitive processes. Keep in mind that some psychologists tend to be more interested in cognition per se, while others are more concerned with how cognition changes with development. Nevertheless, as Neisser (1976) has emphasized, "No theory that fails to acknowledge the possibility of development can be taken seriously as an account of human cognition" (p. 62).

When scientific psychology began a little over 100 years ago, it was very concerned with such mental processes as sensation and perception, association, imagery, and attention—processes that help us acquire and use firsthand information about the world. It was also very interested in using scientific methods of analysis to study these mental processes. Toward this end, early experimental psychologists such as Wilhelm Wundt (see Figure 1.1) and Edward Tichener relied on a technique called **introspection,** which is the observation by the subject of his or

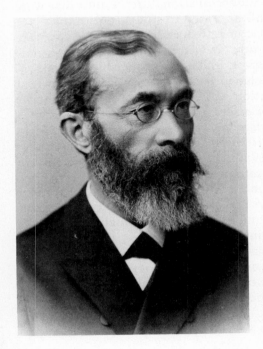

Figure 1.1   Wilhelm Wundt founded the first formal laboratory of psychology in 1879. He felt that psychology should concern itself with the contents of consciousness by using the method of introspection.

Photograph courtesy of The Bettman Archive. Reproduced by permission.

her thoughts and feelings. In our daily lives we often use an informal kind of introspection when we describe what we are seeing, remembering, or feeling. The form of introspection used in the early scientific laboratories was far different than the kind we employ in our everyday lives. In Wundt's laboratory, for example, subjects were trained to make at least 10,000 separate introspections before they were considered ready to participate in an experiment (Lieberman, 1979). Trained introspectors supposedly could report the content of their thoughts and the structure of their thinking system which produced the thoughts.

Although introspection gives some insight into the workings of our internal cognitive processes, it soon fell into disfavor as a scientific method. One reason for this was the impact of Freud's theories about the nature of the **unconscious,** the part of our mental life about which we are unaware. Introspectionism was based on the idea that all mental activity would be available for verbal report. However, Freud's ideas and the introspectionists' findings challenged this belief and raised serious questions about the accessibility of cognitive content and processes. A second problem was getting scientists to agree on the phenomena studied. Unlike other scientific methods which separate the observer from the object being studied, introspectionism depends on the observer's ability to report objectively on his or her own cognitive processes. When the objectivity of an individual's reports could not be verified by scientists through direct observation, further questions were raised about the usefulness of this approach to study cognition.

Scientific opposition to the use of introspection began to grow rapidly around the turn of the century. In place of introspection, a new movement called **behaviorism** arose under the leadership of John B. Watson in the United States. Behaviorism is a school of thought that stresses learning as the explanation of development. For behaviorists learning means the formation of *associations,* or connections between stimuli and responses. Behaviorism emerged as the reigning paradigm in American psychology in the 1920s and remained the dominant theoretical approach well into the 1950s. Behavioristic approaches remain popular today, especially in education and clinical work.

The scientific appeal of behaviorism rested in its insistence on studying observable external behaviors rather than the internal workings of the **conscious,** the aspect of our mental life about which we are fully aware. By ruling out complex intellectual processes, the behaviorist approach engendered a certain narrowness in theoretical focus, which limited its direct relevance to cognitive psychology. On the positive side, the behaviorist emphasis on carefully controlled and reliable research methods underscored the need for more methodological rigor in cognitive studies.

In the meantime, in Europe a second approach, called **Gestalt psy-**

chology, emerged to fill the vacuum created by the demise of Wundt's introspectionist approach. In many respects, Gestalt psychology was the forerunner of modern cognitive psychology, because it took as its subject matter the scientific study of mental events. Unlike Wundt, Gestalt psychologists believed that mental processes could not be analyzed into elementary units because wholeness and organization characterize such processes. In the famous Gestalt phrase, "The whole is greater than the sum of its parts." For example, they recognized that a musical melody is more than a sum of the individual notes.

The methods available to Gestalt psychologists at the time were not well refined. The lack of a rigorous methodology, coupled with upheavals in European society during the era of World War II, soon led to a standstill in the Gestalt psychology movement. In addition, many Gestalt psychologists who came to the United States were not accepted by native behaviorists. Elements of the Gestalt approach, however, still color contemporary theorizing about cognitive processes such as problem solving and creativity, as we will see in Chapter 7.

By the 1950s psychology began to undergo what T. Kuhn would label a paradigmatic shift. There was general dissatisfaction with the behavioristic orientation as a general theory of behavior. Particularly problematic was the behaviorists' tendency to generalize their findings from animal studies to human behavior. Another major problem was that behavioristic theories could not explain as broad a range of phenomena as originally presumed. For example, one of the best-known behavioristic theories is the interference theory of forgetting, which is discussed in Chapter 6. Many psychologists felt that interference theory could be used to fashion a general theory of forgetting, but research has yielded results that flatly contradicted the theory (Postman & Underwood, 1973).

The growing influence of Jean Piaget, the famous Swiss developmental psychologist, also had a great impact on the study of cognition. Piaget is best known for his work on children's cognitive development, and since the early 1920s had been producing a prodigious volume of work on the development of children's thought processes and how children's mode of thinking changes with development. However, psychologists in the United States were slow to accept Piaget's work, partly because his writings were often difficult to read and translate into English, but more importantly because Piaget did not use traditional experimental methodology to test his ideas. He relied instead on a technique called the **clinical method** to probe intensively the cognitive processes of individual children, very often his own three children. Using this procedure, Piaget asked children a series of loosely structured questions and followed up unexpected answers with additional questions. Although they were based on few subjects, Piaget's findings have a high degree of **generalizability,** which means that the results can be applied to individuals or cultures other than those he studied. The enormous impact of Piaget's work will become evident when his contributions are discussed in subsequent chapters.

At least two other intellectual cross-currents contributed to the so-called cognitive revolution in the 1960s. First, technological advancements in the previous decade led to increasing use of digital computers to carry out complex cognitive operations such as solving mathematical equations and playing chess. Psychologists quickly borrowed ideas from computer specialists and applied these concepts to the study of human **information processing**—that is, the acquisition, coding, processing, storage, and transformation of information. The computer technology not only allowed cognitive psychologists to develop working models of how the mind functions but also gave them an objective means of representing these mental events. Although questions have been raised about how closely computer programs mirror the functions of the human mind, the computer technology alleviated some of the subjectivity problems inherent in the introspection method.

The other major influence on the cognitive revolution stemmed from radical changes in the field of **linguistics,** which is the formal study of the structure of language. The behavioristic orientation in linguistics, dating back to the 1920s, started to give way to a more cognitive orientation. The clash of competing theoretical views was seen in the appearance of two books in the mid-1950s, Skinner's (1957) *Verbal Behavior* and N. Chomsky's (1957) *Syntactic Structures.* Skinner, the preeminent behaviorist, argued that language is acquired by learning, like any other behavior, whereas Chomsky proposed an abstract system of innate rules by which language is acquired and produced. By most accounts, Chomsky fared better in this exchange. His arguments, which are discussed in Chapter 5, formed the basis of the new cognitive developmental analysis of language.

Over the past decade, ideas about how cognitive processes are acquired and transformed have continued to be refined and developed. By the 1970s journals devoted to the investigation of cognition such as *Cognitive Psychology, Memory and Cognition*, and *Cognitive Science* appeared and gave impetus to the cognitive revolution. Many universities also established experimental laboratories to study cognitive processes, although some cognitive psychologists (such as Neisser, 1976) have urged that we begin to study cognition in the world outside the laboratory. As mentioned, the cognitive approach has been important in areas such as cognitive developmental psychology as well as in areas outside psychology such as computer science and linguistics. The approach is also having a growing impact on research in social and personality psychology (Sampson, 1981) and in the neighboring disciplines of biology, sociology, and economics. Figure 1.2 summarizes the major developments in the history of the cognitive approach to psychology.

In the brief span of the last 25 years, the cognitive approach has mushroomed into one of the most active and intellectually exciting research branches in psychology. Part of the appeal of this approach lies in its conceptualization of human beings as active seekers of information, who constantly search their environment for new information. This search is guided not only by previous knowledge but also by present goals and expectations (Moates & Schumacher, 1980). The acquisition of new information in turn modifies future searches for information, as you will read in Chapter 6 when we discuss the concept of the cognitive schema.

The cognitive approach assumes that people do not have an unlimited capacity to process novel information. We are limited by the number of items we can hold in memory at one time, the speed with which we can manipulate mental symbols, and our ability to search our memories for stored information (Siegler, 1983). To overcome these processing limitations, human beings develop various cognitive strategies such as rehearsing, organizing, and elaborating to-be-remembered information; using external memory aids (e.g., notes, tape recorders); and adopting problem-solving techniques (e.g., means-ends analysis, as discussed in Chapter 7).

Finally, the cognitive approach assumes the need to study internal mental processes in addition to overt behavior. Although internal cognitive activities cannot be observed directly, strong inferences can be made about the mental rules, organizations, and structures people possess by observing people's performance on various cognitive tasks. Experiments can then be designed to isolate these processes and allow us to explain and predict the type of behavior they will produce (Moates & Schumacher, 1980).

While enthusiasm for a cognitive approach to psychology and related fields continues to grow, another major revolution is under way—the life-span revolution. Because human beings interact continually from

Figure 1.2   Summary of the history of the cognitive approach to psychology.

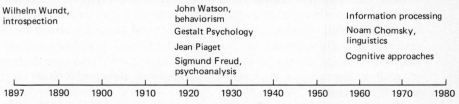

From *The Promise of Cognitive Psychology* (p. 10) by R. E. Mayer, 1981, San Francisco: Freeman. Copyright 1981 by W. H. Freeman and Company. Adapted by permission.

infancy through old age with their environment, their behavior and knowledge must be assumed to change in fundamental ways across the entire life cycle. Thus, to understand something about cognition, we must discuss how organisms learn and develop cognitively over time. To show how the cognitive and the life-span revolutions are related, we must review the history of the life-span developmental approach to psychology.

THE PERIOD OF THE LIFE-SPAN REVOLUTION

To help you appreciate the significance of the life-span revolution in developmental psychology, particularly the branch dealing with cognitive development, let us return to the origins of scientific psychology about 100 years ago. As you recall, Wundt had established a psychological laboratory to study complex mental events, much as a physicist studies the complex behavior of atoms and molecules. At about the same time, G. Stanley Hall, the founder of child psychology, set up the first experimental laboratory in psychology in the United States. Like Wundt, Hall was an experimental psychologist, but he focused his attention mainly on the child's developmental needs. Wundt, on the other hand, was more interested in the structure of the normal adult mind, which he sought to demonstrate by using well-practiced subjects. Hall's ideas, with their emphasis on individual development, were more in keeping with the United States **Zeitgeist**—the prevailing ideology and outlook characteristic of a particular time—and soon led to the establishment of child study laboratories around the country.

With these new laboratories came new paper-and-pencil questionnaire techniques that replaced the introspective methods Wundt had been using with adults. The use of these new techniques was stimulated primarily by a demand for basic descriptive information on children's development. However, there was also a growing demand for objective diagnostic tools that could be used in determining a child's mental level and progress in school. James McKeen Cattell, who had trained under Wundt, led the testing movement in the United States. Cattell introduced the term *mental test*, but his tests were very much in the Wundtian tradition in that they were primarily measures of sensory capacity, precision of discrimination, and reaction speed (Boring, 1950). These tests proved to be very poor predictors of school performance because they did not assess the verbal processing demands that confront schoolchildren.

Alfred Binet of France developed more appropriate tests for measuring school abilities. Binet had been commissioned by the Paris school system to develop an instrument that could be used to study children who were having learning difficulties in school. With Théophile Simon, Binet succeeded in producing the first successful "developmental" intelligence test. This test was called developmental because its items were arranged by difficulty level and were scored in terms of chronological and mental age. Binet and Simon's test was eventually translated into English by Lewis Terman at Stanford Univerity and became known as the Stanford-Binet test.

As the testing movement gained momentum, adults as well as children were assessed. Early tests such as the Stanford-Binet were not designed for adult samples, and this led to conflicting reports on the development of mental abilities across the life span. (Intellectual assessment will be discussed in Chapter 8.)

From 1920–1950, child psychology continued to grow rapidly in the United States. The behaviorist approach gave psychologists a promising means of modifying child development through the systematic application of learning principles. An opposite approach was taken by child developmental psychologist Arnold Gesell, who conducted extensive observational studies of children at the Yale University Clinic of Child Development. He concluded that maturation, rather than environment (or learning), is the most influential determinant of development. The maturation-environment debate is a central one in the history of developmental psychology, and it will be discussed in Chapter 2.

During the 1920–1950 era, the first concerted effort to establish a life-span orientation in psychology also began (Baltes, 1979). Prior to this time, there had been some scattered attempts to study developmental processes from infancy through old age. Most noteworthy are the studies conducted by the Belgian scientist Adolph Quetelet during the nineteenth century on the growth of creativity across the life span. Quetelet (1835) presented evidence that creative talent among English and French playwrights began to develop around age 21, peaked between the ages of 25 and 35, remained stable for several years, and then declined gradually after age 55. Quetelet was also probably the first investigator to employ the **cross-sectional method** of research, an especially important research tool in life-span psychology. In the cross-sectional approach, different age groups are compared on a particular behavior at approximately the same time.

Another way to study developmental change processes from infancy through old age is by using the **longitudinal method,** which investigates behavior changes in a single age group over two or more points in time. During the 1920s, research institutes such as the Institute of Human Development at the University of California, Berkeley, and the Fels Research Institute in Ohio began intensive longitudinal studies of children. As these children grew into adolescence and adulthood, the investigators became interested in studying life-span developmental changes in their mental abilities. Although these long-term longitudinal studies spanning 30–40 years are no longer common because of practical and financial problems, they served to focus investigators' attention on individuals as they grow, mature, and age. These studies also anticipated the current emphasis in life-span psychology on multidisciplinary investigations, since the members of their research teams included psychologists, sociologists, anthropologists, and geneticists.

The life-span movement advanced rapidly in the two decades after World War II, and two factors contributed to these gains. First, child psychologists became less interested in *empirical* studies of child development (studies based only on observation and experimentation) and more concerned with *theoretical* considerations of the concept of development. For example, developmental psychologist Heinz Werner (1957) proposed the **orthogenetic principle** of development, which states, "whenever development occurs, it proceeds from a state of relative globality and lack of differentiation to a state of increasing differentiation, articulation, and hierarchic integration" (p. 126). Inherent in this definition is the notion of *direction*—development involves a transition from very general minimally organized forms to well-organized highly specialized forms. An example of the orthogenetic principle can be seen in children's development of mental concepts. A child's first concept of animals may include only the general category "doggies." Every animal (and sometimes people) the child sees is called a *doggy.* Only later is the concept differentiated and organized in terms of specific categories (doggies, cats, cows) and subcategories (doggies, puppies; cats, kittens; cows, calves). A crucial question in life-span psychology today is whether differentiation of cognitive abilities continues into adulthood and old age, or whether dedifferentiation occurs, so that cognitive skills return or regress to an earlier, more generalized form (see Chapter 8).

Second, interest in the life-span approach to psychology was aided by the rapid development of **gerontology,** the systematic study of the aging process. Gerontologists emphasize that in order to understand aging, we need to examine what happens in earlier periods of development. It is thus not surprising to find that renowned gerontologists such as James Birren, Bernice Neugarten, and K. Warner Schaie advocate a life-span developmental approach to the study of aging.

As discussed, child developmental psychology progressed rapidly from the beginning of the twentieth century, but the psychology of adult development and aging made little progress until the late 1940s. Why were so few psychologists interested in studying aging processes? This lack of interest in the adult phase of the life span can be traced partly to widely shared beliefs among scientists and the general public about the nature of later life development. Traditionally, many people viewed adulthood as a stable plateau and old age as a downhill slide toward physical and mental deterioration. These beliefs are captured in such popular sayings as "Older is slower" and "You can't teach an old dog new tricks." We now know that older dogs *can* learn new tricks (although it may take them a little more time), and development occurs in old age as well as childhood.

The field of life-span developmental psychology became more highly differentiated as it grew and developed in the 1960s and 1970s. Life-span research is now conducted in a variety of areas such as cognitive development, social development, personality psychology, and in related disciplines such as sociology and anthropology. With this rapid expansion has come a recognition of the need to summarize and inte-grate current information. A series of conferences at West Virginia University has helped to clarify some of the major theoretical and methodological issues in the field (Baltes & Schaie, 1973; Datan & Ginsberg, 1975; Datan & Reese, 1977; Goulet & Baltes, 1970; McCluskey & Reese, 1984). And an annual review volume devoted to life-span development first appeared in 1978 (Baltes, 1978).

The recent explosion of interest in life-span theory and research her-alds the arrival of a new revolution in psychology—the life-span revo-lution. Although many psychologists have been won over to the life-span position, some psychologists continue to view development in *age-specific* terms; that is, they assume a static model of behavior and do not consider change across the entire age span. To see how a life-span view compares with age-specific views, three major assumptions of life-span psychology will be considered as they apply to cognitive development. As you read the next section, keep in mind that all of these assumptions are closely interrelated.

COGNITIVE DEVELOPMENT IN A LIFE-SPAN CONTEXT

Although the life-span approach is more of a general orientation to the study of development than a specific, coherent theory of development, several guiding principles or assumptions are shared by the life-span psychologists and serve as a basis for scientific investigations. To illus-trate how these principles pertain to the investigation of cognitive development across the life cycle, we can summarize them in the form of the following three major assumptions:

1. Cognitive development is a continual change process.
2. Cognitive development involves an interaction of person and context.

3. Cognitive development is a multidirectional and multiply determined process.

Each assumption is compared with the assumptions made by investigators who limit their interests to a specific phase or stage of development (see Baltes, Dittmann-Kohli, & Dixon, 1984; Huston-Stein & Baltes, 1976; Lerner, 1982).

Cognitive Development as a Continual Change Process

The first assumption of the life-span developmental approach is that the *potential* for cognitive development and change exists at every age period of the life span. This assumption contrasts with traditional biological growth models of development which assume that cognitive changes progress along a fixed path toward a final *end state* of cognitive maturity reached during adolescence. From the latter viewpoint, child cognitive development is seen mostly in terms of steady growth or progression. After a period of stability in young adulthood, a steady decline or regression begins that coincides with the biological deterioration of our bodies.

In the life-span view, no end state of cognition is assumed. Therefore, cognitive change and other types of development are viewed as continuing throughout life. Furthermore, cognitive growth and decline can occur during any period of development—infancy, childhood, adolescence, or adulthood (Labouvie-Vief, 1982). Considerable controversy surrounds the issue of regressive changes in development at various ages. Children, for example, often show temporary regression when solving a novel problem. They fall back on more elementary rules, a process which appears to be a necessary step in forming a more complex representational system. Of course, temporarily regressing does not necessarily guarantee further cognitive growth.

Older adults too sometimes appear to regress to an earlier level of cognitive functioning on various logical problem-solving tasks. However, much of this regression may be illusory in that older people may have had limited schooling or experience in dealing with certain types of cognitive problems relative to younger adults. We will return to this point when cohort effects are discussed.

Cognitive Development as an Interaction of Person and Context

In addition to the potential for continual change across the life span, cognitive development involves an interaction or intertwining of the person and context (or environment). Just as the person changes continually throughout the life course, so does the sociocultural context of development change. In age-specific models of development, such as the biological growth model, the role of context does not receive major attention. Rather, the emphasis is on universal cognitive changes or stages that occur regardless of the particular context or environment. Fortunately, increasing numbers of psychologists recognize the importance of social and cultural contexts in cognitive development. Contextual variables such as family environment, peer relations, and cultural membership now receive greater attention than they did 20 years ago.

The life-span approach places emphasis not only on immediate (or proximal) contexts of development, but also on past (or distal) contexts. This concern can be seen most clearly in the work on **cohort,** or generational, effects on cognitive development. The term *cohort* describes a group of persons born during approximately the same period of historical time—often a particular year, such as the cohort of 1950. Studies by Schaie (1979) and colleagues show that cohort membership is often more significant than age in explaining cognitive differences between different generations. For example, a 60-year-old person may perform more poorly than a 30-year-old on a test of intelligence because the older individual grew up during a time when such tests were not routinely given to all students in school. (More will be said about cohort effects in Chapter 2.)

Cognitive Development as a Multidirectional and Multiply Determined Process

One of the major objectives of life-span psychologists is to describe how children, adolescents, and adults change as they develop and to explain the determinants of these changes. From a biological growth model perspective, change is described as *unidirectional* and *cumulative.* In other words, cognitive changes occur in a fixed sequence of stages or steps that build on one another like a pyramid. Life-span psychologists regard stages of cognitive development such as those proposed by Piaget as an important set of cognitive changes, but not the only one. They see changes as more *multidirectional* and *variable.* The discrepant developmental patterns between two different types of intelligence—*verbal* and *performance* intelligence—are a good example of a multidirectional change function. Verbal abilities are those we use to define words or describe the similarity between two objects; verbal intelligence increases (or at least does not decrease) over the course of the life span. Performance abilities, which are based on skills such as arranging blocks to form a design or filling in symbols to match numbers, increase with age to adulthood and then show decline in later life.

Figure 1.3 illustrates the differences between a unidirectional and

Figure 1.3   Multidirectional conception of life-span development. Four hypothetical examples of behavior-change processes varying in terms of onset, duration, termination, and directionality over the life course.

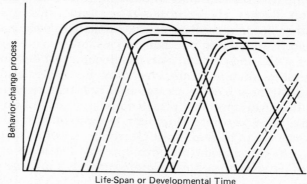

From "Life-Span Developmental Psychology" by P. B. Baltes, H. W. Reese, and L. P. Lipsitt, 1980, *Annual Review of Psychology, 31*, p. 73. Copyright 1980 by Annual Reviews Inc. Reprinted by permission.

multidirectional conception of development. The figure shows that behavior-change patterns for an individual can differ in direction as well as onset, duration, and termination. Thus, a behavior-change process—intelligence, for example—may show various developmental trajectories depending on the intellectual abilities involved. Certain intellectual abilities (such as performance skills) may appear earlier than other abilities (such as verbal skills) in the individual's history; and if intellectual abilities decline, they do so at varying times and rates. No single curve or pathway can adequately capture this multidirectionality of development.

As reflected in Figure 1.3, differences exist within individuals in their cognitive change processes at every age. A comprehensive understanding of life-span cognitive development also requires information about variability between individuals, or *interindividual differences.* As a rule, greater interindividual differences in cognition occur with increasing age and experience. Because interindividual variability characterizes life-span development, explanations of cognitive change processes become more complex than in biological growth models of childhood development where homogeneity and universality of change is assumed. Consider that certain biological and environmental changes closely linked with chronological age (such as maturation of the nervous system, entry into school) may explain how children develop cognitively. On the other hand, adult cognitive development may be better understood by examining life events—such as job promotions, family changes, and serious illnesses—not related directly to chronological age. Thus, life-span cognition is a multiply determined process.

We have examined how a life-span view compares with static, age-specific views of cognitive development. Keep in mind that a life-span approach does not compete with, so much as complement and enrich, age-specific approaches. For example, Piaget's stages of children's cognitive development, culminating in adolescence, are much more meaningful when viewed in a total life-span context.

The next chapter focuses on the theories and methods used by psychologists to study cognitive development. Once again, the usefulness of a life-span framework for describing and understanding cognitive change processes will be underscored.

SUMMARY

1. Cognitive abilities enable us to obtain information about our physical and social environment, and they help us to organize our experience in terms of complex rules and social systems.

2. *Cognition* is defined as a process that allows the organism to know and be aware. It includes topics such as perception and attention, spatial cognition and imagery, language, memory, problem solving and creativity, and intelligence.

3. Because cognitive abilities are important for leading successful lives in a changing society, there is great interest in the study of the nature and development of cognitive processes. Many psychologists believe that the past two decades have witnessed the cognitive revolution.

4. Scientific revolutions or paradigmatic shifts occur when the weight of the scientific data does not conform to existing ways of thinking about the world.

5. Scientific paradigms focus investigators' attention on the most relevant problems and provide a direction for future research. However, they may also blind scientists to other viewpoints.

6. Scientific investigations of cognitive processes date back over 100 years, but interest in how knowledge is acquired is centuries old.

7. Early experimental psychologists such as Wundt used a technique called introspection, which required practiced adult subjects to report on their cognitive processes while performing a laboratory task.

8. Two major problems with introspection are that unconscious processes are not available for verbal report and that there are no objective means of verifying the reports.

9. Behaviorism arose in opposition to the introspectionist approach. Behaviorists insisted on studying observable behaviors, rather than conscious and unconscious cognitive functions.
10. Three major factors have contributed to the cognitive revolution in psychology: (1) recognition of the limitations of the behaviorist approach, (2) the impact of Piaget's work on children's cognitive development, and (3) developments in disciplines such as computer science and linguistics.
11. Another scientific revolution—the life-span revolution—is beginning to have a major impact on the study of cognition as well as other types of development.
12. Prior to the life-span revolution, investigators in the United States focused on testing children's mental development and describing and modifying children's behaviors.
13. Factors contributing to the life-span revolution in psychology include (1) the development of children into adults in long-term longitudinal studies, (2) increased scientific concern with defining the concept of development, and (3) the rapid growth of the field of gerontology.
14. Many psychologists now take a life-span approach to the study of developmental changes, but some view behavior in terms of a specific age group such as children, adolescents, or adults.
15. Life-span psychologists make three principal assumptions about the nature of cognitive development. They view cognitive development as (1) a continual change process, (2) an interaction of person and context, and (3) a multidirectional and multiply determined process. These views complement those held by psychologists who take an age-specific approach to cognitive development.

Key Terms

metacognition

cognition

paradigmatic shifts

introspection

unconscious

behaviorism

conscious

Gestalt psychology

clinical method

generalizability

information processing

linguistics

Zeitgeist

cross-sectional method

longitudinal method

orthogenetic principle

gerontology

cohort

Suggested Readings

Baltes, P. B., Reese, H. W., & Lipsitt, L. P. (1980). Life-span developmental psychology. *Annual Review of Psychology, 31*, 65–110. This first review chapter in the *Annual Review of Psychology* series on life-span development contains a clear, cohesive treatment of the theoretical and methodological assumptions of the life-span approach with illustrations in selected topical areas such as memory and intellectual development.

Flavell, J. H. (1985). *Cognitive development* (2nd ed.). Englewood Cliffs, NJ: Prentice-Hall. A well-written scholarly overview of cognitive development from infancy to young adulthood. The emphasis is on Piaget's work, but other approaches are considered, most from an information-processing view.

Gardner, H. (1985). *The mind's new science: A history of the cognitive revolution.* New York: Basic Books. A fascinating look at the cognitive revolution that has swept through psychology and other related disciplines since the 1950s. The book reviews historical work in individual cognitive sciences such as artificial intelligence and linguistics as well as current work in perception, mental imagery, categorization, and reasoning which may lead to a single unified cognitive science.

Gelman, R. (1978). Cognitive development. *Annual Review of Psychology, 29*, 297–332. In this chapter reviewing the research literature on preschoolers' cognitive capacities, Gelman recommends that we focus more on what young children can do cognitively, rather than limit ourselves to what they cannot do.

Kuhn, T. S. (1977). *The essential tension.* Chicago: University of Chicago Press. A collection of selected essays on scientific tradition and the nature of scientific change. Although fairly technical in development, this work clarifies issues raised in T. Kuhn's (1970) *The Structure of Scientific Revolutions.*

Neisser, U. (1967). *Cognitive psychology.* New York: Appleton-Century-Crofts. The book that perhaps more than any other helped provide an integrated framework for the field of cognitive psychology. Though nondevelopmental and focused primarily on perceptual processes, it clearly describes the basic assumptions of the information-processing model of cognition.

Rybash, J. M., Hoyer, W. J., & Roodin, P. A. (1986). *Adult cognition: Processing, thinking, and knowing.* Elmsford, NY: Pergamon. This recent text reviews research and theory on information processing, knowledge representation, and formal and postformal models of cognitive development. Emphasis is placed on the observable strengths of adult cognition. Well worth reading.

Wolman, B. B., & Stricker, G. (Eds.). (1982). *Handbook of developmental psychology.* Englewood Cliffs, NJ: Prentice-Hall. A comprehensive and up-to-date handbook that covers development over the entire human life span. Among its 50 chapters are chapters on cognitive theory, life-span development, and cognitive development in infancy, childhood, adolescence, and adulthood.

CHAPTER 2

Theories and Methods in the Study of Cognitive Development

OUTLINE

OVERVIEW

Psychologists generate theories to explain and predict specific aspects of human behavior. In this chapter we discuss four different theoretical approaches for studying and understanding the nature of cognitive change across the life span. The close interplay between theories of cognitive development and the methods used to study them will also be examined.

In the first section we consider organismic developmental theories. Organismic developmental theorists such as Piaget and Werner view cognitive development as movement through a series of distinct stages or steps which the organism actively constructs through interactions with the world. A second major approach to cognitive development, information processing, is then discussed. From an information-processing perspective, cognitive development results from changes in the way organisms acquire, store, and respond to information.

Two other approaches for studying cognitive changes are also considered: behavioristic and contextualistic. Behavioristic theorists conceptualize cognitive development as a gradual accumulation of specific learning experiences. The contextualistic approach emphasizes the effect of context variables such as the social environment and culture on cognitive processes. Regardless of their theoretical orientation, cognitive developmental psychologists are increasingly incorporating contextualistic notions into their models.

All four approaches are compared as to how they describe general dimensions of cognitive change. For example, theories may describe change as structural (a change in organization) or behavioral (a change in selected behaviors).

Next nature and nurture are discussed in relation to cognitive development. There is considerable controversy about the role each plays in explaining the causes of cognitive change. As an alternative to the nature-nurture controversy, we consider cognitive developmental changes that possess species-adaptive value, regardless of cause.

The following section considers methodological problems in describing and explaining cognitive developmental changes across the life span. Three developmental research designs—cross-sectional, longitudinal, and sequential—are presented with their relative strengths and weaknesses. The final sections examine methodological issues in sampling subjects and choosing measurement instruments.

VARIOUS PSYCHOLOGICAL THEORIES

Psychological theories are a lot like diamonds. On the surface they often appear alike, with each possessing similar value. However, when their facets are examined, substantial differences emerge. Even the same theory viewed from a slightly different angle may reflect an entirely new meaning to an astute observer.

In this chapter various psychological theories are examined as they pertain to the study of cognitive development. You will discover that the majority of these theories are diamonds in the rough. They have potential value, but need considerable refinement and polish. We will also look at the various methods psychologists use to study cognitive development. Although methodological issues often attract the greatest interest among researchers, students frequently view methodology as peripheral and confusing. Indeed, the famous cognitive psychologist George Miller once remarked that methodological issues are bread and butter to the working scientist, but can be spinach to everyone else (R. Lachman, Lachman, & Butterfield, 1979). An attempt will be made to avoid such problems here by focusing on the methods that are most important in investigating cognitive processes across the life span.

Before we present the various theoretical approaches, some terms should be clarified. In Chapter 1 the term *paradigm* was used to refer to the system of beliefs, concepts, and ideas shared by scientific investigators. Paradigms guide the selection of hypotheses, methodologies, and analysis procedures and help scientists to organize and study the world. In the scientific literature, paradigms are referred to as presuppositions, cosmologies, world views, or world hypotheses (T. Kuhn, 1970; Overton, 1984; Overton & Reese, 1973; Pepper, 1942).

Paradigms are more general and global than **theories.** A paradigm consists of a shared belief system, whereas theories are designed to provide specific explanations for scientific phenomena (Achenbach, 1978). Thus, two scientists who share the same paradigmatic orientation may adopt different theoretical frameworks. Piaget's and Freud's theories can be used to illustrate this point. Both theorists shared similar paradigmatic assumptions about development (e.g., development is stage-like), but Piaget emphasized cognitive development and Freud emphasized emotional development.

At an even more specific level, we encounter **hypothetical constructs,** which are concepts invented to describe and explain relationships among events, objects, properties, or variables (P. Miller, 1983). The cognitive structures (e.g., mental schemes, mental operations) proposed by Piaget are good examples of hypothetical constructs. Although such structures cannot be observed directly, their existence can be inferred by observing external behavior. More will be said about the concept of structure later in this chapter.

The following sections present four different theoretical approaches for studying and understanding the nature of cognitive processes. The (1) organismic developmental and (2) information-processing approaches represent the most important contemporary frameworks for the study of cognition. The (3) behavioristic and (4) contextualistic approaches are also discussed; the former is more representative of psychology's recent past and the latter its possible future. You will find that each of the four perspectives differs in how it accounts for cognitive change processes over time. You will also discover why the first three frameworks—organismic developmental, information-processing, and behavioristic—have become increasingly contextualistic in their orientation.

ORGANISMIC DEVELOPMENTAL APPROACHES

Organismic developmental approaches assume that cognitive change processes are similar to organic processes. Just as biological processes (breathing, eating, sleeping) enable us to adapt and survive in our changing world, cognitive processes (memory, problem solving, intelligence) are organized or structured to perform a similar adaptive function. Indeed, much of our psychological functioning grows out of our biological functioning. In order to understand changes in our cognitive activities, it is necessary to look at the cognitive system as an organized *whole*, rather than as a set of constituent *parts*.

An additional assumption of organismic developmental positions is that the whole is always in a state of transition from one distinct level of organization to the next; and cognitive development, like physical development, progresses in a fixed sequence of qualitatively distinct levels or *stages*. For example, in physical growth, infants crawl before they walk; in cognitive growth, they utter single words before they construct grammatically complex sentences. Each stage builds on the preceding stage(s) and makes subsequent stages possible. Stages cannot be skipped or moved through in reverse order.

From the organismic developmental perspective the organism is structured physically and psychologically to reach a final, *end state* of development. In terms of individual physical growth, the end state is biological maturity reached in late adolescence. In cognitive development, the end state is complex, abstract thought as exemplified by Piaget's stage of formal operations.

The organismic, or organic, view of development can be traced to the early Greek philosophers. It can be found in Plato's idealism and the notion that contemplation (reflective thought) is the ideal goal, or end state, of human existence. This view also can be found in the writings of the German philosopher Immanuel Kant, who spoke of a "natural purpose" to development—a goal toward which organisms are propelled because of their nature. Darwin's theory of evolution of the species, with its emphasis on adaptive characteristics, was another major precursor.

A key tenet of organismic approaches is that human beings are inherently active in their pursuit of the final goal, or end state, of development. Overton and Reese (1973) label this view the *active organism model* of psychology. According to this model, human beings provide the source of their actions in the world rather than the world providing the source of all human action (Lerner, 1986). Through their actions or, more precisely, interactions with the world, humans construct their own experience and knowledge. Philosophically, this is a **constructivist view**; it contrasts with mechanistic views, which consider all knowledge to be copied directly from external experience.

When organisms interact with their environment, two opposing tendencies arise. On the one hand, organisms strive to maintain continuity in order to conserve their organization, but at the same time they transform this organization into novel, or *emergent*, forms. By "emergent" we mean that a higher, more complex stage of organization cannot simply be reduced to a lower, less complex one. Thus, discontinuities or qualitative differences in development emerge at each new stage. For instance, a 1-month-old infant's behavior may be explained on the basis of simple reflexes and stimulus-response connections, whereas a 2-year-old's behavior may be better understood in terms of symbolic, representational ability. This representational capacity may enable the older child to engage in novel behaviors, such as imitating a model over a long time delay, that are impossible for the young infant. Attempting to reduce the 2-year-old's activity to the level of organization shown at 1 month of age would be inappropriate because representational skills are not present at the earlier stage (Lerner, 1986).

Let us summarize the major features of the organismic position:

1. Human beings are seen as organized or integrated *wholes*.
2. Development proceeds through a series of qualitatively distinct *stages*.
3. Development is directed to a final ideal *end state*.
4. Organisms are *active* in their construction of knowledge.
5. Novel, or *emergent*, forms of development result from interactions with the environment.

To remember these five points, think about them as being logically consistent and interrelated. If you accept one assumption, you must be able to accept the entire set of assumptions. In the next sections we review the organismic developmental theories of two prominent psychologists—Jean Piaget and Heinz Werner. Try to become aware that although their ideas are consistent with organismic developmental approaches, their theoretical orientations are somewhat different.

The Impact of Piaget

Piaget's theory is the best known theory of cognitive development. His work has had an enormous impact not only on psychologists but on philosophers and educators. Although Piaget's ideas have been increasingly challenged, they will probably continue to influence cognitive developmental researchers for years to come. We can give only a modest glimpse of Piaget's monumental achievement. In order to fully grasp his theory, one would need to devote a lifetime of study to it. To understand the theory it is helpful to know something about Piaget (see Figure 2.1).

By any standard, Piaget (1896–1980) was a precocious youngster. By the age of 10 he had published his first scientific paper, a one-page article on an albino sparrow he observed in a park. He also developed a keen interest in the study of mollusks (shellfish), which led to several more publications and an offer to serve as curator of the mollusk col-

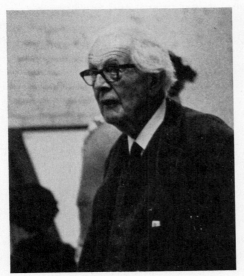

Figure 2.1 Jean Piaget revolutionized our understanding of cognitive development in children.

Photograph courtesy of Bill Anderson/Monkmeyer Press Photo Service. Reproduced by permission.

lection at a natural history museum in Geneva, Switzerland. He declined the offer because he had not yet finished high school!

In 1918, at age 21, Piaget received a doctorate in biology from his hometown university, Neuchâtel. Although he loved biology, he also expressed a deep interest in philosophical issues. During his years as a graduate student, he published a philosophical novel and several articles on philosophy. In these publications one can find seeds of many of his later ideas such as the organization of actions, part-whole relationships, and equilibrium and disequilibrium (P. Miller, 1983).

Finding experimental biology too restrictive and philosophy too speculative, Piaget turned to the field of psychology. His first job in psychology was in Alfred Binet's laboratory in Paris. Piaget worked on standardizing Binet's tests of intelligence, but initially showed little enthusiasm for this task. Piaget was not interested in a child's ability to give the correct answer to a test item, but in the cognitive processes which the child used to produce answers. He noticed that children of similar ages gave the same kinds of incorrect answers and used similar reasons in justifying their responses. It struck Piaget that younger children are not simply "less bright" than older children, but that they understand the world in a qualitatively different way. With this realization, Piaget rejected the entire mental testing approach and set about developing an entirely new approach to studying intelligence.

In pursuing his ideas on cognitive development, Piaget turned to the branch of philosophy called **epistemology.** Epistemology deals with the processes of knowing and the nature of knowledge. Piaget's interests centered on how knowledge is acquired and how changes occur in the relationship between the knower (organism) and the known (environment). To be precise, Piaget can be characterized as a *genetic epistemologist.* "Genetic" here refers not to inborn or innate qualities, but to emergence or development. By studying the development of knowledge and the nature of knowing, Piaget thought he could provide answers to many of the classic epistemological questions dealing with space, time, causality, and quantity. For example, how do children develop the knowledge of themselves as an object bounded by but separate from other objects in space?

In order to study the development of children's thought processes, Piaget renounced the use of standardized intelligence tests. He felt that such tests created "artificial channels of set questions and answers," and (as you recall from Chapter 1) he pioneered the development of the *clinical method,* which "encourages the flow of spontaneous tendencies" (Piaget, 1926, p. 4). Piaget argued that each child understands questions in a different way and to ask questions appropriate to the child's level, the content must be modified accordingly. A sample segment from a clinical interview with a 6-year-old child is shown in Box 2.1.

Box 2.1   A Sample Clinical Interview

Q: How did the sun begin?
A: *It was when life began.*
Q: Has there always been a sun?
A: *No.*
Q: How did it begin?
A: *Because it knew that life had begun.*
Q: What is it made of?
A: *Of fire.*
Q: But how?
A: *Because there was fire up there.*
Q: Where did the fire come from?
A: *From the sky.*
Q: How was the fire made in the sky?
A: *It was lighted with a match.*
Q: Where did it come from, this match?
A: *God threw it away. . . .*
Q: How did the moon begin?
A: *Because we began to be alive.*
Q: What did that do?
A: *It made the moon get bigger.*
Q: Is the moon alive?
A: *No. . . . Yes.*
Q: Why?
A: *Because we are alive. . . .*

From *The Child's Conception of the World* (pp. 258–259) by J. Piaget, 1929, New York: Harcourt, Brace & Company. Copyright 1960 by Routledge & Kegan Paul Ltd. Reprinted by permission.

One of the major reasons for Piaget's success with this technique was his perceptive observational skill. He spent hours observing the behavior of his own children, Lucien, Laurent, and Jacqueline. Other researchers criticized Piaget because he based much of his initial theorizing on his children. Piaget believed that such criticisms were less important than the rich data that he was able to collect on children's thought processes.

Overview of Piaget's Theory

We begin by describing several general features of Piaget's theory of intelligence. More specific aspects will be given later. First, what did Piaget mean by the word *intelligence?* For him intelligence is a form of *biological adaptation*, a kind of biological achievement that allows us to survive and adapt to the environment. Adaptation at a psychological level implies that the organism attains a cognitive balance, or *equilibrium*, with the environment. This notion is similar to the biological notion of homeostasis, whereby the organism strives for harmony with its surroundings. In interactions with the world, an equilibrium is not achieved immediately, but requires a series of successive adaptations, each allowing for more effective interaction. These successive shifts in equilibrium to increasingly higher adaptive levels are called **equilibration.**

The concept of equilibration can be illustrated with Piaget's conservation-of-liquid problem. This problem (discussed more fully in Chapter 7) deals with children's judgments about the amount of liquid in containers of different sizes. Typically, preschoolers say that after water is poured from one container into a taller and thinner one, the taller one contains more liquid. Thus, for preschoolers, amount of liquid is a function of height. Their thinking, though cognitively immature, can be said to be in an equilibrium. Eventually children notice that the new container is not only taller but also thinner; this realization leads to cognitive conflict and disequilibrium. Cognitive equilibrium is restored at a more advanced level when children can consider both height and width at the same time. That is, they can understand that height compensates for width and that the amount of liquid is *conserved* (remains unchanged).

Piaget saw the equilibration process as one of the most important parts of his theory. Indeed, he argued that all significant cognitive developmental advances result from some form of equilibration. However, many development psychologists have criticized the concept because of its vagueness and elusiveness (A. Siegel, Bisanz, & Bisanz, 1983). They argue that Piaget did not describe the nature of the interaction between the developing organism and the environment. Moreover, he was not explicit about the time span covered by the concept. Equilibration appears to encompass both moment-to-moment cognitive adjustments as well as long-term mental reorganization, such as from one cognitive stage to the next.

Another key idea in Piaget's theory is that the organism is the fundamental unit of cognitive activity. Seeking an equilibrated state, the organism actively constructs a model of reality that agrees with its present level of understanding. Thus, the organism discovers knowledge about the world instead of merely passively copying knowledge as behavioristic theories maintain. The organism also tends toward a gradual, not immediate, discovery of knowledge. Fully equilibrated states are only gradually realized, not achieved overnight.

In addition to these general definitions of intelligence, Piaget concerned himself with several more specific aspects, namely, the **content, function,** and **structure** of intelligence. Content of intelligence is similar to the raw, observable data of intelligence. The content of an individual's thinking can be measured by giving him or her an item on a standard intelligence test (e.g., "How are an orange and an apple alike?"). As we have noted, Piaget was not interested in studying the content of a person's answers, but the processes by which the person arrived at them. Still, Piaget did not ignore the importance of content; cognitive processes such as classification and comparison only take on psychological reality when applied to a particular content (D. Kuhn, 1978).

Of equal importance to Piaget was how intelligence functions, or operates. He postulated two inherited intellectual functions—**organization** and **adaptation.** "Organization" refers to the tendency of all organisms to organize and systematize their psychological functioning into integrated wholes. At a physical level, cells become organized into functioning organs (liver, heart, kidneys, lungs) which act together in a complex interrelated way. Similarly, at a psychological level, individuals tend to organize their world into meaningful systems of activity. For example, the young infant gradually develops eye-hand coordination; at first, looking and grasping exist as two separate, uncoordinated activities. The older child begins to classify the world according to organized categories such as animals, people, and fruit. These higher-order organizations permit the child to interact more effectively with the world.

The second function of intelligence is adaptation. All organisms tend to adapt to their environment. There are two complementary sides to this adaptive process—**assimilation** and **accommodation.** By "assimilation" Piaget means that organisms interact with the external environment using the internal psychological organization they already possess. "Accommodation" refers to the tendency to modify one's internal organization in an effort to interact with the environment. These two processes can be best understood with a couple of illustrations. Consider how an infant reflexively sucks the mother's breast to receive nourishment. In initial attempts to suck, an infant will use the actions he or she already possesses (such as mouth movements), but will have to modify these movements to accommodate to the demands of the environment (such as the shape of the nipple). If the mother switches to bottle feeding, the infant may try to use the same sucking behavior (assimilation) and only gradually move his or her mouth differently to adapt to the changed situation (accommodation). When these processes are working equally, an equilibrium results. When one dominates the other, a disequilibrium exists. Both processes are involved in every interaction with the environment.

Next let us examine how assimilatory and accommodative processes may work in an adult's behavior. Consider an adult reading a political opinion in a newspaper that agrees with his or her own opinions. We would say that the person assimilates this belief to already existing cognitive organizations. By the same token, if the opinion runs counter to the person's currently held beliefs, he or she may be forced to accommodate to this new information.

To summarize, organisms inherit the two basic intellectual functions of organization and adaptation, which enable them to interact with and survive in the world. Throughout the life span, organization and adaptation continue to function in the same way. Thus, the functions of intelligence remain invariant across different periods of development. What does change with development are the cognitive structures of intelligence.

Structure is a difficult term to define because of its many different uses in Piagetian theory. At the most general level, "structure" refers to an individual's mental organization or ability (Elkind, 1981). When Piaget refers to the cognitive structures of infants, he uses the term **sensorimotor scheme.** A sensorimotor scheme is any organized pattern of activity or series of actions for dealing with the environment, such as sucking, looking, grasping, hitting, or kicking. Although infants construct these schemes and later mental structures through their own actions, their first schemes are primarily reflexive. Even reflexive activities, however, quickly become part of an infant's self-regulated activity. For example, an infant may suck when not being fed or may anticipate feeding by making sucking movements.

Now let us consider the cognitive structures of older children. They too possess a pattern of organized activity—or schemes—for acting on the world, but at a more abstract intellectual level. From approximately age 7 on, children's structures can be described as mental operations organized as logical mathematical systems. An operation is an internalized action that forms part of an organized structure. For example, think about a child who is trying to classify a set of objects such as toy blocks into shapes, sizes, and colors. Piaget described this activity in terms of the operation of classification. The child groups the objects into several categories and hierarchies of categories, revealing an organized structure of thought. Children, however, are not necessarily fully aware or conscious of these structures. As children develop, their structures become more numerous, organized, and efficient. Changes in the cognitive structures are the essence of cognitive development.

What about the cognitive structures of adolescents and adults? According to Piaget, previous structures become incorporated into new emergent structures at higher levels of organization. By adolescence the structures are organized around a set of formal, logical systems of thinking which represent the highest level of understanding. Thought becomes more logical, abstract, and flexible. Thinking continues to develop throughout adulthood as the structures are generalized to more and more content areas. Changes after adolescence do not constitute true structural change, only changes in content and stability (P. Miller,

1983). As we will discuss in Chapter 8, some writers disagree with Piaget's view of structural change in adulthood and his conception of adult thinking as "postadolescent thought."

Stages of Development

Piaget conceptualized cognitive development as movement through a series of invariant stages, each characterized by a different level of structural complexity. Many psychologists, and lay persons too, use the term *stage* to refer to a person's behavior at a particular age; for example, one might say "He is in the talkative stage." In contrast, Piaget's use of the term implies several things about cognitive growth. First, the stages are *invariant*, that is, they proceed in a regular order. No stage can be skipped, and regression to an earlier stage is impossible. Second, the stages are *universal*; they occur in the same sequence for all individuals in all cultures. Although individuals from different cultures may differ in the content of their thinking and may not reach the final stage of development, their cognitive abilities change in the same general way (Dasen, 1972; Greenfield, 1976). Third, stages imply that cognitive development is divided into *qualitatively different* periods. Each stage represents a distinct level of psychological organization. For example, a qualitative change occurs as the infant moves from the action structures of infancy to the mental operations of middle childhood.

Piaget divided the life span into the following four discrete stages. Remember that each of these stages is logically interconnected with the others and builds on previous stages.

1. *Sensorimotor period (approximately birth–2 years)*
Infants' understanding of the world depends on direct sensory experience and motor actions, hence the term *sensorimotor*. Infants first know the world through reflexive activity and after several substages begin to think before acting. Box 2.2 describes the substages of the sensorimotor period in detail.

2. *Preoperational period (approximately 2–7 years)*
Children develop the ability to use symbols (words, concepts, mental images) to represent objects and events in the world. These symbols become organized in increasingly complex and logical thought systems, although much of children's thought remains unorganized and illogical.

3. *Concrete operational period (approximately 7–11 years)*
Thinking becomes organized into logical systems, which enable children to perform complex mental operations such as carrying out rever-

Box 2.2   Development in the Sensorimotor Period

The sensorimotor period of development begins at birth with genetically programmed reflexes and ends around 2 years of age with the onset of symbolic, representational thought. This period has the following six substages of development, each representing a higher level of adaptation to the environment.

1. *Reflexive stage (approximately birth–1 month)*
The infant's behavior consists mostly of reflexes—involuntary and automatic responses to various stimuli—which are slightly modified as the infant interacts with the world. For example, sucking occurs when the infant's mouth makes contact with a stimulus such as a breast or bottle. Whether the infant is bottlefed or breastfed, gradual modifications in sucking occur. Different bottles and even different breasts require somewhat different sucking patterns, as do other objects such as thumbs, toys, and tables (Piaget calls this adaptation *generalizing assimilation*). Despite these small but possibly significant adjustments in sucking behaviors, Piaget still tends to think of such activities as primarily reflexive. Nonetheless, Piaget observed that infants can spontaneously produce and exercise their beginning sensorimotor schemes (a process he called *functional assimilation*), thereby constructing a world of things to look at, grasp, suck, feel, and so on.

2. *Primary circular reactions (approximately 1–4 months)*
In Stage 1 only minimal modification of the reflexes occurs, and infants' responses can be regarded as schemes in only the most limited sense. During Stage 2, schemes undergo substantial elaboration and refinement, and *primary circular reactions* can occur. These reactions are called "primary" because the action centers on infants' bodily responses rather than on external objects. For example, infants in this stage may bring their hands to their mouths for the express purpose of sucking their thumbs. The thumbsucking that occurred in the reflexive stage was an accidental uncoordinated behavior. By Stage 2, infants have acquired the ability to engage in efficient hand-mouth coordination as well as eye-hand, eye-ear, and other coordinations. We call infants' reactions "circular" because they involve almost endless repetition of an activity. For example, when Piaget repeatedly tried to remove his son Laurent's hand from the child's mouth, Laurent kept returning the hand there.

These repetitions appear to lead to the first signs of memory in the infant. Infants may come to recognize objects that they have sucked, grasped, touched, or dropped before (Piaget referred to this as *recognitory assimilation*). Furthermore, infants recognize objects that are similar to but not identical to those acted upon before. This is an instance of generalization of sensorimotor schemes to novel objects.

3. *Secondary circular reactions (approximately 4–8 months)*
During Stage 2, infants responded mainly to the bodily action or behavior. By Stage 3, or secondary circular reactions, infants respond to events and objects in the external environment. Initially by chance, and later by design, infants perform an action that results in an unanticipated but interesting consequence. For example, a ball rolls off a table and bounces, or a rattle is shaken and produces a noise. In the previous stage the sheer pleasure of rolling or shaking was of primary interest, but now the consequences of the action are. Children may grasp and release a ball just for the pleasure of seeing it bounce, and then repeat this action over and over.

Piaget attached special significance to secondary circular reactions. They are the first signs of intentionality in the behavior of the infant and mark the onset of truly adaptive behavior. However, Piaget was reluctant to interpret these reactions as evidence of unmistakably intentional, deliberate, means-end behavior. For example, whether infants at this stage shake a rattle repeatedly *in order to* hear it make noise is doubtful. Nevertheless, when infants repeat a motor activity to re-create an interesting result, they are separating activity from the results of the activity. In a sense then, infants become "young experimenters" manipulating the environment and constructing their own activities.

During this stage, several other accomplishments occur, including the beginning of genuine imitation. For example, infants seem more likely to repeat their responses if a model mimics them. However, these behaviors must not be novel behaviors, but ones that the infants have spontaneously produced. Furthermore, the behaviors should be ones that can be seen or heard; infants in this stage can imitate vocalizations and manual gestures but not facial expressions. Infants in Stage 3 also show the beginnings of play behavior. They often playfully exercise their sensorimotor schemes, as when they repeatedly vocalize a sound.

4. *Coordination of secondary schemes (approximately 8–12 months)*
In this stage infants coordinate several secondary schemes previously used singly to achieve some goal. By this time there is clear,

unmistakable evidence for means-ends behavior and an identification of cause-effect relationships. Stage 4 infants can take familiar schemes from one situation and apply them to a new situation, but there is no clear evidence that various alternative schemes are considered. For example, an infant may push aside one object (motor scheme) to look for a second object (another motor scheme) (Flavell, 1985). Here the infant is using a scheme learned in a familiar situation and applying it to a new situation. This action shows originality and knowledge of a goal, but not necessarily consideration of possible alternative means of reaching that goal.

Several parallels exist between Stage 4 and Stage 2. As in Stage 2, sensorimotor schemes become coordinated into an integrated pattern. But the sensorimotor schemes of the Stage 4 infant center on external objects in the outside environment, not their own bodies. There is also a parallel in that new sensorimotor schemes are being applied in a relatively invariant, reflexive manner. Toward the end of Stage 4, different characteristics of novel objects are explored by applying different schemes or variations of the same scheme. The infant can thus be seen as a developing, active experimenter.

In Stage 4, infants overcome the limitations on imitation and play noted in Stage 3. Infants now imitate novel actions not visible on their own bodies. This is a tremendously important advance because infants can now learn simply by observing the behavior of others. (As we note later, imitation is a powerful mechanism in cognitive developmental changes at all ages.) In Stage 4, play becomes more clearly differentiated from other means-end activity and is engaged in for its own sake. Thus, play becomes a means and an end in itself.

5.   *Tertiary circular reactions (approximately 12–18 months)*
In Stage 5 repetition again becomes important in a child's interaction with the environment. Children become relentless explorers, vigorously examining pots and pans in cupboards, knickknacks on shelves, electric outlets in walls, garbage pails and wastebaskets. Unlike in Stage 4, children begin to modify their schemes to fit new situations. Stage 4 infants were likely to explore in a fixed trial-and-error manner; Stage 5 infants develop an intentional, systematic approach in their search for goals. They develop a "Let's see what happens" scheme, which is modified in progress toward a goal. Piaget calls these attempts to produce novel unexpected results *tertiary circular reactions.* For example, a child may "experiment" with letting an object fall from her playpen. She may vary the position of her arm, the height from which the object is dropped, and the place on which she drops it. Simi-

larly, a child may discover new means for reaching familiar ends by pulling a blanket through the bars of a crib to reach an object resting on the blanket but out of reach.

As children gain experience by systematically varying their actions, they gradually begin to develop the ability to solve problems by thinking. But at Stage 5, children still attain goals mainly by active sensorimotor exploration.

6. *Invention of new means through mental combinations (approximately 18–24 months)*

Stage 6 provides the first clear-cut evidence of systematic intelligence. Piaget describes this achievement as the *invention of new means through mental combinations,* and sees it as the culmination of the child's first five substages. Eighteen-month-olds are able to adapt solutions to problems without having to experiment overtly with different sensorimotor schemes. External exploration of objects is gradually replaced by internal mental representations. For children in this stage mental representation opens up a whole new way of solving problems and adapting to the world. Piaget calls this newly developed capacity for representation the *semiotic,* or symbolic, function. The child's behavior can be described as inventive or insightful rather than as trial and error.

Piaget (1963) described the Stage 6 behavior of his daughter Jacqueline at age 20 months. She arrived at a closed door with a blade of grass in her hand. As she grasped for the doorknob, she realized she could not open the door without putting down the grass. She placed the grass on the floor, opened the door, picked up the grass, and entered the room. When she went to leave the room, she put the grass down, but realized that opening the door would brush aside the grass. Accordingly, she moved the grass beyond the door's path, opened the door, picked up the grass, and exited.

sals in one's mind (if A $\longrightarrow$ B, then B $\longrightarrow$ A). The use of systematic thinking is restricted to concrete here-and-now objects and activities.

4. *Formal operational period (approximately 11–15 years and older)*

Children are no longer limited to the concrete situation, but can apply mental operations to solve purely abstract and hypothetical problems in the present, past, and future. Children systematically test hypotheses and can revise or abandon hypotheses in the light of new information.

Cognitive stages of development lie at the heart of Piagetian theory. They form the central part of his theory, but have been subjected to the broadest criticism (Brainerd, 1978, 1983). On the positive side, stages help us organize diverse mental phenomena around a few understandable and orderly patterns. They also focus our attention on the qualitative nature of mental development. This focus represents a major break with the earlier behavioristic tradition of viewing children's thought as a similar but incomplete version of adult thought. On the negative side, not every investigator has found that children behave in the way Piaget described. For example, recent evidence suggests that infants and preschoolers may know more than Piaget claimed (Flavell, 1985; Gelman, 1979). Stages also do not appear to capture many of the more interesting aspects of mature adult thinking, such as the ability to reflect on and evaluate the nature of formal operational thinking (Labouvie-Vief, 1982).

Fischer (1980) has suggested that Piagetian researchers abandon all-inclusive stage notions in favor of domain-specific descriptions. He has proposed that they concentrate on particular domains such as problem solving or language rather than on the totality of cognitive development. This emphasis on domain-specific stages characterizes the next theorist we discuss.

Werner's Theory

Although not as well known or sufficiently elaborated as Piaget's theory, Heinz Werner's theory of development has been influential in theorizing about cognition. Like Piaget's, Werner's theory is firmly rooted within the discipline of biology. Werner's theory also proposes a series of developmental stages or levels, although these are not as well specified as Piaget's and are not confined to cognitive behavior.

The cornerstone of Werner's organismic theory of development is the orthogenetic principle (see Chapter 1). This principle cuts across various domains (cognitive, physical, social) and provides a foundation for all developmental functioning. As you may recall, the orthogenetic principle states that organisms have "a tendency to move from a state of relative globality and undifferentiatedness towards states of increasing differentiation and hierarchic integration" (Werner, 1957, p. 126). The idea of differentiation and hierarchic integration can be found in Piaget's notion of classification, with the organism differentiating itself from objects in the world.

For Werner, differentiation and hierarchic integration are highly relevant to understanding cognitive development. Biological development proceeds from the fertilization of a single undifferentiated egg cell with no specialized functioning to a multicelled organism with functionally integrated organ systems. Cognitive development can be similarly characterized along a dimension of increasing differentiation and integration of the various psychological systems. Werner also believed that the orthogenetic principle represented a basic inherited tendency of the organism, similar to Piaget's belief in the inherited invariants of adaptation and organization.

The general outline of Werner's theory is not entirely novel (Thomas, 1985). The theory can be traced to scientific developments in biology in the nineteenth century—in particular, Charles Darwin's ideas on the evolution of nonhuman and human species from simpler to more complex life forms. Embracing Darwinian evolutionism, psychologists began to compare the intellectual powers of animals and children with the more highly "evolved" intelligence of adolescents and adults. Psychologists during this era also showed a great interest in studying diverse mental phenomena associated with primitive cultures and psychological disorders such as schizophrenia. Werner felt that the orthogenetic principle could account for these phenomena along the lines of complexity and differentiation.

In addition to his general principle of orthogenesis, Werner (1957) outlined the following major trends in cognitive development over the life span: (1) syncretic to discrete, (2) rigid to flexible, (3) diffuse to articulated, and (4) unstable to stable. "Syncretic to discrete" refers to the progression of the individual from an undifferentiated to a differentiated organism. An example with regard to intellectual development is holophrastic speech (Thomas, 1985), which occurs when a young child uses one word to refer to or represent an entire situation. Older children and adults show more differentiated speech by employing a variety of words. A 2-year-old may say "milk" to request something to drink, whereas an 11-year-old would say "If there is any milk left, I'd like a glass." This does not mean that older children or adults never engage in global, syncretic thinking. They too may use a single word to describe their desires or impressions.

Werner also proposed that the organism tends to move from a state of *rigidity to flexibility,* whereby new skills and ideas are employed to meet changing situational demands. A good example of this trend can be found in the area of problem solving. When playing a game of cards, young children often fail to think or plan ahead, and they may rely on only one or two strategies. Older children are more adept at planning a strategy, remembering the cards that have been played, and anticipating opponents' moves. Does this imply that adolescents and adults are more flexible in their behavior than children? To a great extent, the answer is "yes." However, there exists considerable controversy about whether the thinking of older adults becomes more inflexible or rigid with age (Botwinick, 1984).

Another trend identified by Werner is the move from *diffuse to articulated,* which refers to the degree of coordination or interdependence among the separate elements of any physical or mental system (Salkind,

1981). For example, in biological development, the organ systems develop independently and function on their own, but with time they become interdependent. A psychological example of this principle is found in language development. As they develop the ability to form complex sentences, children coordinate their separate words into whole units that express a coordinated series of thought.

Finally, Werner describes the trend from *instability to stability* in individual development. By "instability," Werner means that the system has not established an equilibrium. Behavior tends to be momentary and fluctuating, as in young children's rapid attentional shifts from one thing to another. With development, greater stability is achieved, and the system as a whole is strengthened. For example, older children can sustain attention and concentrate on long-term goals (Thomas, 1985).

Let us now summarize these four trends. With development the organism progresses from a syncretic, rigid, diffuse, and unstable state to one of discreteness, flexibility, articulation, and stability. The more cognitively complex the organism, the closer to these end states the individual appears. Finally, these four trends are aspects of the orthogenetic principle of development.

Beyond these orthogenetic trends, Werner identified a number of developmental stages. Unlike Piaget, Werner did not attach specific ages to the stages, nor did he restrict himself to the realm of cognitive behavior. Table 2.1 depicts the organismic stage model of mental development proposed by Werner (J. Langer, 1970). Note the overall similarity between these stages and those described by Piaget. Because Werner is more interested in general features of development, he has not elaborated his stages as much as Piaget. This is one reason why Werner's model has not been as widely accepted. Werner also did most of his work before the organismic view gained widespread popularity.

Box 2.3 shows how a contemporary psychologist has been influenced by both Werner and Piaget.

INFORMATION-PROCESSING APPROACHES

Over the past decade and a half the information-processing approach has emerged as one of the leading strategies for research on cognition, particularly in the area of attention, memory, and problem solving. Its rapid emergence has coincided with a decline in Piaget's influence and a turning away from structural theories of cognition. Although not incompatible with organismic developmental theory, the information-processing approach draws upon alternative models for conceptualizing

Table 2.1
Werner's Organismic Stage Model of Mental Development

Stage	Developments
Sensorimotor Development	The infant's mental activity is organized around motoric, sensory, and affective processes. Objects are understood in terms of their physical movements, and there is a limited differentiation between subject and object. For example, inanimate objects are perceived as animate or possessing inner forms of life.
Perceptual Development	The child forms percepts and concepts of the world. Perception is initially global; wholes are seen rather than individual parts. With development, perception becomes more selective and analytical. The individual parts are integrated to form new wholes.
Contemplative Development	More "primitive" forms of mental life seen in the preceding stages are integrated at a more mature level of thinking. However, less mature patterns of functioning do not simply drop out when the higher-order forms develop. Rather, they become part of a hierarchy, with higher-order forms dominating lower-order forms.

cognitive growth and development (Reese, 1973a, 1973b). Both organismic developmental and information-processing approaches incorporate an active organism model of development, as discussed below. However, organismic models, unlike information-processing models, present developmental changes as qualitative, emergent, directed to a final endpoint, and usually irreversible.

The information-processing approach, much like the life-span approach, is not a single theory of behavior, but a general framework for studying cognition. The major objective is to trace the flow of information across space and time through an information-processing system (R. Lachman et al., 1979; Reitman, 1965). The human processing system, analogous to an electronic computer, is conceptualized as having *inputs, throughputs,* and *outputs.* Input begins when information in the form of a stimulus (verbal, visual, tactile) impinges on the sensory receptors. As the sensory information moves through the system, it is attended to, transformed into a meaningful code, compared to information already in memory, and stored in memory for future use. Output occurs in the form of a verbal or nonverbal response, a decision, or a representation stored in memory.

Box 2.3   Jerome Bruner

Jerome Bruner is a psychologist who has made major contributions to the study of cognitive development in the United States. Among his many publications are *Studies in Cognitive Growth* (Bruner, Olver, & Greenfield, 1966) and *Beyond the Information Given* (Bruner, 1973). His writings are influenced by both Piaget and Werner. Like Piaget, Bruner argues that cognitive development proceeds through a series of stages. And, like Werner, he is concerned with the modes or types of representation people use when they store information in memory.

Bruner has proposed three types of representation modes:

Enactive—the child defines events in terms of the *actions* they evoke. Perceptions and actions are closely linked. For example, an infant who is playing with a rattle and drops it will shake its fist as if the act of shaking will return the rattle. Adults rely on enactive representation in such activities as driving, bicycling, and golf.

Iconic—The child uses mental images or pictures to represent objects that are not physically present. Perception and action can be separated, so that the infant can imagine a lost rattle without having to go through the physical action of shaking. Older children and adults use iconic representation too as in trying to mentally picture a person who they met earlier in the week.

Symbolic—Children represent the world in the form of words and symbol systems such as language. Symbols can be detached from objects and mentally manipulated. These mental manipulations are involved in logical, abstract thinking.

Despite the parallels between Bruner's different modes of representation and the Piagetian stages, Bruner differs from Piaget in significant ways. In contrast to Piaget's rigid stage notions, Bruner believes that children in principle can be taught the fundamentals of any subject regardless of age. Bruner also sees the development of language as a major factor in the emergence of children's complex thinking skills, whereas Piaget viewed language as a consequence of changes in cognitive skills.

Human beings as sophisticated thinking machines or computers is the metaphor in the information-processing approach. Care must be taken not to stretch this metaphor too far, however, because human beings are unlike computers in many important ways. The neural pathways in the brain may not be directly comparable to the electrical circuitry in a computer (Pribram, 1986). The machine analogy is also misleading in that human beings are not seen as passive, motionless entities controlled by external forces. Rather, individuals are viewed as active seekers who search for information in the environment and often construct inferences about this information using present knowledge and past experience. Thus, we cannot classify information-processing theories as purely mechanistic (Kail & Bisanz, 1982; Reese, 1976; Shaw & Bransford, 1977).

Various information-processing approaches differ in how seriously the computer is taken as a model of human thinking (P. Miller, 1983). At one extreme is the *computer simulation* approach, which seeks to develop computer programs that will model human thought processes. At the other end are theorists who use the computer metaphor only as a convenient heuristic device. They use computer terminology (such as *information input, executive control system, subroutines, storage capacity*) to discuss human information processing, but they do not attempt to translate human processes into computer programs. Most developmental information-processing researchers employ the latter approach rather than computer simulation. In between these two approaches are theorists who apply the analogy of the computer as a general-purpose symbol manipulator to human thinking, but without the formal simulation system (R. Lachman et al., 1979).

Now stop for a moment and consider all the information that is bombarding your senses: the written words on this page, a light overhead, the cushioned chair, the traffic outside, and some softly (or perhaps not so softly) playing music all may be competing for your attention. How is your mind able to receive, organize, interpret, and respond to all this information?

To answer this question, consider how your cognitive system is working right now. You are probably trying to ignore all the irrelevant information in an effort to attend to the letters and words on this page. Each word or set of words is recognized as a meaningful unit. The ideas that you read are being compared to what you already know about the subject. Not all the information here is being stored in your memory; much is lost, but we hope enough remains for recall at a later point. Several component cognitive processes are at work here—attention, perception, comprehension, problem solving, memory, and language.

In describing and explaining cognitive development, information-processing theorists seek to understand how each component process or operation is changing with age. In other words, how do the various steps in processing from initial input to final output differ across developmental levels? As you will see in later chapters, age changes are evident in almost every step of information processing. More importantly, how do we identify the mechanism or "transitional system" underlying the progression from one developmental level to the next (Sternberg, 1984)? Are differences due to age changes in memory capacity and the speed of processing or to the growth of control processes and strategies such as semantic organization and elaboration? Knowledge about one's own cognitive capabilities, or metacognition, and knowledge about specific content areas (e.g., chess, physics) also appear to be important factors in explaining cognitive developmental trends (Siegler, 1983).

Until relatively recently, most information-processing studies focused on adult cognition, rather than on cognitive change processes over time. The rationale for this emphasis was that understanding any type of developmental process is easier when we know where the process is heading (Siegler, 1983). By first identifying the commonalities in children's and adults' information processing, the unique features of development can be isolated. This emphasis has had positive benefits. For example, results showing that adults often fail to use formal, rational thinking on complex information-processing and decision-making tasks have led researchers to question Piaget's description of the formal operations stage (Shakelee, 1979).

Researchers did not take long to appreciate the benefits of the information-processing approach in studying developmental processes (Siegler, 1983). The approach offers a generally appealing metaphor of the human being as a limited capacity symbol manipulator. People set goals; processing limitations hinder the goals' attainment; and people develop memory strategies such as rehearsal, organization, and elaboration to overcome the limitations. Overall, this sequence seems to capture closely how humans go about knowing the world. The information-processing approach also provides a precise descriptive vocabulary for characterizing cognition and cognitive processes. Computer programming languages such as tree diagrams, flow charts, and production systems (to be discussed shortly) give researchers a powerful method for describing what transpires between input and output. Similarly, notions such as schema, scripts, frames, and story grammars (see Chapter 6) give us new insights into the way knowledge may be organized (Kail & Bisanz, 1982; Siegler, 1983). Finally, information-processing models offer developmental researchers a whole array of powerful analytic techniques for examining cognitive processes. For example, *chronometric methods* use reaction-time data to develop models of the temporal course of information processing. Detailed *protocol analyses*, which rely on subjects' verbalizations, give precise moment-by-moment descriptions of strategies people use to solve problems.

A good illustration of a developmental information-processing study is seen in Siegler's (1978, 1981) work with the balance-scale apparatus depicted in Figure 2.2. The apparatus is similar to one used by Inhelder and Piaget (1964) in a study of formal operational thinking. On each side of the fulcrum (midpoint) are four equally spaced pegs on which equal-sized metal weights can be placed. The arm of the scale can tilt right or left or remain level and balanced, depending on where the weights are placed. The subject's task is to predict which side will go down. Two pieces of information are relevant to solving the problem: (1) the number of weights and (2) their distance from the fulcrum.

Siegler tested children aged 5–17 years on a series of balance-scale problems. He identified four different rules that children might use to solve the problems:

1. Children using Rule 1 consider only the number of weights on each side of the scale. If the weights are equal, the children predict that the scale will balance. If the weights are unequal, the side having the greater number of weights is always predicted to go down.

2. Using Rule 2, children still consider the number of weights as the major dimension, but if there are an equal number on both sides, distance from the midpoint is considered.

3. Using Rule 3, children take both dimensions—weight and distance—into account, but experience conflict when one side has the greater weight and the other is the greater distance from the fulcrum. For example, if both sides have an equal number of weights but the distances are unequal, children predict that the side with the weights farthest from the fulcrum will tip down. However, if the number of weights and the distances on both sides of the scale are unequal, children resort to guessing.

4. Rule 4 children know how to determine the exact contribution of weight and distance. They multiply the number of weights on each peg by the peg's distance from the fulcrum. By comparing the sums of the products on both sides, they can make an accurate prediction about which side will go down.

Figure 2.2 Balance-Scale Apparatus.

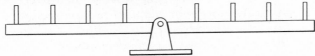

From "Three Aspects of Cognitive Development" by R. S. Siegler, 1976, *Cognitive Psychology, 8,* p. 482. Copyright 1976 by Academic Press. Reprinted by permission.

The results of Siegler's (1978) study show a clear developmental pattern across problem type, with older children more likely to use Rules 2 and 3. Few children of any age used Rule 4. The rule models accurately characterized the predictions of almost 90 percent of the children, with a range of approximately 80 percent for 5-year-olds to 100 percent for 17-year-olds. Thus, these results demonstrate that children employ increasingly sophisticated rules on this task with age. But what mechanism or set of mechanisms can explain these improvements? Siegler (1978) suggests that differences between younger and older children on the balance-scale task may lie in the way they *encode* the problem, that is, how they attend to and store the information in memory. Younger children encode only the weight dimension, but older children encode the dimensions of weight and distance.

How might Siegler's four rules be translated into a computer program? First, they need to be represented as a tree diagram like the one shown in Figure 2.3. Each node in the decision tree represents either a "yes" or "no" answer. Next, using computer language, a **production system** is developed. A production system is a set of procedures or operations stored in memory. Productions are *condition-action rules* for changing the information in the currently activated state of the cognitive system (P. Miller, 1983). As the productions are applied to each step in a problem, they transform the initial problem state to the final state. Consider the following example of a production: if X is present → Y occurs. Thus, if the number of weights on each side of the balance are equal (X), then the child will say that the scale will balance (Y). A model production system for the balance-scale task is shown in Figure 2.4.

Production models are valuable because they give us a very precise and detailed description of an individual's information processing. They make explicit the nature of the task and the strategies people use for solution. They also force investigators to be very explicit in their descriptions of cognitive processes. Too often our understanding of cognition is couched in vague, imprecise language. Of course, information-processing models may quickly become overly complex and unwieldy, and the scientific-sounding language of information processing may be no nearer the truth than more simply stated theories (behavioristic) or more elegant ones (Piaget's).

One of the most exciting recent developments in information-processing theory is the notion of adaptive production systems (Simon, 1979), which have the capacity for *self-modification*. They go beyond the static if → then rule conditions and zero in on how information is learned and modified in the first place. How does a person learn to combine and recombine strategies, abandon unrewarding ones, and plan short-range and long-range goals (Anzai & Simon, 1979)? The notion of

Figure 2.3 Decision Tree Diagrams of Rules for Performing the Balance-Scale Task.

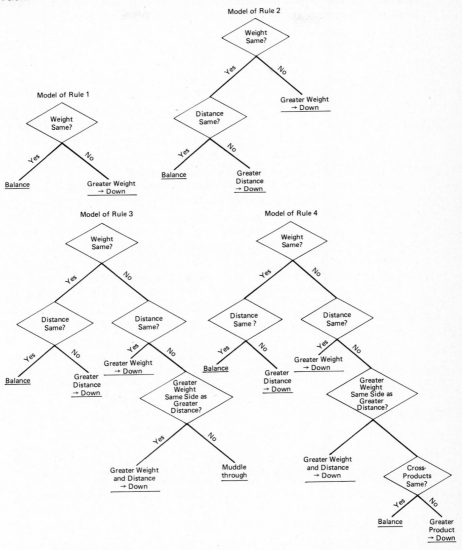

From "Three Aspects of Cognitive Development" by R. S. Siegler, 1976, *Cognitive Psychology*, 8, pp. 484–485. Copyright 1976 by Academic Press. Reprinted by permission.

Figure 2.4   A Model Production System for the Balance-Scale Task. Production systems (P) are presented for the four rule models used to solve the balance problem. Torque = downward force, D = distance, W = weight.

Model I

    P1: ((Same W) → (Say "balance"))
    P2: ((Side X more W) → (Say "X down"))

Model II

    P1: ((Same W) → (Say "balance"))
    P2: ((Side X more W) → (Say "X down"))
    P3: ((Same W) (Side X more D) → (Say "X down"))

Model III

    P1: ((Same W) → (Say "balance"))
    P2: ((Side X more W) → (Say "X down"))
    P3: ((Same W) (Side X more D) → (Say "X down"))
    P4: ((Side X more W) (Side X less D) → muddle through)
    P5: ((Side X more W) (Side X more D) → (Say "X down"))

Model IV

    P1: ((Same W) → (Say "balance"))
    P2: ((Side X more W) → (Say "X down"))
    P3: ((Same W) (Side X more D) → (Say "X down"))
    P4: ((Side X more W) (Side X less D) → (get Torques))
    P5: ((Side X more W) (Side X more D) → (Say "X down"))
    P6: ((Same Torque) → (Say "balance"))
    P7: ((Side X more Torque) → (say "X down"))

| | Transitional requirements | |
	Productions	Operators
I → II	add P3	add distance encoding and comparison
II → III	add P4, P5	
III → IV	modify P4; add P6, P7	add torque computation and comparison

From "The Representation of Children's Knowledge" by D. Klahr and R. S. Siegler, 1978, in *Advances in Child Development and Behavior* (Vol. 12, p. 78) edited by H. W. Reese and L. P. Lipsitt, New York: Academic Press. Copyright 1978 by Academic Press. Reprinted by permission.

a self-modifying or self-regulating system is also present in Piaget's constructs of assimilation and accommodation. Thus far, few developmental psychologists have used production systems, and whether such systems are actual theories of cognition or simply descriptions of cognition in computer programming language remains unknown (Newell, 1973). Still, production systems represent one of the clearest examples yet of how self-modification may occur. For this reason they deserve more attention than they have been given.

OTHER THEORETICAL APPROACHES

We will now discuss two other theoretical frameworks for studying cognitive development—behavioristic and contextualistic. Behavioristic approaches dominated American psychology until the 1960s and still represent a potent force. Contextualistic approaches are becoming increasingly popular and may eventually emerge as the most powerful framework for conceptualizing cognition.

Behavioristic Theories

Behavioristic approaches contrast sharply with more organismically oriented approaches in significant ways. Most behaviorists dispense with the stage notion altogether and see development as the gradual accumulation of various behaviors shaped by experience. Thus, development is seen as continuous, not stage-like. Furthermore, the organism is viewed as passively responding to various experiences, rather than as being cognitively active. People do not act but react to external forces (such as rewards and punishments) that act upon them. Because only observable causes of behavior are considered, complete empirical prediction is considered possible in principle. Although internal factors (such as genetic background and maturational states) are not entirely ignored, behaviorists pay much less attention to them than to external variables.

Theorists who take a behavioristic approach see learning as the key to explaining development. In this view, people learn specific behaviors such as counting, reading, and playing a musical instrument, rather than acquire psychological structures. Although most behaviors are complex, behavioristic theorists attempt to reduce them to their simplest units. The assumption that behavior is reducible is called **elementarism** and derives from the mechanistic model of development (Overton & Reese, 1973). For behaviorists, the most elementary units of behavior are the stimulus response, or S-R, associations, which can be combined by conditioning to produce more complex sequences of behavior, both motor and verbal.

Robert Gagné (1977) has offered a cumulative learning model that posits a hierarchy of learning processes from simple S-R (stimulus-response) associations to complex rule learning and problem solving. According to Gagné, development is the result of acquiring simple associations before learning complex rules. The learning of complex rules depends upon many intermediate processes in the hierarchy, such as motor and verbal chains, multiple discriminations, concepts, and simple rules.

For example, Gagné (1977) describes a cumulative learning sequence for acquiring number operations in mathematics. In Figure 2.5, you can

Figure 2.5   A Learning Sequence for Number Operations.

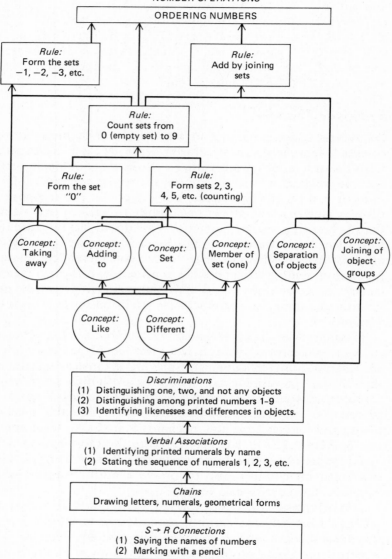

From *The Conditions of Learning* (p. 181) by R. M. Gagné, 1965, New York: Holt, Rinehart and Winston. Copyright 1965 by Holt, Rinehart and Winston. Reprinted by permission of CBS College Publishing.

follow a sample sequence by looking first at the bottom of the figure. The child must first learn to mark the numbers down with a pencil in response to a specific stimulus such as saying the names of the numbers. After such *stimulus-response connections* are formed, the child then learns to connect these S-R associations into *chains.* The child who can draw letters, numerals, and geometrical forms has learned a simple chain of responses and can proceed to the level of *verbal associations.* For example, the child identifies the printed numerals by name or states a numerical sequence (1, 2, 3, and so on). Next the child must master *discriminations* among different numbers of objects, various printed numerals, and similar and dissimilar objects. Following this, the child needs to learn a series of *concepts* such as "like," "different," "taking away," and "adding to." These concepts form the basis of *rules,* such as rules related to forming the null set (0) or sets of 2, 3, 4, 5; counting sets from 0–9; and adding by joining sets. By learning these rules, children acquire the ability to order numbers.

The learning sequence does not always conform exactly to the model shown in Figure 2.5. Children often do not need to learn all discriminations before learning certain concepts, nor do they always need to acquire all concepts before certain rules. The sequence depends, among other things, on the content of the material to be learned. And the relationships among the various levels in the hierarchy are probably more complex than Gagné originally envisioned. For the most part, however, his proposed sequence appears to hold up fairly well.

Another learning theorist whose work has generated a great deal of research is Albert Bandura. Bandura adds a new dimension to the strict behavioral approach by considering the role of cognitive processes in observational learning. By *observational learning,* Bandura means that we acquire many of our behaviors simply by watching others perform. The behavior acquired may be a motor response, a moral judgment, or a cognitive rule. Learning is not, as traditional behaviorists maintain, always a gradual trial-and-error process shaped by its consequences. Since human learning, unlike animal learning, often occurs in social situations by observing others, Bandura's theory is labeled *social learning theory* (Zimmerman, 1983).

Figure 2.6 displays the four subprocesses involved in observational learning. In line with information-processing theory, a person selectively *attends* to incoming information; then, in the *retention* processes, he codes the information, makes a decision, and rehearses it. This "active organism" view contrasts with traditional behaviorist accounts of human beings as "passive responders." The characteristics (developmental level, power, social attractiveness) of both the model and the observer are important determinants of what is attended to and retained in memory. Even if the model is noticed and understood, the individual must still convert the modeled behavior into a symbolic code that can be stored in memory.

The two other processes shown in Figure 2.6—*motor reproduction* and *motivation*—refer to the actual performance of the behavior. Bandura gives both of these processes a cognitive interpretation. For example, he decomposes motor reproduction processes into how a person cognitively organizes the behavior, modifies it as a result of feedback, and judges how closely the behavior matches the observed behavior. Consider the motor processes a child needs to do a multiplication problem: numerals must be correctly written, "carry" marks must be noted, and so on (Zimmerman, 1983). Motivational processes deal with the tendency to behave in order to produce reinforcing consequences. These consequences may be direct (external reinforcement), vicarious (observing others being reinforced), or self-administered (self-reinforcement). Motivation reciprocally affects the processes of attention and retention as well as motor reproduction.

Each of the four processes depicted in the Figure 2.6 model may change developmentally. One critical change is in children's symbolic functioning. The ability to symbolize an observed behavior and store the symbol in memory frees the developing child from having to view a behavior and reproduce it directly. A more sophisticated symbolic ability allows the child to learn a behavior by reading a description of the behavior or being instructed by a model.

In terms of framing a comprehensive theory of cognitive development, Bandura's theory is probably not as useful as Piagetian or information-processing approaches. But it does have several strengths. First, it draws our attention to the "hot" side of cognition, or the motivational and emotional aspects of thinking (Zajonc, 1980). Examples of hot cognition include individuals' confidence in themselves as learners

Figure 2.6   Cognitive and Noncognitive Processes underlying Observational Learning.

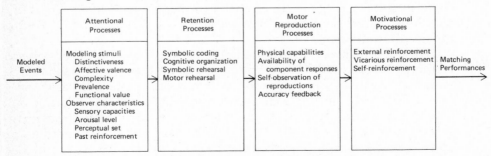

From *Social Learning Theory* (p. 23) by A. Bandura, 1977, Englewood Cliffs, NJ: Prentice-Hall. Copyright 1977 by Prentice-Hall, Inc. Reprinted by permission.

and their estimates of their own abilities. Growing evidence suggests that beliefs about one's personal efficacy or competence can predict cognitive and behavioral functioning (Bandura & Schunk, 1981; M. Lachman, 1983). Piaget and information-processing theorists have been more concerned with the "cold" side of cognition, or cognition without emotion or subjective belief. Bandura's theory also sensitizes us to the situational or contextual dependence of behavior (Zimmerman, 1983). For example, situational factors such as reinforcement and task complexity help determine whether a child shows certain cognitive abilities on Piagetian and information-processing tasks.

Contextualistic Theories

The contextualistic approach to life-span cognitive development was discussed briefly at the end of Chapter 1. A life-span contextualistic perspective sees cognitive growth as a multidirectional and multiply determined process that depends on complex interactions between a constantly changing organism and an ever-changing environment (Labouvie-Vief & Chandler, 1978). Moreover, there is no absolute or fixed end state to development. Now that we have introduced these concepts, let us examine them.

One of the major limitations of organismic as well as information-processing approaches according to the contextualistic view is their failure to predict human performance across a broad range of environments or situations. Whether we are talking about Piaget's cognitive stages or the computer programs of information-processing theorists, the focus traditionally has been on the internal cognitions of the organism, not the external environment or context. Contextualist theorists argue that the environment is inherently active too. The organism's activity arises from its dynamic interactions with an active environment, and these interactions change the environment as well as the organism. From a contextualistic perspective, the organism is described as being "in transaction" with the environment (Sameroff, 1975). The timing of this organism-environment transaction plays a key role in development.

The contextualistic emphasis is increasingly reflected in contemporary versions of organismic developmental theories and information-processing theories as well as in more mechanistically oriented approaches such as Bandura's. With respect to organismic theories, Pepper (1942) states, "contextualism and organicism are so nearly allied that they may almost be called the same theory" (p. 147). Both models emphasize the importance of change, the importance of qualitative rather than quantitative shifts in behavior, and the role of *dialectical contradictions* in producing development. A dialectical contradiction occurs when different developmental dimensions or processes (such as assimilation or accommodation) are out of balance; resolution of the contradiction makes further development of the individual and society possible.

The major difference between contextualistic theories and organismic theories lies in their assumptions about the direction and end state of development. Whereas organismic theorists assume that developmental change is ordered toward some fixed ideal goal or universal end state, contextualists make no assumptions about the directionality of change (Labouvie-Vief & Chandler, 1978). This simple omission has major consequences. Chief among them is that the contextualistic perspective places much stronger emphasis on the plasticity (intraindividual change in structure and function) of development across the life course and the possibility of a variety of developmental outcomes. For example, contextualistic models lead us to question whether formal, logical thinking is the ideal standard or outcome by which all thought should be judged. Box 2.4 gives an example of a life-span contextualistic interpretation of adult thought.

The contextualistic perspective is also being incorporated into modern information-processing theories with a focus on the interaction between an information-processing system and the task environment (Siegler, 1983). Rather than study information processes such as attention, perception, memory, and problem solving apart from their context, contextualists view processing as greatly dependent on the task environment as well as on previous knowledge. For example, the success of problem solving depends on the nature of the problem, the individual's familiarity with it, and the size of the problem space (see Chapter 7). Furthermore, individuals can adapt their problem-solving strategies to suit various problem contexts. Failure to consider this fact substantially reduces our ability to draw general conclusions about cognitive development.

Contextualists feel that the failure to recognize the contextual and social relativity of knowledge creates problems not only in interpreting developmental research but also in conducting cross-cultural research. It is increasingly recognized that laboratory tasks often fail to reveal the extent of mental abilities among different cultural groups, particularly when the material is presented in unfamiliar ways. For example, Irwin and McLaughlin (1970) found that Liberian adults could successfully classify bowls of rice, but not abstract geometrical stimuli varying in color, shape, and number. On the other hand, Irwin, Schafer, and Frieden (1974) later discovered that United States undergraduates showed the same classification difficulties when asked to sort bowls of rice rather than more familiar cards with squares and triangles.

In regard to development, the term *context* may simply imply a

Box 2.4   A Contextualistic Interpretation of Cognitive Development

In a study of language comprehension, G. Cohen (1979) presented young adult college students and older adults with the following prose passage:

> Downstairs, there are three rooms: the kitchen, the dining-room, and the sitting room. The sitting room is in the front of the house, and the kitchen and dining-room face onto the vegetable garden at the back of the house. The noise of the traffic is very disturbing in the front rooms. Mother is in the kitchen cooking and Grandfather is reading the paper in the sitting room. The children are at school and won't be home til tea-time. (p. 416)

When Cohen asked the subjects who was being disturbed by the noise, the college students invariably replied, "the grandfather." Older adults typically failed to make this inference. According to G. Cohen (1979), college students used logical reasoning to draw inferences from the text based on facts about the grandfather in the front room, the traffic noise being disturbing in the front room, and no one else being in the house but the mother. Cohen attributes older adults' failure to draw the "correct" inference to a decline in logical competence in old age.

Is this conclusion justifiable? Labouvie-Vief (1985) contends that older adults may not lack logical competence, but may interpret the context of the situation in a different way than younger adults. In a study using the passage above, Labouvie-Vief (1985) found that many older adults pointed out that the grandfather may have been deaf or that he would have left the room if the noise had been disturbing. From a contextualistic view, these comments appear to be quite sophisticated and adaptive because they consider the complexity of social contexts. By comparison, the young adults' literal interpretation of the passage seems youthful and naive.

mechanistic behavioral orientation, as in the question "How did the situation or context affect the behavior?" (Overton, 1984). However, contextualist theorists clearly mean something quite distinctive by *context*, which they conceptualize at several quantitatively different levels of analysis—biological, psychological, physical, and sociocultural. Moreover, the individual is seen as making an active contribution to the context, rather than being the passive recipient of environmental stimuli. Thus, individual attitudes, thoughts, and behaviors interact continually with the physical, social, and cultural components of various environments. If the person's characteristics "fit" the context, then adaptive behavioral outcomes occur. In contrast, people who are mismatched with their environment may show alternative, and not always adaptive, developmental outcomes.

The contextualistic and life-span perspectives on cognition have much in common. Both perspectives emphasize the potential for cognitive change across the life span and the multidirectionality and multidimensionality of such change. And this potential is thought to derive from the reciprocal interplay between individuals and contexts. To quote Lerner and Busch-Rossnagel (1981), "the life-span view promotes a model of development we have seen described as a contextual or a dialectic one. In so doing, it sees individuals as both products and producers of the context that provides a basis for their development. As such, individuals may be seen as producers of their development" (p. 6). Finally, development is determined by multiple forces which may not act together to produce one developmentally ideal end state.

In contextualistic formulations, cognition is seen as an activity inherently embedded within the social and cultural context in which it occurs. Thus, one of the best ways to study cognition is in a naturalistic setting using familiar, contextually valid materials. (The issue of contextual validity is discussed at the end of the chapter.) In the future, greater numbers of developmental psychologists will probably adopt contextualistic approaches to investigate cognitive functioning in everyday situations.

THEORETICAL DESCRIPTIONS OF COGNITIVE CHANGE

The four theoretical approaches reviewed in this chapter differ sharply in how they conceptualize cognitive development. All four are similar in that they must take a stand on how to best describe cognitive change. In this section we consider how the theories attempt to resolve questions about the nature of cognitive change by considering four different dimensions of change: (1) structural versus behavioral, (2) qualitative versus quantitative, (3) continuous versus discontinuous, and (4) universal versus nonuniversal. Table 2.2 summarizes the theoretical descriptions of change that will be discussed.

Structural versus Behavioral Change

By *structural versus behavioral* change, we are asking whether cognitive development is primarily seen as a reorganization or restructuring

Table 2.2
Summary of Theoretical Descriptions of Change in the Organismic Developmental, Information-Processing, Behavioristic, and Contextualistic Approaches

Approach	Nature of Change
Organismic Developmental	Change is primarily structural, qualitative, discontinuous, and universal.
Information-Processing	Change is mainly behavioral, quantitative, and continuous, but qualitative discontinuous shifts and reorganizations in development can also occur. Changes and processes are universal, although considerable contextual variability exists.
Behavioristic	Change is primarily behavioral, quantitative, continuous, and nonuniversal. Qualitative, discontinuous changes are reducible to prior elementary forms.
Contextualistic	Change can take multiple forms. Changes are mostly nonuniversal and context specific, but universal sequences may exist during certain periods of development.

of our cognitions or as an accumulation or deletion of specific cognitive behaviors. Organismic theorists contend that truly meaningful cognitive development occurs only when the structures of thought undergo a radical transformation such as that between concrete and formal operational stages of thought. Information-processing and behavioristic positions emphasize cognitive change as the product of a gradual build-up of discrete cognitive skills and behavior. Contextualists may classify either type of change as developmental depending upon whether they are more organismically oriented or more mechanistically oriented (Overton, 1983, 1984).

Qualitative versus Quantitative Change

Closely tied in with the structural-behavioral dimension is the *qualitative versus quantitative* distinction. This distinction can be best understood with an example. When a 3-year-old child adds 500 new words to his or her vocabulary, we refer to this as a quantitative change. However, the child's change from using single words to grammatically complex sentences is a qualitative change. In the latter instance, the child is not simply adding something more, but something different. Organismic theorists show more concern for the qualitative aspects of cognitive change from one stage to the next, although they allow for the possibility of quantitative changes within a stage. Information-processing theorists emphasize quantitative changes (such as increases in memory capacity) but also take into account qualitative shifts in information processing (such as changes in memory strategies). Behaviorists argue that development may appear qualitative, but can always be reduced to quantitative change consisting of an accumulation of learning experiences. Contextualists again seem to allow for either possibility, depending on their theoretical bent.

Continuous versus Discontinuous Change

The qualitative versus quantitative issue cannot be separated from the third change dimension of *continuity versus discontinuity*. Here the issue is whether behavioral changes are reducible (continuous) or irreducible (discontinuous) to prior forms (Overton & Reese, 1973). By one definition, qualitative changes are discontinuous because they cannot be reduced to earlier forms and because they are abrupt (Werner, 1957). In other words, we cannot understand a new whole by breaking it into its previously separate parts. The change in organization of the separate parts produces a new, or novel, whole with emergent properties. Remember that "emergent" means that the new properties cannot be completely predicted from the parts. This point of view is consistent with organismic models. Quantitative change can be either continuous (such as adding 5 vocabulary words per day for a year) or discontinuous (such as adding no words in one week and then 20 the next). In the mechanistic model, both types of change can be predicted from the organism's past history. Thus, there are no emergent properties in developmental change. What looks like emergent, qualitative differences—discontinuity—is based on prior elementary forms.

So far, we have concentrated on *descriptive* continuity and discontinuity. But continuity and discontinuity can also exist at the *explanatory* level. An example that highlights this distinction can be found in Piaget's theory. His stages of cognitive development are descriptively discontinuous, but the mechanisms for explaining transitions from stage to stage (assimilation, accommodation) are continuous because they do not vary across the life span (Huston-Stein & Baltes, 1976).

Universal versus Nonuniversal Change

Finally, it is important to consider whether the observed changes, regardless of their true form, are *universal or nonuniversal.* Are the same cognitive changes found in all individuals in every society and culture, or are they context specific? Organismic theorists such as Piaget argue for the universality of cognitive stages. Behaviorists are at the other extreme and see all behavior as context bound and therefore nonuniversal. Information-processing theorists have been frequently criticized for not considering context variables; they have traditionally been more concerned with identifying universal processing mechanisms and stages for specific cognitive tasks. As mentioned, however, information-processing psychologists have become increasingly interested in studying the contextual dependency of cognitive skills. Finally, contextualists tend to side with the nonuniversality position, but admit universal cognitive sequences might occur during certain periods of development.

NATURE, NURTURE, AND COGNITIVE DEVELOPMENT

The previous section dealt mainly with descriptions of cognitive change. In this section the focus shifts to a heated theoretical debate about the explanations of cognitive differences—the nature-nurture controversy.

The Nature-Nurture Controversy

One of the oldest and most heated controversies in developmental psychology is whether the causes of development can be explained on the basis of **nature** (inner biological and physiological processes) or **nurture** (social and physical environmental context). This controversy goes by many different names such as *heredity versus environment, innate versus acquired, instinctual versus learned,* and *nativism versus empiricism.* Because any theory of development must account for the effects of these components, some call this the central issue in developmental psychology today. Others see it as an outdated and dead issue.

Over 25 years ago, Anne Anastasi (1958) proposed a resolution to the nature-nurture controversy. Rather than ask such questions as *which* is more important (heredity or environment) or *how much* does each contribute to behavioral development, Anastasi suggested that we need to ask *how* nature and nurture interact. In other words, how do they jointly contribute to development?

As Baltes, Reese, and Nesselroade (1977) point out, these questions presuppose different paradigmatic views. The how question is more compatible with the organismic world view because it focuses on strong interactions between the organism and the environment. The how-much question reflects greater concern with additive, quantitative properties of development and, therefore, is more consistent with the behavioristic or mechanistic position (Overton, 1973). Interestingly, information-processing approaches say little about the nature-nurture controversy. While information-processing theorists acknowledge the implicit importance of nature (maturation of the sensory receptors, neurological development), they show more concern with how the experimental environment modifies cognitive processing on a moment-by-moment basis on selected laboratory tasks (P. Miller, 1983).

In order to illustrate the differences among the various paradigmatic views on the nature-nurture issue, let us focus on Piaget's organismic position. Piaget is usually classified as an interactionist theorist because he felt that neither heredity nor environment play a greater role in determining development. Rather, he was concerned with how innate and environmental factors interact to produce developmental change.

Piaget claimed that heredity equips the organism with sensory, neurological, and muscular structures to deal with the world at birth as well as providing the individual with an internal, maturational timetable. This timetable serves to open up new developmental possibilities for the creation of novel schemes. For example, when the child develops the ability to coordinate hands and eyes, new possibilities occur for actively exploring objects in the world.

According to Piaget, maturation is necessary but not sufficient to produce developmental change. Piaget is often mistakenly labeled as a maturational theorist, although he believed that maturation cannot be separated from experience. Piaget divided children's experience with their environment into two categories—physical experience and social experience. Physical experience involves unguided and direct physical actions on objects in the world. The child acts upon objects such as a rubber ball and by these actions notes certain properties of the object, such as the ball's ability to roll, bounce, and rebound. Piaget emphasized that the child's reflections on the actions, and not the passive observation of objects, bring about cognitive growth. Thus, it is not merely seeing a ball bounce, but the conclusions the child draws from the action of dropping or throwing a ball that are important.

Although physical experience is important, the child also needs social experience, which involves educational and cultural transmission of information from external sources. For example, teachers transmit knowledge to children via books, recitations, and charts. Of course, children must be maturationally advanced and have sufficient physical experience with the world to benefit from these efforts.

Another factor discussed earlier—equilibration—is necessary to maintain a balance among the above factors. Maturational changes, physical experience, and the influence of the social environment inevitably produce disruptions in a child's equilibrium with the world, forcing her or him to accommodate (develop new structures) to new situations. In summary, the types of cognitive schemes and structures a child constructs depend upon the dynamic interaction of the three factors of maturation, physical experience, and social experience.

Whereas organismic theorists such as Piaget focus on the question of how hereditary and environmental factors interact, mechanistically oriented psychologists are interested in how much each factor contributes to development. As you recall, Anastasi's (1958) paper implied that the questions "How much?" and "Which one?" are meaningless because the contributions of heredity and environment cannot be estimated independently. However, if one accepts the major tenets of the mechanistic position that development is quantitative, linear, and unidirectional, then these questions are no longer meaningless (Overton & Reese, 1973). Usually, such questions are tested by employing individuals who vary in their genetic and environmental similarity. Environmental similarity is determined by whether individuals are reared together or apart. The expectation is that the higher the persons' similarity on both dimensions, the higher the correlation in IQ (intelligence quotient) between pairs of individuals. Thus, identical twins reared together should be most similar in IQ, and unrelated individuals growing up in different environments should be most dissimilar. As expected, the correlations between identical twins exposed to the same environment are high (about .87), while the correlations between unrelated persons reared apart are extremely small (near zero). The correlation in fraternal twins is lower than in identical twins, but much higher than in unrelated persons. Even identical twins reared apart have more similar IQ scores than fraternal twins raised in the same home.

Despite these clear-cut findings, their interpretation is not straightforward. One major difficulty involves our definitions of *similarity* and *dissimilarity*. For example, many identical twins separated at birth and reared in apparently dissimilar environments actually resided in quite similar environments. In many cases, they lived in the same towns, attended the same schools, and were being raised by relatives of their parents (Kamin, 1974, 1981a). In one extreme case, the twins lived next door to one another! It is also important to reemphasize that these studies approach the nature-nurture issue from a mechanistic viewpoint, assuming that the contributions of each variable can be estimated quantitatively. Organismic researchers reject this notion and insist that the two influences cannot be separated.

Regardless of one's theoretical stance, two major problems hamper further progress on the nature-nurture issue. The first problem is definitional: How do we operationalize heredity and environment? As Anastasi (1958) noted, genetic effects on development are always indirect. We do not directly inherit high intelligence, fluent language, or good memory. All hereditary influences must occur within the context of a supportive environment. Without this context, genetic effects cannot be realized. The problem of defining *heredity* is compounded by the fact that the study of genetics has not typically been a province of psychologists.

Matters do not become easier when attempts are made to define *environment*. Anastasi (1958) argued that environmental effects on behavior can vary along a broad-narrow continuum. At the broadest level are environmental factors such as social class, which provide a general supportive context for the developing organism. More narrow environmental factors may be experiences such as travel or entertainment, which can be cognitively stimulating. Still narrower effects affect us on a momentary, day-to-day basis, such as when a professor informs us that we wrote a wrong answer on an examination. Thus, the specific environmental level being considered needs to be made explicit.

The second major problem in resolving the nature-nurture controversy stems from the fact that very few empirical studies on the issue have been developmental studies, and these were confined primarily to childhood development. Twin studies, for example, look at individual differences among children at a single point in time to determine whether heredity or environment accounts for differences. Although separate hereditary and environmental effects can be analyzed within this "individual differences" perspective, the "normative" perspective on development rejects the notion that these effects are separable (McCall, 1981; Plomin, 1983). The normative perspective focuses on average or *normal* developmental changes, such as the average changes in cognition from infancy to childhood. From this latter view, genetic effects do not occur in a vacuum, but within an environment in which the genes can be expressed over time. The failure to distinguish between these two perspectives on heredity-environment effects has been a source of great confusion in the nature-nurture debate (McCall, 1981).

From a life-span perspective, we can speculate about the nature of hereditary and environmental influences. In general, genetically based processes are seen as most influential in early life. This can be illustrated with Waddington's (1957) concept of **canalization**, which McCall (1981) has applied to the study of mental development. *Canalization* refers to the channeling of development along a path or track. The path along which all members of a species tend to develop is known as a **creod.** To the extent that species-typical environments exist, development will follow the creod. If the environment is atypical for a species, development will drift off the creod.

McCall (1981) provides a canalization example for early cognitive development. He proposes that development is highly canalized during the first 18–24 months of life, so that infants, regardless of environment, exhibit many of the same mental behaviors. These behaviors are fundamental characteristics such as acquiring language and symbolic functioning that every member of the species acquires. If their environment is disrupted, infants possess a self-righting tendency which compensates. Thus, if babies are exposed to an atypical environment and then removed, their behavior will tend to return (self-right) to the creod. After this time mental development becomes less canalized, and stable individual differences appear. For example, even though all children acquire language, some are more fluent than others.

Canalization is depicted in Figure 2.7 as a scoop. The diverging paths or tracks pictured in the scoop are the hereditary creods, which allow for individual differences in genetic dispositions. The contrasting designs inside the scoop represent qualitative stages of mental development. Now imagine that a small marble represents an individual whose life span begins at the left side of the scoop. As the marble rolls down the scoop through developmental time, it follows heredity's creod; but environmental forces, which can be represented as strong winds, are indispensable for development. Environmental winds blowing up or down the scoop produce individual differences in the rate of mental development, while those blowing across the scoop may deflect

Figure 2.7   A Scoop Model of Canalization in Mental Development.

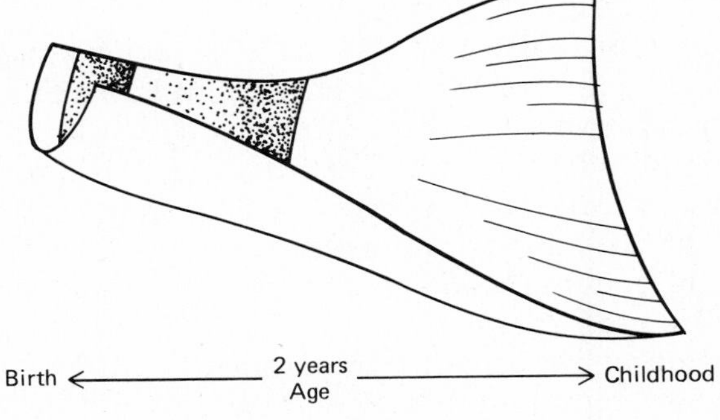

Birth ←————— 2 years ————→ Childhood
Age

development along a different creod. Notice that while unique environmental and genetic circumstances are more likely to influence development after age 2 than before, the organism's behavior can still be modified by strong environmental forces.

Baltes, Reese, and Lipsitt (1980) present a similar view that canalization progressively widens as development proceeds over the entire life course. Their rationale is that genetic control over the adult and aging portion of the life span is less because evolutionary processes (which are assumed to reflect genetic influences) are presumed to affect only the prereproductive years. However, evolutionary and genetic influence may be operating during the postreproductive years in such phenomena as **terminal drop.** Terminal drop, which will be discussed more in Chapter 8, is the rapid and precipitous drop in mental abilities a few months or years prior to physical death. Thus, there may be a second peak in genetic influence at the far end of the life span.

Alternatives to the Nature-Nurture Controversy

Since genetics and environment are involved in every human behavior, continued debate over their relative contributions seems pointless. As an alternative to the nature-nurture controversy, we might try to identify patterns of behavior that have evolved over time and that possess species-adaptive value. This is exactly what researchers known as ethologists attempt to do. Ethologists focus their attention on adaptive behavior characteristics that are common to every member of the same species, rather than on individual differences among members. Although most often applied to animal species, this approach can also be applied to the human species by examining behaviors that are universal across different cultures and societies.

Mergler and Goldstein (1983) have developed an ethological or evolutionary model for describing changes in human cognition during old age. They argue that cognitive aging changes ordinarily seen as negative may serve an adaptive function for society as a whole. For example, older persons often show processing deficits in recalling detailed information, but they appear quite adept at summarizing the gist of information and drawing broad generalizations. Thus, they may be particularly well suited to roles, such as oral historian, which involve the transmission of information in summarized form. Mergler and Goldstein's model represents a new and exciting way to conceptualize cognitive development and should prove more fruitful than continued controversy over nature and nurture.

Critical Periods and Cognitive Development

In ethological approaches to development the notion of *critical periods* is a central one. Ethologists claim that there are certain periods during maturation when the organism is maximally influenced by specific kinds of experience. Just as Freud argued that infancy is a critical time for determining later personality development, ethologists such as Konrad Lorenz talk about a critical period of *imprinting*. That is, shortly after birth ducklings will follow the first large moving object they see— in other words, they imprint. For example, when Lorenz moved in the presence of the ducklings, he became the imprinted object and the ducklings followed him, instead of their natural mother (Hess, 1973). Once the critical period has passed, imprinting is more difficult to establish.

Developmental psychologists who accept the critical-period view emphasize the long-term consequences of early experience for development. As T. G. R. Bower, a well-known expert on infant perceptual development, writes, "I believe that infancy is the critical period in cognitive development—the period when the greatest gains and the greatest losses can occur. Further, the gains and losses that occur here become harder to offset with increasing age" (1974, pp. vii–viii). Eric Lenneberg, an authority on language development, takes a similar view. Lenneberg (1967) believes that a child who is not exposed to language during the first few years of life may not be able to speak.

Until recently, the view that the infant years exert a disproportionate and irreversible effect on the developing organism was rarely challenged. However, evidence now suggests that children can overcome the damaging consequences of early negative experiences. In a celebrated case, a young girl named Genie was not exposed to language until after age 13 (Fromkin, Krashen, Curtiss, Rigler, & Rigler, 1974). Although she had been isolated from age 2 and had heard no speech, she was able to learn certain aspects of language after puberty. Because she had difficulty with her syntax (grammar), we cannot completely discount the critical-period notion.

In their extensive review of studies on early experience, Clarke and Clarke (1976) concluded that the "whole of development" is important, not just the first 5 years or so. Thus, Clarke and Clarke do not think that one developmental stage plays a greater formative role than any other. Jerome Kagan, a Harvard psychologist, has reached a similar conclusion in his studies of the effects of impoverished environments on intellectual development in Guatemalan children (Kagan, 1971; Kagan, Kearsley, & Zelazo, 1978). Such conclusions may be premature until life-span data are available. In Chapter 10, we will return to the matter

of critical periods when we discuss the effects of early childhood intervention (training) programs on later cognitive development.

CURRENT METHODS IN COGNITIVE
DEVELOPMENTAL RESEARCH

The previous three sections have examined how psychologists of varying theoretical orientations attempt to describe and explain changes and
differences in cognitive development. In this section, the methods
researchers use to investigate questions about cognitive development
will be explored. In reality, theory and method go hand in hand.
Depending upon their theoretical orientation, developmental psychologists may be likely to employ certain methodologies; and the methodologies employed may suggest different theoretical questions (Overton & Reese, 1973).

Research Designs

The first methodological issue is the choice of a research design. As discussed in Chapter 1, the two major designs for studying age-develop-
ment relationships are *cross-sectional* and *longitudinal*. The major difference between the two is that cross-sectional designs compare two or
more groups of people at a single point in time, whereas longitudinal
designs compare a single group of individuals at two or more points in
time. Cross-sectional research examines age *differences*, and longitudinal research looks at age *changes* (Schaie, 1967). Because longitudinal
designs directly involve change, researchers generally regard them as
more representative of a true developmental design than cross-sectional
designs.

Cross-Sectional Designs

To give you a clearer idea of a cross-sectional study, let us use the following hypothetical example. Suppose a school system asks you to evaluate mathematical ability differences between second, fourth, sixth,
and eighth graders. You administer a set of mathematical problems to
individuals at each grade level and obtain *group averages*. As predicted,
you find a linear increase in mathematical skill with increasing age.
Eighth graders do better, on the average, than sixth graders, who do better than fourth graders, and so on. At this point, you have described
differences between grade levels, but have not explained them. The differences could be due to age, but they also may be due to other factors
such as practice or experience. Perhaps you hypothesize that the superiority of the older children resides in their greater experience with the

task. You give each group varying amounts of practice on the task to see if the age differences will be reduced. If they are reduced, then the experience variable helps to explain the initial differences observed.

Although the cross-sectional design may give you information about how mathematical performance typically varies with age, and perhaps even why it varies, a number of important questions remain. How do *interindividual* differences among children as well as adults change with age? What is the relationship between earlier and later cognitive development? What environmental or contextual factors affect development? To answer these types of questions, a longitudinal, or *repeated measures*, approach is needed. Even though longitudinal studies sometimes span years or decades, they often involve comparatively short periods (days, months), as in studies of substages in infant cognitive development.

Longitudinal Designs
If the school system discussed above asked you to study mathematical thinking longitudinally, your design might look like the following. Let's say in 1987 you select a group of second graders and test these schoolchildren in 1989, 1991, and 1993. This approach would allow you to examine individual change patterns in mathematical ability as well as group trends. You could also determine whether early mathematical precocity in any way predicts later intellectual performance. Finally, you could examine specific environmental events (such as curriculum changes, new homework procedures) between times of testing which might affect mathematical performance. This design thus provides you with significant descriptive information on mathematical skill development across age (or time).

Because longitudinal designs involve repeated measures they have usually been regarded as superior to cross-sectional designs. However, unless proper experimental controls are instituted, longitudinal results may be open to a wide variety of alternative explanations (Baltes & Nesselroade, 1979; Baltes et al., 1977). For example, repeatedly testing subjects may involve practice or test-retest effects, which lead to inflated results. In fact, a tremendous amount of positive and largely unrecognized biasing occurs because of retesting (Baltes et al., 1977). One potential solution to this problem is to select a different but representative sample from the same original group of subjects at each time of measurement. This approach, known as an *independent measurements* longitudinal design, avoids the problem of repeatedly testing the same subjects.

Subject attrition or experimental mortality also creates problems in longitudinal research, especially if subjects who drop out of a study differ systematically from those who stay in. Typically, those who remain to participate are brighter, healthier, and more highly motivated than those who do not remain, a result that appears to be true for children as well as adults. There is also a problem with testing only a single group (cohort) of subjects. Would your results be the same if you had tested children between 1937 and 1943 rather than 1987 and 1993? If not, then the possibility of a *cohort effect* exists. Mathematical instruction may be radically different now than it was 50 years ago. Finally, have you accounted for specific environmental events (e.g., teachers' strikes, school closings) that might affect mental performance? These historical events might well bias your results.

Sequential Designs

Over the past two decades there has been considerable attention to the development of **sequential methods** involving successions of cross-sectional and longitudinal designs, each covering different birth cohorts (Baltes & Nesselroade, 1979; Schaie, 1965). The major rationale of these designs is that the study of development involves both individual (ontogenetic) changes as well as historical-evolutionary (cohort) changes. In cross-sectional sequences, independent observations are made at all ages and cohort levels. For example, in the cross-sectional sequential study in Figure 2.8*a*, the 1960 and 1980 testings are made with members of different age groups and different cohorts. Longitudinal sequences test at least two different cohorts at different times across the same age range (see Figure 2.8*b*). Both strategies avoid the problem of limited generalizability across time and cohort. As Baltes et al. (1977) point out, simultaneous application of both designs is desirable (though not always practical) because they supplement one another by providing alternative experimental controls. For example, the results of cross-sectional sequences can be used to estimate the magnitude of retest effects in longitudinal sequences (Baltes et al., 1977). Retest effects involving repeated measures are a major problem in sequential research (Botwinick, 1979), as is using different time spans for the age, cohort, and period-of-measurement dimensions in sequential studies. Finally, there is disagreement about whether sequential designs can be used for explanatory purposes as well as descriptive purposes (Schaie & Baltes, 1975). Unless the necessary controls are used, it is probably best to think of sequential designs as descriptive.

How frequently have the various designs been employed in cognitive developmental research? Because they are quick and economical, cross-sectional designs have been the designs of choice among developmentalists. This is certainly true, for example, in Piagetian studies where different aspects of cognitive ability such as conservation, classification, and seriation have been studied in samples of children (Versey, 1980) and adults (Papalia, Salverson, & True, 1973; K. Rubin, 1976)

Figure 2.8 (*a*) **Cross-sectional sequences test members of different age groups and different cohorts at two or more times.** (*b*) **Longitudinal sequences test two different cohorts at different times across the same age range. Different symbols = different persons.**

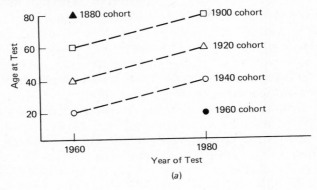

(a)

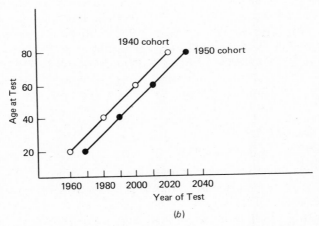

(b)

From *Adult Development and Aging* (p. 20) by K. W. Schaie and J. Geiwitz, 1982, Boston: Little, Brown. Copyright 1982 by K. W. Schaie and J. Geiwitz. Reprinted by permission of Little, Brown and Company.

varying in age. Investigators typically use the results to check the accuracy of Piagetian stages in children or the extent of cognitive regression in adults.

Most longitudinal designs within a Piagetian framework concentrate on the 4–10-year-old range, which covers the preoperational to concrete operational period, and especially the years 5–7, which are believed to be an important transitional period. Few longitudinal studies of formal operational development are available. Karplus and Karplus's (1972) study of the development of proportional reasoning between ages 10–15 is one of the only longitudinal studies in the literature. To date, there have been no sequential studies of Piagetian cognition. For the most part, sequential designs have been used to study age-related changes in adult cognition (see Chapter 8).

Life-span researchers pay more attention to design issues than child developmentalists. One reason is that the study of childhood encompasses a smaller age range. For example, in studying children's cognitive abilities between ages 2–6, cohort effects may not pose a major problem. But comparing 20-year-olds with 60-year-olds is more problematic because of the generational (cohort) difference. But, even in childhood investigations, dynamic changes in society (including changes in educational institutions, child-rearing practices, and family arrangements) may increase the likelihood of cohort effects. Another reason for the differential emphasis on design questions is the nature of the abilities studied. Child researchers often investigate the development of basic cognitive abilities such as perception, attention, and memory—abilities which seem to have a strong maturational component and a uniform developmental sequence. However, many of the abilities assessed by life-span researchers—especially those measured by standardized intelligence tests—do not follow a predictable course, but depend more on particular life events and social experiences. The question of how much cohort factors affect adult age differences in more basic cognitive processes such as perception and attention is still unanswered (Kausler, 1982).

Sample Selection and Measurement Equivalence

We have just reviewed cross-sectional, longitudinal, and sequential developmental research designs. This section focuses first on methodological problems related to sample selection and maintenance. Later, problems connected with selecting equivalent measurement instruments across age groups are discussed.

In longitudinal designs, especially life-span ones, sample maintenance is a major problem because subjects often drop out, a problem referred to earlier as "experimental mortality." However, even initial samples in longitudinal designs may be unrepresentative because subjects who volunteer to participate in repeated testing are likely to be more motivated than people who do not volunteer. Selecting and obtaining a representative sample is not as problematical in cross-sectional studies as in longitudinal studies, but sampling still poses a problem. Perhaps the biggest difficulty, particularly in life-span studies, is the differential availability of subject populations. Some groups (such as schoolchildren, college students, nursing home residents) form captive populations and are more easily accessible to researchers. Thus, much research is based on unrepresentative groups, which limits our ability to generalize our findings to the population at large.

Another problem, not generally recognized by developmental researchers, involves time-related changes in the population as a whole. Demographic studies show that the mortality rate and age structure of the population change over time. These changes can create problems, especially if the study runs several years. The major problem involves a process called **selective survival,** or the biological and psychological survival of particular subgroups of the population. There is evidence that survival rates are related to intelligence, with adult survivors being more intelligent on the average than nonsurvivors (K. Riegel & Riegel, 1972). Life-span researchers must be alert to differential survivorship rates if they are to draw valid conclusions about cognitive changes over time.

One final comment is needed about the selection of age groups for life-span research. Contrary to what you might expect, life-span studies do not necessarily require comparisons of subjects at every age level from infancy to old age. Nor does an age-specific study become a life-span developmental study merely by adding more age groups. The focus must be on a process (such as cognition) that shows "intrinsic life-span perspectives" (Huston-Stein & Baltes, 1976, p. 172), which simply means that the process involved shows systematic or regular changes across the life span.

In addition to sample selection and maintenance, measurement equivalence is a key concern of life-span researchers (Labouvie, 1980). Can we be certain that we are measuring the same intellectual process across different age levels? This issue can be illustrated by returning to our earlier example of mathematical ability among schoolchildren. Suppose you chose a reading problem dealing with computing the area of a triangle as your main dependent (outcome) measure. For young children who have never encountered this type of task, such a measure might assess their problem-solving skill. However, for older children— especially those who have solved dozens of similar problems—this task might measure memory of a formula $(A = \frac{1}{2} bh)$ rather than true problem-solving ability.

Even if you are measuring the same characteristic in different age samples, the measures may not be equivalent in meaningfulness and difficulty level. Does an intelligence test hold the same meaning for a 16-year-old high school student as it does for a 50-year-old businessperson? Will the intelligence test be equally difficult for these two individuals? The first question deals with the problem of contextual validity, an issue to be discussed shortly. One solution to the latter problem involves giving a range of tests varying in difficulty level to different age groups. Each group works through each test until the members encounter their *ceiling*, or point where they miss all the answers.

Our purpose has been to sensitize you to some of the obstacles investigators encounter when conducting research in a life-span framework. Ways of overcoming these obstacles have also been considered. We should emphasize again that life-span approaches do not simplify as much as they enrich our understanding of developmental processes. Now we turn to an issue receiving considerable attention from cognitive developmental psychologists.

Contextual Validity

During the past few years, there has been great interest in improving the **contextual validity** of developmental studies of cognition. Contextual validity refers to the extent to which one can generalize developmental changes observed or manipulated under laboratory conditions to those occurring in the real world (Bronfenbrenner, 1977; Hultsch & Hickey, 1978; Neisser, 1976). Neisser (1976), in particular, has criticized the "artificiality" of many laboratory investigations of cognition.

How do developmental psychologists improve the contextual validity of their research? Several things can be done, including changing tasks, experimental settings, and manipulations. N. Denney and Palmer (1981), for example, administered groups of adult subjects (20–79 years of age) two types of problem-solving tasks—one a standard laboratory task and the other a problem that you might encounter in real life. For example:

> Let's say that one evening you go to the refrigerator and you notice that it is not cold inside, but warm. What would you do?

N. Denny and Palmer (1981) found that the ability to solve the standard problem declined with age, but performance on the real-life problem improved up to ages 40–50 and then decreased. Thus, the cognitive developmental trend observed may depend on the type of task used. It may also depend on the setting of the research. Baddeley (1981) studied memory in everyday life by having people calculate instances of absent-mindedness. He suggests that results for everyday memory may not parallel laboratory findings.

This concern with contextual validity represents an exciting and healthy trend in cognitive developmental research. But developmentalists must avoid simply substituting one task or situation for another without considering how such changes relate to developmental theory.

We have reviewed some of the major theoretical and methodological issues in conducting life-span work on cognition. As you have seen, life-span researchers face formidable obstacles in conceptualizing and studying cognitive developmental changes, but this should not be a cause for despair. Indeed, every approach to human cognition has its limitations. Since the beginning of the cognitive revolution some 25 years ago, significant advances have been made in developing more contextually valid perspectives on cognition, in clearly defining the major theoretical problems, and in designing more sophisticated methodological strategies to solve them (Lerner, 1986). Taken together, these advances are a cause for great optimism about the future.

SUMMARY

1. Two of the most important contemporary approaches to the study of cognitive changes are organismic developmental theories and information-processing theories.

2. Organismic developmental theories assume that psychological change processes are similar to biological processes. Cognitive development, like biological development, proceeds in a fixed series of stages.

3. Piaget's structural theory of intelligence is the best known example of an organismic developmental approach to cognition. Piaget described three specific aspects of intelligence: (1) content, (2) function, and (3) structure.

4. Piaget proposed four discrete stages of cognitive development: (1) sensorimotor, (2) preoperational, (3) concrete operational, and (4) formal operational.

5. Werner's orthogenetic theory characterizes cognitive development along a dimension of increasing differentiation and integration of the different psychological systems.

6. Information-processing theories attempt to account for changes in the way organisms receive, store, and react to sensory information. These theories use the computer as a model for human thinking.

7. Behavioristic theories view cognitive development as the gradual accumulation of specific learning experiences.

8. Recent contextualistic accounts of cognitive development emphasize the reciprocal interactions between the developing organism and the changing environmental context. Contextualistic and life-span perspectives share similar assumptions about the nature and sources of cognitive change.

9. Substantial theoretical differences exist with regard to the description of cognitive change. Change can be described as structural or behavioral, qualitative or quantitative, continuous or discontinuous, and universal or nonuniversal.
10. The nature-nurture controversy concerns whether developmental differences in cognition can be best explained on the basis of nature (biology, maturation) or nurture (environment, experience). An alternative to the controversy involves looking at developmental processes that possess species-adaptive value, regardless of specific cause.
11. Three different research designs—cross-sectional, longitudinal, and sequential—have been used to study cognitive development across the life span. Life-span researchers typically pay more attention to design issues than do child developmental psychologists.
12. Selecting representative samples and choosing contextually valid measures for different age groups are major methodological problems in life-span developmental studies of cognition.

Key Terms

theories	sensorimotor scheme
hypothetical constructs	production system
constructivist view	elementarism
epistemology	nature
equilibration	nurture
content	canalization
function	creod
structure	terminal drop
organization	sequential methods
adaptation	selective survival
assimilation	contextual validity
accommodation	

Suggested Readings

Baltes, P. B., Reese, H. W., & Nesselroade, J. R. (1977). *Life-span developmental psychology: Introduction to research methods.* Monterey, CA: Brooks/Cole. This text provides an excellent general introduction to key methodological issues in research design and theory construction in life-span developmental psychology. Though aimed at an introductory level, the book contains material typically found in more advanced texts on developmental research.

Brainerd, C. J. (Ed.). (1983). *Recent advances in cognitive-developmental theory: Progress in cognitive development research.* New York: Springer. This edited volume is part of the *Springer Series in Cognitive Development.* It covers emerging theories in cognitive developmental psychology including contextualism, the rule-oriented approach, socio-biology, working memory analyses, and ethology.

Flavell, J. H. (1963). *The developmental psychology of Jean Piaget.* New York: Van Nostrand Reinhold. A comprehensive and scholarly overview and evaluation of Piaget's theory, this book has provided an introduction of Piaget's work to psychologists in the United States.

Ginsburg, H., & Opper, S. (1979). *Piaget's theory of intellectual development* (2nd ed.). Englewood Cliffs, NJ: Prentice-Hall, 1979. A shorter and more readable account of Piaget's theory than Flavell's (1963) work. It is generally regarded as one of the best shorter summaries of Piaget's work available.

Klahr, D., & Wallace, J. G. (1976). *Cognitive development: An information-processing view.* Hillsdale, NJ: Erlbaum. An early attempt to apply the information-processing paradigm to the problems raised by research in the Piagetian tradition. The book describes children's cognitive abilities at different levels of development and the mechanisms underlying transitions from one level to the next.

Langer, J. (1969). *Theories of development.* New York: Holt, Rinehart and Winston. This scholarly book presents three general developmental perspectives including psychoanalytic, mechanistic, and organismic theory. It also outlines the steps needed to produce a comprehensive theory of development.

Rosenthal, T. L., & Zimmerman, B. J. (1978). *Social learning and cognition.* New York: Academic Press. This book presents a social learning perspective on the development of children's cognition in the areas of language, moral judgment, conservation, concept attainment, and problem solving. One of the most thorough and comprehensive treatments of social learning theory's contributions to cognitive research available.

Spiker, C. C. (1966). The concept of development: Relevant and irrelevant issues. *Monographs of the Society for Research in Child Development, 31*(5, Serial No. 107). A rather old, but important paper on the general concept of "development." Though much of the paper deals with problems associated with defining developmental changes, there is a section on the relation of the concept of development to cognitive aspects of behavior.

Sternberg, R. J. (Ed.). (1984). *Mechanisms of cognitive development.* San Francisco: Freeman. This book addresses the important but neglected question of how cognitive development takes place. Psychological mechanisms underlying cognitive changes are considered, primarily from an information-processing perspective.

CHAPTER 3

Perceptual and Attentional Development

OUTLINE

OVERVIEW

Perceptual changes are evident across the entire life span, although most theory and research on perception has focused on infancy, childhood, or old age. In this chapter the classic philosophical debates about the nature of perceptual experience from childhood to adulthood will be reviewed, and then some of the major contemporary theories of perceptual development will be examined. Next, we will look at perception at the sensory level of analysis. Changes in sensory processes such as vision and audition are often among the most dramatic aspects of perceptual development, and such changes may have a significant impact on everyday functioning. The coordination between the various sensory systems as well as perceptual illusions will also be discussed.

In the following section, the selective nature of perception will be emphasized. A major part of perceptual development involves learning to focus selectively on important information and to disregard unimportant information. The question of whether there are limits to our attentional capacity will then be examined. Some psychologists believe human beings have limited attentional resources, while others think that no known capacity limitations exist. Attentional processes that require a great deal of mental effort will be differentiated from those that function more or less automatically. In addition, the relationship between attention and arousal will be discussed. Finally, individual differences in the way people perceive, organize, remember, and think about information will be considered. The investigation of these differences forms a useful link between perceptual processes and higher-level cognitive processes.

SOME QUESTIONS ABOUT PERCEPTION

Perceptual development is truly a life-span process. It begins at birth, or even earlier during the prenatal period, and continues to the moment of death. Despite this fact, most investigations of perception have not been conducted within a life-span developmental framework (Pollack & Atkeson, 1978). Instead, theory and research on perceptual processes have been limited primarily to infancy, childhood, or old age or have been confined to experimental laboratory studies in which age has not been included as a variable. This chapter will emphasize the usefulness of a life-span perspective for integrating the empirical information on age-related changes and differences in perception.

Several key questions can be raised about the nature and course of perception across the life span. What can newborn infants see and hear? Are their perceptions organized and interpreted in the same way as those of an older child, adolescent, or adult, or are they the great mass of "blooming, buzzing confusion" described by William James (1890)? What role does experience play in the acquisition of perceptual competencies? Are some perceptual abilities innate? Finally, do we perceive the world objectively, or do we live in a totally subjective world? These are some of the major questions raised in this chapter and the chapter that follows on spatial cognition and imagery.

Although these questions have a history dating far back before the beginnings of psychology, the answers remain elusive. One reason is that the perceptual experience of two individuals is difficult to compare directly and must be inferred from self-reports of their behavior. When you look at the blue sky overhead, for instance, are you really seeing the same blueness as another observer? A second reason is primarily methodological. The limited behavioral repertoire of the infant poses a formidable methodological barrier to developmental studies on perception. We cannot simply ask babies to report on what they see, hear, or feel. Recent investigators have developed ingenious techniques for assessing perceptual capacities during infancy and early childhood; some of these techniques will be discussed in this chapter.

DEFINITION OF PERCEPTION

Let us begin by defining some basic terms. What is **perception?** As E. Gibson and Spelke (1983) define it, "Perception is the process by which animals gain knowledge about their environment and about themselves in relation to the environment" (p. 2). Since it involves the beginning of all acquired knowledge, perception is a fundamental aspect of cognition. In classic psychological theorizing, perception is typically distinguished from an even more fundamental process called **sensation.** Sensation involves the initial contact between the organism and the environment, when sensory stimulation (lights, sounds, colors) first activates the sensory receptors. Thus, sensation provides the raw sensory data for perception. Organizing and extracting meaning from this information is done by the process of perception. Although this distinction between sensation and perception is somewhat arbitrary, and there is often a blurring between the two processes, such distinctions help developmentalists to identify the level at which age-related changes occur.

NATURE-NURTURE REVISITED

Of all the topics covered by this book, the area of perception is most closely tied to the nature-nurture debate. For centuries philosophers turned to the topic of perception as a way of answering basic epistemological questions about the origins and nature of knowledge. Most of their questions centered on infants. What do infants know before they have any experience in the world? How do infants acquire knowledge about the world? Answers to these questions depend on whether one believes in **empiricism,** the theory that all knowledge comes by way of the senses and grows through experience, or **nativism,** the idea that infants are innately equipped to organize rudimentary knowledge.

Empiricism

From an empiricist perspective, the perceptual world of the infant is radically different from that of the experienced adult perceiver. Infants are not naturally endowed with perceptual knowledge at birth, but must acquire perceptual skills through sensory experience. The stimuli in the environment excite the sensory receptors, giving rise to sensations that become *associated* to form higher-order ideas and concepts. Thus, through a process of association, complex perceptions of the world are built up from elementary sensations. For example, in learning to read, we associate the visual features of letters and their sounds to form meaningful words.

The empiricist point of view traces its lineage from the writings of the English philosopher John Locke (1632–1704). Locke described the infant's mind as a *tabula rasa,* or "blank slate," a view that extends back to Aristotle. In Locke's opinion, the mind contains no innate ideas at birth. What is etched on the slate is determined solely by experience. Several other early philosophers such as George Berkeley (1685–1753) and David Hume (1711–1776) also held strongly empiricist views. Berkeley appealed to empiricist concepts to explain perceptual problems such as depth and distance perception. A somewhat modified empiricist view was later expressed by William James (1890), who described the infant's perceptual world as a "blooming, buzzing confusion" of sights and sounds. In his view, experience played an influential role in organizing perceptions into meaningful wholes.

Nativism

In sharp contrast to the empiricist approach, nativists believe that infants and adults share certain perceptual similarities. Infants enter the world with rudimentary notions of time and space as well as with the abilities to perceive visual size, depth, form, and movement. Their minds impose an organization on their sensations, so that the infant's world is not a disorganized chaos, as James maintained.

The nativist view of perception can be seen most clearly in the writings of French philosopher René Descartes (1596–1650) and German philosopher Immanuel Kant (1724–1804). Descartes wrote about the mind's natural ability to infer distance from the angles created by near and far objects. In his *Critique of Pure Reason*, Kant held that notions of space and time are innate. Thus, human beings are not viewed as empty slates.

As can be seen in this chapter and the next, the nativist-empiricist argument is still very much with us. Although some battles have been won by one side or the other, the controversy is not dead. Perceptual developmental psychologists continue to debate such issues as whether form and space perception are innate or learned. However, they now use scientific experimentation instead of philosophical speculation to answer these questions. In this chapter we will review what each view—empiricism, nativism—has to contribute to the study and understanding of perception across the life cycle.

THEORIES OF PERCEPTUAL DEVELOPMENT

Different theories have been proposed to explain the relationship between perceptual and cognitive development. Some psychological theories consider perception to be a primitive organizing process that supplies the basic elements for cognition, but is eventually complemented in more developmentally mature individuals by higher-order cognitive processes. Piaget's constructivist theory of cognition exemplifies this view of perception (see Chapter 2). Other perceptual theories emphasize organisms' increasing ability to detect meaningful features of the environment without relying solely on their cognitive constructions. Eleanor Gibson's differentiation theory illustrates the latter approach. We will now review the Piagetian and Gibsonian positions as well as a model which attempts to reconcile the two positions.

Piaget's Constructivist Position

As discussed in Chapter 2, Piaget has become a towering figure in the study of developmental cognition. However, his theoretical ideas have been much less influential in the field of perceptual development (Walk, 1981). Perhaps this is because Piaget regarded perception as a preliminary organizing process that supplies the basic data for cognition. As you may recall from Chapter 2, Piaget stressed the importance of active experience in gaining knowledge about the world. This emphasis is consistent with an empiricist position attributing an active role to the environment. However, Piaget rejected the notion of the mind as a *tabula rasa* with content limited to perceptual experience. He stressed that all experience is assimilated into the child's sensorimotor schemes such as looking at, touching, or sucking an object. Thus, the experience that matters to the child is not strictly perceptual, but active; it is not based on the infant's ability to passively observe objects, but on his or her ability to act on them. For example, a child does not passively watch an object disappear, but actively tries to bring about the object's reappearance by reaching for it or gazing at the spot where it disappeared.

Piaget agreed with the nativists (or nature point of view) in stressing the contribution of the active, knowing child to the interpretation of perceptual experience. According to this view, the child's understanding of concepts such as space, time, and causality imposes meaning and order on his or her perceptual world. However, Piaget strongly disagreed with the nativists when he argued that these concepts are gradually constructed in the course of development, not innately given at birth. Thus, Piaget's constructivist view of perceptual and cognitive development can be seen as occupying a central ground between strict empiricist and strict nativist positions.

Piaget strongly believed that the sensorimotor schemes of infants do not provide valid objective information about the external world. Initially, infants are restricted to their immediate sensory experience; they only perceive objects in terms of their practical activities toward these objects. Only gradually do infants gain a more objective understanding of the way in which the world is spatially and temporally organized. For example, not until 6 or 7 months of age do infants acquire a concept of the permanence of objects—the idea that objects which disappear from view do not cease to exist (see Chapter 4). By the end of the sensorimotor stage, infants develop a capacity for internal mental representation. External motor actions are replaced by internal mental representations. Although older children do not cease to perceive, they are less tied to their immediate perceptions and more reliant on higher-order cognitive skills such as classifying, comparing, and judging.

Gibson's Differentiation Position

Piaget's account of perceptual development contrasts sharply with the empiricist position of Eleanor Gibson (1969, 1982; J. Gibson, 1979). In accord with empiricist approaches, E. Gibson views the environment as a source of meaningful information that does not require any enrichment or interpretation. In contrast to traditional empiricist approaches, she views the world as so rich in information that no associative learning is needed to impart meaning. Furthermore, the infant is equipped with sensory systems capable of detecting information from birth, and these sensory systems are coordinated with each other. In contrast, Piaget sees the senses as separate and unintegrated in early infancy. Gibson acknowledges that some sensory systems (such as audition) are more mature at birth than others (such as vision), and each system shows enormous change with development (E. Gibson & Spelke, 1983).

In the Gibsonian view, one major function of perception is to detect **distinctive features** from environmental stimulation. This concept forms a cornerstone of her theory. "Distinctive features" can be defined simply as dimensions of difference between two or more objects. For example, look at the nonsense "scribbles" in Figure 3.1. How is scribble A in the center different from the surrounding ones? Note that some scribbles have four coils (also like scribble A), whereas others have three or five coils. The number of coils is a distinctive feature that differentiates one stimulus from another. Other distinctive features in Figure 3.1 are the amount of stretching or compression in the coils and the mirror reversal (left-right) orientation.

J. Gibson and Gibson (1955) used these stimuli to study developmental differences in the process of **differentiation,** or the ability to detect features that distinguish one class of objects or events from others. Children aged 6–8 years and 8½–11 years and adults were shown the standard scribble A and asked to identify it from memory among

Figure 3.1   Scribbles used to study perceptual learning. The standard scribble is the four-coil one labeled A.

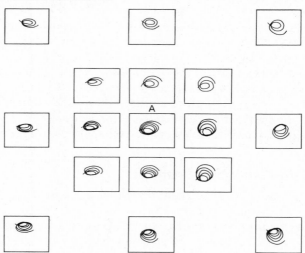

the other scribbles shown one at a time. After each run through the deck of 18 cards, subjects were shown the standard again. The youngest children averaged 13.4 incorrect or undifferentiated items on the first trial, older children 7.9, and adults 3.0. The adults achieved perfect recognition after an average of 3 runs through the deck. The older children did the same after 5 runs, and the youngest children never achieved perfect recognition and were stopped after an average of 7 runs through the deck. With repeated exposure of the stimuli, older children and adults gradually learned more about the basic dimensions of difference between the standard and the other objects, but the younger children did not.

The process of perceptual development thus comes about as a result of learning more and more about the basic dimensions of difference between objects (E. Gibson, 1969; J. Gibson & Gibson, 1955). But the learning process also involves the detection of **invariants,** or objects that will have the same features across individual members despite variations in other features. Note in the Figure 3.1 coils that the curvature of the lines is invariant across the scribbles, even though the looseness or compactness of the coils is not. In explaining the detection of invariants, Gibson highlighted an important difference between her theory of perceptual development and Piaget's (P. Harris, 1983). Piaget maintained that children construct the notion of invariance by acting upon objects to transform them and then reversing the transformations. For example, a child may tilt several blocks on their sides and then move them back into an upright position. By doing this the child finds that certain properties of the blocks (size, shape) remain invariant, despite the blocks being moved. In contrast, E. Gibson argued that invariants are not the end result of a child's active construction, but can be detected in the stimulation in the environment. Thus, a child can observe that certain types of movements leave an object's shape unchanged. Developmental changes in perception result in a better correspondence with objects and events in the world which serve as a source of stimulation.

Another major difference between E. Gibson and Piaget involves the issue of *representation* (P. Harris, 1983). As noted, Piaget believed that the child becomes progressively less reactive to immediate perceptual experience and gradually begins to use representational (symbolic) thought. E. Gibson dissented from such a view by arguing that development brings about a more organized, economical, and selective search for information in the environment. The developmental change is not in becoming less tied to stimulus information in the external environment. For E. Gibson, the major difference between infants at the beginning of the sensorimotor period and the end is in their ability to select information from the environment. This is not to say that the infant fails to develop representational competencies such as imagery or expectations, but the infant does not need to rely on these representations to gain valid information about the world. We will return to the issue of perceptual selectivity later in this chapter when we discuss the topic of attention.

Neisser's Perceptual Cycle Model

Ulric Neisser (1976) has offered an alternative view of perception that combines E. Gibson's differentiation position with Piaget's constructivist position. According to Neisser, the structure of information available in the environment plus the cognitive structures internal to the perceiver determine what is perceived. In other words, perception is an active, constructive process that depends on the type of information available.

Neisser called the structures (or plans) that direct perception the **anticipatory schemata.** These schemata (plural for *schema*) direct exploratory movements of the head, eyes, and hands. Through perceptual exploration of the *optic array*—the pattern of ambient light reflected from objects—the original schemata are modified. Once the perceptual structures are modified, they direct further perceptual search. Thus, perception is inherently active and selective.

Figure 3.2 illustrates Neisser's **perceptual cycle** model, which presents perception as a continuous and cyclic activity. The action of per-

Figure 3.2   The perceptual cycle model.

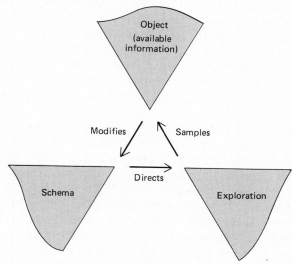

From *Cognition and Reality: Principles and Implications of Cognitive Psychology* (p. 21) by U. Neisser, 1976, San Francisco: Freeman. Copyright 1976 by W. H. Freeman and Company. Reprinted by permission.

ception modifies the perceiver's schemata, which undergo what Piaget labeled an accommodation; this change results in a new perception. These changes in perception do not simply make an internal replica or representation where none existed, but change the perceptual schemata so that the perceptual activity follows a different course (Neisser, 1976). By altering the perceptual schemata, the perceiver engages in an activity involving information from the environment as well as from his or her own cognitive mechanism.

Neisser (1976) has provided several examples of the perceptual cycle. Suppose you are sitting in your room and hear a footstep outside the doorway or catch a glimpse of someone out of the corner of your eye. These sounds and sights indicate that someone is in the immediate environment and guide further perceptual exploration. They allow you to anticipate what an exploratory glance or movement in the direction of the visitor might reveal. To see the visitor, you might have to turn your head or rotate your eyes. But perception is not complete at this point, since you will probably have to shift your gaze repeatedly to pick up additional information. Each eye movement is thus based on "stored information" acquired by experience. It is important to emphasize that the existing schemata, formed by previous experience, determine what is perceived and do not simply add to it. Thus, perception is more a matter of differentiation than of enrichment.

Does this mean that we only see or hear what we expect to see or hear? Not entirely. When a perceptual cycle is carried out, schemata tune or adjust themselves to the information available so that perception is *veridical*, or accurate. For example, pygmies who inhabit dense, tropical rain forests are said to make ridiculous perceptual errors when they first encounter objects at a distance. In one instance, a pygmy who had never seen a buffalo before thought it was an insect when viewed from afar. With greater experience, the pygmies learned to make more veridical perceptual judgments.

Neisser's view of perception has much in common with Piaget's notions of cognitive development. For example, a perceptual cycle is similar to the *circular reactions* described in Box 2.2. An infant who manages to produce an environmental effect (such as shaking a toy that produces a noise) will tend to repeat the act over and over again. These cyclical activities typically involve overt actions such as touching as well as the less overt activities of the eyes and ears. As the cyclic activities continue, children gradually alter the information they pick up (they accommodate to the new information). However, in Neisser's view, children make perceptual errors that require accommodation not because they are in an illogical stage of cognitive development, as Piaget maintains, but because they do not have enough experience in attending to environmental events (see Box 3.1).

Box 3.1   The Gestalt Wholistic Position

The German word *Gestalt* roughly translates as "configuration" or "organized whole." As mentioned in Chapter 1, one of the major aims of Gestalt psychologists in the area of perception was to specify the principles by which individual features of stimuli are combined into larger organized stimulus configurations. According to such famous Gestalt psychologists as Kurt Koffka, Wolfgang Köhler, and Max Wertheimer, the individual features of stimuli are not directly observable from their individual parts. Suppose you look at a circle of *R*s:

```
        R   R
    R           R
    R           R
    R           R
    R           R
      R       R
        R   R
```

In this example the whole has the property of circularity, which is not evident in the individual letters.

Gestalt psychologists described a set of innate principles by which parts become grouped together to form organized wholes. In the Gestalt view people interpret their perceptions according to these natural rules, regardless of previous perceptual experiences. The first rule, as described by Wertheimer, is the principle of *proximity*, which states that the closer two figures are to each other, the more likely they will be to be grouped together. An example of visual perception is shown in Figure 3.3*a*. A subject who looks at these lines tends to see four pairs of parallel lines, rather than eight separate lines. All else being equal, we also tend to group objects according to *similarity*. Thus, in the left half of Figure 3.3*b*, we group the *X*s together in columns and the *O*s together in columns; but in the right half of Figure 3.3*b*, we see rows of *X*s and *O*s. The next principle is *good continuation*, which means that we generally perceive contours of objects as continuing smoothly. This principle is often used in camouflaging objects. For example, in Figure 3.3*c* we could describe the figure as four curvy lines radiating from a single center point, *X*. However, more commonly, we perceive two lines (*AD*, *BC*) running through point *X*. Finally, we have a natural tendency to complete any gaps or missing parts in a figure, a principle called *closure*. Thus, when we look at the square with a gap in the middle (see Figure 3.3*d*), we tend to see it as a whole square, rather than as separate lines.

Gestalt psychologists claimed that the human brain is innately

Figure 3.3   The Gestalt principles of (*a*) proximity, (*b*) similarity, (*c*) good continuation, and (*d*) closure.

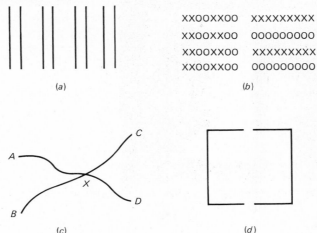

equipped to organize shapes and forms into meaningful wholes. They strongly disagreed with the empiricist notion that humans gradually build perceptions through an association of separate elements. Rather, perceptions were believed to result from a sudden reorganization of the perceptual field based on the innate principles outlined above. As a result of these principles, children were thought to be able to perceive the world much like adults.

Piaget rejected the Gestalt conclusions about children's perceptions. He agreed that the child's initial perception of a picture or object may be based on primitive, organizing rules; but as children grow older, their cognitive processes guide and control their perceptions. To test the Piagetian position, Elkind (1977) gave children aged 4–11 years a series of ambiguous pictures that could be perceived in one of two ways. For example, when you look at Figure 3.4, do you see a pair of silhouetted faces or a white vase? If Piaget is correct, older children should have a greater ability to shift from one stimulus to another (they should reverse the figure and its background) because of their superior cognitive flexibility. The results of Elkind's study supported Piaget's position; older children reported significantly more figure-ground reversals than younger children.

In the adult development literature, some early evidence suggested that older adults also have difficulty in shifting between stimuli when viewing ambiguous pictures (Korchin & Basowitz, 1956; Silverman & Reimanis, 1966). This difficulty could stem from an inability to discriminate perceptually figure from ground

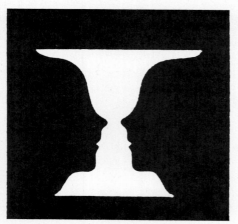

Figure 3.4   Reversible figure-ground pattern.

The pattern can be seen as either a pair of silhouetted faces or a white vase.

or to ignore irrelevant features of the stimulus. More recently, investigators have reported no age differences in the rate of figure reversals between old and young adults (Kline, Culler, & Susec, 1977). Response cautiousness may be one reason why older adults fail to report stimulus reversals in some studies (Botwinick, 1984). The more ambiguous a stimulus, the more uncertain older adults become about their responses.

LIFE-SPAN CHANGES IN BASIC SENSORY PROCESSES

Changes in basic sensory processes over the life span are among the most dramatic aspects of perceptual development. What causes these changes? Most can be traced to physiological changes in the sensory receptors and the nervous system. For this reason, it is important to examine neural and chemical changes in the sensory systems and the effects of such changes on our cognitive functioning. Vision and audition, generally considered to be the two sensory processes that bear most directly on cognition, will be examined in greatest detail. The development of smell, taste, and touch will then be briefly examined. These senses are the earliest to develop and probably play a large role in an infant's acquisition of knowledge of the world. Finally, the coordinations between the sensory systems will be discussed. Our senses do not operate in isolation from one another; they are closely interconnected. For example, we frequently look in the direction of a sound source or identify objects by touch which we have previously only seen.

Vision

The eye is our most complex sensory receptor. Of the various sensory organs, it is the last to fully develop and often the first to show sensory decline. With development and aging, several major structural changes occur in the eye that affect our visual functioning. One major change occurs in the **pupillary reflex**—the contraction of the iris and the pupil in response to bright light—and affects our sensitivity to brightness. Researchers studying visual sensitivity in infants have found that infants respond to brightness changes immediately after birth. During the first 2 months of life as the pupil increases in size, rapid changes occur in brightness sensitivity. In general, the amount of brightness required to elicit a response decreases as the infant matures. Between the second year of life and adolescence, the pupil continues to increase in size. From late adolescence onward, however, the pupillary opening gradually gets smaller, a process called **senile miosis.** Thus, brightness discrimination decreases with age, and these decreases are greater at low and intermediate levels of illumination than at higher levels (Weale, 1963).

A second major structural change in the visual system occurs in the crystalline lens of the eye. Beginning as early as 5 years of age, the lens of the eye builds up inert tissue that reduces the amount of transparency. Unlike the hair, nails, and skin, the cells of the lens are not shed (Fozard, Wolf, Bell, McFarland, & Podolsky, 1977). Cells are compacted so that the lens does not grow too large, and with increased age the lens gets denser. The lens also increases in yellowness with age, which reduces the amount of light reaching the retina. Because of this yellowing, the older eye loses its sensitivity to the shorter wavelengths of the color spectrum (blue, green, violet). These colors are absorbed by the yellowing lens. Sensitivity to longer wavelengths in the visual spectrum (red, orange, yellow) is less affected. The most significant consequence of these changes is their effect on visual acuity and visual accommodation.

Visual Acuity

Visual acuity refers to how clearly the visual system can discern fine detail. In older children and adults, acuity is typically measured by means of a Snellen chart. Perhaps you can recall being tested by an eye specialist. If you can read the big letters at 20 feet away that the average person can also see at 20 feet, you are considered to have optimal "20/20" vision. If you have 20/200 vision, you can read something at a distance of no greater than 20 feet that the average person can read or see at a distance of 200 feet.

Not until 10 or 11 years of age do children achieve the standard 20/

20 vision of adults. Visual acuity for infants under 1 month of age has been estimated to range from 20/150 to 20/290 (L. Cohen, DeLoache, & Strauss, 1979). However, because we cannot give infants a Snellen chart, it has been difficult to accurately determine their visual acuity. In fact, infants once were considered "functionally blind" at birth. With the advent of new methods for testing infant vision, more optimistic estimates of their visual acuity skills have been found (T. Lewis, Mauer, & Kay, 1978). For example, the visual acuity of infants can be tested by measuring their eye movements in response to moving stripes. As children grow, their vision gradually improves, so that the average 6-year-old entering school has vision in the 20/30 to 20/20 range.

Acuity reaches its maximum point sometime in the late teens and remains stationary over the young and middle adult years. By old age poorer vision once again becomes the rule. The incidence of poor vision (worse than 20/50) increases from less than 10 percent to more than 30 percent in the 60–80-year age group (U.S. National Health Survey, 1968). These changes may account for some of the difficulties older people experience on cognitive tasks requiring discernment of fine detail.

Visual Accommodation

Visual accommodation is defined as the ability of the lens of the eye to adjust its shape to bring a distant object into sharp focus. (Piaget also used the word *accommodation,* but with an entirely different meaning. Make sure you don't confuse the two!) Our eyes seem to have a set lens adjustment of approximately 20–30 centimeters. In newborns accommodation is fixed at about 18–19 centimeters and objects nearer or farther away look blurry. Some early research by Haynes, White, and Held (1965) indicated that the average infant cannot focus as well as an adult until the age of 3 or 4 months. More recent research, using high-contrast visual stimuli and advanced measurement techniques, suggests that Haynes et al. (1965) probably underestimated the accommodative ability of very young infants (Banks, 1980; Braddick, Atkinson, French, & Howland, 1979). The latter studies show that the accommodative ability of infants as young as 1 or 2 months of age is accurate enough to focus on objects across a wide range of distances.

Visual accommodation steadily improves during the first few months of life, but decreases gradually from childhood to adulthood, with the biggest decline occurring in the 40–50-year age range (Brückner, 1967). As adults grow older, the ciliary muscles that control the shape of the lens weaken. (This weakening may be adaptive in that the lens becomes increasingly immobile and makes these muscles less effective.) This change, along with changes in the shape of the eye, leads to an inability to focus on near objects, a condition known as **presbyopia,** or farsightedness. Thus by age 40 or 50 most adults require a pair of reading or driving glasses to see near objects. A second set of changes involving the retina and nervous system does not become noticeable until ages 55–65. These changes occur because of reduced blood circulation in the retina and are reflected in changes in the size of the visual field and sensitivity to low quantities of light (Fozard et al., 1977).

Practical Implications of Visual Changes

The visual changes described above have practical significance. For instance, driving a motor vehicle at twilight or at night under conditions of changing illumination may pose a real problem to older drivers. Older drivers are handicapped under such conditions because their eyes adapt more slowly to alternating light and dark conditions than do younger adults' eyes. Similarly, the ability to perform such occupations as clerical worker, air-traffic controller, and astronomer may be hampered because of vision changes.

Fozard and Popkin (1978) cite a study by Hughes which looked at the effect of visual illumination on work produced by two groups of office workers—young adults (19–27 years) and middle-aged adults (46–57 years). Subjects were required to search for 10 target numbers on a sheet containing 420 numbers. Each worker performed several searches under three different illumination conditions (low, medium, high). Both young and middle-aged workers performed better under increased illumination, but this was particularly true for the middle-aged group. Providing an appropriate environment for various activities and occupations (such as increased lighting of work areas, local lighting of steps and ramps) may alleviate some visual problems of older workers. Too much illumination may lead to glare problems, especially among older workers who may be developing or suffering from **cataracts,** a condition in which the lens of the eye becomes opaque. In this case, leaving control of lighting as much as possible to the individual is probably the best practical solution.

Audition

Like vision, audition (hearing) shows substantial changes from infancy to old age. In infancy auditory perception is especially critical in learning and producing language and in detecting the location of people, objects, and events in space. However, until recently it was difficult to determine if babies hear as well as adults. Part of the difficulty in assessing infants' hearing is that they do not give specific signs of having heard anything. Unlike the visual system, the auditory system is devoid of unique behavioral responses such as eye movements or eye fixations; for example, humans are not able to prick up their ears (Aslin, Pisoni, & Jusczyk, 1983).

Over the past decade and a half investigators have developed a wide array of ingenious assessment methods for testing infants' hearing capacity. Among the most frequently employed are measures of electrical brain responses, heart-rate changes, nonnutritive sucking, and behavioral reflexes. In all of these procedures, the infant is typically presented with a familiar stimulus for a period of time and his or her reactions are measured to a series of novel or change stimuli (Morse & Cowan, 1982). Using such response measures, investigators have produced some exciting findings on infants' basic hearing capacities.

At one time, fetuses and newborns were thought to be functionally deaf. We now know that a gelatinous fluid in the inner ear may hamper proper assessment of hearing among newborns. Once the fluid is drained, infants have a remarkably good capacity to localize and discriminate among sounds of varying duration, loudness, and pitch (Eisenberg, 1976; Leventhal & Lipsitt, 1964). In general, auditory acuity improves up to adolescence and then seems to level off. It is difficult to determine how much of this improvement is due to developmental changes in the auditory system and how much is due to nonsensory factors such as attentional changes and differences in response criteria. In other words, older children may show greater auditory sensitivity than infants because the former are more attentive and more likely to respond selectively to auditory signals. It is not surprising that many contradictions about developmental changes in auditory perception exist in the literature (Aslin et al., 1983).

With increasing age in adulthood, several auditory changes occur, beginning in the early 30s for men and the later 30s for women. Szafran and Birren (1969) summarize these changes as follows:

1. Most impairment occurs at the upper sound frequencies, with the 4000–6000 Hz (abbreviation for *hertz,* the number of cycles per second) range showing the greatest loss. The losses for the upper sound frequencies are greater for men than for women, but the losses for lower sound frequencies are equal for both sexes. For most everyday activities, deafness for upper frequencies (above 3000 or perhaps 4000 Hz) is not of any practical significance (Botwinick, 1984). A frequency range above 4000 Hz (the highest note on a piano) falls outside of the range of most normal conversation.

2. The left ear shows more pronounced loss in the majority of cases, and the differences in threshold between the right and left ears are

greatest at the highest frequencies. (A *threshold* is the smallest change in stimulus magnitude required to produce a sensation.)

3. In many adults there is a shortening of the loudness scale, a process called **recruitment**. Recruitment causes older adults to perceive a change in stimulus intensity of the auditory signal as much greater than the change actually is.

The causes of hearing loss in old age are multiple, encompassing sensory changes of the inner ear (cochlea) and of the cochlear nerve to the auditory cortex. Hearing loss may also be due to age-related changes in attention and concentration. If older people suffer from attentional lapses, as the evidence suggests, then they may be less likely to concentrate on a sound source in the environment. Finally, the environment plays a role in the development of auditory problems, as in cases of "noise pollution." Older people who have been exposed to hazardous auditory environments (such as working with loud machinery) are poorer hearers than those who have not been exposed to such environments (Botwinick, 1984). Even among young adults, exposure to high loudness levels (e.g., listening to loud music) may produce temporary or even permanent hearing loss.

What effect do hearing losses have on cognitive abilities in various age groups? In what is probably the most systematic approach to this question, Hans Furth (1966) performed a series of studies comparing deaf and hearing children on traditional Piagetian tasks. Furth discovered that deaf children perform as well as hearing children on these tasks, although they may occasionally lag behind. Hearing children, for example, may solve problems at 11 years of age that are not solved by deaf children until 15 or 16 years of age. Hearing loss among adults has also been studied in relationship to cognitive performance. Granick, Kleban, and Weiss (1976) investigated the effects of hearing loss on cognition in the elderly. They found that hearing loss was strongly related to reduced cognitive performance. However, cognitive changes such as declines in attention may have influenced hearing, rather than vice versa.

Hearing loss can also negatively affect our ability to effectively hear conversation and communicate with other people (see Chapter 5). In particular, consonant sounds with high frequency characteristics and low acoustical power (such as /f/, /g/, /s/, /t/, /z/, /th/, and /sh/) may be difficult to perceive when hearing acuity is diminished. Hearing aids help amplify higher frequencies and allow people to listen to conversation better. But hearing aids that amplify all sounds equally may be less useful when more hearing loss occurs at some frequencies than at others, as is typically the case in old age. One solution to this problem is to use a hearing aid whose amplification across particular frequency ranges is adjusted to the individual wearer's needs.

Touch, Taste, and Smell

The senses of touch, taste, and smell have been much less studied than the senses of vision and audition, but we have some basic information. From studies on infant reflexes, we know that babies are sensitive to touch. For example, if we brush our fingers against the side of their cheek or around their mouth, they will turn their head in the direction of the touch (called the rooting reflex), and if we stroke the soles of the feet, their toes will curl outward (called the Babinski reflex). Infants' sensitivity to tactile stimulation is important for their learning about the stimulus properties of objects (shape, size, texture). Theories of social attachment also emphasize the significance of touch for promoting the development of an emotional bond between infants and parents (Cairns, 1979).

The sense of taste serves an important function by providing information about substances that may be ingested. And, as is well known, taste sensitivity is intricately related to the sense of smell. When your nose is stuffed because of a cold, you may complain that your food is "tasteless." If your sense of smell is inactive, you may no longer be able to distinguish between a potato and an apple, or between red vinegar and red wine.

Most investigators believe that there are four primary taste qualities: sweet, sour, salty, and bitter. All other taste sensations are produced by some combination of these. The specialized receptor cells for sensing taste, the *taste buds,* are more widely distributed on the tongues of infants than on the tongues of older children or adults. Newborns are sensitive to strong tastes and can distinguish among three of the four basic flavors—sweet, sour, and bitter. They will also explore objects— toys, blankets, tables—through taste and touch, as any parent knows. Visual exploration becomes more prominent after the visual system develops further.

Over the life span, the distribution of taste buds on the tongue decreases from all but a few areas, although the greatest loss in taste buds does not occur until old age (Cowart, 1981). This finding may explain why many children find their food too spicy, and many older adults complain that their food tastes flavorless. Despite the fact that taste sensitivity declines from childhood to adulthood, adults may compensate for such decline through learning. Thus, many adults become skilled wine tasters or gourmet cooks, even though they have, on the average, fewer taste buds than children.

The sense of smell is especially difficult to study in early life because so many other variables affect the olfactory (smell) threshold, including temperature, humidity, sex, genetic background, and cognitive and emotional factors (Birren, Kinney, Schaie, & Woodruff, 1981). Much of the information on the infant's sense of smell is based on anecdotal reports or observational data, but there have been some empirical studies. Lipsitt, Engen, and Kaye (1963) showed that infants from 1–4 days old are sensitive to strong odors and can differentiate among various smell sensations. In one of the few life-span studies of olfactory sensitivity, Rovee, Cohen, and Shlapack (1975) reported no age differences among subjects ranging in age from 6–94 years. This finding suggests that senses which develop earliest in life, such as olfaction, may also be among the last to decline.

Although smell is usually considered a minor sense, it serves several important functions. For example, it may warn us of a dangerous situation such as leaking gas or other poisonous chemicals. The sense of smell may also be influential in the formation of early social attachments. For example, by 6 to 10 days of age infants learn the unique smells of their mothers' breasts (Macfarlane, 1975). In addition, smell is closely associated with certain emotional experiences. Smelling a favorite food or perfume may resurrect memories of a long-forgotten earlier experience. Indeed, olfactory memories are often among our most powerful recollections.

Sensory Coordination

So far we have talked about the different senses as separate systems, but the senses do not work in isolation from each other. For example, coordination exists between vision and hearing, as when we see the movements of a speaker's lips and hear the sounds produced. If you have ever watched a film in which the soundtrack is poorly synchronized, you know how important this coordination is. Or consider the coordination between our eyes and hands. As adults we assume that our hands will reach the proper distance to grasp an object within our visual field (see Box 3.2). Of course, not every sensory event is equally well coordinated. For example, the sound of the wind is not accompanied by a visual input.

Vision and Hearing

How soon does the ability to coordinate the eyes and the ears develop? Mendelson and Haith (1976) hypothesized that infants come into the world equipped to learn about the relations between sights and sounds. To test their hypothesis, Mendelson and Haith studied infants less than 1 week old. They measured the infants' glances by the position of reflected infrared lights on the pupils of the infants' eyes. They found that the sound of a male voice increased the amount of time babies kept their eyes open, increased their eye control, and caused them to look more at the center of the visual field and to scan with smaller eye movements. The sounds thus appeared to make the babies alert to possible visual stimulation.

When Mendelson and Haith (1976) played a repeating tape recording of a man reading an excerpt from a children's poem by A. A. Milne, the

Box 3.2   The Empathic Model

How does the environment look, sound, smell, and feel to older people? To answer this question sociologist Leon Pastalan has developed "the empathic model," a simulated environmental model for anyone who wants to experience the world as a person over 70 years of age would. Pastalan, Mautz, and Merrill (1973) used things like coated glasses, ear plugs, and a gluelike fixative for fingertips to simulate age-related changes in the sensory system. Students who participated in testing the empathic model reported dramatic changes in their everyday activities. For example, going to the supermarket became a real problem because they could not identify signs above the shelves identifying the location of the storegoods (see Figure 3.5 for a view of a supermarket under unsimulated and simulated conditions). Students also had difficulty in the checkout line because they were unable to distinguish a nickel from a quarter and were pushed by impatient shoppers.

Pastalan's work has been useful in many applied contexts. Builders of a large rehabilitation center in Chicago and designers of a 200-bed home for the aging in Detroit, Michigan, have tried to incorporate his ideas into their construction projects. In addition, the empathic model has been used to train bus drivers, telephone operators, and nursing home personnel to be aware of the special sensory problems of older people. The model has also been used in older driver retraining programs to sensitize elderly people to their own sensory changes.

Not all investigators agree with Pastalan's approach. They argue that his simulation procedures overestimate the amount of sensory loss in old age and do not account for gradual adaptations to such loss over time. It has also been pointed out that the simulation experience is only temporary, unlike the irreversible changes experienced by the elderly person. In spite of these criticisms, Pastalan's empathic model is a useful first step in understanding how our sensory systems change as we get older.

Figure 3.5 View of a supermarket under unsimulated and simulated conditions

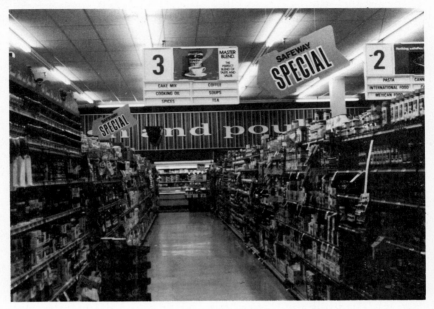

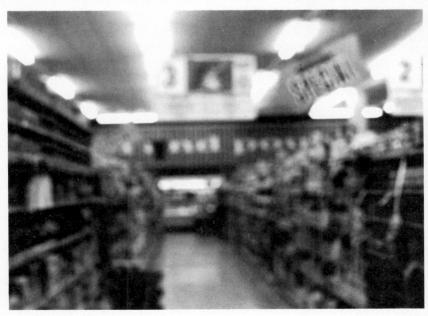

Photographs courtesy of Dr. Lynn R. Offerman. Reproduced by permission.

babies looked in the direction of the voice when the poem began; but as the poem continued, their attention gradually tended to wander away from the sound. These results indicate that infants are biased to respond in one sensory modality with increased alertness or activity in another. In other words, the infants' auditory modality seemed to affect the way their visual modality received information.

In an interesting series of experiments, Elizabeth Spelke showed that infants' ability to detect sight-sound correlations is present as early as 4 months of age. In one study Spelke (1979a) had 4-month-old infants watch two events, one a film of a woman playing peekaboo, the other a film of some percussion instruments being played. Infants viewed these films side by side. A speaker located between the films played the soundtrack appropriate to one film and then to the other. The main experimental question was whether the infants would notice the correlation between the sound and one of the films and look at the appropriate film. A control group of infants viewed the film with no accompanying soundtrack. The results indicated that when a soundtrack was available, infants tended to watch the appropriate film. This was especially true for the film with the percussion instruments.

In a subsequent study, Spelke (1979b) showed 4-month-old babies movies of a yellow kangaroo and a gray donkey bouncing across the grass. The films and their soundtrack were run in several combinations, both in and out of synchrony. Their visual searches showed that babies detected a connection between simultaneous sound bursts and visible events. Spelke concluded that at the first sight of a strange object, infants perceive a unity in motion and sound by detecting temporal synchrony.

Spelke's studies support E. Gibson's theory of perceptual development. The infant does not appear to depend on learned associations between sights and sounds, but can detect similarities in their patterning, whether they occur together in the natural world or not.

Vision and Touch

Another important coordination that develops during the first year of life is between vision and touch. The importance of this ability can be seen in the writings of Piaget (1954), who saw the origins of intelligence in the sensorimotor coordinations of the child. Piaget believed that infants must learn eye-hand coordination, but some psychologists dispute this claim. In some early research, Bower, Broughton, and Moore (1970) claimed that neonates (newborns) exhibit an innate ability to shape their hands as they reach toward objects, showing that vision guided their tactile expectations and thus the shaping of their hands. Bower et al. (1970) fitted infants under 2 weeks of age with a special set of stereoscopic glasses. These glasses allowed the researchers to produce a visible, but not tangible, object known as a **virtual object** in the third dimension. The infants reached accurately for the virtual object, modeling their hands correctly to accommodate to its specific shape and showing distress and surprise when the object could not be grasped. These findings contradict Piaget's assumption that infants gradually learn to coordinate vision and touch during the first 3 or 4 months of life. As will be pointed out in Chapter 4, subsequent attempts to replicate these findings have not been altogether successful (Yonas, Oberg, & Norcia, 1978).

Although there is little to support Bower's claims of the innateness of eye-hand coordination, evidence shows that infants can translate tactual information into visual information during the first year of life. Bryant, Jones, Claxton, and Perkins (1972) took advantage of the natural interest young infants exhibit toward noisy objects. They placed a small semiround object in the hand of infants without its being visible, and they made the object produce an attractive noise. Subsequently, infants were offered a choice between the potentially noisy object that they had felt in their hands and a differently shaped object. Most infants unhesitatingly reached for the object they had felt, presumably in order to get it to make a noise. Because the infants' experience with the object had been only tactile, this reaching indicated an ability to translate information from a tactual to a visual mode.

Other studies on eye-hand coordination have led researchers to conclude that this is an important ability for cognitive development. Rose, Gottfried, and Bridger (1981) showed that infants can form a visual representation of an object and relate the representation to an object's tactual appearance. They presented 1-year-olds with a geometric object that could be visually explored, or in darkness, so that it could only be tactually explored. Afterwards, they presented the familiar object and a novel one in darkness. Infants preferred to touch the novel object, a result suggesting that they could recognize the familiar object, regardless of whether they had seen it or only touched it before and that they could discriminate the novel object from the familiar one.

These studies do not reveal exactly how early intersensory coordination emerges in the first year of life and how this process is acquired developmentally. By age 6 months, infants seem to spend a lot of time in visual-tactual inspection of objects. By this age infants have had considerable opportunity to engage in visual-tactual exploration (such as reaching out for toys), so experience is undoubtedly an influential variable. However, one cannot entirely rule out maturationally based factors. Maturation of the visual system and changes in the central nervous system may contribute to an infant's visually directed reaching for objects. As infants become older, their intersensory coordinations tend to show steady improvement (Abravanel, 1968; Zaporozhets, 1965).

Illusions

Studies on basic sensory processes are geared toward understanding the way that we see, hear, feel, taste, and smell the world as it really is. Occasionally, we misperceive reality and experience an **illusion**, which occurs when the perceived properties of objects (shape, size, texture, sound) differ from their actual properties. Figure 3.6 illustrates three geometric illusions commonly used in studies of children and adults. In Figure 3.6 the line segments or circles to be compared are equal, but because of the surrounding figures or lines, they are perceived as different.

Geometrical illusions such as the Müller-Lyer illusion (see Figure 3.6a) and the Ponzo illusion (see Figure 3.6c) can be understood if we envision the object projected into a third dimension. For example, we can interpret the arrows at the top and bottom of each vertical line in Figure 3.6a as defining a three-dimensional corner, with the corner on the right appearing to be closer to us than the one on the left. The vertical line that appears more distant (the left one) is perceived as larger, even though both lines produce equal retinal images. In this case, we unconsciously infer that the farther line must also be larger. Similarly, Figure 3.6c can be thought of as a flat projection on a three-dimensional space, with the vertical lines converging in the distance, much like railroad tracks. From experience you know that distant railroad ties are actually the same size as the near ones, even though they project a much smaller retinal image. Again we unconsciously enlarge the more distant lines.

No single theory can explain illusions in terms of their stimulus properties or the age-related differences in responses to them (Fozard et al., 1977; Kline & Schieber, 1985). Life-span changes in response to illusions seem to depend on the age of the person tested, the type of illusion, and the procedure for measuring their effects (Coren & Porac,

Figure 3.6   Geometric illusions: (a) Müller-Lyer illusion, (b) satellite circles or Tichener circles, (c) Ponzo illusion.

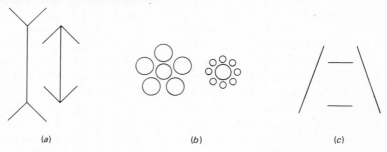

(a)   (b)   (c)

1978). Several investigators (Comalli, 1965; Eisner & Schaie, 1971; Wapner, Werner, & Comalli, 1960) report that susceptibility to the Müller-Lyer illusion (see Figure 3.6*a*) is high in early childhood, remains stable in adulthood, and increases in later adulthood. The findings for the satellite circles, or Tichener circles, illusion (see Figure 3.6*b*) are more contradictory. Some investigators (Wapner et al., 1960) found increased susceptibility during childhood, stability in middle adulthood, and some decline in susceptibility in old age (cf. Eisner & Schaie, 1971). Studies using the Ponzo illusion (see Figure 3.6*c*) also yielded conflicting results (Leibowitz & Gwozdecki, 1967; Leibowitz & Judisch, 1967).

Why is the study of illusions important in cognitive development research? As Coren and Porac (1978) state, "illusions afford a unique opportunity to assess age changes in sensory-physiological functions and cognitive–information processing strategies, since evidence indicates that these percepts are a composite of both types of mechanism acting together" (p. 193). The notion that both sensory and cognitive processes may be involved in illusions has led to a distinction between **Type I illusions** and **Type II illusions**. Originally proposed by Piaget, and later modified by Pollack (Pollack & Atkeson, 1978), this distinction is based on whether changes in illusion magnitude with age depend on physiological changes in the sensory receptors (Type I) or intellectual mechanisms (Type II). According to Pollack, susceptibility to Type I illusions, such as the *simultaneous* Müller-Lyer illusion (simultaneous because both vertical lines are presented for visual comparison at the same time; see Figure 3.6*a*), should decrease during childhood as the eye matures physiologically, level off in adulthood, and then increase in old age as physiological processes in the eye deteriorate. Similarly, susceptibility to Type II illusions, such as the *successive* Müller-Lyer illusion (successive because the left vertical line is presented first followed by the right vertical line), should decrease in childhood as the individual matures intellectually, remain stable in adulthood, and then increase as a consequence of intellectual losses in old age. Because each line segment of Type II illusions is presented separately, subjects must integrate the information over time and space, a process that uses higher levels of cognitive functioning.

So far research on Pollack's predictions has produced conflicting results. There is evidence that Type I illusions are correlated with the efficiency of the receptor system and not intelligence, as Pollack hypothesizes. Further, as predicted, a significant correlation exists between intelligence and the perception of Type II illusions. However, the results for the developmental predictions of Pollack's model are not so clear-cut. Susceptibility to Type I illusions seems to level off in adulthood, but—contrary to Pollack's predictions—does not worsen in old age. Type II illusions show greater accuracy through childhood and a reversal in old age, as predicted by the model. Whether this reversal is due to an inability to integrate stimulus information in later life is unknown. Additional work is needed to determine the empirical relationship between specific changes in cognitive processes across the life span and susceptibility to visual illusions.

Although most developmental studies involve age-related susceptibility to visual illusions, there have been some studies of auditory illusions involving the **verbal transformation effect.** This effect occurs when an auditory stimulus such as a word or sound is presented repeatedly, and the stimulus is perceived as having changed. For example, if you hear the word *police* said over and over again, it may begin to sound like *please*. Children less than age 6 and older adults report fewer verbal transformations than other age groups in this type of study (Warren, 1961). The lack of transformation, at least among older adults, might represent a more generally cautious approach to sensory input as a result of sensory and cognitive losses. Among young children neurological immaturity could account for a failure to reorganize or transform the stimulus input.

THE SELECTIVE NATURE OF PERCEPTION

In everyday activities such as listening to a conversation, driving a car, or watching a basketball game, we cannot consciously attend to the myriad stimuli impinging on our sensory receptors. Rather we must learn to *attend,* or focus, on the most relevant or important aspects of the stimulus situation. E. J. Gibson (1969) referred to this as a process of "optimization of attention" (p. 456) in her theory of perceptual learning and development.

Developmentally, the ability to selectively perceive or attend seems to depend on the age as well as the experience of the observer. Very young children are attracted to the most salient, or noticeable, feature of the sensory stimulation, such as bright colors and loud noises. As children get older and more experienced, they learn to focus their perceptions on the most relevant aspects of the stimulus information. They learn to notice information because of its importance in relation to their activity (E. Gibson & Spelke, 1983; A. Pick, Frankel, & Hess, 1975). Thus, active perceptual exploration is a key ingredient in the developmental process.

Attention in Young Infants

A great deal of research on attention in young infants has focused on the following questions: Do infants attend? What does the young infant prefer to look at? Do innate mechanisms guide the infant's attention? Studies seeking to answer these questions have usually been guided by broader concerns involving the nature of infant cognition. Because the infant's response repertoire is limited in comparison to those of older children and adults, investigators have had to rely on responses that infants make. Of all their responses, the one most commonly used in laboratory investigations is the tendency of infants to look at, or *fixate* on, visual stimuli. By studying visual fixation, investigators hope to draw some inferences about the earliest stages of cognitive development (such as formation of a memory representation, interest in novelty).

Robert Fantz and colleagues (Fantz, 1966; Fantz, Fagan, & Miranda, 1975) introduced the research technique most often used by investigators today to study infant attention. In their procedure, an infant is placed inside a "looking chamber" and shown a series of two-dimensional, flat pictures. An experimenter observes the reflections of the pictures on the infant's cornea and judges which picture the infant is attending to. The experimenter also measures the total amount of fixation time for each picture. If fixation times differ, then infants can be said to have a visual "preference" and to discriminate between the two pictures.

The types of pictures used by Fantz in his research are shown in Figure 3.7. Fantz found that infants as young as 2-3 months of age could discriminate among these stimuli. Subjects preferred to look longer at the face, newspaper, and bull's-eye than at the nonpatterned stimuli. Generally, as infants get older, they prefer to gaze longer at more and more complex stimuli. Changes in the underlying physiological organization of the eye may explain some of these preference shifts (R. Hoffman, 1978; Karmel & Maisel, 1975). R. Hoffman (1978) suggested that the switch from subcortical to cortical processing at about 2 months of age may account for changes in visual preferences.

Although Fantz's technique has been extremely useful as a gross measure of looking versus nonlooking behavior, it does not give much information on the specific parts of a stimulus to which infants attend. In a now classic study, Salapatek and Kessen (1966) used a corneal photography technique to record infants' visual gazing patterns. This technique enabled Salapatek and Kessen (1966) to photograph the exact points of infants' eye movements on an equilateral triangle target. They found that under 2 months of age, an infant's attention is limited to the vertices (or edges) of the triangle and not distributed over the whole

Figure 3.7   Pattern perception in infants. Importance of pattern rather than color or brightness was illustrated by the infants' response to a face, a piece of newsprint, a bull's-eye, and plain disks colored red, white, or yellow. Even the youngest infants preferred patterns. Dark bars show the results for infants from 2 to 3 months old; light bars show results for infants more than 3 months old.

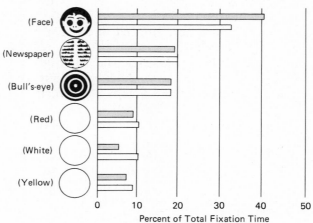

From "The Origin of Form Perception" by R. L. Fantz, 1961, *Scientific American*, p. 72. Copyright 1961 by Scientific American, Inc. Reprinted by permission.

form. Maurer and Salapatek (1976) examined the way in which 1- and 2-month-old infants scanned a human face. Like Salapatek and Kessen (1966), they found that the 1-month-olds scanned only a few parts of the entire face and concentrated on areas involving the outer contour such as the chin and the line of the hair. However, by 2 months of age, the infants' eye movements scanned a greater number of features. Two-month-olds were more likely to fixate on the internal portions of the face—the eye, the nose, or the mouth—and to look at a greater amount of contour. Thus, the developmental changes in infants' scanning patterns apply to geometric figures as well as to meaningful figures such as a human face (L. Cohen et al., 1979).

Why do infants look at more internal features of stimuli with increasing age? One recent hypothesis suggests that it is an artifact of the stationary stimuli used in these experiments. Even at birth infants seem to prefer moving rather than stationary representations of objects (see Acredolo & Hake, 1982). Addition of movement to stimuli, such as moving eyes on a face, seems to enhance infants' internal scanning. In the absence of movement, infants limit their scanning to the external contours of stimuli. The reasons for this are unclear but may be related to limited perceptual processing capacity; infants may be limited by the number of features they can attend to simultaneously. Another possibility is that the larger size of external forms makes outer contours more attention grabbing (i.e., more salient). The explanation of this externality effect, however, remains controversial.

There is also a controversy about whether infants prefer to look at novel stimuli or familiar stimuli. Stimuli that are totally familiar are not likely to provide much new information for cognitive growth. On the other hand, stimuli that are too novel or unfamiliar may be so discrepant from an infant's schema (the sensory representation of stimuli) that they become difficult or impossible to assimilate. Thus, stimuli at an intermediate level of discrepancy are likely to be most optimal for eliciting an infant's attention development.

Harvard psychologist Jerome Kagan calls this preference for moderately new stimuli the **discrepancy principle.** In his review of several lines of evidence, Kagan (1972, 1978) concluded that from 2 or 3 months of age, babies seem to show a preference for moderately novel stimuli; he also noted that this attentional shift is accompanied by several other major changes in the brain and behavior. For example, electrical potentials of the infant's brain elicited by visual stimuli become more like those of an adult, with alpha rhythms appearing for the first time. On the behavioral level, cooing begins to increase. By the time an infant reaches 2 or 3 months of age, informational properties of objects (discrepancy, novelty) become as important as physical properties (movement, complexity) in grabbing and maintaining the child's attention.

Recall from Chapter 2 that Piaget, like Kagan, emphasized the importance of moderate discrepancy in cognitive development. Children assimilate new information to existing cognitive structures. When faced with new objects, relations, and events, however, children are forced to accommodate in order to reestablish cognitive equilibrium.

Many questions have been raised about the characterization of infants as "preference creatures" who prefer to attend to certain types of stimuli more than others. In *Rules That Babies Look By*, Marshall Haith (1980) discusses several inadequacies of preference studies. Haith points out that in studies such as Fantz's, babies spend only about half of their time looking at the preferred stimulus and only about 5–10 percent less time gazing at the nonpreferred stimulus than the preferred one. Why does the baby look at the preferred stimulus only half the time? What is the baby doing with the nonpreferred stimulus? For Haith the central question is not how long the baby looks at stimuli, but what the child is doing or trying to do with the stimulus array.

Haith's (1980) position is that stimuli do not produce behavior as much as they constrain it. The baby pursues a biological agenda which maintains the firing of neurons in the visual cortex in the brain. Focusing on external contours and contrasts stimulates the infant's visual system and causes the neurons to fire. Haith characterizes these innate dispositions for dealing with different visual circumstances as "rules." Although the baby is not consciously aware of these innate rules, or principles, they help maintain neural pathways and establish new ones. Haith (1980) concludes, "early visual activity cannot be understood in terms of infant reflexes, infant preferences, or in terms of stimulus organization alone. The newborn must be thought of as a biologically organized creature who behaves visually in a continuous rather than a discrete preferential or attentional fashion" (p. 13).

What conclusions can we now draw about the nature of infant attention? In a famous statement, William James (1890) claimed that the infants' sensory world is a "blooming, buzzing confusion." If this were true, we would not expect infants to be able to pick out specific aspects of sensory stimulation. But we have seen that infants appear to attend selectively to stimulus features in their immediate environment and by doing so actively organize their perceptual experience (A. Pick et al., 1975). Furthermore, as Haith (1980) has indicated, infants are biologically equipped to search for information and are able to adapt to changes in information during the search. Infants are not passive information responders; they are active information seekers.

Attentional Changes in Children and Adults

After infancy, attentional processes become increasingly interwoven with other cognitive processes such as memory, learning, and intelligence (Flavell, 1977). Selective attention becomes possible not only for external stimuli but also for internal stimuli. In Flavell's (1977) words, as children mature, they "can mentally attend to things before and after, as well as during, their perceptual presence" (p. 167). For example, a child can mentally attend to the contents of his or her memory in order to remember something (see Chapter 6). And what is stored in memory becomes more abstract and less tied to specific sensory modalities such as vision or audition.

Even young infants can systematically scan the features of a stimulus, but they do not necessarily direct their attention to the most relevant or critical pieces of information. The development of this discriminatory ability appears to involve at least two skills: (1) the ability to attend selectively to the most relevant aspects of stimuli and (2) the ability to ignore irrelevant or extraneous stimuli.

Different methods have been used to study attentional deployment in children and adults. One popular procedure involves measures of **central learning** and **incidental learning.** In a frequently employed version of this procedure, a subject is shown a series of cards containing two pictures (a familiar animal, a common household object) and told to remember one of the pairs of objects (the animal). After this *central* recall task is completed, the subject is unexpectedly shown one of the objects in each pair and asked to remember the object with which it had been paired. The latter manipulation supposedly reflects the amount of attention that subjects allocate to the central recall task. The more that subjects attend to the central (i.e., relevant) objects, the poorer their recall of the *incidental* (irrelevant) objects should be.

These studies reveal that both central recall and incidental recall increase with age through approximately 10 or 11 years, indicating that children are not differentiating between relevant and irrelevant information. By age 13, the learning of central information continues to increase, but incidental learning undergoes a dramatic decline. These results presumably indicate that older children are better able to focus on the dimensions that are relevant to the solution of the task (see Hagen & Hale, 1973; P. Miller & Weiss, 1981). In other words, older children become more competent at selective attention.

In the adult developmental literature, a wide variety of central and incidental learning procedures have been employed, and the results have been equivocal. Wimer (1960) found a larger deficit for central recall than for incidental recall with increasing age. Mergler, Dusek, and Hoyer (1977) employed the incidental learning paradigm developed by Hagen and Hale (1973) to examine central and incidental recall in two age groups—young (mean age 28.4 years) and old (mean age 70.9 years). Young adults performed better than old adults on both the central and incidental recall tasks, suggesting that results were not simply due to deficient selective attention skills. Rather, the results support Eysenck's (1974) suggestion of an age-related processing deficit which influences total recall performance. A processing deficit involves the overall amount of attentional resource available rather than the way in which attention is allocated. In other words, old adults in the Mergler et al. (1977) study appeared to have less attentional capacity than did young adults. We will discuss processing deficits in greater detail later in this chapter and again in Chapter 6 when we present the depth-of-processing approach to memory.

Perceptual Salience

Another important factor affecting age differences in selective attention is the **perceptual salience** of the task dimensions. "Perceptual salience" refers to the relative sensitivity of the perceptual system to dimensions, relations, and categories in the stimulus environment. The higher the salience of a dimension, the greater the likelihood it will be perceptually processed. Figure 3.8 illustrates how salience is typically assessed

Figure 3.8 Perceptual salience task. The task is to pick the stimulus that is most similar to the stimulus in the large card. The choice of card A reflects a color preference, whereas card B indicates a position preference.

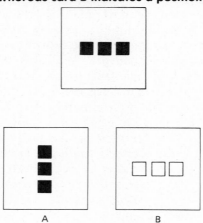

in research studies on attention. The subject is presented with pairs of stimuli that differ on dimensions such as form, color, number, and position. From these pairs the subject is to pick the stimulus object that is "most like" the stimulus in the top card. For example, in Figure 3.8, the choice of card A reflects a color preference, while the selection of card B shows a position preference.

Several studies have supported the perceptual salience position. Odom and colleagues (Odom, 1972; Odom, Cunningham, & Astor-Stetson, 1977) have shown that perceptual salience determines recall accuracy of both the central and incidental dimensions on incidental learning tasks. In a study on kindergarten, third-, and sixth-grade children, Odom (1972) observed fewer errors in recall of the central dimension when it was relatively high in salience than when it was relatively low. West, Odom, and Aschkenasy (1978) also explored the effects of perceptual salience on problems requiring subjects to coordinate different relevant dimensions. Three different age groups—children (mean age 11.9 years), young adults (mean age 19.7 years), and old adults (mean age 69.4 years)—solved a series of conceptual coordination problems. Each subject was shown a series of items, each consisting of three cards containing stimulus values from two relevant dimensions. The task was a coordination problem because the correct card (a red square) contained one dimensional value that matched a second card (a *red* circle) and another dimensional value that matched a third card (a blue *square*). In each age group, problems that contained subjects' most salient dimensions were solved faster and more accurately than problems containing their least salient dimensions. These results suggest that perceptual preferences continue to play an important role in adulthood. In a study comparing middle-aged (mean age 41.6 years) and elderly (mean age 72.2 years) adults on conceptual coordination problems, Rebok (1981) also found evidence for the effects of perceptual salience on problem solving.

Focusing on the most relevant features of stimulus information is not the same as actively ignoring irrelevant information. In complex problem-solving situations, the ability to screen unimportant or extraneous information may become essential. Consider how critical this ability is when someone is driving a car through a crowded street or intersection, or trying to read a complicated bus schedule.

Developmentally, the trend is in the direction of an increased ability to ignore irrelevant information from childhood through adulthood. However, old age may be accompanied by a decreased ability to ignore irrelevant information (W. Hoyer, Rebok, & Sved, 1979; Rabbitt, 1965). In the W. Hoyer et al. (1979) study, the effects of various increased amounts of irrelevant information on the speed and accuracy of problem solving in three different age groups—young adults (mean age 20.6 years), middle-aged adults (mean age 52.4 years), and elderly adults (mean age 72.6 years)—were investigated. Subjects solved problems modeled after the one in Figure 3.8, which required them to match one of two stimulus objects to a standard stimulus. Each problem contained either zero, one, two, or three dimensions which varied across the stimulus objects and were irrelevant to the solution (variable irrelevant dimensions). As shown in Figure 3.9, all subjects responded more slowly and made more errors as the amount of irrelevant information increased, but the elderly were disproportionately affected by increased irrelevancy. These findings suggest that declines in problem solving with advancing age may be due in part to an inability to ignore irrelevant information. Rabbitt (1965) also reported that the number of irrelevant dimensions adversely affected young as well as old adults on a card-sorting problem, but older subjects showed a greater decrement in card-sorting times in the presence of irrelevant information.

AUTOMATIC PROCESSES AND THE LIMITS OF ATTENTION

Most of the earliest work that led to the development of contemporary cognitive psychology was concerned with the investigation of the limits of human skills and abilities (Salthouse, 1982). These limits were most evident in situations in which two tasks had to be performed simulta-

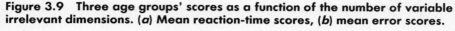

Figure 3.9   Three age groups' scores as a function of the number of variable irrelevant dimensions. (*a*) Mean reaction-time scores, (*b*) mean error scores.

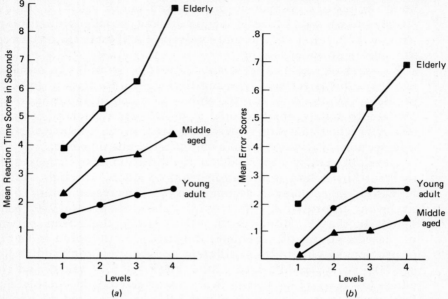

From "Effects of Varying Irrelevant Information on Adult Age Differences in Problem Solving" by W. J. Hoyer, G. W. Rebok, and S. M. Sved, 1979, *Journal of Gerontology, 34*, pp. 556 & 558. Copyright 1979 by the Gerontological Society of America. Reprinted by permission.

neously. For example, if someone asked you to carry on a conversation, type a letter, and listen to the radio at the same time you would probably have great difficulty managing these three activities together, especially if you were just learning to type. The mechanism most often used to explain poor performance under such conditions is limited attentional capacity or processing resources (see Box 3.3).

Considerable controversy surrounds present notions of attentional capacity and processing resources. Some investigators believe that limitations on performance may not reflect attentional limitations as much as underdeveloped skills. If this is the case, we should be able to learn to carry out several activities simultaneously by acquiring specific skills. Another issue is whether we have one common pool of attentional resources or whether each sensory modality has a certain amount. In order to perform certain tasks we may use our visual modality; on others we employ our auditory modality. Finally, does the total amount of attentional capacity remain fixed or does it vary across age groups, tasks, and situations? We will look at some of these issues in the next section.

Box 3.3   Attention Deficit Disorder

In recent years a growing body of research has focused on children with attentional problems. Although most children develop normally, about 3 percent of elementary school–aged children display attentional and behavioral characteristics that are serious enough to interfere with their learning and achievement (American Psychiatric Association, 1980). Many diagnostic labels have been given to this disorder, including hyperactivity, hyperkinesis, minimal brain damage, and maturational lag (D. Ross & Ross, 1976; G. Weiss & Hechtman, 1979). In the most recent version of the American Psychiatric Association's (1980) *Diagnostic and Statistical Manual of Mental Disorders* (or *DSM-III*), this condition is referred to as "attention deficit disorder with hyperactivity" rather than "hyperkinetic reaction of childhood" syndrome, as it was called in the second edition (or *DSM-II*). The switch in diagnostic labels was made to highlight the prominent feature of children with this disorder—their attentional deficits.

An attention deficit disorder is never diagnosed on the basis of a single characteristic or symptom. Clinicians employ several different criteria, including inattention, impulsive behavior, hyperactivity and motor restlessness, onset before age of 7, and duration of at least six months. A difficulty in sustaining attention may manifest itself in various ways. The child may fail to finish things that he or she starts or may fail to stick with a school or play activity. Impulsive behavior may be shown by a child who often acts before thinking or who frequently speaks out of turn in class. Excessive general hyperactivity, although not always present in children with attentional deficits, is relatively common. In the preschool and school years, the child may have difficulty sitting still or staying seated. He or she may incessantly run about and climb on things unless closely supervised.

The etiology of attention deficit disorder is unclear. Genetic factors, neurological impairment, physical abnormalities, high lead concentrations in the blood, diet, and family and school environments have all been cited as potential causative factors. At this time it seems that the disorder is caused by interactions of biological, psychological, and social variables. Sex appears to be another important variable, with boys being much more affected by the disorder than girls. Sex ratios in the range of 3:1 to 9:1 have been reported, but the reasons for this sex difference are not known.

From a life-span perspective a major question about children diagnosed as having attention deficit disorder with hyperactivity is "What happens to them as they grow older?" Although clinical observation suggests that the condition improves with age, children do not simply outgrow these difficulties. In later childhood, children continue to show problems of inattention, lack of concentration, impulsivity, and underachievement. Upon reaching adolescence, the most serious problems relate to school failure and to the frequency of antisocial behavior (G. Weiss & Hechtman, 1979). Relationships with teachers, peers, and parents are hampered by these problems. Longitudinal studies indicate that relatively few children or adolescents with attentional and hyperactivity problems become grossly disturbed as adults, but they continue to show signs of impulsivity, poor social skills, and lower occupational achievement.

Different treatment approaches—medical, behavioral, and educational—have been employed with hyperkinetic children. The ultimate goals of these approaches are to increase attention spans, to reduce excessive activity levels, and to improve ability to profit from classroom instruction. As Zentall (1975) pointed out, traditional treatment approaches assume that children with hyperactive disorders suffer from minimal brain damage, are unable to filter out irrelevant stimuli, and are in a constant state of overarousal. Accordingly, treatment seeks to reduce the amount of stimulation in the child's environment. A recent proposal is that hyperactive children with attentional deficits may be underaroused rather than overaroused. According to this view, hyperactive children engage in high levels of activity in order to increase stimulus input and increase their arousal levels. Support for the underarousal hypothesis awaits further empirical testing.

Divided Attention

One of the clearest experimental demonstrations of attentional capacity limits can be found in studies of **divided attention,** in which subjects are asked to pay attention to more than one task. (Studies on selective attention require subjects to pay attention to only one thing at a time.) To illustrate this concept we will examine a well-known study by Neisser and Becklen (1975) on selective looking. Neisser and Becklen (1975) videotaped two different events. The first involved a game in which one player tries to slap his opponents' hands without getting slapped; the second showed three men throwing a basketball to one another. Subjects were asked to press a button whenever something significant happened in either episode. Even when the two scenes were superimposed on one another, subjects had no difficulty following a single episode. This would be like watching two television programs on the same television screen and trying to pay attention to only one of them. However, subjects experienced great difficulty trying to attend to both episodes simultaneously, suggesting that if we can follow a particular flow of information, it is difficult to follow an unrelated one.

In a ground-breaking study, Cherry (1953) employed an experimental technique in which subjects listened to two spoken messages being played simultaneously through a set of headphones. Subjects were instructed to pay attention to a single message (left ear or right ear). In addition, subjects were told to repeat everything they heard in that ear as they heard it. If the words were spoken slowly, the task was not difficult; but if the words were spoken rapidly, the task became extremely difficult. This technique is called **shadowing** and assumes that directing processing resources in one direction (attending to one message) will reduce the amount of processing available for the other source.

Cherry's (1953) subjects remembered very little about the unattended message in the shadowing task. They could tell if the voice in the unattended message was male or female and if the sex of the speaker changed. However, they did not notice a change from one language to another; nor could they repeat any of the words spoken, even if the words were repeated several times. Performing this task is similar in many ways to being at a party, where one tunes into one conversation (message) and tunes out others. You may pay attention to another conversation if you hear your name being mentioned or a subject of interest to you being discussed, but fail to notice other aspects of the conversation.

Are there age changes in selective looking or listening abilities? In an early series of studies, Maccoby and Konrad (1966, 1967) asked children of several ages to repeat one of two messages they heard simultaneously. In general, the children became more accurate in repeating the message as they became older, and instructions to attend to one message (the relevant one) improved the children's recall accuracy. In other research, older children and adults seemed to be less distracted in their auditory attention by competing voices than younger children (Doyle, 1973; Sexton & Geffen, 1979). Numerous studies have reported that older adults also perform more poorly on dual listening tasks (see Craik, 1977, for a review).

Different theoretical models have been proposed to account for the fact that certain information is attended to while other information goes unnoticed. Usually these models use a filtering or *bottleneck* device that regulates the flow of information and prevents information overload. Broadbent's (1958) single-channel model of attention is a **filtering model** because it postulates that our sensory organs consistently process sensory information, but information from only one input gets processed at a single time. Thus, if you are listening to a message with your right ear, you cannot simultaneously attend to information with your left ear. In Broadbent's model the bottleneck occurs at the beginning stages of perceptual processing; in other filtering models, it is located "deeper" in the system (Deutsch & Deutsch, 1963; Johnston & Heinz, 1978; D. A. Norman, 1968). An alternative **attenuation model** has been proposed by Treisman (1964). This model postulates that we can operate multiple channels of processing at one time, but the more channels we process, the weaker (or more attenuated) the incoming signals become. For example, if you try to take notes and listen attentively to your professor, you may find that you cannot concentrate fully on either activity. Although not intended to account for developmental changes in children's and adults' attention, the above models have been influential in our conceptualizations of attentional limitations.

In *Cognition and Reality*, Neisser (1976) argues against the notion of limited attentional capacity. He points out that there are no known physiological or psychological limits to the amount of information we can pick up at one time (see also Neisser, Hirst, & Spelke, 1981). Neisser (1976) believes that one reason why we can have difficulty in divided attention situations is because the activities "have no natural relationship to each other" (p. 101). For example, writing a letter and throwing a baseball require incompatible responses. However, in other cases, such as attending to two conversations simultaneously, one task masks a signal from a different one. In this instance, a person may have an excruciatingly hard time following both conversations.

Neisser (1976) points out that we can learn through practice to perform simultaneously many activities such as walking and talking or driving and talking. In one study, Spelke, Hirst, and Neisser (1976) had two college students work on an experiment one hour a day for the entire semester. The subjects were asked to silently read stories while trying to copy words dictated by an experimenter. As you can imagine, the students first found the task to be quite difficult, and they read very slowly. With practice, however, their reading levels eventually returned to normal. The experimenters then introduced a twist into the study. Instead of presenting words to the subjects at random, as had been done, they selected words from a category such as 20 plural nouns or 20 words that composed meaningful sentences. The results showed that subjects had copied down words without noticing the categories. When later alerted that (unspecified) categories and sentences would occasionally be embedded in the word lists, subjects were able to detect them, although at first their reading performance was impaired.

Practiced subjects can do what novice subjects often cannot do. According to Neisser (1976), the superior performance of practiced individuals cannot be based on a limited amount of fixed capacity of attention. Instead performance level depends on the *skill* of the performer. Our level of skill helps free our attention to engage in other behavior. Actions that once required effort become *automatic*, and behaviors appropriate to the beginning stages of skill acquisition drop out. In many ways, automaticity of a skill can be likened to a reflex; skilled performers often comment that they acted without conscious realization until after the act.

Reading is a prime example of this process. Reading skill has many different components—having adequate visual acuity to read; coding and ciphering letters; distinguishing the distinctive features of letters from each other; systematically relating letters to sounds, combining sounds into words, and identifying meaning in sentences (Downing & Leong, 1982; LaBerge & Samuels, 1974). Each of these activities requires considerable attention, so that beginning readers limit their input by reading slowly. As their reading skills improve, readers may speed up their reading and learn to vary their speed as a function of the situation (difficulty level of the material, their familiarity with the material, the relevancy of the text information). In a recent review of studies on reading, A. Brown, Bransford, Ferrara, and Campione (1983) conclude that as children become more efficient readers, they are better able to allocate their attention and effort in a more economical and flexible manner.

Automaticity

The concept of automaticity in relation to practice has become an important one in both the childhood and adult developmental literatures. The concept goes by many different names including *automatic*, *involuntary*, and *systematic processing*. These automatic processes are contrasted with controlled, deliberate, or effortful processes. **Automatic processing** can be defined as "a fast, parallel process . . . that requires little subject effort and that demands little direct subject control" (A. Brown et al., 1983, p. 111), whereas **controlled processing** is a slow serial process that requires a good deal of mental effort and allows the subject a large degree of control. Automatic processing is described as a *parallel* process because subjects examine all the items in their short-term memory at once, whereas in controlled processing they examine the items as a part of a *series*, one at a time (see Chapter 6).

Shiffrin and Schneider (1977) sought to determine the limitations on attention that predict the use of parallel and subject-controlled processes. In one of their studies subjects were shown a rapid sequence of 20 frames on each trial (see Figure 3.10). Before the trials, subjects were told to search for certain digits from a set of digits. Sometimes they were told to search for one target, at other times for four targets simultaneously. Subjects indicated their detection of the target by pressing a button. The two experimental conditions were *consistent mapping* and *varied mapping.* In the consistent mapping condition, subjects were shown memory set targets from one category (such as digits) and distractor items from another category (such as letters). In the varied mapping condition (see Figure 3.10*a*), the targets and distractors were all either letters or digits. The results under the two conditions were quite different. Under consistent mapping conditions (see Figure 3.10*b*), subjects learned after many trials to search for four targets almost as quickly as one. Shiffrin and Schneider (1977) contended that these subjects used **automatic detection,** which does not require attentional control from the subjects. In contrast, under varied mapping conditions, as the number of target items increased, the subjects' performance steadily worsened. Even after more than 2000 practice trials, subjects required more time to search for a set of four targets than for only one target. Schneider and Shiffrin (1977) suggested that the varied mapping condition produces **controlled search.** In controlled (serial) search, subjects compare each member of the target set individually with each frame until a match is found. Attentional effort and time is needed to make each comparison.

Perhaps you have experienced these two processes in your cognitive activities. Many adults have developed automatic methods of distinguishing numbers and letters after many years of controlled search. Thus, a number embedded within a string of letters (CTG4JE) may

Figure 3.10   The two search conditions in Schneider and Shiffrin's experiments. (*a*) Varied mapping condition and (*b*) consistent mapping condition. For each trial the sequence of events was presentation of (1) memory set, (a) a fixation dot, (b) two dummy frames not containing the target, (c) the target frame, (d) two dummy frames not containing the target.

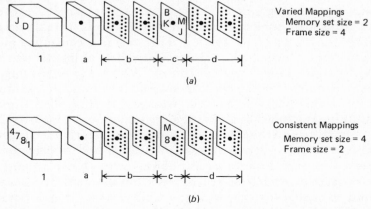

(*a*)

(*b*)

"pop out" of the display. You recognize that the letter series contains a number before you are able to identify the exact digit. Perhaps with many years of experience on certain jobs (such as quality control inspector, copy editor, brain surgeon), a person becomes capable of automatically spotting certain things. Moreover, this experience may offset some of the age-imposed limitations on such skills.

The automatic-controlled distinction has several ramifications for developmental research. First, it suggests that much expertise that comes with age and experience results from processes that were initially controlled and effortful (W. Hoyer, 1985). Further, it implies that processes that are relatively automatic should be efficient even in young children and should undergo fewer dramatic developmental changes (A. Brown, 1975; Hasher & Zacks, 1979). More will be said about automatic and controlled processes in Chapter 6.

ATTENTION AND AROUSAL

Selectivity is a major component of attention. Another dimension of attention is **arousal,** which psychologists define in a variety of ways. In our discussion the term will be used to describe a general level of alertness that serves to keep our attentional system activated to receive perceptual inputs.

Differences in arousal level are related to performance differences in various perceptual and cognitive tasks by an inverted U-shaped function, which is called the Yerkes-Dodson law (Yerkes & Dodson, 1908). Easterbrook (1959) and D. A. Norman (1976) have suggested that the relationship between arousal level and performance can be explained by the utilization of attentional cues. At very low levels of arousal, selectivity of attention is low; both relevant and irrelevant cues are attended to uncritically. Performance is optimal at moderate levels of arousal. Selectivity increases, and the subject focuses on relevant cues and ignores irrelevant cues. However, at high levels of arousal, performance ceases to improve and begins to decline, presumably because the nervous system is responding to too many stimuli at once. The attentional span is narrowed, and relevant cues are overlooked. Because simple tasks require fewer cues, they are not as affected by high arousal levels as are more complex tasks which require more attentional capacity (Broadbent, 1971; Solso, 1979). For example, during a time of high arousal, you would probably be able to recite the alphabet, but might be unable to play a game of chess. However, the more practiced or more automatic the task—even if it is fairly difficult—the less likely it is to be disrupted under high levels of arousal.

Kahneman (1973) has proposed a model of attention that incorporates our "limited capacity" attentional system and fluctuating arousal levels. Kahneman's model provides an alternative to filter theories of attention, which explain information-processing limitations in terms of structural bottlenecks. Kahneman assumes that there is a general limitation on people's capacity to perform mental work, and this capacity can be allocated among various concurrent activities. His model of the allocation of capacity to mental activities is shown in Figure 3.11. The two major elements of the model are the "allocation policy" and the "evaluation of demands on capacity." The evaluation of demands is the executive of the system that causes mental capacity or effort "to be supplied as needed by the activities that the allocation policy has selected" (Kahneman, 1973, p. 11). The allocation policy is controlled by four factors: (1) *enduring dispositions*, which reflect the rules of involuntary attention (switching attention to a conversation in which your name is mentioned); (2) *momentary intentions*, such as listening to a voice on the right earphone; (3) *evaluation of demands*; and (4) effects of *arousal*.

The last factor in Kahneman's model, arousal, is closely related to available capacity, as shown by the wavy line that separates them in Figure 3.11. Arousal and attention can increase or decrease according to the changing demands of ongoing activities. More capacity is available when arousal levels are moderately high than when they are low. Thus, attention (or mental effort) and arousal can vary together. Finally, arousal levels can be increased by such factors as anxiety, fear, anger, sexual excitement, and drugs.

Figure 3.11   Kahneman's model of attention allocation.

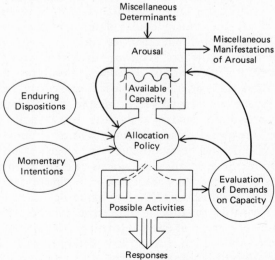

From *Attention and Effort* (p. 10) by D. Kahneman, 1973, Englewood Cliffs, NJ: Prentice-Hall. Copyright 1973 by Prentice-Hall, Inc. Reprinted by permission.

INDIVIDUAL DIFFERENCES IN
PERCEPTION AND ATTENTION

Individuals differ in the way they approach perceptual and cognitive tasks. Some people attend to the smallest, minutest details of a problem. Others prefer to get the "big picture." Similarly, many people carefully inspect all the elements of a problem, work slowly, and verify their answers before responding. Other individuals quickly scan the information at hand, arrive at a rapid solution, and are less concerned about responding incorrectly. These individual variations in organizing, attending, processing, remembering, and thinking about a problem are known as **cognitive styles** (Kogan, 1982). Cognitive styles form a useful bridge between the (mostly) perceptual processes discussed in this chapter and the higher cognitive processes discussed in later chapters. They reflect stable tendencies among individuals in organizing and dealing with information in the environment. In this chapter, we will look at three of the at least nine cognitive styles that have been identified.

Field Dependence and Field Independence

One of the most extensively studied cognitive style differences is that between **field dependence** and **field independence.** Field-dependent people "depend on" or are influenced by the surrounding contextual cues of the perceptual field. They may either be helped or misled by attending to these cues. In contrast, field-independent people are able to function relatively independently of the context.

Several different instruments have been devised to measure these styles. The most commonly used measure is the Embedded Figures Test, which consists of a series of complex geometric shapes (see Figure 3.12) in which a simple shape such as a rectangle, triangle, or diamond is embedded. The subject is asked to identify the simple shape contained in the larger, more complex one. Performance on the test is measured by how much time the subject takes to locate the embedded figure and by the subject's number of correct identifications of the figures. Subjects who require more time and make fewer correct choices are labeled field dependent. Those who can disembed the figures quickly without making errors are field independent. This distinction is not absolute because the scores lie along a continuum.

The Rod-and-Frame Test is an alternative test of the same cognitive style. In this procedure subjects are required to adjust a luminous rod to an upright position in a darkened room. The rod is suspended within a tilted frame. Field-dependent people have difficulty ignoring the cues

Figure 3.12　Sample item from the Embedded Figures Test. The subject's task is to identify a simple shape that is embedded in a larger, more complex pattern.

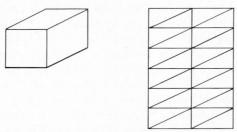

From *The Embedded Figures Test* Figure 8-E, Form B by H. Witkin, 1969, Palo Alto, CA: Consulting Psychologists Press. Copyright 1969 by Consulting Psychologists Press, Inc. Reprinted by permission.

from the frame and tend to line up the rod parallel with the sides of the frame. Field-independent people are able to overlook the contextual cues given by the frame and use their own bodily cues to adjust the frame to a true vertical position.

The two tasks described above have been given to children as well as to adults. On the Embedded Figures Test, simpler geometric shapes are usually employed to test children. On the Rod-and-Frame Test, a human figure is sometimes superimposed over the rod to make the task more interesting to children. On both tasks, the generally reported finding is that children become increasingly field independent as they get older, but at any given age both field-dependent and field-independent styles exist (Kogan, 1983; Witkin & Goodenough, 1981). Findings on changes in field independence across the adult life span are more inconsistent. Lee and Pollack (1978) studied female subjects ranging in age from the 20s to the 70s who were matched on visual acuity and IQ. They obtained significant age differences for mean solution times on the Embedded Figures Test, with older women taking more time to locate the figures (thus showing greater field dependence) than younger women. In a recent study, Panek (1985) similarly reported that older adults were more field dependent than younger adults, even after statistically controlling for the effects of IQ. In contrast, Lee and Pollack (1980) administered the Rod-and-Frame Test to females in their 40s, 50s, and 60s. No significant age differences were found, suggesting that field dependence–independence may not be a unitary construct in the latter portion of the life span. In studies on cognitive styles among older adults, it is especially important to control for sensory difficulties, health, and cohort-related factors such as educational and occupational differences.

Some psychologists not only attempt to describe the differences between field-dependent and field-independent cognitive styles, but also to relate such styles to personality variables. Witkin and his research group (1954) pointed out personality differences between people with one or the other style. Field-dependent people are described as having a more interpersonal focus; field-independent people are considered more autonomous in their relations with others. In addition, cognitive style may influence occupational choice: Field-dependent people tend to enter fields such as social sciences, humanities, and education, which demand a global interpersonal perspective. Field-independent people gravitate to fields such as mathematics, the natural sciences, engineering, and architecture, which require highly developed analytical skills. The evidence here is not strong, but the notion of individuals going into certain occupations because of their cognitive styles is intriguing.

Another variable related to individual differences in cognitive styles, particularly in the domain of field dependence and independence, is sex (Kogan, 1983; Maccoby & Jacklin, 1974). Women have been shown to be more field dependent than men on a variety of cognitive measures, whereas men exhibit greater field independence. These sex differences are also apparent in childhood, although some investigators report that girls are more advanced in field independence than boys during the preschool years (Coates, 1974, 1978). This stylistic difference in preschool may be related to the fact that girls are biologically more mature than boys during the early years of life (Kogan, 1983). However, findings from cross-cultural studies raise doubts about whether sex differences in field dependence and independence are an inherent part of our biology. In studies of preliterate hunting-and-gathering cultures, negligible sex differences in field dependence and independence are reported (Witkin & Goodenough, 1981). Few authors have attempted to examine biological and cultural contributions to sex-related differences in cognitive styles within a single study.

Reflectivity and Impulsivity

Individuals can differ on perceptual and cognitive tasks in the way they approach problem-solving situations. Some people look at a problem very carefully and consider all the alternatives before giving a solution. Kagan, Rosman, Day, Albert, and Phillips (1964) term this a *reflective cognitive style.* Individuals who are quick to respond before they consider all the alternatives and tend to make many careless errors are described as *impulsive.*

Individual differences in **reflectivity-impulsivity** are most often measured with the Matching Familiar Figures Test (Kagan et al., 1964). On this test the subject is shown a picture and asked to find an identical match from among six other pictures (some versions employ more than six pictures). The six picture choices are similar to each other, so that mistakes are easy to make (see Figure 3.13). Reflective individuals tend to inspect all the alternatives for a few seconds before making a choice. They are more likely to make the correct selection on their first attempt. Impulsive individuals respond quickly, often without considering all the alternatives, and their first choices are more frequently incorrect.

Research has shown that stable individual differences in this style appear among children at a very early age. Further, there are gradual increases in reflectivity up to at least age 10, as measured by increases in response times and decreases in errors on the Matching Familiar Figures Test. After age 10, response times begin to decrease and errors stabilize (Salkind, 1978; Salkind & Nelson, 1980). Thus, children become increasingly efficient on this test with development.

Not surprisingly, stylistic differences are related to school performance differences. Reflective children tend to do better than impulsive children on reading, memory, and reasoning tasks. Such findings have often led to the conclusion that reflectivity is the preferred cognitive style, at least among children (in old adults, reflectivity is often negatively interpreted as slowness). But reflectivity may not always be the most optimal conceptual style, as some important research by Zelniker and Jeffrey (1976) suggested. Zelniker and Jeffrey (1976) found that reflective children do better on tasks that require analyses of fine inter-

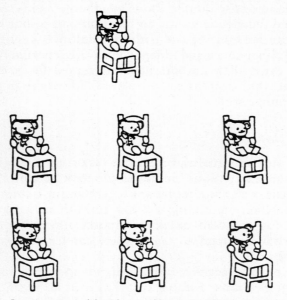

Figure 3.13 Sample item for reflectivity-impulsivity from the Matching Familiar Figures Test. Reflective individuals tend to scan all the alternatives before deciding which exactly matches the standard (top) item.

From *Learning and the Educational Process* (p. 135) by J. D. Krumboltz (Ed.), 1965. Chicago: Rand McNally. Copyright 1965 by Rand McNally & Company. Reprinted by permission.

nal detail; impulsive children do better on tasks requiring attention to outer contours of objects and global comparisons.

Do differences in reflectivity-impulsivity correlate with behavioral or personality differences among children? In preschool children, they appear to be related to play and social relations. Reflective children appear to consider each toy carefully, play longer with one toy, and show less dependence on the teacher. Impulsive children dart from one toy to another and are easily distracted by other playthings. However, they are more responsive in social relations than reflective children. At the elementary school level and beyond, there is weaker evidence for the real-world behavioral correlates of reflectivity-impulsivity (Kogan, 1983). Hence, we should be careful not to generalize this construct beyond the differences observed on measures such as the Matching Familiar Figures Test.

Until recently, all of the research on reflectivity-impulsivity was limited to the preadolescent years (Kogan, 1973). Now a few studies on life-span changes along this dimension can be found in the literature (Kogan, 1982). But the little evidence we have on this stylistic difference is contradictory. N. Denney and List (1979) tested five different age groups ranging from the 30s to the 70s using the Matching Familiar Figures Test procedure. The older subjects took longer to respond and committed more errors than the younger subjects. Thus, older adults cannot be simply classified as reflective or impulsive. Education, sex, occupation, and retirement status were unrelated to performance. Coyne, Whitbourne, and Glenwick (1978) compared a young adult group (aged 18–27) with an old adult group (aged 61–87) and found, surprisingly, that the older adults were more likely to be impulsive and to make more errors. Further research is needed to resolve these discrepant findings.

Categorization and Conceptualization Styles

Stylistic differences have also been reported on tasks requiring subjects to sort stimulus objects into different categories. The objects employed have been either geometric shapes, pictures of everyday objects, or words describing them. Though a variety of different objects are employed, common bases for categorization and conceptualization have been identified. Kogan (1982) has summarized the findings of this research in terms of the distinction between **similarity groupings** and **complementary groupings**. Similarity groupings categorize objects according to similarity in *function* (a knife and scissors are both used for cutting) or *category* (beans, corn, and spinach are all vegetables). Complementary groupings are formed with objects that show complementarity in function (a match and a stove are grouped together because the match is used to light the stove). Kogan (1974) and Cicirelli (1976) reported a predominance of similarity groupings in samples of young and old adults, but the old adults also showed more complementary groupings than young adults. Greater complementarity has also been reported in samples of young children (Kogan, 1982), but this evidence does not mean that older adults regress to the categorization ability level of young children. Unlike young children, old adults are able to explain the logic behind their groupings. In fact, complementary groupings may be adaptive for old adults in that this is the way objects "naturally go together" in the real world. Further, the number of complementary groupings in later adulthood decreases among those with higher educational levels and more professional occupations.

As Kogan (1982) recently pointed out, the future study of cognitive styles could benefit from a greater integration of stylistic differences with other perceptual and cognitive processing abilities. For example, the measures of field dependence–independence and reflectivity-impulsivity have a large selective attention component. Research on selective attention should be systematically related to these cognitive style differences. Cognitive styles may also be important in various spatial tasks such as spatial perspective taking. In the next chapter we will discuss the subject of spatial cognition, and you should think about how one's cognitive style might influence one's organization of spatial concepts.

SUMMARY

1. Perceptual development is a process that shows considerable age-related change across the entire life span. No single theory can account for these changes.
2. Sensation involves the initial activation of the sensory receptors, whereas perception involves the organization and extraction of meaning from sensory information.
3. For centuries philosophers turned to perception as a way of answering basic epistemological questions about the nature of knowledge. Philosophers differ over whether perceptual knowledge is learned (empiricism) or innate (nativism).
4. Psychologists such as Piaget consider perception as a primitive organizing experience that provides the raw elements for higher cognitive processes. Other psychologists such as E. Gibson emphasize the meaningfulness inherent in the environment. Neisser's perceptual cycle model reconciles these two viewpoints.

5. The most dramatic changes in perception occur at the sensory level. Sensory changes, especially negative changes, can have a major impact on everyday cognitive functioning.

6. The major changes that occur in the eye with age include changes in the pupillary reflex, crystalline lens, and retina. These have significant effects on visual acuity (the ability to discern fine detail) and visual accommodation (the ability to focus on near objects).

7. In general, auditory acuity improves with age until adolescence, levels off until the 30s, and then gradually declines. Most age-related loss in hearing occurs at the highest frequencies.

8. The different senses are not separate systems, but are intercoordinated with each other. Sensory coordination is present during the first year of life.

9. Occasionally, people misperceive reality and experience an illusion. Illusions may involve sensory (Type I illusions) and cognitive processes (Type II illusions).

10. An important aspect of perception is the ability to selectively attend to relevant information and to disregard irrelevant information. Selective attention is found among young infants, although they do not always focus on the most relevant stimuli.

11. In older children and adults, attentional processes increasingly intertwine with other cognitive processes such as memory. The ability to selectively attend to important information and to ignore unimportant information improves though adulthood, but shows some decline in later life.

12. The perceptual salience of information on cognitive tasks is important because more salient stimuli are processed before less salient stimuli.

13. Poor performance on divided attention tasks—in which we pay attention to more than one task at a time—can be explained in terms of a limited attentional capacity. However, some psychologists argue that the amount of information that can be attended to simultaneously has no upper limits.

14. An important distinction in developmental research is the difference between automatic and controlled processing. Automatic processes require little attentional effort, whereas controlled processes are self-regulated and demand much effort.

15. Arousal is an important component of attention. It has been hypothesized that the relationship between arousal and performance is due to the utilization of attentional cues.

16. Individuals differ in the way they perceive, organize, and remember information. These differences are called cognitive styles, and they include field dependence–field independence, reflectivity-impulsivity, and categorization and conceptualization styles.

Key Terms

perception	discrepancy principle
sensation	central learning
empiricism	incidental learning
nativism	perceptual salience
distinctive features	divided attention
differentiation	shadowing
invariants	filtering model
anticipatory schemata	attenuation model
perceptual cycle	automatic processing
pupillary reflex	controlled processing
senile miosis	automatic detection
visual acuity	controlled search
visual accommodation	arousal
presbyopia	cognitive styles
cataracts	field dependence
recruitment	field independence
virtual object	reflectivity
illusion	impulsivity
Type I illusions	similarity groupings
Type II illusions	complementary groupings
verbal transformation effect	

Suggested Readings

Bornstein, M. H. (1984). Perceptual development. In M. H. Bornstein & M. E. Lamb (Eds.), *Developmental psychology: An advanced textbook* (pp. 81–131). Hillsdale, NJ: Erlbaum. This chapter illustrates the relevance of the developmental approach to the study of perception. It covers philosophical, methodological, and substantive issues in investigations on perceptual development with an emphasis on the importance of perceptual research across the life span.

Comalli, P. E., Jr. (1970). Life-span changes in visual perception. In L. Goulet & P. B. Baltes (Eds.), *Life-span developmental psychology: Research and theory* (pp. 211–227). New York: Academic Press. Comalli's chapter focuses on age changes in susceptibility to visual illusions. He cites evidence to support a progressive-regressive pattern of perceptual ability changes across the life span.

Haith, M. M. (1980). *Rules that babies look by: The organization of newborn visual activity.* Hillsdale, NJ: Erlbaum. This book summarizes five ground-breaking studies on early infant visual behavior and the rule systems that infants possess for learning about their visual environment. Although written primarily for the graduate student and academic researcher, the book contains enough general information on early visual competencies to interest the undergraduate reader.

Hoyer, W. J., & Plude, D. J. (1980). Attentional and perceptual processes in the study of cognitive aging. In L. W. Poon (Ed.), *Aging in the 1980s: Psychological issues* (pp. 227–238). Washington, DC: American Psychological Association. This chapter highlights some important recent trends in the study of perceptual and attentional processes in adulthood and old age. The authors suggest that perceptual aging research is rapidly progressing in three major areas: (1) sensory aging processes, (2) selective attention, and (3) higher-order cognitive processes controlling sensory and attentional mechanisms.

Kahneman, D. (1973). *Attention and effort.* Englewood Cliffs, NJ: Prentice-Hall. This classic volume deals with how individuals selectively allocate attentional resources in a limited capacity information-processing system. Kahneman's model holds that we can flexibly use our limited resources to meet the demands of various attentional tasks.

Pick, A. D., Frankel, D. G., & Hess, V. L. (1975). Children's attention: The development of selectivity. In E. M. Hetherington (Ed.), *Review of child development research* (Vol. 5, pp. 325–383). Chicago: University of Chicago Press. A comprehensive overview of the empirical findings on infants' and children's attention. The authors also identify problems that need to be investigated in order to better understand attentional development in children.

Spoehr, K. T., & Lehmkuhle, S. W. (1982). *Visual information processing.* San Francisco: Freeman. This book reviews the full range of visual processing and the methods psychologists use to study processing. It provides a broad, integrative view of how the visual processing system works and also considers the relationship between sensory and cognitive processes.

Walk, R. D. (1981). *Perceptual development.* Monterey, CA: Brooks/Cole. This book provides an excellent and highly readable in-depth survey of the field of perceptual development. It includes information on infant visual perception, perceptual deprivation and enrichment, attention, and perceptual development in special populations such as the blind, the deaf, and the aged.

CHAPTER 4

Spatial Cognition and Imagery

Questions about the fundamental nature of space have held great interest for scientists and philosophers. In this chapter various conceptions of space are considered in relation to the origin and development of spatial cognition. We will consider the controversy over whether spatial concepts are biologically endowed, gradually constructed through active experience, or specified by information in the stimulus environment. We will also present several examples of infant spatial knowledge in an effort to solve how infants perceive and organize space. The development of search behavior for hidden objects is one of the most crucial aspects of this early knowledge.

The next problem is how individuals mentally represent spatial information. We will examine how we form images in our minds, rotate or manipulate these images, and use them to find our way through the environment. Also considered are developmental changes in the use of spatial reference systems. Young children define spatial positions in reference to their own bodies (or egocentrically), whereas older children and adults define the frame of reference by positions external to their bodies (or allocentrically). The implications of these developmental changes for everyday spatial behavior are presented.

The last section deals with individual differences in spatial ability and skills. An attempt is made to understand why males, on the average, perform better than females on spatial tasks. In addition, we examine cross-cultural differences in spatial cognition.

DIFFERENT CONCEPTIONS OF SPACE

What is the nature of space? Is our knowledge of space innate or learned through experiencing the environment? These seemingly simple questions have fascinated and perplexed scientists and philosophers for centuries. Conceptions of space, like those of time, have shifted radically, and we are still revising our definitions. As Forman (1975) states:

> For yet another time, man has found himself underestimating the fundamental nature of space. First Newton demonstrated the limitations of Aristotle, then Einstein showed the limitations of Newton. The possibility of a third comprehensive revision in cosmology has caused us to doubt the reliability of the observer. The study of the cosmos becomes as well a study of the thinking process. (p. 111)

The third revision Forman is referring to is a post-Einsteinian revolution, with a broad outline that can only be speculated on at the present time. Each of the first three theories about space—Aristotelian, Newtonian, Einsteinian—departed more and more from childhood spatial concepts, but was limited by other intuitions and assumptions. Thus, to understand space, we must understand something about the nature of our cognitions and thought processes as observers.

Our conceptions of space are closely related to all other forms of knowledge. Regardless of the cognitive process involved, we use spatial concepts. They serve as tools in memory and problem solving, as in remembering a familiar route or in finding our way around an unfamiliar environment. They also are fundamental to language acquisition, for example, in concepts such as *up-down, right-left, above-below,* and *front-back.* In addition, spatial concepts often have affective meaning, so that spaces, such as churches and battlefields, are endowed with special emotional significance. Thus, spatial cognition is an important topic.

Absolute versus Relative Space

To discuss different conceptions of space, we must make some important distinctions to give you an appreciation of the diversity of ways space can be defined. One such distinction—implicit in Forman's statement above—is that between **absolute space** and **relative space.** By absolute space we mean "a framework that exists independently of anything contained within it" (Liben, 1981, p. 4). Objects are contained within the space, but if they are removed, the space remains fundamentally unchanged. The Newtonian view is a good example of an absolute conception of space.

You might recall from a high school physics class that Newton tried to describe mathematically the forces that keep the planets in motion. He concluded that the natural paths of planets (and other objects) were on a straight line through a uniform empty space; gravity deflected the planets from this would-be straight line. Only the distance between two objects determined the strength of the force they exerted upon each other. Because space was thought to be uniform and unchanging, the position of the observer became largely irrelevant.

A contrasting view is that space is relative and does not exist independently of the objects within it. As the position of objects and the observer changes, space is transformed. Einstein's general theory of relativity is a relativistic conception of space. Little of what can be said here about relativity theory can be grasped on a purely intuitive level. Through mathematical models, particularly non-Euclidean models (discussed below), Einstein showed that the shape of motion through space depends on the perspective of the observer. What two observers perceive at a given time depends on their motion relative to one another and to the event.

To cite Einstein's famous example, imagine you are traveling on a speeding train. If you could measure the relations of objects in the train and those outside the window, you would be able to produce a body of data. However, these data would be grossly inaccurate if the train came to a sudden halt, and you were suddenly able to account for the motion bias. In other words, your data would be affected by the fact that your measurements were not fixed, but changing constantly (Sinnott, 1981).

Euclidean versus Non-Euclidean Space

Paralleling the distinction between absolute and relative space is the distinction between **Euclidean** and **non-Euclidean** models of space. The Euclidean model is a three-dimensional concept of space (height, width, distance). Each of these dimensions can be easily visualized as part of a framework or coordinate system. The non-Euclidean model, in contrast, allows for the possibility of more than three dimensions and is not so easy to visualize. The four-dimensional space-time model of Einstein, which describes motion in a curved space, is a non-Euclidean model. In this model space and time form inseparable dimensions, whereas in the Euclidean model space and time are seen as independent.

Much of the developmental work on spatial cognition assumes that the Euclidean model is the most cognitively mature conception of space (Piaget & Inhelder, 1967). This assumption persists despite more pluralistic conceptions of space, as exemplified in Einstein's multidimensional model of space and time. However, it can be argued that the relativistic notions employed by physicists can be used by adults in complex everyday situations and may represent a more advanced form of spatial thinking (Sinnott, 1984). We will return to this point in Chapter 8, when we discuss postformal operational development.

Practical versus Representational Space

One final distinction is **practical space** versus **representational space**. In many respects, the distinction is similar to the one between enactive, iconic, and symbolic representation proposed by Bruner (see Box 2.3). Practical space refers to the capacity to act or move in space (Piaget & Inhelder, 1967). Locomoting the self from one point in space to another or manipulating an object in one's hands is an illustration of practical space. According to Piaget, such activity requires sensorimotor knowing or intelligence, but not necessarily a knowledge of representational space—the mental represention of spatial objects and relations. Young children avoid bumping into the walls of their homes by direct perception and sensation, even though they may not be able to represent mentally the interior of their homes.

A major issue is whether children's navigational competencies reflect an underlying representational system. Many psychologists disagree with Piaget, claiming that behavior in space indicates an underlying representation, even though it may be difficult to measure. Of course, practical space and representational space are not independent, as most psychologists, Piaget included, would readily admit. Spatial concepts may influence behavior in space, just as spatial activity may lead to better spatial representations.

The Origins of Spatial Concepts

There is considerable debate not only about the various conceptions of space but also about the origins of spatial concepts. Some writers have maintained that our concepts of space, like those of time, are innate biological givens. For example, the nineteenth-century philosopher Immanuel Kant believed that infants possess basic a priori knowledge of the categories of space and time that makes all subsequent learning possible; infants could not sense an object as an object unless they first know it is separate and in space (Forman, 1975). More recently, scientists have shown that organisms are equipped with highly specialized brain cells designed to receive information in certain ways. Some cells respond best to depth information, while others respond best when a stimulus is a certain color (Spoehr & Lehmkuhle, 1982).

Other writers such as Piaget and A. Siegel and White (1975) have argued that biological endowment and environmental factors interact to produce our conceptions of space. In this view, individuals actively construct their conceptions of space through their own activities. Biological factors (such as neurological maturity, physical coordination and mobility, sensory capacity), however, set the limit for certain types of spatial activities and sensations. For example, an infant standing in a playpen may enjoy dropping toys on the floor outside the playpen. Through this activity, he or she learns something fundamentally important about spatial concepts such as depth. Nonetheless, the infant's ability to conduct and interpret these spatial "tests" is constrained by his or her grasping abilities, mobility, and neurological maturity.

In Chapter 3, we contrasted Piaget's views on perception with those of E. Gibson. Gibson's theory of direct visual perception leads her to view space in a very different way than Piaget. She argues that all the information needed for spatial perception is contained in the optic array, and the infant does not need to construct an idea of space. The information in the optic array is sufficient to *specify* depth, movement, change of the position of objects, motion of the observer, and so on. By "specifying" an object or event, Gibson means that the information in the stimulation must correspond to our perception of it. For example, when the whole visual field is transformed, we say that the motion of the observer in space is specified. More will be said about these ideas later in the chapter.

Although we do not intend to discuss all the possible uses of the term *space* (there is simply not enough space for such a discussion), we will use the term in a variety of ways. We will argue that an understanding of space cannot proceed without considering the cognitive level of the observer. Therefore, we will present more of a relative as opposed to an absolute conception of space. We will also limit ourselves primarily to representational or conceptual space, although practical space will be discussed next.

SPATIAL ORGANIZATION IN INFANTS

For many years developmental psychologists grossly underestimated the perceptual and cognitive abilities of infants. Recent methodological advances and the work of innovative researchers have brought about a rediscovery of the infant and an emphasis on initial competencies. As Chapter 3 reveals, we now attribute, perhaps too much so in the opinion of some psychologists, an impressive range of perceptual and cognitive abilities to infants. No longer are infants seen as mere bundles of primitive reflexes existing in the "blooming, buzzing sensory confusion" that William James (1890) described. What is the nature of the cognitive competencies infants reputedly possess? For the most part, we can argue that spatial cognition characterizes the infant's early knowledge about the world.

What does it mean to say that an infant can perceive space? In the most general sense, it means that infants can perceive where things are, their direction and distance, and the relationships of objects to each other and to themselves (Yonas & Pick, 1975). The next four sections present several examples of infant spatial knowledge. Because the research on infant spatial perception is so voluminous (for reviews, see Acredolo, 1981; L. Cohen & Salapatek, 1975), we will restrict ourselves to the following areas: head and eye orientation, depth perception, object constancy, and object concept.

Head and Eye Orientation

One of the first signs of infant spatial knowledge is head and eye orientation to a sound source in the peripheral visual field (P. Harris,

1975). In an ingenious study, Aronson and Rosenbloom (1971) asked mothers to look at their infants (aged 30–55 days) through a sound-proof window. Loudspeakers were positioned so as to make the mother's voice appear to come either from her mouth or from the left or right side of the room. When the sound source moved from the mother's mouth to 90° left or right, infants became very upset, grimacing and sticking out their tongues. One interpretation of these behaviors is that infants have *expectancies* about the nature of visual stimuli in space and that the mother's voice coming from a location different from the mother's mouth violated these expectations. An alternative interpretation is that the infant's attempts to orient in two directions at one time produces the distress (Bower, 1982; Yonas & Pick, 1975).

We can see the importance of infant expectancies about spatial locations more clearly in a fascinating study performed by Bower, Broughton, and Moore (1970). In this study, 6-day-old to 6-month-old infants were presented with both real objects and virtual objects. (As you recall from Chapter 3, a virtual object is an image that appears to be real but is not.) The illusion is produced by having the infants wear Polaroid goggles and projecting an image through a rear projection screen with a stereoscopic device. The results showed that infants as young as 7 days reached out for both the real and virtual objects, but they became violently upset when they could not grasp the virtual object. They did not become upset when they touched the real object. These findings suggest that infants are able to orient their hands and arms in the direction of a visible stimulus, much in the way they are able to orient their head and eyes in the direction of an auditory stimulus (P. Harris, 1983). However, attempts to replicate the Bower et al. experiment have not been totally successful (F. Gordon & Yonas, 1976; Ruff & Halton, 1978), and different explanations of the results are possible. F. Gordon and Yonas (1976), for example, found that infants, 5–6½ months of age, reached toward the virtual object, but did not become upset when the object was not real. The authors indicated that this result was not surprising, given the inaccuracy with which the infants reached. Since infants often attempt to grasp for an object (real or virtual) at places other than its usual location, the absence of tactual information should not be unusual to them. We do not know whether this lack of accuracy is due to a lack of motor control or an inability to determine depth (F. Gordon & Yonas, 1976).

Depth Perception

A 6-month-old who is in the presence of a real object will not only reach toward it, if it is close enough, but will also move in the direction of the object if it is out of reach (Yonas & Pick, 1975). Walk and Gibson took advantage of this fact in their classic studies of **depth,** or distance, **perception** (E. Gibson & Walk, 1960; Walk & Gibson, 1961).

Depth, the third dimension of space, has been regarded as the true problem of spatial perception because only flat images can be formed on humans' two-dimensional retinas. Nevertheless, the flat retinal image does provide some depth cues (Spoehr & Lehmkuhle, 1982). One cue is provided by the slightly different views our two eyes have of the world. The two images from our eyes form to produce one image that has depth in a process called **stereopsis.** Depth cues are also given monocularly (with one eye). These cues include *interposition* (near objects cover or obscure more distant objects), *aerial perspective* (distant objects contain less detail), *linear perspective* (parallel lines converge with increasing distance), and *motion parallax* (nearer objects appear to move faster and farther than distant objects when the head turns).

In their studies of depth perception, Walk and Gibson (1961; E. Gibson & Walk, 1960) employed an apparatus called the **visual cliff** (see Figure 4.1). The experimenter places the infant on a center board. On one side of the visual cliff's center board (the shallow side), a visual pattern appears directly underneath a glass or plexiglas surface. On the other side (the deep side), the pattern is several feet below the glass. In the standard method, the mother stands on one side and then the other,

Figure 4.1 The visual cliff used by Walk and E. Gibson to test depth perception.

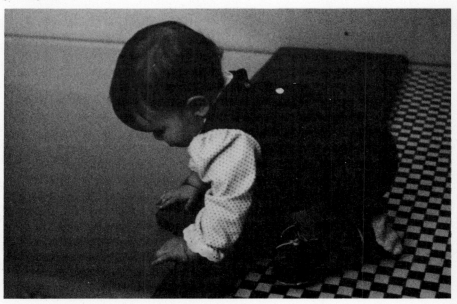

Photograph courtesy of Dr. Richard Walk. Reproduced by permission.

calling to the infant. If the infant crawls to the mother across the shallow but not the deep side, it can be concluded that the infant can discriminate depth. In a variation of this method, the infant is placed directly on the wide end of a center board that gets progressively narrower. The mother stands at the narrow end, and the infant must get off the board on either the shallow or the deep side to reach her.

Results of studies using the visual cliff apparatus with 6–14-month-old infants indicate that they can discriminate depth. Even when coaxed, most of the infants tested refused to cross the deep side to reach their mothers. However, the infants did cross the shallow side.

One problem in using the visual cliff with infants younger than 6 months is that they cannot crawl. Thus, questions about the nature-nurture issue and depth perception cannot be studied using the two procedures outlined above. A newer procedure is to place the infant directly on the shallow and deep sides and monitor its heart rate. The presumption is that any change in heart rate from one side to the other indicates depth discrimination. Using this procedure, Campos and associates (Campos, Hiatt, Ramsay, Henderson, & Svejda, 1978; Schwartz, Campos, & Baisel, 1973) showed that infants younger than 6 months can discriminate depth, but do not appear to fear depth. In other words, their heart rate slowed on the deep side, indicating attention and interest. Older infants (9–10 months) manifested fear of depth as shown by heart-rate acceleration, which varied as a function of crawling experience: The more experience the infant had, the greater the fear of depth.

Campos emphasized the importance of infants' learning experiences—perhaps as the result of falling—in the development of the fear of depth, but recent research by Nancy Rader and colleagues supports a maturationally based explanation (Rader, Bausano, & Richards, 1980; Richards & Rader, 1981). These investigators found that the best predictor of visual cliff avoidance was age of onset of crawling; neither age of testing nor amount of crawling experience predicted avoidance. Infants who learned to crawl late avoided the deep side of the cliff, and infants who learned to crawl early tended not to avoid it. This finding runs directly counter to what learning theory would predict.

Rader explains her findings on the basis of an internal, maturationally governed program that is activated only by visual information specifying a support. This program, which emerges around age 6 or 7 months, purportedly guides infants to shift their weight forward onto their hands when they encounter a support and inhibits their forward weight shift when a drop is detected. Thus, Rader sees avoidance of the cliff not so much as a fear response, but as an inactivation of a motor program that occurs only in the presence of certain stimulus information. If infants develop the ability to crawl rather late, the motor program may already be activated, and they should avoid the cliff even though they have little crawling experience. If infants develop the ability to crawl before the program develops, they may rely on tactile feedback more than visual feedback to direct their crawling. When the deep side of the cliff feels solid to the touch, infants will crawl over it, but if it feels like an empty space, they will avoid it.

As evidence for this interpretation, Rader et al. (1980) report that few infants avoid the deep side of the cliff when they are locomoting in a walker rather than crawling. If avoidance of the cliff reflects a learned fear response, then one would expect it to operate, regardless of the form of locomotion. Rader's results suggest that avoidance may not be mediated by conditioned fear, but by a motivational program specific to one form of locomotion—crawling. Although this is a provocative suggestion, infants are unlikely to gain nothing from the active experience of crawling. Perhaps they learn to make fine adjustments in the maturational program, if one exists.

Object Constancy

When infants learn that a third dimension extends beyond their own bodies, they become capable of making crucial distinctions about their immediate surroundings. One such distinction is between an apparent change in state and a real change in position (Forman, 1975). For example, an infant learns that despite changes in position, certain properties of objects such as size and shape remain constant. This occurs even though the size of the retinal image is different at different viewing positions. How does the infant accomplish this feat?

The major focus of investigation has been **size constancy.** Bower (1982) has reported that size constancy occurs as early as the second month of life. In one of his well-known studies (Bower, 1966), infants aged 6–8 weeks were trained to turn their heads in the presence of a large cube. To reinforce the head-turning response, an experimenter jumped up cooing and smiling and said "peekaboo." (Peekaboo is a favorite game of infants.) When the infants' head-turning response was well established, Bower modified the situation by presenting (1) the same cube three times as far away (thus maintaining the objective size but changing the retinal size); (2) a cube three times as large as the first cube at the same distance (thus maintaining the retinal size but changing the objective size); or (3) a cube three times as large as the first cube at a distance three times the original distance (thus changing both the objective size and the retinal size); these relationships are shown in Figure 4.2. The infants responded much more frequently to the stimulus when its objective size remained the same (size constancy) than when the stimulus size increased so as to maintain the same retinal image.

Figure 4.2   Bower's size constancy experiment. The true size and retinal size of stimuli used in different test conditions were varied.

Conditioned stimulus	Test stimuli		
	1	2	3
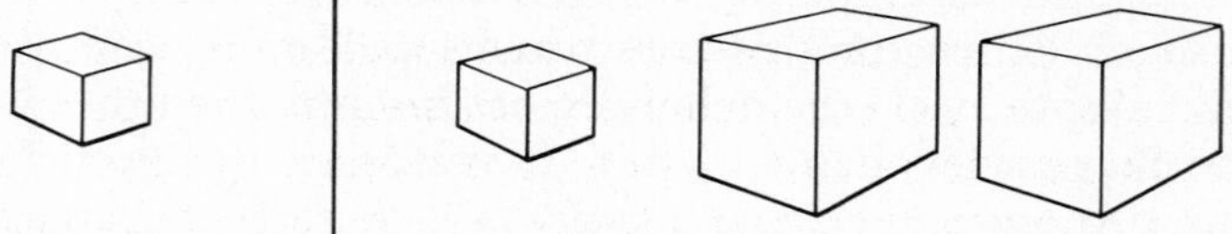 True size			
True distance 1	3	1	3
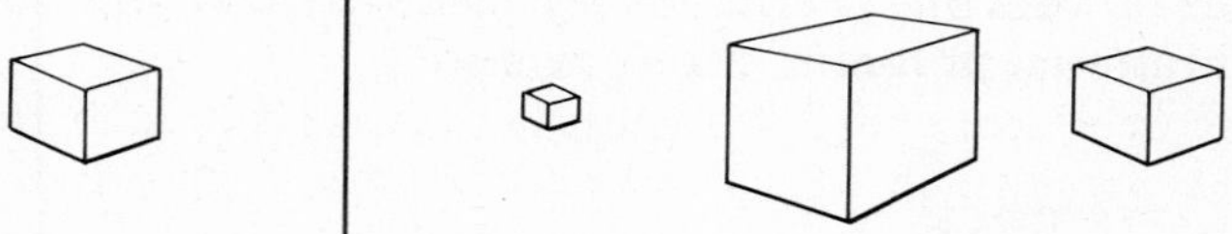 Retinal size			
Retinal distance cues	Different	Same	Different
Average number of responses elicited 98	58	54	22

From "The Visual World of Infants" by T. G. R. Bower, 1966, *Scientific American*, p. 82. Copyright 1966 by Scientific American Inc. Reprinted by permission.

These results suggest that size constancy is present at a very early age and may be a biologically prepared response.

Not all recent research confirms Bower's results. In their review of the literature on size constancy in infants, Day and McKenzie (1977) concluded that the evidence on this question is mixed. Follow-up studies by McKenzie, Tootell, and Day (1980) found evidence of size constancy in older infants (about 6 months), but not as early as Bower reported (2 months). These studies indicate that some capacity for size constancy appears very early in life, but do not indicate how precise infants' size constancy is (E. Gibson & Spelke, 1983).

Object Concept

Another major development related to the infant's perception of the third dimension is the development of an **object concept**. Object concept, or the concept of object permanence, is the knowledge that objects that have gone out of sight still exist. To the infant, various aspects of objects such as size and shape may be constant, but what about the objects themselves? As adults, we know that something that disappears from our immediate view does not cease to exist. Although some philosophers have questioned whether this is indeed the case, the independent existence of objects is a working assumption of our daily lives. Do infants show the same knowledge?

The development of an object concept is one of the most intriguing aspects of infant cognitive growth and has been studied by hundreds of developmental researchers, most notably Piaget and Bower. According to Piaget (1954), there is little evidence of object concept during the first half-year of life. Piaget (1954) described the lack of object permanence in his son: "Laurent's reaction to falling objects still seems to be nonexistent at [5 months]: he does not follow with his eyes any of the objects which I drop in front of him. . . . When I drop the object outside the bassinet Laurent does not look for it (except around my empty hand while it remains up in the air)" (p. 14). To Piaget the fact that Laurent did not search for an out-of-sight object showed that the child lacked a mature object concept. Like other sensorimotor abilities, an object concept develops in a series of gradual stages, which are described in Box 4.1.

The usual interpretation of object concept studies is that infants experience difficulty because they cannot represent objects that have gone out of sight. In other words, infants lack representational space. However, Bower (1975) points out that the infant's problem stems not from representation, but from "the concept of an object and the possible spatial relations between objects that are permitted by that concept" (p. 45).

To explain Bower's statement, we need to look at some additional object concept studies. One of these is described in Piaget's (1954) *The Construction of Reality in the Child.* A 5-month-old infant who is presented with a toy will grasp for it. However, if the toy is placed on top of another toy in *full view* of the infant, he or she will stop all attempts to grasp the object and will act as if the object no longer existed. Thus, for a 5-month-old infant, one object placed upon another ceases to exist in the same way that an object covered by a cloth ceases to exist (Bower, 1975).

A similar phenomenon can be seen in the behavior of a baby at Piaget's Stage 4 of the object concept (see Box 4.1). Here, the experimenter hides an object under one of two visible, opaque cups, called A and B. Infants at this stage can retrieve the object hidden under cup A, but if the object is then hidden under cup B, they will try to retrieve it from where they found the object before. The pattern of search is called the "Stage 4" or "A, not B" (A$\bar{\text{B}}$) error and is one of the most intriguing aspects of object concept development. In Piaget's view, the A$\bar{\text{B}}$ error can be interpreted in terms of a lack of representational ability. That is,

Box 4.1   The Development of an Object Concept

Piaget described the sensorimotor period of development in terms of the infant's ability to adapt to changing environmental circumstances and events, but he also discussed changes in the infant's understanding of objects, space, time, and causality. Here we will focus on the six stages of the development of an *object concept*. These stages parallel the broader stages of sensorimotor growth discussed in Box 2.2.

1. *Lack of an object concept—Stages 1 and 2*
   (approximately birth–4 months)
   Infants show no understanding that an object has a reality extending beyond their immediate visual field. If an object is removed from their visual field, it ceases to exist for them. They may continue to look at the location where the object disappeared, but they will make no attempt to search for it.

2. *Brief, single-modality search for an absent object—Stage 3*
   (approximately 4–8 months)
   In Stage 3 infants actively search for an object removed from their visual field, but the search is limited to the modality in which they perceived its disappearance. For example, an infant who sees a parent drop a rattle will search for it visually but will not reach for it. During this stage children also visually search for a familiar object covered by a cloth, provided they can see parts of it exposed. However, if the cloth completely obscures the object, infants behave as if the object has ceased to exist.

3. *Prolonged multimodality search—Stage 4*
   (approximately 8–12 months)
   Stage 4 is probably the most critical in the development of an object concept and the concept of space. By stage 4, infants actively search for and retrieve objects that have completely disappeared from their view. However, if the object is hidden behind one place, A, retrieved, and then hidden, with the infant observing, behind place B, he or she will search only in place A. Apparently, the action of retrieving the object hidden in place A overrides the infant's perception of seeing it hidden at B. (Gratch, 1975, provides a fuller discussion of this "A, not B" [A$\bar{\text{B}}$] search error.) This error has been well studied by researchers because it appears to support Piaget's claim that infants are egocentrically concerned with their own actions and cannot represent objects in space.

4. *Follow sequential displacements if object is visible—Stage 5 (approximately 12–18 months)*

Infants begin to retrieve objects hidden in more than one place if they witness the transfer of the object from one place to another. Initially, infants can follow only two movements, or displacements, of objects, but eventually they can follow several visible displacements (e.g., an object moves from one hand to another and then behind a screen). Infants remain unable to deal with invisible movements, or displacements, of objects from place to place. They cannot infer that if an object is not in one place, it must be in another.

5. *Follow sequential displacements if object is hidden; symbolic, mostly internal representation of objects—Stage 6 (approximately 18–24 months)*

By Stage 6, children can follow successive displacements of an object even if they do not observe its movement. They can represent objects internally, which enables them to form a systematic search strategy. Using such representation, they can mentally follow the object's route and infer where it must be hidden.

young infants cannot conceptually represent spatial relations and rely on external actions for their knowledge about space. Thus, the action of previously retrieving an object from location A overrides the infant's perception of seeing the object hidden in the new location B. Bower, however, argues that we can produce the same AB̄ behavior by using transparent cups, where the object is not hidden from view, but remains fully visible inside the cups. Bower's interpretation of this result and the one cited earlier is that the infant conceives of objects in terms of a "bounded volume of space" having a top and bottom, front and back, and a right bound and a left bound. When an object is placed on top of, inside of, behind, or beside another object, it loses its boundedness and becomes part of the other object. For the infant, the object no longer exists as a unique entity but is seen as a single object.

A different view of the AB̄ error has been proposed by Bjork and Cummings (1984), who argue that the error may be an artifact of the way infants are tested. Bjork and Cummings (1984) point out that almost all the studies reporting this phenomenon have been conducted with a two-choice hiding task, which limits all the errors on the B-hiding trials to the A location. In order to find what would happen when more than two locations are used, Bjork and Cummings (1984) tested 8–12-month-old infants on a five-choice hiding task. In two experiments using five possible hiding locations, they found little evidence that infants search incorrectly at the A location; most of the search errors occurred at locations that were closest to B. They interpreted these results to mean that the infants' search errors result from a memory problem rather than a conceptual one. The fact that the majority of search errors occur nearer to B indicates that infants understand something fundamental about relations of objects in space and that they store some of the information about the current spatial location of the object in memory. However, infants do not always engage in the most effective processing and storage operations that will allow them to remember an object's precise location.

The results of the Bjork and Cummings (1984) study are difficult to reconcile with Bower's (1975) findings. Clearly, in a situation involving transparent cups, memory problems would appear to be ruled out, since the object remains visible inside the cup. It thus remains to be seen whether the memory explanation of infant search errors can better account for infants' Stage 4 behaviors than alternative explanations such as Piaget's and Bower's.

What happens when infants are presented with a moving object to follow rather than a stationary one? Several studies have examined the effect of temporary occlusion (covering) of a moving object on the child's expectations of its continued permanence and reappearance (see P. Harris, 1975, 1983, for general reviews). The standard procedure here is to employ an occluder (such as a tunnel) and observe the infants' anticipatory eye movements as they follow a moving object's (such as a toy train) disappearance and reemergence. If infants can anticipate the future positions of objects, then some psychologists assert that the infant has the beginnings of object permanence.

A well-controlled study carried out by Meicler and Gratch (1980) illustrates this approach. The researchers tested infants of 5 and 9 months of age on an apparatus consisting of an object mounted on a flatcar which moved along a track behind a cardboard screen. Infants were shown one of two trial sequences, either a *stop trial* (on several trials the object remained out of sight six times longer than on other trials) or a *transformation trial* (a different object emerged from behind the screen). These trial sequences, which violated normal expectations, were designed to determine whether infants can anticipate the reappearance of objects. The results showed that anticipation occurred rarely among the 5-month-olds and occasionally among 9-month-olds. These results appear to support Piaget's claim that 5-month-old infants have only a limited sense of the permanence of objects, and this sense is not well developed even at 9 months of age (Meicler & Gratch, 1980).

Piaget's constructivist view of object permanence contrasts sharply with that of J. Gibson (1979) and other more traditional empiricist approaches. J. Gibson is interested in the study of event perception involving continuous changes in the stimulus array over time. In his view events provide information about transformations in objects as well as invariant properties that persist over changes in sensory stimulation.

Consider the temporary occlusion of objects, which has been frequently studied in infant perception research. As an object gradually disappears from view, progressively more of the surface area is hidden, or occluded. According to J. Gibson (1979), the sensory stimulation that is available as the object disappears provides valid information about its continued existence. Rather than having to construct an object concept out of an uninformative visual environment, as Piaget argues, children have all the information specified to them by the event. However, children must learn to distinguish between two types of disappearance—one when the object is gradually occluded by being screened or covered, and the other when an object suddenly disintegrates, or "implodes" (J. Gibson, 1966). The visual information specifying these two events is quite different because in the first case the object can be expected to reappear, whereas in the second case it cannot be. In summary, J. Gibson's account provides a radical alternative to Piagetian interpretations of object concept development.

So far we have dealt with infants' growing understanding of the permanence of single objects. As infants mature, their understanding of the relations between two (or more) objects also grows. This understanding can be inferred from the behavior they direct toward objects during activities such as play. Many developmental investigators have noted that during the early sensorimotor stages, infants direct their behavior toward single objects before they establish relations between objects (see Gesell & Thompson, 1934). Even when young infants establish relations between objects, it frequently is at the most rudimentary level. For example, a 9-month-old playing with blocks may simply bang one block against another, often without releasing them or placing them next to each other.

A change in understanding, however, occurs toward the end of the first year. This change can be seen clearly in children's behavior on the Bayley Scales of Infant Development (Bayley, 1969), which are commonly used to measure infants' perceptual, motor, language, and spatial development. One test from the Bayley scales measures an infant's understanding of *in* and *on* relationships. Initially, the infant's understanding of *in* and *on* is rather poor. At about 9½ months, an infant will place a cube in or over a cup, although the cube might not be released. By approximately 13 months, an infant is able to put small beads through a hole. And around 25½ months, the infant can correctly place three different shaped objects in a form board, even if the objects are not directly adjacent to their appropriate forms. Understanding of the *on* relationship shows a similar developmental trend. Not until after the second year can the infant correctly align one object surface with another. For example, at approximately 26 months the child is able to place a doll's head correctly on the neck with the head facing forward in relation to the body (H. Pick & Lockman, 1981).

After 1 year of age, a child's physical actions begin to reflect a developing *representational* capacity. The child becomes capable of systematically approaching two objects in space and anticipating their relationship. In one famous Piagetian example, a child opens a door slowly in order to avoid disturbing a piece of paper lying on the floor on the other side. The child apparently has formed a mental image of the two objects and what would happen if he or she opened the door quickly.

SPATIAL REPRESENTATION

For many years, psychologists have been interested in the development of spatial representation. Understanding the representation of object relations is essential for all sorts of everyday activities. Some examples are judging distances covered in a walk; identifying depth, size, and position in cartographic maps and photographs; and sailing a boat from one point to another.

In part, people's spatial representations can be defined by the kinds of cognitive operations that can be performed on their spatial information (H. Pick & Lockman, 1981; Wellman, 1985). For example, knowing how to go from point A to point B implies knowing how to go from point B to point A. Piaget calls this cognitive operation **reversibility.** Similarly, knowing how to go from point A to point B and from point B to point C implies knowing how to go from point A to point C, a cognitive operation called **transitivity** (reversibility and transitivity are discussed further in Chapter 7). How early do these abilities develop?

In his studies on the development of visually guided manipulation of objects, Piaget observed that as early as 9 months of age, infants possess an elementary spatial understanding of reversibility in this manipulative (practical) space. For example, his son Laurent could rotate a bottle to obtain the nipple even when the nipple was originally out of sight. Questions about other aspects of infants' understanding of spatial representation, such as transitivity, have not received the attention they deserve.

In addition to operations such as reversibility and transitivity, spatial representation involves performing mental operations such as *mental rotation* and *perspective taking.* We will talk about each later. But first we must introduce the topic of mental imagery.

Mental Imagery

Suppose I asked you the following question: How many windows are in your living room? To answer this question, most people attempt to mentally picture their living room and then scan each wall, counting the number of windows on each (Shwartz & Kosslyn, 1982). Or I ask you to imagine going to a baseball game. You may "see" the ball diamond, scoreboard, and players; "hear" the crack of the bat and the cheer of the crowd; "feel" the sun beating down on your head; and "smell" hot dogs, popcorn, and beer. The study of **mental imagery** involves how people form and transform these so-called mental pictures in their minds in the absence of any external stimuli. Although imagery processes are in many ways similar to the perceptual and attentional processes discussed in Chapter 3, there are some major differences between imagining and seeing (or hearing or touching) an object.

Although everyday experience may tempt us to call an image a "mental picture," there has been considerable historical controversy over the nature and form of images. More than a century ago Galton (1883) administered a questionnaire to 100 people in which he asked them to recall their breakfast table. He then asked them several questions about their images of the table. The main result did not shed much light on the nature of imagery, but showed that some people form very vivid, clear images while others report only faint images of their original perceptions. Galton later developed a measure of imagery that was related to age, sex, and other individual differences.

In a classic study on imagery performed by Perky (1910) at Cornell University, subjects were asked to imagine an image of a common object, such as a banana, on a white screen. The subjects were unaware that a pale image of the object was being projected onto the back of the screen. Subjects described their image in terms of what they were seeing, but they did not notice that they were looking at an actual picture. In short, they could not distinguish between the perceived and the imagined. Though these results are provocative, we cannot rule out the possibility that subjects may have done what the experimenter wanted them to do (called an experimenter demand effect) or that they simply did not perceive the projection on the screen because it was very faint.

Interest in imagery quickly dwindled with the advent of behaviorism, which shortly followed the Perky experiment. Such behaviorists as John B. Watson denounced "mentalistic" concepts such as imagery, consciousness, mental states, and the mind. You will recall that behaviorists favor an objective analysis of behavior with a focus on observable behavior. Within the past 15 years, however, the rise of interest in cognitive processes has been paralleled by a resurgence of interest in the psychological study of imagery. Much of the 1960s research simply tried to establish the existence of imagery, perhaps in reaction to the behaviorist attacks. Currently, the existence of imagery is not questioned so much as its form. What is a mental image? What do we "see" or "hear" when we have a mental image? Is a mental image "real" or is it stored in information contained in a different sensory modality? Is an image based on an actual object different than the one conjured up in one's imagination? And, of greatest interest to developmental psychologists, when does imagery originate and how does its form change with increasing age? Box 4.2 considers imagery and cognitive development.

At the heart of the controversy over mental imagery is whether the same representations are used for imagery and visual perception. Do we form mental pictures of what we see? A series of experiments by Shepard and associates (see Shepard, 1978) had results that suggest a *second-order isomorphism* between imagery and perception. An "isomorphic relationship" implies a direct, one-to-one correspondence between the elements of two entities. According to Shepard (1978), "the proposed equivalence between perception and imagination implies a more abstract or 'second-order' isomorphism in which the functional relations among objects as imagined must to some degree mirror the functional relations among those same objects as actually perceived" (p. 131). To understand this statement, we must examine some of Shepard's work.

Consider the following experiment. You are shown the arrangement of connected squares in Figure 4.3a. Your task is to use the shaded square as a base and to fold the other squares along their edges until they form a cube; once you form the cube, the arrows should be aligned. (You may wish to construct a paper figure similar to the one in Figure 4.3a to confirm this.) Let's also suppose that for each arrangement, I ask you to decide whether the arrows meet. The more folds you need to make, the longer your decision time should be. For example, in Figure 4.3a, you would have to complete the whole cube before deciding, but in Figure 4.3b, you could decide after only three folds (ignore the three squares at the bottom of the figure because they are irrelevant to your decision). Figure 4.3c also would require only two folds, though it results in a mismatch of the arrows.

If Shepard's expectation about a second-order isomorphism between an image and a perception from the real world is correct, then the number of folds required ought to affect decision times regardless of whether the alignment of the arrows is done mentally or is physically carried out with the object present. In either case, the more mental or physical folds needed, the longer the decision time should be. You could verify this for yourself by constructing other figures like those in Figure 4.3 and folding them manually until the arrows match.

Box 4.2   Imagery and Cognitive Development

The notion that children use mental imagery in their thinking to a greater degree than adults is not new in the developmental literature (Bruner, Olver, & Greenfield, 1966; Piaget & Inhelder, 1971). For many years it has been widely recognized that children engage in visual thinking in their play activities and games. Children are notorious for having "imaginary companions" who populate their fantasy play; and many favorite children's games (e.g., video games) have significant visual components. Why do children tend to use imagery more than adults?

Kosslyn (1983) provides a simple but compelling explanation of the phenomenon in his recent book *Ghosts in the Mind's Machine*. Consider the question: What shape are a German shepherd's ears? According to Kosslyn, adults who are asked this question typically generate a mental image of the dog's head and mentally scan the image for the answer. However, if the same question is repeated over and over again, adults no longer need to rely on imagery; they can retrieve the answer from their verbal memory. Thus, adults use imagery to answer queries about unfamiliar properties of objects. Because children find that many things are unfamiliar, they may be more likely to depend on imagery as a source of information. As children grow older and become more knowledgeable, they may still rely on visual memories, but increasingly convert information into verbal representations.

To explore the claims that children employ imagery more than adults, Kosslyn (1983) performed a reaction-time experiment in which 6-year-olds, 10-year-olds, and young adults received two different trial blocks. In the first block, subjects heard the name of an animal, followed five seconds later by a possible property of the animal. Subjects were simply told to "think about the properties of the whole animal" and then decide as quickly as possible whether the property belonged to the animal. Subjects responded by pressing one button if the property was appropriate and another button if the property was inappropriate. At the conclusion of the trial block, subjects were asked how they evaluated the properties of the animal: by mentally picturing an animal and "looking" at it? by having a mental picture but not needing it? by not having a mental picture, but "just knowing"? or by some combination of these strategies?

The second block of trials was preceded by a set of imagery instructions. Subjects were instructed to form a visual image of an animal upon hearing its name and then to "look" at the animal in the image to evaluate a particular property. As before, subjects were requested to respond as quickly as possible by pushing a button to indicate whether the property was appropriate or inappropriate for the animal.

The results showed that subjects required more time to evaluate imaged properties than nonimaged properties, and the effect held across all three age groups. Overall reaction times decreased with age, but this effect was primarily due to evaluations made under the no-imagery (trial block 1) instructions. Adults were slightly faster than children when imagery was required, but they were much faster than children under the no-imagery condition. This finding suggests that adults could access information stored in nonimaginal, verbal forms more easily than they could generate and scan images. Moreover, under the no-imagery instructions, the number of subjects who reported using imagery varied systematically with age. Only one 10-year-old and one young adult reported using imagery predominantly, while almost half of the 6-year-olds did. Together, these results offer convincing evidence for the claim that young children use imagery more than older people.

Since initial experimental investigation, Kosslyn (1983) has considerably expanded his theory on how imagery develops with age. Rather than claim that children use imagery more than adults regardless of the context, the theory aims to identify the situations in which individuals are likely to use imagery and those in which they are not. Adults may be more likely to use imagery when thinking about an attractive member of the opposite sex; children may be more inclined to use imagery when thinking about toys, birthday parties, or ice cream cones (Kosslyn, 1983).

Identifying the situations in which imagery occurs is an important direction for future research, and such research could have practical as well as theoretical value. For example, if we knew the situations in which children are naturally motivated to employ imagery, we could design more effective instructional techniques that incorporate visual stimuli. The existing cognitive strengths of children could be capitalized on by such applications.

Research by Shepard and Feng (1972) confirmed the above expectation (see Figure 4.4). Decision times were linearly related to the number of folds necessary to make a decision. This finding has been replicated in studies of mental rotation using different sets of visual stimuli such as views of three-dimensional objects, random polygons, alphanumeric characters, and pictures of human hands.

Figure 4.3   Stimuli used in the mental paper folding experiment.

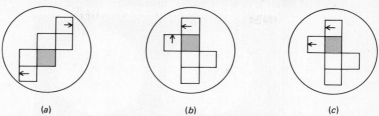

(a)   (b)   (c)

From "A Chronometric Study of Mental Paper Folding" by R. N. Shepard and C. Feng, 1972, *Cognitive Psychology, 3,* p. 230. Copyright 1972 by Academic Press. Reprinted by permission.

Figure 4.4   Mean reaction times for the mental paper folding experiment. The mean times increased linearly as the number of folds necessary to make a decision increased.

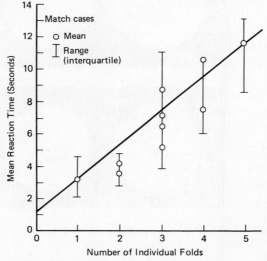

From "A Chronometric Study of Mental Paper Folding" by R. N. Shepard and C. Feng, 1972, *Cognitive Psychology, 3,* p. 232. Copyright 1972 by Academic Press. Reprinted by permission.

Mental Rotation

One difference between **mental rotation** studies and Shepard and Feng's (1972) study is that the relative positions of the stimuli being rotated remain constant in the former studies. That is, the structural relations between the parts of the object do not change, as in the mental-folding experiment. Shepard and Metzler (1971) performed the first study on mental rotation. Using complex three-dimensional stimulus pairs such as those depicted in Figure 4.5, they asked eight subjects of unspecified ages to decide whether the two objects were the "same" or "different."

Figure 4.5   Stimulus pairs used in the mental rotation experiment. Which of these pairs of objects are the same, and which are different?

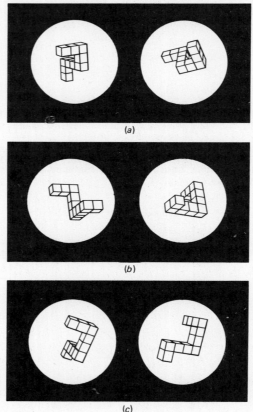

From "Mental Rotation of Three-Dimensional Objects" by R. N. Shepard and J. Metzler, 1971, *Science, 171*, p. 702. Copyright 1971 by the American Association for the Advancement of Science. Reprinted by permission.

Notice that in Figure 4.5*a*, the left-hand figure can be mentally turned or rotated on its vertical axis to yield the "same" figure as the right-hand one. In Figure 4.5*b*, the angle of rotation is greater. To compare these figures, you must mentally turn over the left-hand figure on its horizontal axis before you can answer "same." The pair in Figure 4.5*c* cannot be rotated into congruence, no matter how you rotate them, so you would answer "different."

If images are isomorphic to the physical objects they represent, then the decision times based on image rotation should vary as a function of the angular separation between objects—the greater the angular separation between two objects, the longer the decision time. The results of Shepard and Metzler's (1971) research showed that as the angle of rotation increased, decision times also increased. Subjects took longer to mentally rotate a figure 180° than they did 20°. However, the results showed very little difference between the amount of time to mentally rotate objects in the picture plane (see Figure 4.5a) versus those in the depth plane (see Figure 4.5b).

Are there developmental differences in mental rotation ability? To study this question, Marmor (1975) gave a mental rotation test to 5- and 8-year-olds. She asked children to decide whether two panda bear forms were the same or different (had the same or opposite hands raised). The stimuli were presented either in the same orientation or one stimulus differed from the other by up to 150°. Like Shepard and Metzler (1971), Marmor (1975) found that decision times increased linearly as a function of the angular discrepancy between stimuli, and the effect held for both age groups. In a similar experiment, Marmor (1977) reported that children as young as 4 can use mental rotation and this ability does not depend on the attainment of concrete operations. Piaget and Inhelder (1971), in contrast, proposed that mental rotation as indicated by **kinetic imagery** (images of movement) does not emerge in a child's thinking until age 7 or 8 because concrete operational ability is required to mentally represent the transformation of an object from an initial state to a final state. A preoperational child can represent the initial state and final state of an object in motion, but not the intermediate states.

To test Piaget and Inhelder's proposal about the relationship between cognitive development and kinetic imagery, Kerr, Corbitt, and Jurkovic (1980) partially replicated Marmor's (1977) study. They divided 47 children, ranging from about 4–7 years, into three groups—preoperational, transitional, and concrete operational—according to their scores on two Piagetian tasks. The children were then administered a test of kinetic imagery that required them to mentally rotate stimulus figures, two pairs of wooden monkeys, presented at different angles. In contrast to Marmor, Kerr et al. (1980) found a clear relationship between children's performance on the mental rotation task and their level of cognitive development, but no significant relationship between age and mental rotation. Children in a transitional stage to concrete operations and fully concrete operational children were able to mentally rotate the objects, as shown by a linear relationship between their reaction times and the angle of rotation—a relationship not found in the preoperational children's data. However, young children may be able to use mental rotation, but not in the systematic way that older children and adults do.

There are relatively few studies of changes in spatial rotation skills after age 7 or 8, presumably because, according to the Piagetian account, there is little to study. But the available evidence points to developmental changes in mental rotation skills after age 7 (Kail, Pellegrino, & Carter, 1980; Marmor, 1977). Both Kail et al. and Marmor reported significant increases in *speed* of mental rotation with age, with adults rotating stimuli more than twice as fast as children. Few or no significant age-related differences in *accuracy* of mental rotation have been reported in studies comparing children and adults. Developmental improvements in mental rotation ability may have practical importance in school subjects, such as geometry and science, and in occupations, such as engineering, drafting, and design, which require high levels of spatial ability.

Are there adult age changes in the speed of mental rotation? Because of the decline of nonverbal (spatial) abilities relative to verbal abilities on the Wechsler Adult Intelligence Scale (Wechsler, 1955) (see Chapter 8), some investigators of adult development have hypothesized that spatial skills such as mental rotation should also decline with age. Gaylord and Marsh (1975) tested 10 young adult males and 10 elderly males using the depth rotation figures employed by Shepard and Metzler (1971). As in Shepard and Metzler (1971), subjects were asked to decide whether pairs of stimulus items were the same or different (mirror images of each other). Figure 4.6 shows that both age groups' decision times increased as the angle of orientation increased. However, the older group was significantly slower than the younger age group at all angles of orientation, and also showed greater variability, especially with increasing difference in angle of orientation. Gaylord and Marsh (1975) explained their results in terms of a generalized age-related slowing of cognitive processes.

Jacewicz and Hartley (1979) took issue with Gaylord and Marsh's conclusion. The former argued that one difference between age cohorts is their differential experience with timed tasks involving unfamiliar stimuli such as those used in both the Shepard and Metzler (1971) and Gaylord and Marsh (1975) experiments. Accordingly, Jacewicz and Hartley (1979) used stimulus items (letters of the English alphabet) with which both age groups are familiar. Younger and older college students were asked to judge whether letters rotated 0°–180° away from a normal upright position were standard letters or mirror images of standard letters. For example, subjects saw rotated figures such as ⅍ and were asked "Is this a regular *F* or a reversed *F* if the figure were upright?" No age differences appeared in the rate at which letters could be rotated mentally, a finding that refutes the generalized slowing hypothesis. When different samples of young and old adults were then tested using basically the same procedure with unfamiliar lowercase Greek letters, the speed of reaction of older subjects was slower than younger subjects', but again there were no significant differences in rate of mental rotation.

The evidence for adult age changes in speed of mental rotation is contradictory. A well-designed study by Berg, Hertzog, and Hunt (1982) using a broader age range and different stimulus materials has

Figure 4.6 Mean reaction time of each subject in each age group as a function of angular orientation. The groups show little overlap; the spread of scores tends to increase with increasing differences in orientation; and the older group shows the increase to a greater extent.

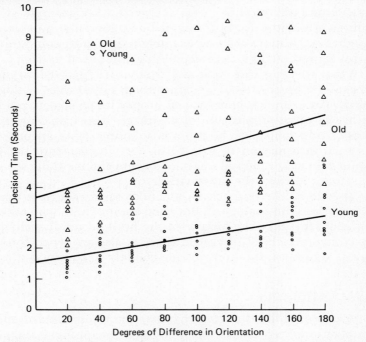

From "Age Differences in the Speed of a Spatial Cognitive Process" by S. A. Gaylord and G. R. March, 1975, *Journal of Gerontology, 30,* p. 676. Copyright by the Gerontological Society of America. Reprinted by permission.

helped clarify the picture. Berg et al. reported that the mental rotation rate increased linearly across a 20–60-year age range. Their results are compelling because the same trend was found across four days of practice involving almost 2000 total trials. Consistent with Gaylord and Marsh (1975), Berg et al. interpreted their results as evidence of an age-related slowing in the speed of spatial information processing across the adult life span.

Analogical and Propositional Representation

Before we review imagery studies further, we should clarify the nature of representation in imagery. We have seen that a correspondence exists between images and physical manipulation processes. Does this mean that we represent images as an actual "picture in our heads," or do we store images in a different representational form? This question has been hotly debated. Shepard (1978) and others maintain that images appear as **analogical** representations, or analogs, of corresponding physical processes. That is, a continuity or correspondence exists between images and real physical objects. One real-life example of an analog is a flight simulator used to train airline pilots; it simulates actual flying conditions. A more abstract example is an analog computer; each number is represented by a corresponding amount of voltage.

Other investigators such as Pylyshyn (1973; 1981) argue that some images are **propositional,** or conceptual, rather than analogical, or pictorial. For example, many visual properties of objects can be stored as either a verbal proposition or an image. Thus, we store in memory a proposition such as "The zebra is an animal with stripes" and we can retrieve information in that form. Or we can store the information about zebras as a mental image of a zebra and mentally scan our mental picture to retrieve the information.

In general, the research on mental rotation suggests that many representations are analogical. But even among those who take the analogical side, few take the picture-in-the-head notion literally (see Kosslyn & Pomerantz, 1977). Because there is also evidence for the propositional argument, this controversy is likely to continue.

Cognitive Mapping

One area of study that clearly shows the interaction of analogical and propositional representation is cognitive mapping. A **cognitive map** is an internal spatial representation. Suppose someone asks you the distance from your dormitory to your class in psychology. You might imagine a mental picture of your campus, noting important landmarks and routes. If another student stops you and asks directions, you would most likely state these directions in verbal form—turn left at the bottom of the hill, go past the second building, turn right, and follow the sign for the psychology building. You would be less likely to draw the student a map.

Recently, psychologists have shown great interest in studying cognitive maps, perhaps as a consequence of the current concern with the environment and ecology. But the notion of cognitive maps is fairly old. One of the earliest investigations was conducted by Trowbridge (1913), who was interested in explaining why some people become more easily confused about their location than others. He suggested that the source of the confusion lay in the "imaginary maps" of the environment which people carry around in their heads. To study these cognitive maps, Trowbridge had subjects draw the directions from a point in New York City to several other more distant points. He discovered that most subjects could correctly estimate relative distances, but they shifted the various locations clockwise or counterclockwise several degrees.

Another study that stimulated much of the current interest in cognitive maps was K. Lynch's (1960) classic investigation of urban design. Lynch interviewed residents of Boston, Jersey City, and Los Angeles and asked them to describe and sketch images of their city. He concentrated on the elements of individuals' cognitive maps which give structure and meaning to a city. Lynch found that individuals use certain types of elements to mentally represent their environment. These representations include *paths* (routes of passage through the environment), *edges* (boundaries such as rivers, walls, or canyons), *districts* (large identifiable parts of a city such as Greenwich Village in New York City or Chinatown in San Francisco), *nodes* (strategic points such as crossroads or junctions), and *landmarks* (prominent physical objects such as buildings, hills, or statues). People have a unique memory of the elements that make up their cognitive maps.

Both Trowbridge's (1913) and K. Lynch's (1960) studies focused on examining the content of adults' mental maps. Several changes in content, however, appear to occur developmentally. Young children differ from older children and adults in the number and types of landmarks represented (A. Siegel, 1981). The former's cognitive maps also seem more spatially constrained. Kindergartners, for example, have fairly differentiated or detailed representations of their immediate environment, but a more global, "everywhere schema" for areas beyond their familiar surroundings (see Hardwick, McIntyre, & Pick, 1976).

A major problem that plagues investigation of the content of people's cognitive maps is how to externalize the internal representation. Frequently used techniques such as verbal reports (K. Lynch, 1960; Piaget & Inhelder, 1967), sketch maps (Piaget, Inhelder, & Szeminska, 1960), and small-scale models (Piaget et al., 1960; A. Siegel & Schadler, 1977) confound developmental level with the "externalizing" abilities being measured. This is particularly a problem with young children. For example, asking young children to do freehand sketches of their environment confounds their spatial knowledge of the environment with their drawing ability (Moore, 1976; Piaget et al., 1960; A. Siegel, 1981). Another problem is using a small-scale space (such as a piece of looseleaf paper) to represent a large-scale environment (such as a neighborhood). We will return to this particular problem later in the chapter.

What types of spatial knowledge or information comprise the cognitive maps of children and adults? A. Siegel and White (1975) have suggested that spatial knowledge is primarily made up of **landmarks** and **routes**. Landmarks are the salient locations, objects, and points in the environment around which people organize their spatial ability (Herman, Kail, & Siegel, 1979; A. Siegel & White, 1975). Landmarks on your campus might include a building, statue, courtyard, or clock. Routes are the patterns of action that guide an individual's travel between landmarks. Routes are spatially and temporally organized around landmarks.

Developmentally, landmarks are first to be noticed and recalled (A. Siegel, 1981). By going between landmarks, individuals eventually develop a representation of routes. Finally, routes are integrated into an overall framework called a **configuration,** or survey map. Configurations represent a higher-order integration of landmark and route information into a well-organized structure. They are important because they allow people to infer routes to distant landmarks to which they have not traveled.

In the majority of developmental studies of spatial cognition in cognitive mapping, the focus has been on the development of route knowledge and configurational knowledge. In one study of route learning, Allen, Kirasic, Siegel, and Herman (1979) had second and fifth graders and young adults view a simulated walk and select 9 scenes from a series of 50 slides that would most help them remember where they were along the walk. The children did not select the same features as real-world landmarks that the adults did. For example, second graders and, to a lesser extent, fifth graders tended to pick colorful awnings and displays as landmarks, even though the slides contained many similar awnings as reference points at various locations. In contrast, adults tended to select richer and more distinctive perceptual cues such as changes in heading (direction) involving a left or right turn at an intersection.

Allen et al. (1979) also had other children and adults view the same slide presentation and rank distances between test scenes identified by the first sample of children and adults as having high landmark value. As Figure 4.7 shows, Allen et al. (1979) found that fifth-grade children were able to produce almost as accurate distance ratings as adults when tested with adult-selected scenes, but were as inaccurate as second graders when tested with peer-selected scenes. Second graders were little affected by type of test scene selected. The major developmental implication of this finding is that the ability to use landmark information from scenes precedes the ability to recognize scenes on the basis of their potential landmark value.

Using a similar approach, Kosslyn, Pick, and Fariello (1974) looked at preschoolers' and adults' memories for distances between different pairs of objects in a 17–square-foot space. The investigators arranged objects in a quadrant and separated them with either two opaque or two transparent barriers. Preschool children inaccurately perceived objects separated by both types of barriers as farther apart than objects separated by the same distance without a barrier. Adults' estimates were

Figure 4.7 Effects of adult- versus peer-selected test scenes on the accuracy of cognitive maps. Higher congruence scores indicate more accurate cognitive maps.

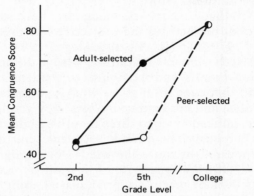

From "Developmental Issues in Cognitive Mapping: The Selection and Utilization of Environmental Landmarks" by G. L. Allen, K. C. Kirasic, A. W. Siegel, and J. F. Herman, 1979, *Child Development, 50*, p. 1067. Copyright 1979 by The Society for Research in Child Development, Inc. Reprinted by permission.

distorted only when the objects were separated by opaque barriers, not when separated by transparent barriers or no barriers. These results support the notion of the development of an integrated cognitive map. Adults integrated the spaces in the adjacent quadrants together, while children treated the space as separate poorly integrated subspaces. This finding is similar to H. Pick's observation (cited in Hardwick et al., 1976) that children organize information about their houses into poorly integrated individual representations and often have difficulty describing what is on the other side of walls separating rooms. Piaget et al. (1960) likewise reported that 8- or 9-year-olds are unable to describe their neighborhoods as a unified whole, but "fix their landmarks in subgroups, based on a number of independent vantage points" (p. 17).

Once landmarks and routes are learned, they are integrated into configurational knowledge (A. Siegel & White, 1975). In children this knowledge occurs late in the developmental sequence; in adults it occurs over a shorter period. Curtis, Siegel, and Furlong (1981), for example, reported that although route knowledge was quite high even among first graders, configurational accuracy improved greatly between first and fifth grade and continued to improve between fifth and eighth grade. Curtis et al. (1981) used a "projective convergence" technique first used by Hardwick et al. (1976). This technique is similar to the technique of triangulation commonly used for navigational purposes. Subjects are asked to point a sighting tube to different unseen targets at various locations to give bearing estimates. They are also asked to give distance estimates to the same targets. A major advantage of the projective convergence technique is that it does not confound measures of spatial knowledge with developmental differences in drawing, verbal, and representational abilities.

Adults' configurational knowledge has been studied in many ways, including slide projections and projective convergence techniques (Herman et al., 1979; Kirasic, Allen, & Siegel, 1984). Herman et al. (1979) tested college freshmen's spatial knowledge of their campus after three weeks, three months, and six months of residential experience. Herman et al. found that even after three weeks, subjects' knowledge of landmarks, routes, and configurations was very good; and this knowledge increased significantly up to three months. Male students showed more landmark knowledge than female students, but no significant sex differences appeared in route knowledge or configurational knowledge. Kirasic et al. (1984) also reported few sex differences in configurational knowledge in their recent study of spatial ability in college freshmen and upperclassmen. Sex differences in spatial ability will be discussed in greater detail later in this chapter.

In summary, a considerable amount of evidence indicates that the development of spatial cognition proceeds from landmark knowledge and route knowledge to knowledge of configurations. Cognitive maps of both children and adults reflect these changes as they become manifest over long periods (in children) or over relatively short periods (in adults). Although these representations are reasonably accurate, they are also subject to much distortion. For example, people tend to overestimate distance between various locations, particularly in cities that cannot be easily visualized such as Tokyo, Japan (Matlin, 1983).

Small-Scale and Large-Scale Space

In considering developmental changes in spatial cognition, we have not differentiated between various types of space. When we talk about a college campus, you might infer that we are dealing with a large-scale, as opposed to a small-scale, space. On the other hand, a model train layout complete with toy buildings might seem like a small-scale environment to you. But size alone does not determine the type of space. What are the defining characteristics of large-scale and small-scale spaces?

One defining property is the notion of **surroundingness**. Large-scale space surrounds individuals, forcing them to explore and construct the environment (Acredolo, 1981). Thus, people can be inside of a large-scale space, but not a small-scale space. Another important characteristic is the number of vantage points. To observe a large-scale space completely, people must perceive it from several different vantage points. Many small-scale spaces can be viewed from a single perspective, although some require multiple perspectives. Thus, large-scale space requires both surroundingness and multiple perspectives, but small-scale space lacks the first property.

Some more examples may clarify the difference between the two types of space. In research on the development of spatial concepts in children, Piaget and colleagues (Piaget & Inhelder, 1967; Piaget et al., 1960) employed mostly small-scale spatial materials. In one famous study, they presented children with a model of three mountains and asked them to indicate how the mountains would appear to an observer from various vantage points (see Figure 4.8). The children viewed the mountains from the outside looking in. The observed space thus did not surround the children, although they could view it from different

Figure 4.8   Piaget's three-mountain task. From his position at A, the child is asked how the scene appears to an observer (a doll that the experimenter seats in positions B, C, and D around the table). The child's task may be to describe the scene viewed by the doll, reconstruct the scene from pieces of cardboard, or pick the correct picture from a collection of several pictures.

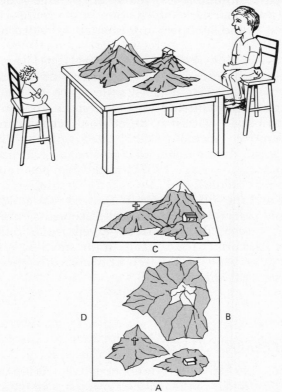

From *The Child's Conception of Space* (p. 216) by J. Piaget and B. Inhelder, 1967, New York: Norton. Copyright 1956 by Routledge & Kegan Paul Ltd. Reprinted by permission.

vantage points. The three-mountain problem will be discussed more fully in the section on spatial egocentrism.

A series of experiments by Acredolo (1981) illustrates the use of large-scale spatial materials. In one of these studies, Acredolo (1976) took children into a small room containing four walls with salient features (pictures, a door, stripes) but only one piece of furniture—a table along one wall. As children stood by the table, Acredolo blindfolded them and took them for a walk around the room. Each child's task was to return to the starting position. The experimenter made this task more difficult by silently moving the table to the other side of the room while the children were still blindfolded. This change made the choice of the table as the starting position incorrect. The results indicated that 10-year-old children were able to return to the starting position by using the landmark features on the walls, whereas many preschool children returned to the table in its new position. In this example, the child was surrounded by the space as he or she moved around the room. Recall that surroundingness characterizes large-scale spaces. Preschool children used landmark information in the room—the table—but did not attend to the landmark information provided by the surrounding walls.

As both Acredolo (1981) and A. Siegel (1981) have pointed out, great caution must be exercised in generalizing developmental findings on people's performance in small-scale space to their performance in exploring and constructing large-scale space. In many instances behavior in small-scale space may differ from behavior in large-scale space. As an example, Acredolo (1981) cited work by Piaget and Inhelder (1967) on the development of knowledge of horizontal and vertical axes. Piaget and Inhelder (1967) had children position small trees on the side of a real sandhill and also asked the children to draw pictures of the trees and the hill. The results showed that children at a particular stage could perform correct vertical placements of the trees on the side of the hill, but still drew the trees perpendicular to the hill. Inability to construct the correct relationship in the small-scale space of the drawing did not prevent the children from correctly operating in the larger space of the real hill.

SPATIAL REFERENCE SYSTEMS

Piaget and Inhelder (1967) interpreted the children's failure to draw trees perpendicular to the inclined ground as an indicator that they had not yet constructed a coordinated reference system of horizontal and vertical axes. We will use the term **spatial reference system** to refer to "a locus or set of loci with respect to which spatial position is defined" (H. Pick & Lockman, 1981, p. 40). Such systems are very similar to configurations because both involve abstract coordinated representations of the environment.

Two types of spatial reference systems are **egocentric** and **allocentric** (or geometric). In an egocentric reference system, spatial positions are defined in relation to the person's body. For example, a child might encode the spatial location of a landmark in relation to where he is standing. In allocentric systems, the frame of reference is defined by positions external to the person. The individual can locate landmarks in relation to other objects in the environment.

A major developmental difference between a child's and an adult's spatial ability lies in the type of reference system used. Children's early representations of space are organized using an egocentric, or self-reference, system. The child locates objects at various distances and directions, using himself as the origin of the reference system. Adults, in contrast, can conceive of themselves as objects in an allocentric system, consisting of a set of spatial relations existing among objects. This ability enables adults to do well on tasks such as perspective taking, which require multiple vantage points.

Piaget described spatial reference systems in terms of geometric concepts (Piaget et al., 1960; Piaget & Inhelder, 1967). He argued that the developmental ordering of these concepts corresponds to the logical order of the generality of such geometric concepts. For example, the first concepts the child develops are very general **topological** concepts such as proximity, order, enclosure, and continuity. These concepts correspond closely to the basic perceptual relationships of Gestalt theory discussed in Chapter 3 (see Box 3.1). Later in childhood, around age 9 or 10, more specific concepts relating to **projective** geometry develop. Projective spatial concepts involve the idea that properties of objects (such as rectilinearity) remain invariant with different changes in perspective. About the same time, even more specific Euclidean geometric concepts emerge. Euclidean concepts are organized in terms of complex relationships that preserve parallels, angles, and distances. For example, adolescents possessing Euclidean knowledge can imagine a straight line extending indefinitely through space parallel to another line. They also can estimate the angles of many similar triangles according to a system of "one-many correspondences" (see Piaget and Inhelder, 1967, p. 474, for a detailed discussion).

In Piaget's theory, topological concepts emerge in the preoperational period of development and integrate into a spatial reference system around age 7. Projective and Euclidean concepts develop almost simultaneously during the concrete operations stage (around age 9-10). Their development is not necessarily complete by this age. Although concrete operational children are able to use a spatial reference system to locate objects in space, they cannot think about the assumptions of the coordinate system (Forman & Sigel, 1979). For example, comprehending the concept of infinite extension—parallel lines drawn on a flat surface will never intersect—goes beyond concrete operational thinking. Similarly, the notion of parallel lines intersecting at some point in a curved space-time interval requires formal operational thought, and perhaps even postformal thinking, about relativity. To what extent Euclidean knowledge and non-Euclidean knowledge are fully developed in adults is difficult to determine because the limits of adults' spatial concepts have rarely been tested. To date most studies of spatial cognition in both children and adults have involved relatively familiar environments and highly differentiated landmark information.

To investigate developmental changes in spatial cognition among children, Piaget used a task consisting of two identical models of a landscape. He showed children the two models and put an object (a doll) on one model. He then asked the child to put the doll "in exactly the same spot" on the other model. The duplicate model was then rotated 180°, and the child had to place the doll on the model under the rotated condition. In the nonrotated condition, the child did not have to differentiate between an egocentric reference system and a more objective, allocentric system. However, under the 180° rotation condition, the child had to make a differentiation in order to place the doll in the correct location and orientation. In general, young children showed an egocentric orientation to the task, which Piaget interpreted as a first attempt to order objects topologically. Piaget and Inhelder (1967) stated that the young child "appears rooted in his own viewpoint in the narrowest and most restricted fashion so that he cannot imagine any perspective but his own" (p. 242).

Eventually, egocentric responding is incorporated into a more coordinated system of projective relations. Now children can shift their frame of reference across variations in perspective. Thus, perspective-taking ability seems to depend on projective knowledge of spatial relations.

Although some investigators do not agree with certain aspects of Piaget's theory of spatial development (see E. Gibson & Spelke, 1983), numerous studies (Acredolo, Pick, & Olsen, 1975; Hardwick et al., 1976; Herman & Siegel, 1978; Smothergill, 1973) support Piaget's conclusions about the prominence of topological concepts before age 7 and the emergence of projective and Euclidean concepts after age 7. Evidence also suggests that Piaget's notions of spatial development are applicable to both small-scale and large-scale spatial materials (Acredolo, 1981).

Spatial Egocentrism

In response to Piaget's claims that young children are egocentric, many studies on childhood spatial egocentrism have been conducted. There has also been great interest in studying whether spatial egocentrism appears again in old age as part of a generalized process of cognitive regression. We will now examine several studies of spatial egocentrism across the life span. Later in Chapters 5 and 9 we will look at communicative egocentrism and examine the relationship between the two types of egocentrism.

Let's begin by reviewing what Piaget said about egocentrism. In several studies, Piaget used the three-mountain problem (see Figure 4.8). In one version, the child's task is to choose from a set of photographs of the mountain landscape the one that best represents the view of the observer. Their findings with 4–12-year-old children led Piaget and Inhelder (1967) to propose a four-stage developmental model of the acquisition of spatial perspective-taking skills. In the first stage, pure egocentrism, children do not recognize that a differently positioned observer will have a different view of a set of objects from their own. In the next stage, children recognize that the observer will have a different perspective, but they cannot overcome their own perspective. In the third stage, not only do children recognize perspective differences but they also are less dominated by their own perspective. However, they do not take into account before-behind and right-left relationships among objects. In the last stage, children can fully take the perspective of the observer and coordinate before-behind and right-left relationships.

Have other investigators found the same stages? Not exactly. In their research on spatial perspective-taking ability, Coie, Costanzo, and Farnill (1973) tested 5–11-year-old children on a task roughly comparable to the three-mountain problem. Their results suggested that success on this problem involves much more than overcoming egocentrism. Even older children who can reconstruct the view of another person continue to make errors such as deciding which objects are seen on the left or right side in another viewer's visual field. These errors, the authors suggest, are spatial errors which are not purely egocentric. These findings support Flavell, Botkin, Fry, Wright, and Jarvis's (1968) view that the transition to successful perspective taking in childhood involves not only quantitative decreases in egocentrism but also qualitative shifts in spatial knowledge.

In another study of the issue, Borke (1975) maintained that the three-mountain task is too difficult and unfamiliar for many children below 9 years of age. Borke modified the task by using small toy objects such as a fire engine and by having Grover, the character from *Sesame Street*, act as the observer. Borke also allowed the children to rotate the three-dimensional landscape to decide on the observer's perspective, rather than have them select a view from a set of flat, two-dimensional photographs. Using these methods, Borke (1975) found that even 3- and 4-year-olds could correctly select another's perspective.

The Coie et al. (1973) and Borke (1975) studies both suggest that we have to be careful about inferring that children use an egocentric frame of reference instead of an allocentric or geometric frame. This point was illustrated in an experiment by Smothergill, Hughes, Timmons, and Hutko (1975) using the following procedure with 5-year-old children: Subjects were given two Y shapes mounted on easels, one of which had an upper arm marked with a yellow dot (the experimenter's Y). On some trials the two Ys were adjacent, and on others back to back. The up-down position of the Ys was also varied. The subjects' job was to place a yellow dot on the upper arm of the Y corresponding to the one on the experimenter's Y. The results showed that subjects used an external topological frame of reference, rather than their own bodies, for placement responses. In the adjacent condition, subjects performed above average when their Y was upright, but below average when it was rotated 180°. Similarly, in the back-to-back condition, they performed below average when their Y was upright, but above average when it was rotated 180°. These results highlight the importance of distinguishing between egocentric and objective frames of reference on spatial tasks.

How do spatial ability changes in adulthood compare to those in childhood? Do adults become more spatially egocentric as they age? In a life-span investigation of spatial egocentrism, K. Rubin, Attewell, Tierney, and Tumolo (1973) gave a perspective-taking task to five different groups with mean ages of 7.6, 11.5, 21.1, 44.1, and 76.3 years. The task was modeled after the one used by Flavell et al. (1968) and consisted of four different stimulus displays of increasing complexity. The elements of the displays consisted of colored wooden blocks and cylinders arranged in various spatial configurations on a small board. The subjects were given a duplicate set of elements and asked to reproduce the display as seen from the perspective of an experimenter who sat approximately 45° to the subject's right. Each succeeding display placed a new demand on the subject by adding a new feature (differences in height, circumference, or color) that had to be taken into account in trying to reproduce the experimenter's perspective (Flavell et al., 1968). K. Rubin et al. (1973) found that the elderly group was superior in perspective-taking ability to the youngest children and equivalent to the oldest children. However, elderly subjects were inferior to the college-aged and the middle-aged groups. These findings suggest a curvilinear relationship between age and spatial egocentrism.

K. Rubin et al. (1973) did not analyze age differences in egocentric versus nonegocentric spatial errors. In a study that made this distinction, Schultz and Hoyer (1976) reported that older adults committed more nonegocentric errors than egocentric errors. These investigators used matrix problems such as the one in Figure 4.9. The subject's task was to select from among the alternatives A–D in Figure 4.9 the one that correctly matched the experimenter's view (as seen from the opposite side of the table) of the larger matrix. On this task, nonegocentric errors involved matches (cards A and C) that were variations of the larger matrix. A correct objective response was a match of the larger matrix rotated 180° (card B), and an egocentric error was an exact (unrotated) match of the larger matrix (card D). Perspective-taking feedback given after each problem led to fewer nonegocentric errors, but did not reduce spatial egocentrism. This failure might be due to the low number of egocentric responses given by older subjects across all experimental conditions (Schultz & Hoyer, 1976). These results suggest that elderly adults' errors on spatial ability tasks may not reflect egocentrism as much as perceptual judgment (nonegocentric) errors.

A later study by Ohta, Walsh, and Krauss (1981) examined spatial perspective taking in young and elderly women. In this study, as in Schultz and Hoyer (1976), both egocentric and nonegocentric errors were analyzed, but the latter were analyzed into their components, including *interposition errors* (failure to recognize that objects are partially or totally hidden when viewed from different positions), *aspect errors* (failure to recognize changes in apparent shape or orientation of

Figure 4.9 A representative spatial egocentrism test problem. Subjects selected from matrices A–D the one that revealed the experimenter's view of the large matrix.

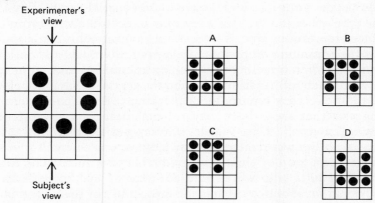

Adapted from "Feedback Effects on Spatial Egocentrism in Old Age," by N. R. Schultz, Jr., and W. J. Hoyer, 1976, *Journal of Gerontology, 31,* p. 73. Copyright 1976 by the Gerontological Society of America. Adapted by permission.

objects when viewed from another position), and *right-left errors* (failure to recognize different right-left relationships among objects when viewed from another position). Ohta et al. (1981) reported that different aspects of spatial perspective-taking ability decline with age. For example, elderly women made more egocentric errors and more nonegocentric errors (e.g., right-left reversals) than young women. The greater number of errors on right-left identifications is consistent with reports in the childhood literature suggesting that right-left reversals are the most difficult perspective-taking skills (Coie et al.,1973; Laurendeau & Pinard, 1970). However, elderly women did not make more interposition or aspect errors than young women. This finding contrasts with Coie et al.'s (1973) report that egocentric errors are eliminated before interposition or aspect errors in the development of children's perspective taking. Usually, egocentric errors are considered a more primitive type of perspective-taking error.

Ohta et al.'s (1981) reported age differences were substantially reduced in a follow-up experiment in which subjects did not have to preview a visual display, but only had to imagine it after viewing separate elements of the display in detail. The reduction of errors under this new condition was attributed to reduced memory storage and retrieval demands. Memory and retrieval abilities, the authors contend, may show more rapid age decline than the ability to reconstruct unviewed spatial information.

Everyday Spatial Behavior

The findings discussed above have important implications for the spatial behavior of elderly adults in their daily environment. If elderly adults (and young children) have poorer spatial perspective-taking ability than other individuals, they may be less likely to form highly integrated representations of large-scale environments. This could account for the common complaints of elderly individuals and children of getting lost when traveling into new or unfamiliar environments.

Not much information exists on the spatial behavior of elderly adults in their everyday environment (Kirasic, 1985). The evidence available suggests that the elderly may restrict their own geographical experiences (Lawton, 1970). Walsh, Krauss, and Regnier (1981) found that spatial ability was related to knowledge of one's neighborhood environment in a group of elderly individuals living in the Los Angeles area. Elderly adults who were more accurate on spatial perspective-taking tasks in the laboratory also made greater use of their neighborhoods, as indicated by the greater average distance they traveled to obtain goods and services. Declines in spatial accuracy can probably be attributed to declines in spatial mobility as well as in physical, perceptual, and cognitive abilities. We need more studies of the relationship of spatial abilities and everyday spatial cognition in elderly and other age groups.

A few developmental studies of spatial knowledge in everyday contexts have been reported. In a recent study, Evans, Brennan, Skorpanich, and Held (1984) found that older adults were less accurate than younger adults in recalling urban landmarks and the location of buildings within a familiar downtown area of their city. And the types of buildings recalled differed between the two age groups. Older people relied more than younger people on such building attributes as high public use, major symbolic significance, unique architectural style, and greater naturalness of the surrounding landscape. Buildings lacking these characteristics were recalled much less often by older adults, but buildings with them were recalled equally well by older and younger adults. Kirasic (1985) reported preliminary data on young and old adults' spatial behavior in simulated shopping trips through a familiar and an unfamiliar supermarket. Both age groups showed poorer spatial performance in the novel supermarket than in the familiar setting (they planned less efficient routes and had difficulty remembering item locations). However, old adults had greater difficulty than young adults in recognizing scenes from the unfamiliar setting. The above findings suggest that more attention should be given to the planning and design of environments that can enhance spatial competence among the elderly.

INDIVIDUAL DIFFERENCES IN SPATIAL ABILITY

The study of individual differences in spatial task performance has a long history in psychology (see L. Harris, 1981; McGee, 1979). However, most studies were based on paper-and-pencil measures rather than more real-life measures. As mentioned, such methods may be inappropriate for externalizing the spatial knowledge of children. We are now going to review two major individual difference variables—sex and culture—as they affect spatial ability.

Sex Differences in Spatial Ability

One of the most consistent findings in the psychological literature is that males are superior to females on spatial tasks (L. Harris, 1981; Maccoby & Jacklin, 1974). A few studies show female superiority on selected spatial tasks, but the vast majority of research favors males. This does not mean that every male will outperform every female in all situations; we are talking about average differences between the sexes.

Among the spatial tasks showing a male advantage are the following:

1. *mental rotation*—males have a faster rate of mental rotation than females (Tapley & Bryden, 1977);
2. *mental "folding"*—males solve folding tasks faster and more accurately than females;
3. *sense of direction*—males are better able to find a route or path through a maze than females. This result is also found in maze studies using male and female rats (McGee, 1979);
4. *perceptual disembedding*—males are better able to disembed or find a simple geometric form hidden in a complex geometric design (Witkin, Dyk, Faterson, Goodenough, & Karp, 1962).

An important question about the above examples is whether these sex differences show up in real life. Does the female who has trouble finding her way through a laboratory maze experience problems in a real-world environment? Similarly, is the male who excels at spatial tasks superior in everyday spatial behavior such as direction finding? We do not have much data on these questions. Anecdotal reports state that males seem to have a better sense of direction than females. An early study by Howe (1931) which asked kindergarten and elementary school students to point to the north, south, east, and west showed that male students were significantly more accurate than female students. In a more recent study, A. Siegel and Schadler (1977) had 4½–6-year-olds construct a small-scale three-dimensional model of their kindergarten classrooms. Boys were more accurate than girls in correctly placing classroom objects such as desks, chairs, tables, and chalkboards in their correct positions. But in Herman et al.'s (1979) study of students' spatial knowledge of a college campus, male and female students showed equally accurate route and configurational knowledge.

Other examples and counterexamples could be cited, but these will suffice. The important issue is explaining why sex differences exist, rather than simply describing or cataloging them.

Two global explanations are usually given to account for observed sex differences in spatial ability: (1) differential socialization and life experience; (2) genetic, neurological, and hormonal differences. In many respects, these two arguments are identical to the nature-nurture explanations used to account for age differences in perceptual and cognitive development (see Chapters 2 and 3).

According to the differential experience argument, males receive more social encouragement, support, and training in spatial activities than females. Parents tend to encourage male children to explore and manipulate objects in space, while they provide fewer opportunities for girls. Girls are encouraged to be more passive and to seek help with a task. Parents also provide different types of toys for their children. Boys are given active toys such as vehicles, sports equipment, machines, and military objects; whereas girls are given dollhouses, play dishes, and other domestic objects (Rheingold & Cook, 1975). Differences can be found in outdoor play activities as well. Boys are more likely than girls to spend time playing outdoors, to use large amounts of space, and to wander away from home (Harper & Sanders, 1975).

Although sex differences in spatial ability may originate in early childhood, most do not appear until adolescence. Perhaps this is because sex-role socialization pressures are particularly strong at this time. If this is the case, we might expect fewer sex-related differences in spatial abilities in adulthood as sex-role socialization pressures ease. Several studies, however, failed to confirm this expectation. For example, Kail, Carter, and Pellegrino (1979) found that young adult women show greater variation than young men do on psychomotor tests of spatial orientation. In an investigation employing several different age groups ranging from teenagers to middle-agers, Wilson and his colleagues (1975) reported that sex differences persist on Shepard and Metzler's mental rotation task, with the male advantage being large and consistent. Similarly, D. Cohen and Wilkie (1979) reviewed several studies and found sex-related differences in spatial task performance among the elderly in the expected direction (see also Walsh et al., 1981).

The existence of sex differences in spatial task performance across the life span implies that factors other than socialization and life experience may be operating. Granted, various life experiences can affect one's spatial performance. Intensive training on spatial problems improves spatial performance, and, in some instances, eliminates sex differences (L. Harris, 1981). But the fact that certain training experiences reduce performance differences between the sexes does not mean that the differences were initially caused by a lack of training. This would be like saying that because aspirin cures a headache, headaches are caused by a lack of aspirin. Acknowledging that experience plays a role in spatial development does not rule out other potential causal variables such as physiological factors. In fact, the effects of training and socialization will always be mediated by physiological mechanisms.

Several theorists have hypothesized that sex-related differences in spatial ability are caused by physiological factors such as sex differences in the amount of information contained on the sex chromosomes, the degree of cerebral specialization, or hormonal levels. A few years ago, a hypothesis that spatial ability is determined by a recessive gene on the X chromosome received initial support, but more recent evidence from studies using larger samples and more refined statistical procedures has not been as positive (Boles, 1980). The basis of the argument was that males are superior in spatial ability because of the positive influence of an X-linked recessive gene. Because males only have one X chromosome, they should be more likely to express the spatial advantage than females whose second X chromosome may offset the effects of the recessive gene.

The X-linked hypothesis has been tested by examining patterns of intrafamily correlations associated with this genetic transmission. If a gene is linked to the X chromosome, a higher correlation should be obtained between sons and mothers (who donate an X chromosome) than between sons and fathers (who donate a Y chromosome). So far research has failed to uncover the expected pattern of correlations.

A second hypothesis attributes sex differences in spatial ability to hemispheric specialization in the human brain. Anatomically, the brain is divided into two hemispheres. The right hemisphere is specialized for spatial processing, and the left hemisphere is specialized for language processing. To what extent do hemispheric differences account for male superiority in spatial tasks? Recent evidence suggests that males have greater right hemisphere specialization than females, and females are more bilateral (less well lateralized) in their spatial and language functioning (see McGee, 1979). L. Harris (1978) believes that this bilateralization in females impedes their spatial processing. As evidence, he cites studies of left-handers, who were assumed to be more bilateral than right-handers in verbal and spatial skills. Left-handers, like females, tended to score lower on spatial tasks because they were less well lateralized (handedness and sex, however, were not always controlled for in these studies).

Another explanation of observed sex differences in spatial ability involves hormonal differences. Only a few studies have examined this issue. In early research, Broverman, Klaiber, Kobayashi, and Vogel (1968) found that females with high androgen levels (more masculinized) had higher scores on spatial ability tests than females with low androgen levels. However, highly masculinized males had lower spatial scores than less masculine males. Furthermore, these patterns have been found with more "psychological" measures such as peer ratings. Boys rated as less masculine by their peers scored higher in spatial ability than boys rated as more masculine (Maccoby & Jacklin, 1974).

The interpretation of the above findings remains unclear. Some minimal level of androgen may be required for normal spatial skills, and perhaps an ideal androgen-estrogen balance exists in males and females. We need more research in this area. One interesting approach might be to study varying androgen levels within each sex in relationship to spatial abilities. If hormonal levels account for differences across the sexes, then the same variable should produce differences within the sexes.

In summary, no one has been able to isolate the causes of sex differences in spatial ability. Further testing and clarification will be needed to determine if these differences are due primarily to experiential factors or to biological differences in genetic, hormonal, and cerebral organizational factors. The differences will most likely be a function of multiple causes, as is true for most other developmental differences.

Cross-Cultural Differences in Spatial Ability

Cross-cultural differences are another source of variation in spatial task performance. In one of the few truly cross-cultural studies on spatial perception, Berry (1966) compared Canadian Eskimos and members of the Temne tribe of Africa on various visual discrimination and spatial ability tasks. The Eskimos scored much higher than the Temne on these tasks, a result that might be due to the relatively featureless environment of the Eskimos. Across land and sea, the Eskimos must travel in a rather barren, icy, colorless environment which lacks distinctive environmental landmarks. These experiences presumably force the Eskimos to develop more refined spatial skills. Males in the Temne tribe performed significantly better than Temne females, but there were no significant sex differences among the Eskimos. This latter result may be due to the fact that Eskimo females, unlike Temne females, share equally in the experience of hunting.

A later study by D. K. Norman (1980) supports Berry's interpretation of environmental demand factors in spatial development. Children from rural Appalachia and from urban and suburban New England centers were compared on spatial mapping ability. The children from a more "barren" environment (Appalachia) were expected to perform better than children from a spatially "richer" environment such as a city or suburb. Consistent with expectations, children from Appalachia were superior in mapping ability to the urban and suburban children. We need to be careful in how we rate barrenness of the environment, however. Cultural biases may lead us to label certain environments as impoverished, when they are not. This problem will appear in Chapter 5, on language development. Moreover, we need to make sure that these results are valid for spatial behaviors on daily tasks.

SUMMARY

1. Historically, there have been many different conceptions of space. Psychologists distinguish between absolute and relative space, Euclidean and non-Euclidean space, and practical and representational space. A controversy exists over whether spatial concepts are innate, constructed through experience, or present in stimulus information.

2. Infants appear to possess a good deal of spatial knowledge. Among their spatial skills are the abilities to orient to a sound source in the visual field, to perceive depth, and to recognize the constancy of objects.

3. One of the most significant aspects of spatial cognition is the development of an object concept, which is the knowledge that objects that have gone out of sight continue to exist.

4. People use mental imagery to represent spatial objects and their relations. Spatial representation is essential for many activities in the everyday environment.

5. The ability to mentally rotate images appears as early as 4 years of age and increases through adulthood. Age differences exist in the speed of mental rotation.

6. There has been considerable controversy over the form of representation in mental imagery. Some investigators suggest that images are analogical, or pictorial, while others suggest that they are propositional, or verbal.

7. One area that shows the interaction of analogical and propositional representation is cognitive mapping. Cognitive maps are composed of landmark and route representations that later become integrated in a framework called a configuration.

8. Developmental studies of spatial cognition employ both small-scale and large-scale spatial material. Large-scale space both surrounds the observer and requires multiple perspectives; small-scale space lacks the first property.

9. Two types of spatial reference systems are egocentric and allocentric. In egocentric systems spatial position is defined in relation to the person's body, whereas in allocentric systems the frame of reference is external to the person.

10. Piaget described spatial reference systems in terms of geometric concepts. He proposed that children first develop topological concepts, followed by projective and Euclidean concepts. To what

extent Euclidean concepts are fully developed in adolescents and adults has not been determined.

11. Spatial egocentrism is the inability to take the perspective or view of another person. Although Piaget's research and research based on his theory indicate that children and elderly adults are egocentric, such claims have been challenged by other investigators using more contextually valid and refined procedures.

12. Research on sex differences in spatial ability consistently shows a male superiority effect. This effect has been explained in terms of sex-related socialization differences as well as genetic, neurological, and hormonal differences. Cultural environment also plays a vital role in people's spatial cognition.

Key Terms

absolute space	mental rotation
relative space	kinetic imagery
Euclidean	analogical
non-Euclidean	propositional
practical space	cognitive map
representational space	landmarks
depth perception	routes
stereopsis	configuration
visual cliff	surroundingness
size constancy	spatial reference system
object concept	egocentric
reversibility	allocentric
transitivity	topological
mental imagery	projective

Suggested Readings

Cohen, L. B., & Salapatek, P. (Eds.). (1975). *Infant perception: From sensation to cognition.* New York: Academic Press. This scholarly volume is a synthesis of research and theory on infant perceptual and cognitive systems. The first three chapters place considerable emphasis on infants' perception of space and their perception of objects and people. The final two chapters deal with infant audition.

Cohen, R. (Ed.). (1982). *Children's conceptions of spatial relationships.* San Francisco: Jossey-Bass. This paperback volume reports on several research programs on large-scale spatial cognition. The researchers discuss spatial cognition as a complex interaction of cognitive, social, and emotional factors. Highly readable and current.

Cox, M. V. (Ed.). (1980). *Are young children egocentric?* New York: St. Martin's Press. This book provides a critical appraisal of Piaget's concept of egocentrism in light of recent research evidence. Chapter 3, on the infant's understanding of space, and chapter 4, on visual perspective taking in children, should be relevant to students interested in egocentrism and spatial cognition.

Kosslyn, S. M. (1983). *Ghosts in the mind's machine.* New York: Norton. This book conveys the current interest and excitement in the study of mental images. It illustrates the kind of work being done on imagery in the field of cognitive science and raises some fascinating questions about the way our minds work. However, only a few pages are devoted to cognitive development and imagery.

Pastalan, L. A., & Carson, D. H. (1970). *Spatial behavior of older people.* Ann Arbor: University of Michigan Press. This book discusses the adaptation of older people to their environmental space from an interdisciplinary perspective. It also discusses the importance of cognitive abilities for learning and using spatial information. Somewhat dated, but worth reading.

Pick, H. L., Jr., & Acredolo, L. P. (Eds.). (1983). *Spatial orientation: Theory, research, and application.* New York: Plenum Press. This volume presents different approaches to the study of spatial orientation from both naturalistic and laboratory studies of spatial behavior. Chapters deal with developmental aspects of spatial orientation, spatial orientation in special populations, map reading, linguistic aspects of spatial cognition, and information processing and spatial cognition.

Siegel, A. W., & White, S. H. (1975). The development of spatial representations of large-scale environments. In H. W. Reese (Ed.), *Advances in child development and behavior* (Vol. 10, pp. 9–55). New York: Academic Press. One of the first systematic treatments of the problem of spatial cognition in large-scale environments describes sequences in the development of spatial concepts in children and adults from a constructivist viewpoint.

Language Development

OUTLINE

OVERVIEW

The development of a complex language system is one of our most remarkable cognitive achievements. Yet despite its obvious importance for our everyday lives, language development is not well understood, particularly after 5 years of age.

This chapter explores the interrelationship of language and cognition. Language is a well-ordered system of rules for speaking, listening, and communicating with other people. Three aspects of language development will be considered: (1) phonological development (production and reception of basic sound units), (2) syntactical development (rules used to combine words into complex phrases and sentences), and (3) semantic development (how words and sentences are combined to express meaning). In recent years, the study of semantic development has attracted the greatest attention among cognitive developmental psychologists.

Many theories attempt to explain the puzzle of language development. Learning theories emphasize the importance of the linguistic environment and various learning mechanisms, whereas biologically oriented theories stress the role of innate predispositions toward language. Today, increasing numbers of psychologists focus on the interaction between the linguistic environment and the maturing child's cognitive learning activities.

The final section of the chapter deals with individual and group differences in language development. As in the preceding chapter on spatial cognition, sex differences in linguistic skills are explored. Social and cultural variables in language acquisition are also considered in the context of bilingualism and Black English.

THE STUDY OF HUMAN LANGUAGE

Language development is one of the most remarkable, yet least understood, aspects of cognitive development. In a short four or five years, a person progresses from an *infant* (Latin for "not speaking") to a full-fledged member of the language community. Although language development is not fully completed at this age (contrary to the impression created by many textbooks), the basic elements of sound production and reception, grammar, and understanding of meaning have been mastered. This rapid progression is all the more remarkable in that children exposed to many different linguistic environments and with a minimal amount of language training from parents go through the same sequence of acquisition at approximately the same time. Even the most sophisticated electronic computer cannot be programmed to do linguistically what 5-year-old children can do with relative ease.

Perhaps because language development occurs so rapidly and predictably, we tend to take it for granted. However, understanding the nature of human language has been a vexing problem for centuries. Only in the last 25 years has substantial progress been made in unraveling some of the most puzzling questions about language. Are infants biologically equipped to produce and comprehend language? What environmental inputs must infants have to become fluent language users? What accounts for the communication failures that children as well as adults sometimes experience? Do children the world over go through the same sequences in learning their native tongues? How do toddlers and children map their words onto preexisting conceptual knowledge? Do language abilities remain stable in the postchildhood stages of life? These are some of the many questions addressed in this chapter.

Progress in attacking these questions can be traced to the revolution that occurred in the field of linguistics during the 1950s. In 1957 Noam Chomsky set forth his insights on how language is understood in his classic *Syntactic Structures.* In this remarkable book Chomsky pointed out that a theory of language learning based solely on operant conditioning principles, as proposed by Skinner (1957), could not possibly account for all the grammatically correct sentences in the English language. Instead N. Chomsky (1965) and other theorists (McNeill, 1970) proposed that human beings (unlike animals) have an innate propensity or predisposition to acquire language. They called this inborn tendency a **language acquisition device** (LAD) to emphasize the automatic nature of the process. Through this device, children infer rules for understanding others' speech and for producing their native language.

Despite questions about the adequacy of LAD for understanding language acquisition (Derwing, 1977; Levelt, 1975) and substantial revisions in the original theory (see N. Chomsky, 1965), Chomsky's ideas have been enormously influential. They have stimulated research on language by both psychologists and linguists, establishing a new hybrid discipline called **psycholinguistics.** An even newer field has since emerged, called **developmental psycholinguistics,** which focuses on the developmental study of language acquisition. Chomsky's ideas also led to rejection of the behavioristic approach that had dominated linguistics in the earlier twentieth century (see Bloomfield, 1933), thus paving the way for a more cognitively oriented approach.

During the 1970s and the first half of the 1980s, the study of language retained its cognitive emphasis, but became increasingly multidisciplinary. New insights have come from fields such as anthropology and sociology. Studies in these diciplines have reawakened investigators to the fact that language use depends on the social and cultural context. The environment a child grows up in has a large impact on the child's use of language rules, the meaning of the child's sentences, and the manner in which the child speaks. The new field resulting from these studies has been called **sociolinguistics** to stress the social nature of all language.

LANGUAGE AND COMMUNICATION

Probably the single most important function of language is to help us communicate effectively. As Tamir (1979) has stated, "Communication is essential to human development. It enables the individual to understand others and the social world as they change throughout the life cycle" (p. 36). **Pragmatics** is the name given to the appropriate use of language in its physical and social context. Various pragmatic rules of language govern communication and make everyday interaction possible. One basic rule of interaction is that participants in a conversation take turns speaking; the amount of time each speaks may vary as a function of the speaker's age, status, and so on. Another rule is referred to as the "adjacency pair" (Tamir, 1979). If I say, "Hey, can you guess what happened?", your reply should be "No, what happened?" In this situation, a second utterance from the listener must follow the speaker's first utterance. Failure to follow this rule interrupts the normal flow of conversational dialogue, as when a person blandly says "Yes" when asked "Do you know the way to the psychology building?"

Pragmatic rules of communication are first seen in the interactions between prelinguistic children and their caretakers. Very early in life infants begin to exchange glances, touches, and caresses with others. These exchanges provide the basis for the development and organization of later forms of social communication. Bruner (1983) describes several game-like situations such as "peekaboo," in which each participant "takes a turn" and responds to the other, much like in a conversation. With development infants play increasingly active roles in such "conversational" sequences. Figure 5.1 presents developmental data for Richard, one of Bruner's (1983) subjects. The data are for an object exchange game in which Richard and his mother handed an object back and forth. Prior to 9 months and 3 weeks of age Richard initiated few exchanges, but after this age he began to participate actively in the exchanges to the point of initiating the game about half the time.

Figure 5.1   Percentage of time spent by mother (adult) or child as agent in the object exchange game.

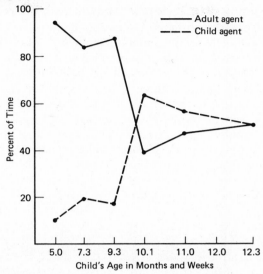

From *Child's Talk: Learning to Use Language* (p. 61) by J. Bruner, 1983, New York: Norton. Copyright 1983 by J. Bruner. Reprinted by permission of W. W. Norton & Company, Inc.

Intentional Communication

From the earliest years of life, human beings are strongly motivated to communicate, a tendency animals do not show (R. Brown, 1973). At first, people communicate with built-in signals such as crying. Even though crying noises reliably elicit reactions from adult listeners, there is little evidence that infants intend such behaviors to have a particular effect. These signaling behaviors occur even in the absence of a listener or observer.

Later in development, infant communication becomes more intentional. Bates (1979) defines *intentional communication* as "signaling behavior in which the sender is aware a priori of the effect that a signal will have on his listener, and he persists in that behavior until the effect is obtained or failure is clearly indicated" (p. 36). An example of intentionality in communication can be seen in the nonverbal gestures an infant uses to signal a desire to parents, such as pointing in the direction of a cookie jar on the top shelf while alternately looking at the parents and the jar.

Bates and colleagues (Bates, 1979; Bates, Camaioni, & Volterra, 1975) have proposed that an infant passes through (1) **perlocutionary,** (2) **illocutionary,** and (3) **locutionary** stages in the development of intentional communication. During the perlocutionary phase, the communicative acts of the infant have an intentional or unintentional effect on listeners, but the infant is unaware of the effect. This phase occurs during the early stages of sensorimotor development, prior to the time when infants differentiate between themselves and objects around them. Besides crying, perlocutionary behaviors include babbling, smiling, and differential responding to human faces.

In the illocutionary phase, the child begins to use signals to make nonverbal requests and initiate social interaction. These behaviors lay the foundation for the child's understanding how his or her actions have a communicative effect on others. Finally, in the locutionary phase, the child begins gradually to use speech sounds together with nonverbal signals, especially gestures, to convey requests and interact socially (see Molfese, Molfese, & Carrell, 1982). The major developmental features of each of these three communication phases along with approximate ages are shown in Table 5.1.

Table 5.1
Three Phases in the Development of Intentional Communication

Phase	Infant's Behavior
1. Perlocutionary Phase (approximately 0–9 or 10 months)	The infant cries and reaches toward a goal object. Changes in the infant's crying and fussing depend upon changes in the availability of the goal object.
2. Illocutionary Phase (approximately 9 or 10–13 months)	While crying or reaching, the infant begins to alternate eye contact between the goal object and the adult. Changes in infant crying and reaching depend on the adult's behavior toward the goal, rather than on the goal itself. Reaching and grasping become more abbreviated, while fussing sounds become more "ritualized" and conventional.
3. Locutionary Phase (approximately 13–24 months)	The infant begins to use conventional names for goal objects along with nonverbal gestures such as pointing and reaching. Naming also begins to occur in solitary play. The first evidence of nonverbal symbolic activity is seen in infants' "pretend" play activities.

Bates (1979) has described these phases in terms of the development of "social tool use," and she has proposed that movement through them depends on achieving a certain level of sensorimotor functioning, or "nonsocial tool use." Three key sensorimotor achievements—object relations, means-end coordination, and deferred imitation—are seen as crucial to the development of intentional communication. For example, unlike a younger infant, a 9-month-old who cannot reach a toy resting on a cloth will pull the cloth toward him and then take the toy (Bates, 1979). Piaget referred to this period of cognitive development as Stage 5 of sensorimotor development, or "tertiary circular reactions" (see Box 2.2). This period is marked by the invention of "new means to familiar ends." A positive relationship between Stage 5 means-ends behaviors and intentional communication has been reported by several investigators (Harding & Golinkoff, 1979; Sugarman-Bell, 1978), although not all infants at Stage 5 use intentional communication. In contrast, the development of object permanence and a knowledge of spatial object relationships are not significantly correlated with communication and language development. Thus, intentional communication seems to depend on certain aspects of sensorimotor development and not others.

Egocentric Communication

As children move through the phases shown in Table 5.1, they become increasingly able to take on the perspective of both the speaker and the listener in communication; that is, they become less egocentric. In chapter 4, we discussed the controversy surrounding spatial egocentrism in young children. To be effective communicators, children (and adults) must understand how the listener's perspective differs from theirs and be sensitive to feedback cues in the course of conversation. R. Krauss and Glucksberg (1969, 1977) have developed an ingenious technique for studying egocentric communication in children. They ask two children to sit at opposite ends of a table separated by an opaque screen in the middle of the table. The experimenter places a row of six wooden blocks in front of one child. Nonsense forms that are difficult to describe are printed on each block. The other child sees a duplicate set of six blocks, but arranged in a different order.

The objective is for one child (the speaker) to stack his or her blocks on a peg and, at the same time, describe the form on each block so that the other child (the listener) can determine the block being described and make an identical stack. No restrictions are placed on types of verbal communication between the speaker and the listener. Prior to the task, children are given practice trials with familiar animal-shaped blocks in full view of each other. After the practice trials, they are separated by the screen and given eight trials with the unfamiliar blocks.

Preschool children do very poorly on this block-stacking task. As Table 5.2 reveals, young speakers frequently use an egocentric frame of reference in their description (e.g., "the one that looks like my mother's hat"), not realizing that the listener has never seen the object being described. As a result kindergarten and first-grade listeners make many stacking errors, and their performance does not improve much across trials (see Figure 5.2). Third-grade and fifth-grade children succeed in reducing their errors so that they are performing with few mistakes by the last four trials.

In an interesting extension of the R. Krauss and Glucksberg (1969) research, K. Rubin (1974) studied communicative egocentrism as well as spatial egocentrism in four age groups: second graders, sixth graders, young adults, and elderly adults. To measure communicative egocentrism, Rubin used the R. Krauss and Glucksberg communication problem; spatial egocentrism was measured in a manner similar to Flavell, Botkin, Fry, Wright, and Jarvis (1968), as described in Chapter 4. Rubin

Table 5.2
Typical Idiosyncratic Descriptions Given by Five Preschool Children in the R. Krauss and Glucksberg Communication Game

		Child				
Form		1	2	3	4	5
1		Man's legs	Airplane	Drapeholder	Zebra	Flying saucer
2		Mother's hat	Ring	Keyhold	Lion	Snake
3		Somebody running	Eagle	Throwing sticks	Strip-stripe	Wire
4		Daddy's shirt	Milk jug	Shoe hold	Coffeepot	Dog
5		Another Daddy's shirt	Bird	Dress hold	Dress	Knife
6		Mother's dress	Ideal	Digger hold	Caterpillar	Ghost

Note: From "Social and Nonsocial Speech" by R. M. Krauss and S. Glucksberg, February 1977, *Scientific American, 236*, p. 104. Copyright 1977 by Scientific American, Inc. Reprinted by permission.

Figure 5.2 Mean number of stacking errors in communication by grade.

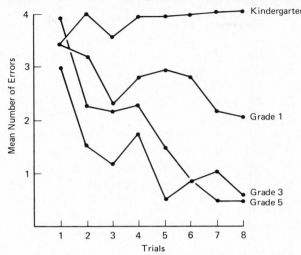

From "The Development of Communication" by R. M. Krauss and S. Glucksberg, 1969, *Child Development, 40,* p. 260. Copyright 1969 by The Society for Research in Child Development. Reprinted by permission.

reported that second graders performed worst on both tasks, sixth graders and the elderly performed equivalently, and young adults performed best. The two egocentrism measures were related only for the sixth-grade and young adult subjects. K. Rubin (1974) interpreted these results as evidence of cognitive regression in later life.

Part of the problem in using measures like the communications task and the spatial egocentrism task involves their nonnaturalistic, laboratory-like quality. For example, a child who has no trouble describing a new toy to a friend over the telephone may be unable to deal with abstract, nonsensical shapes. As a listener, a child needs to be able to spot ambiguities in speech, a process made all the more difficult by ambiguous-looking objects. Similarly, elderly people seem to be able to take the perspective of another in social communication when the situation demands it (see Looft & Charles, 1971), but often fail to see the need for such perspective taking on laboratory tasks like those described above.

Recent research in the area of communication and other aspects of cognitive functioning suggests that investigators may have overestimated the egocentricity in children's speech. This research takes a different approach from that discussed above in that more real-life communication situations are employed, and communication is interpreted more broadly than simple transmission of information about strange-looking objects from speaker to listener. Communication in this research tradition includes the child's ability to use language to make requests, give commands, greet friends, or offer a challenge. One of the most reliable findings is that children can adjust their communicative behavior to the age and status of the listener (Shatz, 1983). In probably the best-known study, Shatz and Gelman (1973) showed that 4-year-olds "talk down" to 2-year-old listeners by using shorter and less complex sentences than they do with age-mates or adults. It has now been demonstrated that children as young as age 2 are sensitive to listener differences. Wellman and Lempers (1977) reported that 2-year-olds choose to communicate to adults more so than peers and are more likely to tailor their messages to their listener's needs when the listener is an adult rather than another 2-year-old.

Despite these impressive demonstrations of communicative skill in young children, some genuine limitations appear in their cognitive functioning and behavior in communication situations. Most of these limitations involve what Flavell calls *metacommunication*—people's knowledge and cognitions about the communications they send and receive. Young children aged 4–6 will occasionally notice that a speaker's message is referentially ambiguous (Beal & Flavell, 1983; Pratt & Bates, 1982). However, they are less likely than older children (7–10-year-olds) to detect the inadequacies of the ambiguous message or to request more specific information from the speaker. For instance, if children are shown two red blocks, one square and one round, and are asked to pick "the red block," younger children are less likely than older children to ask the speaker for clarification, even though they know they can ask questions at any time. What accounts for improvements in children's communicative and metacommunicative skills? In general, children improve their communication skills because they acquire the cognitive and metacognitive abilities that enable them to monitor and evaluate the clarity of their own and others' speech. School and other real-life social experiences which place demands on children to communicate clearly to others and to comprehend the communications they receive may facilitate the acquisition of language-relevant cognitive and metacognitive skills. Experiences in reading and writing may also play an instrumental role in metacommunication (Flavell, 1985).

The shift in emphasis to metacommunication and the integration of cognitive and social processes represent an exciting and healthy trend in language development research. One can readily envision the applicability of this approach to life-span research on language. For example, the development and awareness of communicative intent among members of different generations could be studied. Questions about who initiates intergenerational communication and what gets communicated or miscommunicated would be fruitful areas for further research.

LANGUAGE AND COGNITION

Language is an important vehicle for communication. It enables us to express our thoughts, feelings, and ideas to other people as well as to ourselves. For some time, a central issue in language development research has been the relationship between language and cognition (Matlin, 1985). Most investigators agree that language and cognition are closely related, especially in the early stages of development. During adulthood, language seems to function more independently of thought (Riegel, 1973b). Even with cognitive declines, an older adult may continue to use language effectively (D. Cohen & Wu, 1980). Psycholinguists have, therefore, viewed language as a stable function in later adulthood, unlike cognition, which changes developmentally. Nevertheless, language cannot easily be separated from other cognitive activities, a point underscored by the high correlations between poor language performance and poor performance on tests of attention, learning, and memory (see D. Cohen & Wu, 1980).

What is the relationship between language and cognition? Bates, Benigni, Bretherton, Camaioni, and Volterra (1979) discuss at least six models of the relations between language and thought, three of which will be considered here. The first model views language and thought as independent of one another in early childhood, but interconnected in later childhood. The second model states that language makes the emergence and use of higher-order cognitive skills possible. The third model holds that cognitive operations precede and guide the development of language, with language serving as one representational medium among many. Let us now consider the various viewpoints that have been offered on this topic.

Lev Vygotsky

Lev Vygotsky (1962), a famous Russian psychologist, takes the position that language development affects the course of cognitive growth. In his view language provides a powerful medium for representing abstract experience, more powerful than such representational systems as imagery or mental operations, which develop more slowly. For example, a 3-year-old child who is already forming complex sentences with abstract clauses is only at the beginning of preoperational thinking. While children's cognitive operations are limited and inflexible, their language shows great flexibility and creativity.

According to Vygotsky (1962), language and cognition initially develop along separate pathways; later in development, they become connected to each other, resulting in more complex forms of speech and thought. A key feature of Vygotsky's position is **inner speech,** which is quite different from external, social speech. Inner speech, or self-speech, is internalized, highly abbreviated, and consists mostly of predicates rather than subjects. When we carry out a silent dialogue with ourselves, we are engaging in inner speech. This internal dialogue helps to organize and direct our thoughts. Vygotsky (1962) states:

> Inner speech is not the interior aspect of external speech—it is a function in itself. It still remains speech, i.e., thought connected with words. But while in external speech thought is embedded in words, in inner speech words die as they bring forth thought. Inner speech is to a large extent thinking in pure word meanings. It is a dynamic shifting, unstable thing, fluttering between word and thought, the two more or less stable, more or less firmly delineated components of verbal thought. (p. 149)

Thus, in Vygotsky's system, language and thought are inextricably bound together, although not identical.

Vygotsky was particularly interested in the social or interpersonal origins of language development. Social or external speech from adults regulates very young children's behavior, much as other physical stimuli do. As children grow, they tend to engage in **egocentric speech,** or speech that occurs in social circumstances, but not for communicative purposes. Children are apt to employ such speech when they encounter difficulties in a problem situation. Vygotsky cited the example of a 5½-year-old boy who was drawing a streetcar when his pencil broke. The boy tried to continue drawing, but was unable to because of the broken point. While muttering "it's broken," he began to paint a broken streetcar, all the while talking to himself about the picture. Vygotsky saw this behavior as a telling example of how external speech guided the boy's behavior. Gradually, children's ability to use egocentric speech to plan their actions becomes more fully developed. Around ages 6 or 7, the child's external vocalization disappears and egocentric speech goes "underground" to become inner speech.

Vygotsky's ideas about the development of inner speech differ sharply from Piaget's, especially in regard to the importance of egocentric speech. Piaget observed that the amount of and egocentricity of egocentric speech decline with age and that such speech disappears entirely by ages 6 or 7. He felt egocentric speech reflects a general egocentrism in the child and serves no unique developmental function. Children eventually learn to communicate by taking other people's points of view into consideration. Vygotsky, on the other hand, theorized that egocentric speech becomes increasingly egocentric through childhood as the child learns to adapt such speech to self-regulatory functions. Only later, when the speech is fully internalized, does egocentricity decline. What is more important, according to Vygotsky, egocentric speech is critical for the development of planning and self-guidance skills.

Benjamin Whorf

Another view reflecting the belief that language affects thought has been proposed by linguist Benjamin Whorf (1956). Whorf based many of his ideas on writings by Sapir (1921) and proposed two interrelated hypotheses about the relation between language and thought: **linguistic determinism** and **linguistic relativity.** In its strongest version, linguistic determinism states that the structure of language determines all other forms of perception and thinking. The corollary linguistic relativity hypothesis states that one's thinking will be relative to the forms of language characteristic of one's culture. This relativity hypothesis predicts that speakers in cultures with dissimilar languages will come to conceive of the world in fundamentally distinctive ways.

Whorf based much of his theory on the categorical nature of language. Different cultural groups use different words and constructions to arbitrarily classify various objects and events. There are many examples. Arabs have over 6000 different names for *camel.* This reflects their greater experience with these animals and supposedly allows them to perceive camels differently than someone who has only seen a camel at a zoo. Similarly, Eskimos have many different terms for *snow,* which vary according to its texture, recency, density, and so on, whereas most English speakers have only the single word *snow.* According to the linguistic relativity hypothesis, the Eskimo's perceptions of snow should be different from the average English speaker's (see Chapter 4 for a similar example of spatial concepts in Canadian Eskimos).

Does this mean that people who are not part of the Eskimo or Arab cultures are incapable of making such fine distinctions? Probably not. As Dan Slobin (1979), a well-known psycholinguist, has pointed out, concepts or relations in one language can be translated relatively easily into other languages. Consider the concept of color. The English language has 11 basic color words: *black, white, red, green, yellow, blue, brown, purple, pink, orange,* and *gray.* These words are called basic colors because they are commonly used, in contrast to terms such as *chartreuse, scarlet,* and *mauve,* and because they refer to colors only. In contrast, the Dani of Indonesian New Guinea use two words to describe the entire color spectrum—*mili* for dark, cold hues and *mola* for bright, warm hues (J. R. Anderson, 1985). If the Whorfian hypothesis is correct, the Dani should be less able to distinguish among colors than English speakers.

In an important series of experiments, Rosch studied the ability of the Dani to perceive colors. In one study, Rosch (1973) examined whether the Dani perceive *focal colors* differently than English-speaking subjects. Within the range of each of the 11 basic color terms in English, there is generally one agreed-upon *best* color—a best red, a best blue, and so on. These so-called best colors are known as focal colors. English speakers have been shown to learn arbitrary labels for focal colors more readily than nonfocal colors. In Rosch's (1973) experiment, the Dani also found it easier to learn arbitrary names for focal colors than for nonfocal colors, despite not having names for these colors in their language. This result suggests that the Dani processed the colors in much the same way as English speakers. Contrary to Whorf's linguistic relativity hypothesis, language does not seem to determine the way colors are perceived. Although the hypothesis may eventually prove true for other domains, it does not appear to hold for color categories.

Whorf's (1956) far-reaching proposal generated a good deal of debate and some empirical research, but has been extraordinarily difficult to validate. Language certainly can influence our thinking, as when children learn to use vocabulary words to form categories characteristic of their society. And some ideas can be more easily communicated via some languages than others. In these cases, thought reflects language rather than being determined by it. But whether language limits our ability to perceive and conceptualize reality in certain ways, as Whorf proposes, is open to question. Indeed, some have argued that language makes thought more flexible rather than less flexible (Bruner, 1973).

Jean Piaget

Unlike Vygotsky and Whorf, Jean Piaget sees language as subordinate to cognition; language does not determine cognition, which is to be found in action (Beilin, 1980). Language is only one symbolic vehicle among many (e.g., perception, imagery, mental operations) for the expression of thought. Children who cannot express themselves verbally can engage in symbolic thought, as shown by the object concept. In Piaget's view, a child's sensorimotor activities are essential for the development of semiotic, or symbolic, representation near the end of the second year. The **semiotic function** (ability to symbolize) has important implications for thinking about and remembering objects, people, and events in their absence. Moreover, children with symbolic representational abilities become capable of distinguishing between symbols and their referents (i.e., the things the symbols stand for).

Piaget (1967) observed that the semiotic function is expressed in the form of personal symbols such as *deferred imitation, symbolic play, drawings,* and *mental maps.* These symbolic representations precede the emergence of language and are derived from the development of imitative skills. Piaget (1951) cited many instances of deferred imitation among his own children. For example, when his daughter Jacqueline was 16 months old, she observed an 18-month-old boy throwing a temper tantrum in a playpen. The next day Piaget's daughter screamed in the playpen and tried to move it by stomping her feet—something she had never done before. Piaget explained this behavior as evidence of imitative ability. Because the behavior occurred a full day after being observed, Jacqueline must have stored a representation of the behavior in her mind.

With regard to imitation and language, children use words and sentences long after they have heard them. Such symbolic ability presupposes an ability to store internal images of sounds and sights. The development of the symbolic function makes the emergence of language possible, not vice versa. Piaget therefore concluded that thought is a prerequisite to language.

P. Harris (1983) has recently argued that the cognitive prerequisites hypothesis of Piaget is actually much closer to what Bates (1979) and associates refer to as the "shared base" model. According to this model, certain cognitive and linguistic abilities share common components without one necessarily being prerequisite for the other. Hence, language as one type of symbolic activity has much in common with other representational activities and should emerge around the same time developmentally. To test this model, investigators have looked at the temporal correlations between language and cognition, but they have not tried to demonstrate that certain cognitive achievements invariably precede the attainment of certain language abilities.

Zachry (1978) conducted a cross-sectional study of 24 infants aged 1–2 years. He assessed infants on both sensorimotor abilities and language in order to test Piaget's hypothesis that representational thought precedes "true" language. Sensorimotor Stages 4, 5, and 6 were assessed by means of the Uzgiris and Hunt (1975) scales, a commonly used Piagetian-based testing instrument for infants. Language development was assessed by recording spontaneous verbalizations during a free play session with either the parent or a caretaker present. The results indicated that the attainment of Stage 6 performance was related to the number of different language categories employed by each infant. However, there was no systematic relation between the emergence of specific sensorimotor skills and particular language categories. Moreover, there was a high positive correlation between cognitive development and age. Because language development also correlated with age, the correlation between cognition and language simply may be based on their shared relationship with age, much as motor skills and language skills emerge in roughly parallel fashion (P. Harris, 1983).

Other investigators have focused on a specific aspect of cognitive development—object permanence—and language acquisition. Object permanence has long been thought to be important in language development because it involves the ability to represent an absent object or action (Bowerman, 1978; Corrigan, 1978). Attempts to demonstrate this have not yielded clear evidence of a systematic relationship. For example, Corrigan (1978) performed a longitudinal study of three children ranging in age from approximately 10–29 months. The results showed that performance on a language scale and an object permanence task were correlated with age and with each other. But once the age variable was statistically removed, the correlation between object permanence and language dropped for each of the three children. Thus, research on early language development and infant cognition has failed to show that they are anything more than two independent factors, each linked with age.

According to Piaget, as the child moves into the preoperational and concrete operational stages of cognitive functioning, language still plays no major role in higher-order reasoning or problem solving. One line of research supporting Piaget's view involves studies of deaf children (Furth, 1966, 1971). Although deaf children do not proceed beyond the initial phases of spoken language, their cognitive development goes through the same sequence of stages as hearing children's, albeit at a somewhat slower pace.

This is not to say that language is unimportant to cognitive development. As Piagetian researchers such as Sinclair-de Zwart (1969) have indicated, children who successfully solve concrete operational problems use more advanced language than children who fail to solve them. For example, on a task known as the liquid conservation task (see Chapter 7), children who can solve the task (conservers) are more likely than children who fail to solve the task (nonconservers) to use terms such as *more, less,* and *same.* Piaget himself points out that the use of language in social interactions helps foster cognitive growth by forcing children to take the perspective of another person. As children try to explain their point of view to another, they become aware of their own inconsistencies (Piaget, 1926).

Piagetians (Beilin, 1980; Piaget, 1967) feel that language assumes a greater role in the development of formal operational thought, which involves reasoning about hypothetical problems (see Chapters 2 and 8); the child is no longer limited to representations with concrete referents. Piaget concluded that even though language becomes important in dealing with hypothetical problems, formal operations have their roots in sensorimotor actions, not linguistic achievements.

Language and Cognition Reconsidered

Little evidence has been found for a systematic relationship between language and cognitive development, at least when the latter is conceived in Piagetian stages. One of the major problems in trying to establish such a correlation is the lack of a clear definition of *thought*. None of the current theories of cognitive development can adequately characterize all forms of mental activity and knowledge representation. As noted in Chapter 4's discussion of imagery, knowledge can be represented in various forms, both linguistic and nonlinguistic, which can interact in many complex ways. This leads us to conclude that "language is an integral component of thought, but neither language nor speech can be equated with thought" (Slobin, 1979, p. 153).

Recently, P. Harris (1983) proposed that rather than look at cognition as a prerequisite to language or vice versa, psychologists should focus on the ease with which a translation can be made between available cognitive concepts and language. That is, can a concept be easily stated in conventional verbal form? P. Harris's proposal is too detailed to consider here, but it does highlight the probability that no simple link exists between the development of cognition and the acquisition of language.

DESCRIBING LANGUAGE DEVELOPMENT

Language is a system of well-ordered rules for speaking, listening, and communicating with other individuals. The number of rules is quite large, though not infinite. Through these rules, people can produce and comprehend an almost infinite variety of meaningful word combinations and sentences. N. Chomsky (1957) referred to this ability to generate endless novel sentences from a finite set of rules as the **generative** aspect of language. To give you some idea how remarkable this ability is, if you selected words from an unabridged English dictionary and formed all possible 20-word sentences, you could speak or write for the next 10,000 billion years without repeating yourself! Most of what we hear—other than clichéd expressions such as "How are you?" and "Take it easy"—consists of novel utterances. How, then, are human beings able to communicate? To answer this question, we will look at various developmental stages in the acquisition of the rules of language. We will talk about different types of rules (e.g., phonological, grammatical) separately, but in reality they are inseparable.

Phonological Development

Phonological development is the development of the basic units of sound used to distinguish one utterance from another by producing a change in meaning. For example, changing the initial phoneme in *sat* to *cat* produces a different meaning. These basic sound units, or **pho-**

nemes, are combined to produce words and sentences. The English language is comprised of about 45 basic phonemes or classes of sounds— 36 consonant phonemes and 9 vowel phonemes. The phonemes in other languages range from as few as 20 (in some Polynesian languages) to as many as 60.

Originally, the English alphabet was constructed so that there would be one letter for every given phoneme. In practice, however, letters have many different phonemic sounds associated with them. This is especially true for vowel sounds, such as the long and short /i/ in *bit* and *bite*. The occurrence of so many different phonemic sounds does not seem to pose a problem for infants, who learn to produce the sounds rapidly and at about the same period in their development. Typically, vowel sounds such as the phoneme /u/ are mastered first, beginning with vowel-like *cooing*. This is followed at around 6 months of age with alternating vowel and consonant sounds in the stage of *babbling*. In the earliest phases of babbling, vowel sounds still predominate, but consonant sounds begin to increase in frequency. Although these babbling sounds do not appear to convey meaning, they allow the infant to experiment playfully with sound production.

Until roughly 1 year of age, the number of phonemes produced by the infant continues to expand dramatically, a process called **phonemic expansion.** Some linguists used to believe that infants between 6–12 months of age eventually produce all the sounds found in all human languages, so that African, American, Chinese, and French infants all sound very similar (Dale, 1976). These linguists also argued that because infants in all cultures produce the same sounds, infants have the capacity to learn any language. However, research now suggests that infants do not babble all the world's speech sounds, nor even all those of their native language. Many speech sounds must be added after the infant has begun to talk. The converse also appears true: many of the babbling sounds of the young infant cannot be reproduced by the child a year later.

Toward the end of the first year of life, babbling begins to change. A process called **phonemic contraction** occurs as children's linguistic environment shapes the permissible sounds in their language. Children in an English-speaking environment start to lose the German gutturals and the French nasals, assuming they uttered these sounds. Furthermore, children learn that sounds such as /tw/ in *twice* and /br/ in *brick* can occur in the English language, but not /fw/ as in *fwice* or /bn/ as in *bnick*. All languages employ such phonological rules. Although we may not be able to list them all, we use such rules constantly in our everyday conversation.

For adults, acquisition of the appropriate phonemes can be a major obstacle in learning a second language. Although adults master most aspects of language as quickly or more quickly than children, there appears to be a critical period for phonemic production (Lenneberg, 1967; see Snow & Hoefnagel-Höhle, 1978, for counterevidence on the critical period hypothesis). As you learned in Chapter 2, during a critical period an individual has a special facility for learning, which is not available before or after this time. Sounds that can be produced effortlessly by infants often elude the painstaking efforts of adults. This author can remember trying with great dismay to trill the Spanish /r/ sound in the words *perro* ("dog") and *ferrocarril* ("railroad") in his college Spanish course. Non-English-speaking people have an even worse experience in learning the English language, because there is not always a close correspondence between phonemes and letters.

So far, we have considered sound production. In normal, everyday conversation adults produce about 500 phonemes per minute. The different articulatory organs (vocal cords, palate, lips, tongue) are involved in producing these sounds. How are we able to receive and decode this massive amount of information? What makes *sound reception* possible? The answer is our **categorical perception** of speech. People hear sounds categorically when they perceive them as discontinuous, even though they lie along a speech continuum. If I asked you to listen to *ma* and *na*, you would undoubtedly be able to tell them apart, even if I varied them to make them sound very similar.

Research shows that even very young infants can perceive speech categorically (Eimas, 1975; Aslin, Pisoni, & Jusczyk, 1983). In a recent review of research in this area, Jusczyk (1981) concluded: "Judging from the existing data, it appears that infants are innately endowed with mechanisms necessary for making phonetic distinctions in any natural language, at least to a first approximation" (p. 156). Habituation techniques have been used in these studies to measure infants' sensitivity to sound changes. Infants are habituated to a phoneme (*pa*) and then the sound is changed to a slightly different phoneme (*ba*). At the same time the experimenter looks for changes in the response being monitored. Heart rate, sucking, and head turning are three of the most commonly measured responses. Studies show that babies as young as 1–4 months respond to these subtle phonemic changes and will even respond categorically to speech sounds to which adults do not. For example, when exposed to chirping noises that sounded like birds, adults treated the chirping noises as one continuous sound, but babies treated them categorically.

How can infants perform such feats? Eimas (1975) has suggested that infants have built-in feature detectors, which tune into certain stimuli and tune out others. Experience apparently plays a role, too. Eilers, Wilson, and Moore (1977) reported that infants do not seem to discriminate between *s* and *z* at the ends of syllables or between *sa* and *za*. In addition, with increasing linguistic experience, infants may lose some of their ability to detect phonemic change. Thus, both inborn ability and experience seem to be involved in the categorical discrimination of speech sounds. Young infants also seem to possess many of the same phonetic perceptual abilities as adult listeners.

Several writers have noted that infants seem to show a preference for speech sounds in the frequency band of the human voice (see T. Field, 1982, for a review). In a study designed to demonstrate neonates' auditory preferences for their mothers' voice, DeCasper and Fifer (1980) presented infants 3 days of age or less with tape-recorded versions of Dr. Seuss's *And to Think That I Saw It on Mulberry Street.* On one version of the tape infants heard their mothers' voice, while on another version they heard another mother. By sucking on a non-nutritive nipple in a certain way, infants could produce either the mothers' voice or that of the other mother. The results of this well-controlled study showed that infants could discriminate among voices and that they demonstrated a preference for their own mothers' voice, having had only limited maternal exposure.

Equally impressive findings indicate that young infants can detect subtle changes of voice made by a single individual. Infants show marked behavioral changes when parents become silent in the middle of an interaction or are still-faced (see T. Field, 1982). Of course in the real world, infants are more apt to experience a voice and a face simultaneously than either alone. A talking face may be a more complex, abstract stimulus, and (as discussed in Chapter 3) more likely to be noticed.

Morphological development is the next step up the ladder of complexity from phonological development. **Morphology** is the study of the basic units of meaning in a language. The smallest units of sound that convey meaning in a language are called **morphemes.** Morphemes are comprised of fixed sequences of phonemes and are similar to the units of speech we call *roots, stems, prefixes,* and *suffixes.* The English language has over 100,000 morphemes. Some morphemes such as the plural /-s/ are called *bound morphemes* because they cannot stand alone. However, they can be combined with *free morphemes* (those which can stand alone) such as *pen, bat,* or *top* to form meaningful two-morpheme words such as *pens, bats,* and *tops.* All languages have morphological rules that specify the ways in which morphemes can be combined.

Syntactical and Semantic Development

The study of **syntax** (the rules by which morphemes and words are combined to produce more complex clauses, phrases, and sentences) and

semantics (the ways in which words and sentences are put together to form meaning) have been the two most active areas of research on language development and are closely related. To illustrate this relationship, consider the following sentences:

Colorless green ideas sleep furiously.
Furry jewelers create distressed stains.

Both sentences are syntactically correct but meaningless. Other sentences are syntactically incorrect but fairly meaningful, such as the following:

Furry fight furious wildcats battles.
Sudden melting cause floods snows.

Not surprisingly, people are better able to recognize and remember "normal" sentences, which are both syntactically and semantically correct, than "anomalous" sentences like the examples shown above (Marks & Miller, 1964). Thus, the syntactical structure and semantic meaningfulness of a sentence are intrinsically related.

First Words and Sentences

The study of syntactical and semantic development commences with the utterance of a child's first word. Before this time, little can be inferred about language development in these two domains. Of the two, semantic development is seen as more fundamental by most cognitive developmental psychologists and, accordingly, has received most attention.

One of the most frequently studied aspects of language acquisition involves first words and sentences. Parents eagerly await their infant's first word. Benedict (1975) reported an age range of 9–14 months in the production of an infant's first word. These first utterances are not likely to be perfectly clear and intelligible, but rough approximations of adult speech. For example, the child may say *mih* when referring to *milk.* First words are usually uttered in connection with a child's action or manipulation of an object, as when a child says *bla* to refer to *block* or *kuh* to refer to *cookie.* The words are also likely to be tied to the appearance and disappearance of objects such as *bah* when a ball rolls under the sofa or *mama* when mother appears at the bedroom door. In addition, children use their earliest words to describe actions or to demand attention (e.g., *bye-bye, go*) and to refer to properties or quantities of things (e.g., *more, hot*).

Although a child's first words may be ambiguous, they often convey rich meaning. The term **holophrase** is used to describe the single-word utterances children use to stand for whole phrases or sentences. Parents frequently rely on the child's actions and the surrounding context to interpret his or her holophrases. The child whose ball has rolled under a piece of furniture may point or gesture to the parent while saying *bah*. The child may also employ different stress or intonational patterns. Think of how you might pronounce the word *ball* differently in playing a game of tennis ("Ball?" meaning "Is this your ball?" or "Have you seen my ball?"). Children use similar intonational patterns to communicate.

Considerable debate surrounds the issue of what meaning the child is attempting to convey by using holophrases (R. Brown, 1973; Dale, 1976; Greenfield & Smith, 1976). Does the child who says "milk" have a full sentence in mind—"I want more milk," "This is milk," or "This is milk?" Quite possibly. However, we must look at the entire context in which the word is uttered. As children near the end of the one-word period, they are more likely to use nonverbal gestures and grammatical devices such as inflections or intonational cues to signal their intentions. We can then more confidently interpret the meaning of the holophrase.

The one-word stage of development roughly covers the ages 12–18 months and signals the beginning of a child's vocabulary acquisition. What types of words do infants have in their vocabularies? First words often refer to basic categories such as animals (*dog, cat* or *kitty, duck* or *hen*), food (*cookies, milk, bread*), and toys (*blocks, doll, ball*). By 18 months the child has acquired about 50 words (K. Nelson, 1973a). Children vary in the time they take to achieve a 50-word vocabulary, but they all show approximately the same patterns of development. Slow initial growth up to 10 words is followed by a spurt of new words. Interestingly, studies done on children's vocabulary 50 or more years ago show exactly the same patterns and to a large extent the same vocabulary (see Clark, 1979).

A more important semantic issue than the number of vocabulary words is how the child associates words with objects, events, and relations. Two competing explanations were initially offered for this phenomenon. The first explanation, the **semantic feature hypothesis,** was proposed by Eve Clark (1973). Clark argued that the meaning of a word depends on the semantic components or features attached to the word (for example, *four-legged, barks, tail, furry*). The child notices the most salient features of the item through the senses and applies the correct word (*dog*) when one or more of these is present.

A rival explanation was offered by Katherine Nelson (1973b, 1974). According to her **functional core hypothesis,** the child initially names objects or events in terms of their functional relation to the child's actions (e.g., a ball can be thrown, bounced, caught, rolled, kicked). As evidence for her hypothesis, K. Nelson (1974) found that words referring to objects that could be acted upon (such as *ball*) or moved in some way (such as *car*) appeared more often than other types of words (such as *table, tree, grass*) in children's early vocabulary. Such findings led to heated controversy over the classes of first words produced. Huttenlocher (1974) and Macnamara (1972) contended that nominals, or object words, are the most frequent first words. In contrast, L. Bloom (1973) and Piaget (1962) argued that action or function words are produced more often.

As investigators began to test these rival hypotheses, their shortcomings became more apparent. Most objects, situations, and states are difficult, if not impossible, to characterize in terms of semantic features (Rosch & Mervis, 1975). For example, a word such as *chair* cannot be readily decomposed into a set of common features or components of meaning. Think of the features that all chairs share and that nonchairs do not have. As a start, try to generate a list of common features for a beanbag chair and a deck chair. Problems in doing this kind of semantic feature analysis suggest that such an approach cannot be applied to vocabulary as a whole.

Clark (1983) has abandoned semantic feature theory in favor of a new approach called **lexical contrast theory.** She now proposes that children follow two basic principles in their acquisition of word meaning— **contrast** and **conventionality.** "Contrast" refers to the fact that any pairs of words in a language have contrasting meanings. Clark (1983) illustrates this principle with an analogy to writing a dictionary for an unknown language. In making this dictionary, the writer would select words that have different meanings, each of which would contrast to some extent with words previously selected. Contrasts in word meanings, in turn, depend on the *conventional meanings* assigned by the language community. Words only contrast over time if speakers agree on the conventional meaning of the word.

Clark (1983) feels that the two principles of contrast and conventionality play a central role in language use. For example, in talking about events, children begin to contrast an original term such as *open* with *shut;* or in talking about states, they will contrast *in* and *on* with *to, from, out, off,* and *up.* This process of using contrasting words is motivated by children's need to fill in lexical gaps in their vocabularies. Adults also frequently rely on contrasts and comparisons, as in the use of similes (e.g., X is like Y) or metaphors (e.g., X is a Y), when learning new terms. Although still in the process of being developed, lexical contrast theory promises to provide a more comprehensive framework for studying the acquisition of word meaning than either semantic feature or functional core theory.

Most investigators seem to agree that speech comprehension develops earlier and faster than speech production (Benedict, 1979; Goldin-Meadow, Seligman, & Gelman, 1976; Huttenlocher, 1974). In Benedict's (1979) study, infants could understand 50 words before they were able to produce 10. Although young children are limited in their productive vocabulary, they show a strong desire to communicate. They will often employ a single word, usually a noun, to cover much more than the conventional meaning of the word—a phenomenon coined **overextension.** For example, a child may use the word *doggie* to refer to all four-legged animals or the word *papa* to refer to all males (much to the embarrassment of *mama*). A less-studied phenomenon is **underextension,** in which the child uses a word to refer to less than is generally conveyed by the word. For example, the child says the word *car* to refer only to a toy car, not to cars on the street or cars in television commercials. Because it involves the absence of appropriate word usage, underextension is more difficult to observe and understand.

Adults show the same tendencies as children in speech comprehension and production. For example, we understand many different varieties of English (Australian English, North American English), even though we may be incapable of producing them verbally (Clark, 1983). We also have a huge *receptive vocabulary* of words that we recognize when we hear, but seldom produce.

Ages 2–5

After the one-word stage, new developments in semantics and syntax occur rapidly. Toward the end of the second year of life, children begin to use two-word utterances but pause noticeably between words, as in "Mommy" (pause) "car" (L. Bloom, 1973). These pauses do not appear later in language development. Holophrases are still used to some degree.

By approximately age 2, children start to produce multiword utterances on a more regular basis, beginning with two-word combinations. R. Brown (1973) has described the major characteristics of these two-word utterances. He has suggested that the child's speech at this stage is characterized by semantic completeness because it expresses a complete idea, though it may lack less informative or communicatively nonessential words (e.g., articles, conjunctions, prepositions). R. Brown has called this type of speech **telegraphic speech** because it sounds like the abbreviated speech we hear in a telegram (e.g., *Mom. Broke. Send money.*). Parents may hear the child say "me tired" or "more milk."

Many investigators feel that the study of syntax is possible only when words are combined, as in two-word combinations. Early attempts to describe the syntactical structure of the child's speech used a gramatical system called **pivot–open grammar** (Braine, 1963), which argues that children's speech can be broken into *pivot* words and *open* words, and certain syntactical rules determine how these words are combined. Pivot words consist mostly of adjectival words (e.g., *allgone, on, bye-bye*) and are only a small proportion of the child's vocabulary. Pivot words are attached to the larger class of open words, which are mostly nouns (e.g., *milk, sock, dada*). Children combine these two classes of words into sentences such as "all-gone milk," "sock on," and "bye-bye dada." Formation of these sentences follows specific syntactical rules: pivot words never occur alone; open words can occur alone or in combination with a pivot word; pivot words can occur in the first or second position, but not both.

The pivot–open grammar system came under heavy attack because it appeared to oversimplify the complexity of a child's speech. As R. Brown (1973) has pointed out, even at age 2, children are not restricted to two-word sentences. Using an index called the MLU (mean length of utterance), R. Brown has shown that children intermingle three- and four-word utterances with their single-word and two-word utterances. And Brown has charged that pivot–open grammar fails to capture the semantic richness of these utterances. A famous example is the utterance of a 21-month-old, "mommy sock" (L. Bloom, 1970, pp. 5–6). Bloom indicated that this utterance was produced in many different contexts, apparently with different meanings. In one context, the utterance referred to the mother's sock, but in another context the mother was putting the child's sock on the child's foot.

A more productive approach than pivot–open grammar uses semantic categories such as agent-action, agent-object, and action-object. These semantic relations are present in the two-word utterances of children, as Table 5.3 shows.

Between ages 2–5, the length and complexity of children's sentences increase. Children become capable of regularly forming sentences with four or five words using the subject-verb-object form that characterizes the sentence structure of adults. One major change that occurs during this time is the mastery of several forms of *inflectional morphemes.* Inflections include plural endings, verb tense, and possessive forms.

R. Brown (1973) studied the order in which three children, whom he called Adam, Eve, and Sarah, acquired inflections. He recorded segments of spontaneous speech between these children and their mothers (an audio recording of spontaneous speech is called a *corpora*). In analyzing the data, R. Brown noted the occurrence of inflections, prepositions, articles, and auxiliary verbs. As Table 5.4 shows, children added 14 grammatical morphemes to their speech in much the same order. Children first acquired the present progressive verb form—"I eating," "I walking," "I playing." Next came the prepositions *in* and *on*, which

Table 5.3
Semantic Relations in Two-Word Sentences

Semantic Relation	Form[a]	Example
1. Nomination	that + N	that book
2. Notice	hi + N	hi belt
3. Recurrence	more + N, 'nother + N	more milk
4. Nonexistence	allgone + N, no more + N	allgone rattle
5. Attributive	Adj + N	big train
6. Possessive	N + N	mommy lunch
7. Locative	N + N	sweater chair
8. Locative	V + N	walk street
9. Agent-Action	N + V	Eve read
10. Agent-Object	N + N	mommy sock
11. Action-Object	V + N	put book

Note: From *Psycholinguistics* (p. 220) by R. Brown, 1970, New York: Free Press. Copyright 1970 by the Free Press, a division of Macmillan, Inc.
[a]N = noun, Adj = adjective, V = verb.

are both early spatial concepts, followed by the plural ending /-s/. Irregular past tense endings were mastered next—"I came," "It broke," "I ate." This order progressed through the contractible copulas or connecting verbs, such as the verb *be* ("That's mama") to the contractible progressive auxiliary ("I'm talking").

Why these stages unfold in a nearly uniform order is not know. R. Brown (1973) has suggested that perhaps the morphemic forms mastered early in the sequence are grammatically less complex than those mastered later in the sequence. There may also be a difference in the semantic difficulty of the 14 levels. For example, use of the present progressive verb form (e.g., "I walking") requires only that children understand that an action can endure over time. However, understanding the third-person irregular (e.g., "He has walked") requires a comprehension of present-past relationships and subject-object differentiation.

MacWhinney (1978) has offered **functionality** as an alternative explanation for the regularity of this sequence. "Functionality" refers to the degree to which the child wishes to express an intention. According to this argument, it is more important (i.e., more functional) for a child to express plurality, location, and possession than the copulas or third-person verb inflections. This argument fits nicely into the stages in the development of intentional communication described earlier.

As Table 5.4 shows, children acquire morphemes with irregular

Table 5.4
Grammatical Morphemes in Customary Order of Acquisition

Morpheme	Meanings Expressed or Presupposed	Examples
Present progressive	Temporary duration	I walk*ing*.
In	Containment	*In* basket.
On	Support	*On* floor.
Plural	Number	Two ball*s*.
Past irregular[a]	Earlierness[b]	It *broke*.
Possessive inflection	Possession	Adam*'s* ball.
Uncontractible copula[c]	Number; earlierness	There it *is*.
Articles	Specific-nonspecific	That *a* book. That *the* dog.
Past regular	Earlierness	Adam walk*ed*.
Third person regular	Number; earlierness	He walk*s*.
Third person irregular	Number; earlierness	He *does*. She *has*.
Uncontractible progressive auxiliary	Temporary duration; number; earlierness	This *is* go*ing*.
Contractible copula[d]	Number; earlierness	That*'s* book.
Contractible progressive auxiliary	Temporary duration; number; earlierness	I*'m* walk*ing*.

Note: From *A First Language: The Early Stages* (pp. 274 & 369) by R. Brown, 1973, Cambridge, MA: Harvard University Press. Copyright 1973 by Harvard University Press. Reprinted by permission.
[a]Formation of past tense by means other than *-ed*.
[b]Denotes understanding that an actor or state may occur before the time of utterance.
[c]Use of the verb *to be* as a main verb without contraction.
[d]Use of the verb *to be* as a main verb with contraction.

forms before those with regular forms. Much of the language used around the child—*broke, ate, drank, hit, threw*—is irregular past tense. Children probably learn these forms by rote memorization. Once children begin to use regular verb tense endings—*jumped, walked, played*—they tend to extend these endings inappropriately. The phenomenon of overextending rules for forming past tense is known as **overregularization,** or overgeneralization. Suddenly, children who correctly said "I broke," "I ate," and "I went" begin to say "I broked," "I eated," and "I goed." Children experience similar problems when learning the plural endings of nouns. The plural of *foot* becomes *foots* and *mouse* turns into *mouses.* These errors eventually disappear, but may occasionally be heard even in elementary school.

From ages 3–3½ years, children's simple sentences continue to develop through the addition of auxiliary verb forms that make their questions and negatives sound more adult-like (Whitehurst, 1982). Questions have been extensively studied because of their importance to a child's comprehension of the world. Initially, children use rising intonation at the end of a sentence to signal a question, such as "Dada sleepy?" Later, an auxiliary verb is added, such as "Why dada is sleepy?" However, the auxiliary verb is not inverted until later, when we hear the correct phrase "Why is dada sleepy?"

As question length and complexity increase, children begin to generate wh- questions (where? what? who? why? when? in this order). Notice that the first three questions refer to location (where?), objects (what?), and agents (who?). Questions about causality (why?) and time (when?) seem to be more difficult for children to master. Word order inversions are also commonplace, such as "Why you are thirsty?"

By 5 years of age, a child has succeeded in mastering most of the essential syntactical and semantical elements of the English language system. Sentences become longer and more complicated as children add connectives, relative clauses, passives, and indirect objects. For example, instead of stating two ideas separately, the child uses compound or coordinate sentences (e.g., "I gave Jimmy my toy, and he broke it"). Children tend to put events together in the temporal order in which they occurred.

Later Developments

It has become customary to view a child's language development as essentially complete by age 5. Most writers see language development after this time as mainly characterized by grammatical refinement, addition of a sophisticated vocabulary, and growing semantic awareness. Despite the importance of early language accomplishments, considerable language development occurs after age 5 (Karmiloff-Smith, 1979; Palermo & Molfese, 1972). This should not be surprising because many fundamental cognitive changes occur throughout later childhood and, from several theoretical perspectives, language depends on cognition. In this section, some of these changes are examined, starting with phonological development and proceeding to syntactical and semantic development.

Phonological development after age 5 has been a neglected topic in the developmental literature. Most of the available literature focuses on phoneme production. Templin (1957) found significant increases in the articulation of sounds after age 5 in response to pictures, written words, and an experimenter's oral example. Children showed improvement in their ability to combine clusters of consonants in a series, such as /lfth/ in twelfth. The phonological rules for these consonant blends are more complex than those involving consonant-vowel clusters. In addition, Templin (1957) reported that children become better able to enunciate consonants appearing late in a consonant series. These late consonants usually are the most difficult to pronounce and even give adult speakers trouble, especially when people speak rapidly. By age 8 children's articulation is essentially like adults'.

Two explanations have been offered for age differences in phonological ability: (1) children fail to discriminate among the acoustic cues; (2) they have difficulty with the articulatory gestures. The little evidence available points to articulation problems, not acoustical cue difficulties (see Eimas, Siqueland, Jusczyk, & Vigorito, 1971). The fact that children have little trouble producing sounds in the initial position, but may have trouble making sounds later in a sound sequence seems to indicate articulatory difficulties. Adults too show greater variability in their articulation of consonants in medial (middle) and final positions.

Other phonological developments after age 5 were demonstrated in Berko's (1958) classic investigation of inflectional endings (e.g., plurals, past tense, possessives, third-person singular). Berko presented children aged 4–7 with pictures that were referred to by a nonsense word. She presented a picture of a nonsense animal and said "Here's a *wug.*" Then she presented two more pictures and said, "Here are two others, now there are two _____." She found that the majority of children at all age levels could add the correct plural ending, or *allomorph* /-z/, to form *wugs,* but that the oldest children gave a higher percentage of correct responses than the youngest children. However, when she used a more complicated plural ending /-əz/ as in "This is a gutch. Now there are two _____," children's performance dropped dramatically to less than 40 percent correct. Thus, children may improve their ability to extend some plural endings to new, unfamiliar words, but this does not necessarily prove that they possess a general morphological rule for forming all plural endings. They still need to perfect their knowledge of simple plurals and other inflectional endings.

Deep Structure–Surface Structure Relations

Turning to syntactical development beyond age 5, we find a large number of studies. For the most part, these studies are within the framework of transformational grammar proposed by N. Chomsky. **Transformational grammar** is concerned not only with the surface arrangement of words in a sentence but also with the abstract structures that underlie sentences (Slobin, 1979). It consists of a set of transformational rules for converting the **deep structure** of sentences into **surface structure.** Deep structure involves the abstract relations between words, such as between nouns and verbs, as well as the intended meaning of a sentence. Surface structure refers to the phonological features of words and their order in a sentence. Transformational grammar thus is a syntactical device for relating the underlying deep meaning of a sentence to the surface sounds. The following two sentences should help clarify the meaning of these concepts.

1. Mary threw the ball.
2. The ball was thrown by Mary.

These sentences have different surface structures—sentence 1 is active past tense, and sentence 2 is in the passive voice. But both convey the same meaning and therefore have identical deep structures. Now consider this sentence:

They are eating apples.

Here we have a case of one surface structure with two different deep structures—either some people are eating apples, or the apples are intended for eating. Some other examples are "Visiting relatives can be a nuisance" and "They are shooting psychologists." According to N. Chomsky, the capacity to understand deep structure is prewired into the human brain and gives us the ability to learn language.

A few studies have examined developmental changes in mastery of deep structure–surface structure relations (C. Chomsky, 1969; Kessel, 1970; Morsbach & Steel, 1976). For example, Kessel (1970) employed an imaginary hide-and-seek game in which 6–12-year-old children had to decide which of two dolls would be hiding and which seeking. The decision was made on the basis of eight declarative sentences read to each child. Half of the sentences had the form "Lucy was eager to see," and half had the form "Lucy was easy to see." Both sentences have identical surface forms (subject-verb-adjective-infinitive verb), but they convey very different messages. In the first case *Lucy* is the subject of the infinitive verb *to see* and *eager* is an adjective qualifying *Lucy*. In the second case *Lucy* is the object of *to see*, and there is an implicit subject. Kessel's results showed that 6-year-old children made more errors by assigning the incorrect subject to the infinitive verb in this latter case—that is, *Lucy* was interpreted as the subject of *to see* rather than the object. By 9 years of age, children could make the eager-easy distinction without error.

Why do children have so much difficulty in comprehending the underlying meaning of the second sentence above? According to Carol Chomsky (1969), it is because the sentences violate the **minimum distance principle** (MDP). In sentences that conform to this principle, the noun (or pronoun) phrase immediately preceding the infinitive is the subject of the verb. Consider the following sentences:

1. John wanted Bill to leave.
2. John promised Bill to leave.

Sentence 1 conforms to the MDP because the subject of the verb *wanted* is the immediately preceding noun *John*, and the subject of the infinitive *to leave* is the preceding noun *Bill*. Sentence 2, however, violates the MDP because *John* is the subject of both the verb *promised* and the infinitive *to leave*, even though *Bill* is the noun immediately preceding the infinitive. In her research, C. Chomsky (1969) has shown that children aged 5–9 inappropriately apply the MDP to verbs (such as *promises*) that break the grammatical rule. Thus, they will interpret sentence 2 to mean the same as sentence 1 (i.e., Bill will be leaving in both instances).

Developmental psycholinguists have traditionally assumed that children master most of the elements of syntax by age 5. Although 5-year-olds make deep structure–surface structure distinctions this early (see Morsbach & Steel, 1976), the children are incorrect about as often as they are correct. Not until age 9 or 10 do children consistently comprehend the underlying surface ambiguities.

Expanding Vocabularies

Let us now consider some major trends in later semantical development. To begin, there are increases in vocabulary from age 5 throughout the life span. Because the average adult may have 30,000 or more vocabulary words, the child has a long way to go. In one of the most comprehensive studies of children's vocabulary growth, M. Smith (1926) reported that vocabulary increased from no words at 8 months to almost 2500 words by 6 years. Research on adult development shows that vocabulary continues to grow. Kausler and Puckett (1980) collected vocabulary test scores from subjects 20–70 years of age as part of their study on paired-associate learning (see Chapter 6). Their results reveal progressive increases in vocabulary ability through age 70 (see Figure 5.3).

While most other adult developmental studies show similar trends, evidence suggests that not every aspect of vocabulary continues to improve across the life span. Botwinick and Storandt (1974b) examined definitions given to vocabulary words on the Wechsler Adult Intelligence Scale by young (17–20 years) and old (62–83 years) adult subjects. Botwinick and Storandt scored the responses in the traditional quantitative way, but also analyzed qualitative differences. The age groups did not differ overall in quantitative test scores, but young adults gave qualitatively superior definitions of the test words compared to the old adults.

Figure 5.3   Mean scores (maximum score equals 40) on a vocabulary test for groups of young, middle-aged, and elderly subjects.

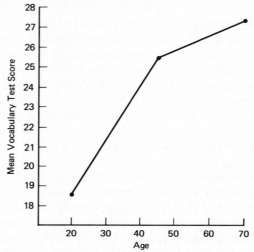

From *Experimental Psychology and Human Aging* (p.55) by D. H. Kausler, 1982. New York: Wiley. Copyright 1982 by John Wiley & Sons, Inc. Reprinted by permission.

Other Semantic Developments

Developmental studies on changes in vocabulary across the life span reveal little about changes in the semantic system. In general, development of semantics parallels other changes in the cognitive system. As the child gets older, the two systems of cognition and language become more interconnected. Language begins to refer not only to present concrete objects and events but also to hypothetical, abstract ones in the past, present, or future.

Exploration of later semantic development has proceeded along several routes. One line of investigation uses word association studies in which an experimenter says a word, and the subject is supposed to say the first word that comes to mind. When children under age 6 perform this task, their word associations are typically **syntagmatic;** that is, response words fit into a common sequence and are a different part of speech than the stimulus word (e.g., the child responds to the word *deep* with the word *hole*). Children beyond age 8 most often give a response word that is the same part of speech as the stimulus word and could replace it in a sentence, such as *deep* and *shallow* (Ervin, 1961; K. Nelson, 1973a). Word associations that are the same part of speech as the stimulus word are called **paradigmatic associations.**

This syntagmatic-paradigmatic shift may coincide with a child's acquisition of rules governing form classes such as nouns and verbs. Older children, like adults, classify words in terms of grammatical categories such as parts of speech or other categories such as animate-inanimate, large-small, and bright-dull. This semantic organization helps children and adults quickly and efficiently retrieve information from memory when needed (see Chapter 6). If I ask you to name the "large powerful mammal of the cat family found primarily in Africa and considered king of the beasts," you will quickly answer "lion." You don't have to search your entire semantic memory system to recall this information.

Some investigators have wondered whether changes in semantic organization in old age are accompanied by a return to a use of syntagmatic word associations (D. Denney, 1972), but not much research has been directed to this question. In some early work, K. Riegel and Riegel (1964) reported that the number of syntagmatic responses in an older adult group (above age 55) showed a slight increase relative to a younger comparison group (aged 17–19). However, both age groups preferred paradigmatic over syntagmatic associations. Because this was a cross-sectional comparison, the effects of cohort factors are difficult to rule out.

Another area of investigation of later semantic development concerns a person's knowledge or awareness of the rules of language, which is called **metalinguistic knowledge** (deVilliers & deVilliers, 1974). Although children master basic grammar by age 5, they do not show a conscious awareness of grammatical rules and relations until later. In their study, deVilliers and deVilliers asked eight children to play a game with two puppets. Children were asked to teach one puppet to speak properly who "said things all the wrong way round." The puppet spoke imperatives with correct (e.g., "Eat the cake") or reversed ("Cake the eat") word order, which the child had to judge as "right" or "wrong." Most of the children who offered corrections knew that something was wrong with the reversed word-order sentences. When required to correct what was wrong, however, they focused on the semantics of the sentence. Thus, one cannot conclude from these results that children necessarily know the grammatical structure of the language. Metalinguistic knowledge continues to increase throughout childhood and adulthood. Box 5.1 discusses children's development of literacy.

We have spent considerable time describing the sequence of early and later language development. This material should give you an appreciation of the scope and complexity of language acquisition. By no means have we exhausted the subject, and the interested reader should refer to the "Suggested Readings" at the end of this chapter.

Box 5.1   The Development of Literacy

How children learn literacy skills such as reading and writing is of major concern to cognitive developmental psychologists. The literature on literacy is vast, but psychologists know relatively little about how the ability to read and write relates to more general trends in cognitive development. David Olson and Nancy Torrance (1983) have argued that the cognitive consequences of literacy stem from the child's learning to treat language as an object in its own right, which has a certain structure; is comprised of sounds, words, and sentences; and has a complex semantic structure or meaning. They refer to these aspects of language as *metalanguage*, and claim that the acquisition of a metalanguage is related either directly or indirectly to literacy. (The notion of metalanguage is similar to the notion of metalinguistic knowledge, but the former does not assume that awareness is a conscious psychological process.)

Children's mastery of metalanguage in the early school years has some important intellectual consequences. One is the ability to distinguish between what words or sentences say and what they mean. In discussing their research program, Olson and Torrance (1983) have pointed out that children and adults who can distinguish between the structure of language and its content can solve problems which are not solvable by persons who fail to make this distinction. For example, Hildyard and Olson (1982) gave preschoolers and schoolchildren an inference task involving complex verbs. Children were presented with sentence pairs such as the following:

John forced Mary to eat the worm.
John forced Mary to eat the ice cream.

Notice that the verb *force* implies that Mary did not wish to eat either item, but she did eat them. The results revealed significant age differences in the types of inferences drawn from the sentences. The preschoolers' inferences seemed to be largely based on their real-world expectancies. In response to the first sentence, they reasoned that Mary did not eat the worm because "nobody eats worms." To the second sentence they responded that Mary ate the ice cream because "everybody likes ice cream." Children with a few years of school answered quite differently. They treated the sentences literally and differentiated between the sentences' actual meaning and spoken meaning. Apparently, through activities such as reading and writing, children come to realize that language has its own structure. Reading and writing seem to draw attention to the form and surface structure of language in a way that speaking does not. These two literacy skills are only one source of knowledge about metalanguage. Conversations with literate adults, class discussions, and preschool literacy activities may also be important determinants of metalinguistic concepts (Olson & Torrance, 1983).

EXPLAINING LANGUAGE DEVELOPMENT

We now turn to an even more demanding task—explaining language development. All theories of language development must account for the remarkable rapidity and uniformity with which children acquire such an abstract linguistic system. The difficulties encountered by theorists who try to explain language development illustrate how complex language is. In this section, three major theories of language acquisition will be examined: (1) learning theories, (2) biological theories, and (3) cognitive theories. Each of these theories can explain some, but not all, aspects of language development. An interactional synthesis that blends the best of the three approaches into one multidimensional, multicausal linguistic system will then be proposed.

Learning Theories

A commonsense approach to language development is that language is learned like many other behaviors (e.g., sitting, jumping, swimming). And the language learned is the language of one's culture. Children growing up in English-speaking families learn to speak English, not Chinese or Spanish. Thus, various learning mechanisms appear to be at work. What are some of these mechanisms?

Imitation

In early learning theory accounts, the linguistic environment was assigned a major role. Parents and others served as linguistic models, and children learned language through processes such as *imitation* and *reinforcement*. Children probably learn some of their language directly or indirectly by observing verbal models and trying to imitate them. Most likely, many vocabulary words and noun and verb forms (especially irregular ones) are acquired in this manner.

While imitation may account for the acquisition of a number of utterances, it cannot explain the fact that children utter thousands of novel phrases and sentences they never heard nor spoke previously. It is unlikely that parents model phrases such as *bye-bye sock, all-gone mommy,* or *set chair,* yet these are the utterances we hear children using.

Another difficulty with imitation explanations is that children do not imitate many language forms, in spite of repeated attempts by parents and others to model such forms. The following example gives you an idea of the frustrating attempts to correct the sentence of a 2-year-old named Ben.

BEN: I like these candy. I like they.
ADULT: You like them?
BEN: Yes. I like they.
ADULT: Say *them.*
BEN: Them.
ADULT: Say "I like *them.*"
BEN: I like them.
ADULT: Good.
BEN: I'm good. These candy good too.
ADULT: Are they good?
BEN: Yes. I like they. You like they? (Kuczaj, 1982, p. 48)

Despite repeated attempts by the adult, Ben continues to use his own rules of speech. And most attempts by parents to model language in the above way stop long before the child achieves linguistic competence.

Reinforcement

In his behavioristic account of language learning in *Verbal Behavior,* B. F. Skinner (1957) used reinforcement as the major explanatory principle: "A child acquires verbal behavior when relatively unpatterned vocalizations, selectively reinforced, assume forms which produce appropriate consequences in a given verbal community" (p. 31).

Skinner's assumption is that the child initially produces speech sounds such as cooing and babbling which the parents selectively reward by talking back, smiling, stroking, and so on. Consequently, babies make the same sounds again. In their eager anticipation of their child's first word, parents will even reinforce rough approximations, such as *daw* for *dog,* but not *baw.* Through gradual shaping and reward, children acquire an initial vocabulary. Later, parents reinforce grammatically correct word orders and meanings by repeating sentences to children and rewarding them for imitating. In this way, children gradually acquire more and more complex stimulus-response chains.

Like the imitation explanation, reinforcement theory accounts appear plausible. But for such accounts to be true, it must be shown that parents selectively reinforce childhood utterances and their attempts have a faciliatory effect on the process of learning phonetics, syntax, and semantics. Most available evidence suggests that this is not the case. In his landmark study, R. Brown (1973) pointed out that parents are more likely to reward children for the *truth value* or *accuracy* of their sentences than for their grammatical correctness. A toddler who points to the sky and says "The sky is green" is not likely to be rewarded, in spite of having uttered a grammatically correct statement; whereas a child who puts down an empty glass and says "I drinked all my milk" receives approving nods. Ironically, these early reinforcement patterns seem to produce adults who can use correct grammar, but who are not always known for being truthful!

Even more damaging to reinforcement theory is the fact that attempts to reward a child do not have a great impact on later language development. K. Nelson (1973a) observed such attempts in her comprehensive study of early language acquisition. She found that mothers who systematically corrected mispronunciations of words and rewarded good pronunciations had children who acquired vocabulary more slowly than parents who were more tolerant of speech errors.

Some evidence suggests that language can be acquired through reinforcement under limited circumstances. For example, various reinforcement programs have been successful in dealing with delayed language in autistic children (see Lovaas, 1977). But these programs are not really convincing proof that language is acquired this way under natural circumstances.

One final criticism of the reinforcement approach to language development is its failure to account for the sequential regularity and rapidity in language acquisition. If each child has a different reinforcement history, then the pattern of language development should vary with each individual child. Although the timing of language learning varies to some extent (e.g., children acquire first words at 9–14 months), the sequencing is the same (e.g., first words are acquired before two-word utterances, the active voice is acquired before the passive voice). Perhaps even more importantly, children tend to make the same mistakes at about the same point, such as when they overgeneralize rules for forming plural and past tense endings. The rapidity of language acquisition does not necessarily rule out reinforcement explanations. A great deal of learning can occur in a short time; for example, children aged 2–6 learn an average nine new vocabulary words per day (Carey, 1978). However, it seems unlikely that so much could be learned so quickly unless the organism has some predisposition to language learning.

Biological Theories

Biological approaches to language assume that human beings have an innate predisposition or predetermination to acquire and use language. (Animals' communication is discussed in Box 5.2.) This assumption is

Box 5.2   Animal Language

From infancy, human beings show a strong tendency to communicate through language. Animals also communicate with each other—cats meow angrily at other cats, bees dance to signal the direction and distance of nectar to other bees, birds chirp noisily at other birds. Are these communications signs of language?

Several early investigations attempted to teach our closest animal relative, the chimpanzee, to speak. Because chimpanzees possess a larynx, similar to human beings, for centuries chimpanzees were thought capable of articulating human speech (we now know that the vocal apparatus for speech is located in the supralaryngeal tract, which is not well developed in infrahuman primates). Of the numerous attempts to teach chimpanzees to talk, only one enjoyed even modest success. Keith Hayes and Cathy Hayes (1951) taught a young chimpanzee, Viki, to utter human speech sounds by manipulating her mouth and lips. After six years of extensive training, Viki could produce very rough approximations of the words *mama, papa,* and *cup.* Such results suggest that chimpanzees cannot learn to talk, but this does not necessarily mean they are incapable of acquiring language.

Chimpanzees may be able to learn a sign language. R. Gardner and Beatrice Gardner (1978) used a version of American Sign Language (ASL, or "Ameslan") to teach vocabulary words to an 11-month-old chimpanzee named Washoe. David Premack (1976) taught a chimpanzee named Sarah to communicate by choosing among a set of physical objects used as symbols for words. Both studies obtained remarkable results. After four years of training, Washoe learned about 160 ASL signs and could occasionally combine signs to generate new sentences. Sarah performed various linguistic tasks with a 75–80 percent accuracy rate and showed an understanding of complex relations.

These studies offer impressive evidence that chimpanzees can master some aspects of language learning. Nevertheless, many investigators have noted that such accomplishments resulted from painstaking training, not from the natural course of language evolution. One of the harshest critics of this research has been Herbert Terrace (1979), who began as a supporter of chimp language. Terrace and colleagues at Columbia University taught a male chimpanzee Neam Chimpsky ("Nim" for short) to use ASL. Unlike many other investigators in this area, Terrace videotaped all the training sessions and analyzed the videotapes. He found no evidence that Nim could combine symbols to form new sentences in spite of his ability to learn vocabulary words. Rather, most of

Nim's multiword utterances had been prompted by the gestures and actions of a trainer. Terrace concluded that chimpanzees' ability to learn language can be explained in terms of simple conditioning principles. The animals do not demonstrate a knowledge of more complex language forms such as syntactical relations, semantic organization, or pragmatical rules.

Some psychologists believe that even if chimpanzees could learn to master basic linguistic forms, they would not use language to communicate with other chimpanzees or to teach their offspring language. However, R. Fouts and Fouts (1985) have reported on a young chimpanzee named Loulis, who has learned from another chimp to communicate with sign language. Loulis's teacher was Washoe, the chimp with whom R. Gardner and Gardner (1978) had worked. Over a five-year period, Loulis learned 55 signs from Washoe and spontaneously "conversed" with Washoe and other chimpanzees using sign language, even when the experimenters were not present. These findings imply that chimpanzees may have the capacity to master a communication system with many of the same basic features as human language, although the scope and flexibility of this system remain in doubt.

expressed in Noam Chomsky's (1957) notion of a "language acquisition device," or LAD. Probably the most detailed treatment of the biological approach has been given by linguist Eric Lenneberg. In his theoretical essay, *Biological Foundations of Language*, Lenneberg (1967) presented his thesis that language is an integral part of the biological and evolutionary heritage of the individual. His theory contends that not only do biological determinants predispose human beings to language development but they also shape the course of language acquisition in children. As evidence, Lenneberg pointed to the sequential regularity in language learning in all normal children around the world. In spite of wide environmental and cultural variations, children begin to babble at about 6 months, utter their first word at 1 year, make two-word utterances by the end of their second year, and master the basic syntax of their native language by the time they are 4 or 5 years old. Lenneberg sees this whole process as maturationally determined and likens it to other maturational processes such as motor development. Where motor development is slowed, as in Down's syndrome children, language unfolds in the regular sequence but is slow to develop. In normal children as well, motor development is more predictive of language development than mental level, at least up to 18 months of age (L. Siegel, 1981).

As further support for the biological basis of language, Lenneberg suggested that there may be a critical period of language acquisition, roughly from ages 2–12. For instance, children appear to acquire language rather effortlessly, but adults must expend great effort. Think of how difficult it is for an adult to acquire even 1000 new vocabulary words in a second language. Furthermore, in cases where speech is disrupted by brain damage, the prognosis is poor if the damage occurred after puberty; prior to puberty individuals seem to recover completely and fully most of their lost speech functions (Lenneberg, 1967).

While much of Lenneberg's biological position is highly speculative and conjectural, there is limited evidence of a critical period in language learning. In a well-publicized case in California, a 13-year-old girl named Genie was discovered after having been deprived of language for all the years of her life (Curtiss, 1977). After six years of intensive training, Genie was able to speak in simple sentences. However, she failed to master certain aspects of language such as *proforms* (e.g., *which*, *that*), passive voice, and auxiliary verbs. Her language level remained at the telegraphic two- and three-word speech of the young child. Apparently, a child has to be exposed to language well before age 13 if language is to develop normally.

If a critical period of language learning exists, what mechanisms underlie it? Lenneberg (1967) suggested that the critical period of language development may be related to *brain lateralization.* In his view, the left hemisphere of the brain is lateralized for language function around age 2. He based his conclusion on clinical data collected from patients such as infants who have lost their left hemisphere. Lenneberg theorized that prior to age 2, neither hemisphere is more involved in verbal processing.

Lenneberg's observations have gotten support in studies on brain-damaged individuals. Figure 5.4 shows that certain areas of the cerebral cortex are devoted to language function. These areas are found in the superior temporal cortex and the frontal cortex. If the brain is damaged in these areas (located in right-handers' left hemispheres and in left-handers' right hemispheres), a condition known as **aphasia** may result. Persons with aphasia show a variety of language dysfunctions including an inability to talk, to understand language, or both. Their articulatory organs (lips, tongue, larynx) remain functional, but they lose their ability to use these organs for speech purposes.

Studies on aphasic individuals leave little doubt that certain areas of the brain have evolved for language function, but the role of the brain in language use remains uncertain. For example, not everyone suffering damage in the areas shown in Figure 5.4 experiences speech impairment. Moreover, language function may be disrupted even if damage is not linked to speech areas. Considerable controversy also surrounds the

Figure 5.4 Parts of the brain associated with language-related activities (speech and language functioning).

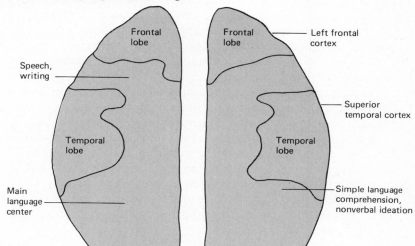

question of brain lateralization and language development. Lenneberg's ideas about lateralization at age 2 have been challenged by findings of lateralized brain function in early infancy (see Eimas, 1975). As children develop, language becomes increasingly lateralized, but this process is not complete until late childhood. Some writers (see D. Cohen & Wu, 1980) have suggested that language lateralization is a process that continues across the life span.

The impact of aging on aphasia is another controversial issue. Although no research exists on monolinguals, evidence on bilinguals and polyglots (those speaking more than two languages) indicates that the form of aphasia depends on the age of onset. Alpert (cited in D. Cohen & Wu, 1980) reported that younger patients are more vulnerable to motor (or expressive) aphasias, older patients to sensory (or receptive) aphasias. Alpert suggested that memory processes in the aged may play a major role in language retrieval failures (see Chapter 6).

Cognitive Theories

As a reaction to biologically based theories of language, some investigators have proposed that language acquisition can be explained on the basis of the principles of cognitive psychology. The cognitive approach assumes that the course of language development is interpretable by the general mechanisms governing cognitive development. Piaget made a similar claim in describing the relation between language and cognition. As you will recall, he felt that cognitive structures emerge before language and guide subsequent language development. However, Piaget was not very explicit about how our cognitions influence language learning.

Several studies on cognitive approaches to language have appeared (L. Bloom, 1970; McNeill, 1970). In a paper on the cognitive basis of language learning in infants, Macnamara (1972) argued that infants first try to understand the meaning of words spoken to them and only later work out the relation between meaning and language, so that "the infant uses meaning as a clue to language, rather than language as a clue to meaning" (p. 1). Thus, Macnamara, like Piaget, distinguishes between children's linguistic systems and their cognitive intentions. This interpretation has been called the "strong cognition hypothesis." The findings cited earlier for the overextension-underextension phenomena support this hypothesis. Children's own concepts, not the words spoken by parents, seem to dictate whether they use a wide or narrow range of words to describe an object or event.

Several writers have noted that using cognition as the basis for all language learning oversimplifies the complexities involved. One major problem that cognitive theories brush over is the *mapping problem* (M. Rice, 1982), or the lack of perfect correspondence between linguistic and nonlinguistic forms of knowledge, and the difficulties in going from one kind of knowledge to the other. For example, children learn certain linguistic rules about grammatical acceptability. "Put the hat on," "put it on," and "put on the hat" are grammatically acceptable, but "put on it" is not (M. Rice, 1982). The "weak cognition hypothesis" (Cromer, 1981) is that cognitive theories can explain the meaning of these sentences, but not the acquisition of the formal linguistic rules.

Can we use cognitive learning principles to accelerate language development? William Fowler has addressed this question in a series of important experiments with Amy Swenson (Fowler & Swenson, 1979). Their approach assumes that language acquisition is a product of cognitive learning, rather than a result of biological maturation or simple operant conditioning. Children are taught by parents to learn a series of abstract language rules in a standard sequence. Numerous teaching techniques are used, including having the parents model certain words, engage in language play with their infants, and look at books together. Fowler and Swenson's (1979) results show rapid gains in the speed of language acquisition in the training group compared with a control group. Even more impressive is their finding that the training works for parents of various educational and linguistic backgrounds (English, Italian, Chinese). Thus, treating language acquisition as a cognitive learning process can lead to accelerated gains in linguistic skill.

Toward an Interactional Synthesis

We have now reviewed three potential explanations of language development—learning theories, biological theories, and cognitive theories. Our review should make clear that each approach has something important to contribute to our understanding of language. Some aspects of language (e.g., vocabulary) may be acquired by means of simple learning principles, but other aspects (e.g., word order) probably require more abstract cognitive rules. Language learning must build on a biological base that equips the organism for understanding and producing speech. Thus, an extreme view of language development as strictly environmental or strictly maturational seems untenable. A more productive alternative is an interactional approach combining elements of learning theories and biological theories with cognitive developmental principles. The form of such a synthesis can be seen in research on parental speech toward children.

According to traditional learning theory, parents selectively reinforce babbling sounds and gradually shape infant speech toward more adult-sounding utterances. However, the findings that parents reward truth value rather than correct speech, children create many novel sentences, and infants progress through identical stages of language contradict the learning position. On the other hand, the extreme biological view neglects the important help in language learning that the parents provide to children. When adults speak to other adults, they speak rapidly, using complex clauses and sentences to refer to events and objects, many of which are not present. However, when interacting with children, adults frequently modify their speech patterns by speaking at a slower rate, pausing between sentences, repeating key phrases, and using much simpler syntax. This style of speaking has come to be called baby talk, or **motherese** (Newport, 1976). Children as young as 4 and 5 use motherese when addressing children younger than themselves (Shatz & Gelman, 1973), and baby talk is sometimes addressed by adults to the elderly (see Box 5.3).

The earliest studies on motherese concentrated on describing the characteristics of mothers' speech (Molfese et al., 1982). These studies concluded that the speech of the mother was quite well adapted to the linguistic level of the infant. However, it was unclear exactly what mothers were reacting to in their infants—age, cuteness, linguistic inability, cognitive level? Snow (1972) found that mothers were not capable of producing fully formed motherese unless the child was present to cue them. This finding suggests that the use of motherese

Box 5.3   Baby Talk to the Elderly

To underscore its teaching function, researchers have called the simplified baby-talk register "motherese" and the speaker the "mommy linguist." However, baby talk is frequently directed to adults in a way not intended to teach them language. For example, in institutions such as nursing homes, caregiving staff members often address elderly residents using baby talk. This simplified speech to the elderly could be used to convey negative messages of dependency and childhood status to the elderly (Ferguson, 1977; Tamir, 1979); or it could be used to communicate warmth, nurturance, and affection. There is not a great deal of empirical information on this important topic.

Linda Caporael (1981) conducted a field study to investigate the language environment of the institutionalized elderly and to explore the relationship between baby-talk usage and characteristics of the elderly as rated by caregivers. For one month she tape-recorded interactions between caregivers (and visitors to the nursing home) and elderly residents during lunch time in the nursing facility's dining room. Three different categories of speech were transcribed and coded: (1) the speech from one caregiver to another (or between a caregiver and a visitor); (2) speech to elderly residents that was not baby talk; and (3) speech in baby talk. Of the almost 2000 sentences recorded, about 22 percent were classified as baby talk to the elderly. Interestingly, the caregivers' ratings of the elderly's characteristics (e.g., sociability, alertness, likability) did not correlate with the percentage of baby talk addressed to subjects. This finding suggests that baby talk to the elderly may be a sociolinguistic speech register rather than a fine-tuning mechanism used to adjust to the competencies of the listener (Caporael, 1981).

Caporael also had college students rate their impressions of baby talk and nonbaby talk on dimensions such as pleasantness, "comfortingness," irritation, and arousal. Contrary to predictions, students rated baby talk *more* positively than nonbaby talk, suggesting that baby talk to the elderly is perceived as conveying a nurturant message. Many questions remain unanswered. Do elderly adults perceive baby talk in the same way college students do? Perhaps a healthy and competent elderly person may see baby talk as demeaning, rather than nurturant. An even more fundamental question is why baby talk is used at all in nursing homes. If an older person is hard of hearing or has experienced cognitive losses, the simplified speech of baby talk may be necessary and adaptive (Tamir, 1979). Conversely, such speech may be used with subtle nonlinguistic cues to reinforce residents' feelings of dependency and powerlessness. Future research on these questions would have great practical and theoretical significance.

depends, in part, on the context of the mother-child interaction, including the linguistic cues provided by the child and the mother's responsiveness to them.

Recent studies have focused on what the mother is actually *doing* in conversational interactions with her infant. One striking finding is the extent to which a mother's speech is directed by a child's activities. Activities such as gazing, reaching, yawning, vocalizing, smiling, and even burping appear to evoke reliable responses from the mother. In fact, the mother's reactions have been described as "an attempt to establish a conversation and to keep the conversation going by giving the child the maximum opportunity to function as a conversational partner and by accepting even the most minimal of the child's behavior as an adequate 'turn'" (Molfese et al., 1982, p. 311). Snow (1978) has shown that mothers strike up "conversations" with infants as young as 3 months, and the nature of these interactions changes significantly over time. Mothers ask questions such as "What is it?" and "What can you see?" as a way of gaining 3-month-old infants' attention. With 7–12-month-olds, the same questions are used in the context of games and routines to direct the infants' attention to what the mothers are interested in. By the time the infant is 18 months, these questions begin to serve more of a tutorial or informational function.

Another thing that mothers do when carrying on a "conversation" with infants is to expand and continue their utterances. Mothers often do this by providing a **recast,** a sentence with the same core meaning as the original but with a simplified, limited structural change. For example, if the child says "daddy shoe," the mother might say "Yes, that's daddy's shoe" if the relationship is possessive, or "Yes, daddy is putting on his shoe" if the relationship seems to be an action-object form. Though mothers (and fathers, too) recast children's speech, the effects of recasting remain unclear. The small body of evidence suggests that by recasting utterances, parents are not trying to provide language lessons for the child, but are attempting to communicate with a linguistically immature individual. Thus, the effectiveness of what the mother does depends on her own activities and language-specific feedback as well as on the cognitive maturity level of the child. In a recent study, Gleitman, Newport, and Gleitman (1984) examined the relationship between the complexity of maternal speech and language growth among groups of 1½-year-old and 2-year-old children. For the younger children, they found a positive correlation between most aspects of mothers' speech (e.g., frequency of expansion, length of utterance, sentence complexity) and the increase in children's use of verbal auxiliaries across a 6-month period. Few significant correlations were found between maternal speech and older children's language development, except for a positive effect of maternal yes-no questions on auxiliary growth.

Gleitman et al. (1984) conclude that language is learnable if the input includes complex sentences, but is more difficult to learn if the input is restricted to the simplest sentences. This conclusion runs directly counter to the motherese hypothesis, which states that the child should receive the simplest input first, followed by more complex input later—the simpler the input, the faster and more error-free language learning will be. To explain this counterintuitive position, Gleitman et al. (1984) emphasize the simplicity of learning rather than the simplicity of grammar. They suggest that at the earliest stages of language learning children focus on stressed syllables, much like when they attend to certain salient aspects of a visual stimulus, and that they search for canonical (well-formed) sentences. Maternal input only affects the child insofar as it matches these "processing biases" of the learner. At later stages, children progressively attend to more complex stimuli, and maternal input becomes less effective. Contrary to the motherese hypothesis, the mother's input does not change, but the child's processing skills and the opportunities for learning provided by the native language do change.

The notion that the mother carries the greatest responsibility in the early learning of linguistic skills but that children reach a point developmentally where they perform these skills on their own is consistent with Vygotsky's (1962) view of language and cognition. As you recall, for Vygotsky, the transition from regulation by others to a regulation by self is a crucial developmental transformation. This transition can be best understood by examining the things that parents, caregivers, teachers, and other adults do to instruct children in using language and solving cognitive tasks.

According to Bruner and colleagues (Wood, Bruner, & Ross, 1976), adults support children's language learning by providing a **scaffold** for their activities. In building construction, a scaffold is designed to support a worker and to allow the worker to accomplish activities not otherwise possible. Similarly, in language learning, "instructors" selectively use a scaffold to extend the skills of the child and to simplify the child's task in the learning process. Scaffolding can be seen in the mother-child interaction during such activities as picture book "reading." Initially, the reading process is under the mother's control, and she encourages any participation from the child (Ninio & Bruner,

1978). Eventually a dramatic shift in responsibility occurs when the child acquires the ability to use labels. At this point the mother increases her expectation that a well-formed word will be produced instead of an unintelligible, babble-like sound. As is evident in this example, scaffolding is not the result of the mother's action, but represents an interaction between parent and child. The child's responses play a key role in shaping the nature and amount of scaffolding provided.

The emerging view is that the initial biologically prepared biases of the learner interact with the structural complexity of language to determine what, when, and how children learn from their mothers' speech. Environmental input is important, but only to the extent that it matches the initial biases of the learner and only within the limits of the conventions of each language. Most current theories emphasize the active role children play in acquiring and processing language. The role of social agents as active facilitators of children's language development is also being increasingly recognized. To play this role well requires that parents and caretakers function as more than passive language models.

INDIVIDUAL AND GROUP FACTORS INFLUENCING LANGUAGE

Remarkable regularity and uniformity are manifested in a child's language development. Regardless of family environment or culture, children seem to acquire language in much the same way. However, several writers have recommended that psycholinguists direct more attention to individual and group differences among children and adults in language abilities (Fillmore, Kempler, & Wang, 1979; K. Nelson, 1981). In their view, the environmental and cultural context of language use will ultimately determine its form and function. Because people are differentially exposed to different contexts, individuals will use different types of linguistic constructions.

In a study of adult-child interactions, Lieven (1978) collected longitudinal data on two pairs of children named Kate (age 18 months at the start of the study) and Beth (20 months). Although the children were similar in terms of their average sentence length or MLU, they seemed to use language for different purposes. Kate spoke slowly and pronounced words clearly. Her words usually referred to objects and events in the immediate environment (e.g., *dog, pretty, dolly*). In contrast, Beth appeared to speak more as a way of engaging her mother's attention; her speech was difficult to interpret, highly repetitive, and not very informative. Lieven (1978) related these differences to differences in the mothers' speech. Kate's mother responded to what her infant said with utterances that were closely related to those of her child. Beth's mother, on the other hand, was unresponsive and her speech was semantically unrelated to her child's speech, yet Beth eventually learned to speak normally. Thus, environmental input alone cannot explain children's language acquisition. Besides parental speech, what other factors might produce individual differences in language?

Sex Differences

One of the most common beliefs about language abilities is that women and girls are more verbally advanced than men and boys. Even in infancy, female babies seem to be more responsive to speech patterns, more easily startled by loud noises, and more spontaneously vocal than male babies. Moreover, it has been reported that girls begin to speak earlier and talk more than boys. Girls have been found to express themselves more frequently, switch from one-word to two-word utterances more rapidly, and develop a vocabulary of 50 words more rapidly than boys (see Klann-Delius, 1981). However, when the mean length of utterances is examined, there is no conclusive evidence of the superior verbal productivity in girls.

Later in development girls seem to take the lead in several areas of language, while in other areas consistent sex differences are not found. In phonological development, girls show better articulation skills and learn to read faster, at least in Western cultures. In addition, articulation difficulties such as stuttering occur with greater frequency among boys than among girls. Much less research has been done on sex differences in the acquisition of syntax, and the evidence reveals no clear trends. There are no obvious indications that girls acquire a syntactic rule system faster than boys. The same conclusions hold true for semantic development. No consistent sex differences have been observed either in the extent of vocabulary development or the conceptual structure of the lexicon (i.e., people's vocabulary). Finally, in the acquisition and use of pragmatic rules of language, girls have been observed to have more frequent and long-lasting conversational turns with their mothers (see Klann-Delius, 1981). However, there do not appear to be any demonstrable sex differences in communicative competence.

The current findings on sex differences and language development do not permit simple conclusions either for or against the verbal superiority of one sex. A major reason for the current state of confusion is that serious methodological shortcomings characterize the bulk of the research. Most studies are cross-sectional, not longitudinal, so that they tell us little about sex-related changes in language development processes. Moreover, they fail to control properly for confounding variables such as differential rearing patterns, cultural opportunity, developmental level, and experimenter sex. When these variables are controlled and adequate sample sizes employed, many observed sex differences disappear. As one reviewer of the current literature has concluded, "In the present state of language assessment the only tenable position is that there is NO significant difference between the sexes in linguistic ability" (Macauley, 1978, p. 361). This conclusion, while a reasonably accurate description of the findings concerning sex differences in language acquisition in infants and children, probably does not tell the whole developmental story. Psychologists in this area need to refine their methodology and take more of a theoretical point of view, examining areas where sex differences may be expected to occur. The domains of semantics and pragmatics appear to be especially fruitful areas for future research on sex differences in language among children.

What about sex differences in language in adulthood? Here again, the literature allows no clear-cut conclusions, but fewer studies seem to find sex differences in language in adolescence and adulthood than in childhood (Maccoby & Jacklin, 1974). Studies that report a sex difference find that women, on the average, are more advanced than men on reading comprehension, some forms of verbal reasoning, and spelling and punctuation.

Bilingualism

Some children grow up in an environment in which they learn and use two languages. At one time, children from such *bilingual* homes were widely reported to show retardation in their language and cognitive development (e.g., see W. Jones, 1960). However, reanalyses of these studies revealed that factors not directly associated with bilingualism (e.g., family income, educational level) were important. When these factors are controlled for, bilinguals do as well, if not better, than monolinguals on both verbal and nonverbal tests.

In a comprehensive review of bilingualism in children, McLaughlin (1977) concluded that children learn a second language with the same cognitive strategies and processes used for the first language. Some "lexical borrowing" (using a word in the first language if one cannot remember the correct word in the second language) may occur, and vocabulary development may be slow. But there is no conclusive evidence that the second language seriously interferes with the first. Furthermore, bilingualism does not appear to have a negative effect on cognitive development or educational achievement. Indeed, bilingualism may be advantageous in expanding a person's opportunities for conversational interactions in an increasingly multicultural society.

Black English

Many studies conducted on Black children living in inner-city ghettos have shown that these children speak a dialect called **Black English,** which differs substantially from middle-class Standard English (generally referred to as "correct English"). As happened with bilingual children, the interpretation first given to this research was that children speaking Black English were linguistically and mentally deprived, compared to those who spoke Standard English.

In several highly influential publications, William Labov (1970, 1972) concluded that Black English is a distinctive, but not a deficient, dialect. In studying Black adolescent gang members, Labov (1970) found that Black English has its own complex language structures complete with logical rules. It is not a random or sloppy collection of linguistic mistakes. For example, Black English is often criticized by teachers for an apparent lack of the verb *to be* (Slobin, 1979). Labov has shown that this verb form appears in Black English and follows regular linguistic rules. Whenever Standard English can contract the verb *to be,* Black English can omit the same verb. The contracted form of the Standard English sentence "She's the first one" can be expressed in Black English as "She the first one." This is not simply an omission of a standard part of English grammar because in cases where *to be* cannot be contracted in Standard English, it cannot be omitted in Black English. Just as one cannot say "That's what they're" in Standard English, it is impossible to say "That's what's they" in Black English (Labov, 1970). Furthermore, when *to be* is needed for special grammatical functions such as marking emphasis (e.g., "I *am* tired.") or imperatives (e.g., "*Be* patient, brothers."), it appears in both dialects. Labov has concluded that the differences between Black English and Standard English may be more apparent than real. The former is not an illogical and irregular version of the latter.

Other writers have pointed out that Black children are in effect bilingual. Houston (1970) showed that Black children employ two different modes of communication—a "school register" and a "nonschool register." The school register, which is used in interactions with persons in authority such as teachers, is characterized by unintelligibility, nonfluency, short utterances, and lack of expressiveness. However, in interacting with friends in natural contexts, Black children engage in expressive language, improvisation, and language play. Because of these different speech registers, Black children may be at a severe disadvantage later in life when they interact in academic and business contexts. Thus, some educators have emphasized a *bidialectical* approach to teach Standard English as well as Black English.

This brings us to the end of our discussion of language. Although substantial progress has been made in understanding language development over the past quarter of a century, much still remains to be done. Psycholinguists and developmental psychologists need to link language function more closely to other aspects of cognitive development. In the next chapter we will examine memory development, an area where language plays an influential role.

SUMMARY

1. In the short span of four or five years, children master most of the essential aspects of their native language. However, language continues to develop after age 5.

2. Developmental psycholinguistics focuses on the developmental study of language acquisition. An even newer field called sociolinguistics stresses the social, communicative function of all language.

3. "Pragmatics" refers to the appropriate use of language in its social and physical context. As children develop, they learn to take on the perspective of both the speaker and listener in communication.

4. Language and cognition are complexly related processes. Some investigators feel that language affects our thought processes; others think that our cognitions affect the language we use. A third view is that language and thought function independently of each other in early childhood, but interconnect in later childhood.

5. Language is generative in the sense that we use a finite set of linguistic rules to generate an almost infinite variety of novel utterances.

6. Three of the major aspects of language acquisition are phonological development, syntactical development, and semantic development. "Phonology" refers to the basic patterns of sounds in a language. "Syntax" and "semantics" refer to the grammatical structure and underlying meaning of a language, respectively.

7. Under normal circumstances children progress through the following invariant sequence of language stages: crying, cooing, babbling, one-word utterances, two-word utterances, and multiword sentences with inflectional morphemes.

8. From age 5, children articulate consonant-vowel clusters more clearly and master deep structure–surface structure relations. The major semantical developments after age 5 include an expanding vocabulary size, a shift to paradigmatic word associations, and an increase in metalinguistic knowledge.

9. Three different theoretical frameworks have been used to explain language development: learning, biological, and cognitive. A more reasonable approach to language development adopts an interactional synthesis in which a biologically prepared and cognitively active organism interacts with the environment to learn language.
10. Adults often use a simplified speech register called "motherese" to converse with children. The activities of the parent and the child's cognitive level are important determinants of the effectiveness of motherese.
11. Language learning shows great regularity, but individual and group differences affect its course. Individual differences related to sex, bilingualism, and Black English have an influence on language, but not as significant as once believed.

Key Terms

language acquisition device

psycholinguistics

developmental psycholinguistics

sociolinguistics

pragmatics

perlocutionary

illocutionary

locutionary

inner speech

egocentric speech

linguistic determinism

linguistic relativity

semiotic function

generative

phonemes

phonemic expansion

phonemic contraction

categorical perception

morphology

morphemes

syntax

semantics

holophrase

semantic feature hypothesis

functional core hypothesis

lexical contrast theory

contrast

conventionality

overextension

underextension

telegraphic speech

pivot–open grammar

functionality

overregularization

transformational grammar

deep structure

surface structure

minimum distance principle

syntagmatic

paradigmatic associations

metalinguistic knowledge

aphasia

motherese

recast

scaffold

Black English

Suggested Readings

Bruner, J. (1983). *Child's talk: Learning to use language.* New York: Norton. In this remarkably insightful book, renowned psychologist Jerome Bruner discusses how young children are assisted in learning to use language by adult speakers. To explain this learning process, Bruner postulates a "language acquisition support system" (LASS) that organizes the interactions between children and adults in a way that enables the child to master language. Filled with many interesting real-life case examples.

Chomsky, N. (1975). *Reflections on language.* New York: Pantheon. An incisive non-technical personal analysis of the current controversies among psychologists, philosophers, and linguists on the growth of language and cognition. Chomsky argues that language, similar to bodily organs, is predetermined by genetic factors.

deVilliers, J. G., & deVilliers, P. A. (1978). *Language acquisition.* Cambridge, MA: Harvard University Press. This highly readable and scholarly overview of children's linguistic knowledge at various stages of early language development contains 10 chapters, including chapters on early and later grammar, the development of word meaning, discourse and metalinguistics, language processes and constraints, and language in developmentally disabled children. Highly recommended.

Hakes, D. T. (1980). *The development of metalinguistic abilities in children.* New York: Springer. This thin volume reports on a study of metalinguistic abilities in children aged 4–8 years. It will stimulate your thinking about how superficially different meta-linguistic skills and different aspects of cognitive development have a common developmental basis.

Obler, L. K., & Albert, M. L. (Eds.). (1980). *Language and communication in the elderly.* Lexington, MA: Lexington Books. This book introduces issues of language and communication over the life span. The experimental section, probably of most general interest, is devoted to the relation of language and cognition in the elderly, discourse style, comprehension problems, and language lateralization over the life span. The clinical section covers medical and psychiatric communication with the elderly, language patterns in normal and dementing elderly, and language rehabilitation in dementia cases. Background chapters aid understanding.

Seiler, T. B., & Wannenmacher, W. (Eds.). (1983). *Concept development and the development of word meaning.* New York: Springer. This volume covers the latest advances in the study of concepts and word meanings in language development. It includes chapters by leading researchers in the areas of word recognition, the acquisition of word knowledge, overextensions and underextensions in children's speech, and a theoretical approach to cognitive development. These topics are approached from very different points of view, which sometimes make it difficult for the reader to see the "big picture."

Shatz, M. (1983). Communication. In J. H. Flavell & E. M. Markman (Eds.), *Handbook of childhood psychology: Vol. 3. Cognitive development* (pp. 841–889). New York: Wiley. A comprehensive up-to-date review of communication skills and behaviors in children. The five major sections consider characteristics of conventional communication systems, theoretical issues in communication research, knowledge bases of communication, implications of children's variability in communication performance, and implications of the findings for future research.

Wanner, E., & Gleitman, L. R. (Eds.). (1982). *Language acquisition: The state of the art.* New York: Cambridge University Press. This volume provides students and researchers with a timely overview of language development from a variety of different theoretical perspectives. It shows the increasingly complex and technical nature of the field.

Memory Development

OVERVIEW

Memory is a familiar and essential component of cognition. Some theories define "memory" as a process or activity; other theories define it as a structure or location. In order to study memory, developmental psychologists have borrowed concepts from information-processing models as well as from other theoretical frameworks including organismic, behavioristic, and contextualistic.

In Piaget's organismic model, memory development is conceptualized as one aspect of a broader set of changes in cognitive operations. Information-processing theorists view memory in terms of specific structural features (sensory register, short-term store, long-term store) and control operations (rehearsal, chunking, elaboration). According to the latter view, developmental differences in memory may be due to differences in the processing capacity of short-term store, efficiency of strategy use, growth of a general knowledge base, or some complex interaction among these factors. Many memory problems appear to result from faulty encoding or ineffective retrieval strategies instead of storage difficulties.

One of the most important current distinctions in memory research is between episodic and semantic memory, although most researchers now stress the continuity between these two aspects. Another important conception is the levels-of-processing framework, which was supposed to replace the two-store theory of short- and long-term memory. According to this perspective, information entering the cognitive system is processed in a hierarchical fashion—in a series of continuous processing stages—rather than passing through discrete memory stores. Current memory researchers also distinguish between automatic and effortful processing. Automatic processing is assumed to occur without attentional demands, whereas effortful processing demands deliberate activation of attention.

In recent years there has been great interest in studying constructive memory, by which people transform or elaborate meaningful information presented to them. Research on how people reconstruct and remember remote events in their lives will be examined.

"Metamemory" refers to people's awareness or knowledge of their own memory processes and how they operate. Developmental changes in memory may be due partly to changes in various aspects of metamemory, such as memory monitoring or memory knowledge. Finally, individual trends in memory development within the wider context of societal and cultural changes are discussed.

SOME USES OF MEMORY

Trying to remember something is a familiar cognitive activity. If asked, almost everyone, young children included, can give examples of the role memory plays in day-to-day life. Their examples may involve remembering a friend's telephone number, the name of the person they talked to last night at a party, the words of an old song, or the answers on a test that they spent the previous week studying for. Memory is not only important in recalling past experiences, objects, or events but also in planning future actions. For example, we may remind ourselves to return an overdue book to the library, or we may place a note on the refrigerator to remove a chicken from the freezer in the morning so we can cook it for dinner that evening.

Memory is critically important to our ability to survive in our world, yet we seldom think about its significance. Perhaps this is because memory is utilized during all familiar thinking activity, even for tasks that people do not commonly consider as memory tasks. For example, tasting the chicken we cooked for dinner involves in part our *expectations*, or memory of what it will taste like. Thus, much of our remembered knowledge has a natural and nondeliberate quality.

Only when we experience the frustration of forgetting do we pay much attention to our memory. Years ago psychologist James McKeen Cattell made the interesting observation that people are ever ready to complain about their memories, but seldom about their common sense or decision-making ability (Wechsler, 1958). Thus, we become accustomed to hearing about memory failures, and perhaps even learn to expect them, particularly in very young children or old adults. However, we rarely pause to consider when our memory system is functioning properly and the amazing feats it can perform. Take a moment to try the memory exercise in Box 6.1. You will probably be greatly surprised at the things you can recall.

Because memory is central to human functioning, developmental psychologists have long been interested in it. Until about 1970, however, most of the developmental research on memory was descriptive and did not deal with theoretical issues. For example, a standard topic in memory experiments involved the number of items (digits, letters, words) that could be freely recalled without cueing or prompting. Suppose I told you to remember the following set of digits: 5-1-7-4. When asked to recall them, you would immediately say 5174. Then I give you a five-digit number, a six-digit number, and so forth, and each time ask you to recall the digits in sequence.

How far could you go on the above memory-*span* task before you would begin to make errors? If you are like most other adults, you could probably immediately recall approximately seven digits in a row, per-

Box 6.1   Remembrance of Things Past

When I lecture on the topic of memory, I often begin my presentation by posing the following question to the class:

> What were you doing on Monday afternoon the third of September two years ago? (after Lindsay & Norman, 1977, p. 372)

The first reaction to this question is usually an incredulous "You've got to be kidding!" After reassuring the class that I am serious, I encourage them to attempt to remember that afternoon. Before you read any further, try to recall what you were doing that day.

Now that you have attempted this memory exercise, how did you proceed? If you are like most of the students in my classes, you probably tried to *reconstruct* the memory by first recalling general information about time, place, and events. Then you might attempt to remember more specific details:

> Let's see. September two years ago. I would be in Philadelphia just starting my senior year in high school. Hmm. That afternoon I would be in class. I would be in either trigonometry or advanced biology. I would probably be doing some trig problems or working on a lab exercise. Wait a minute. I think I had a test that day in trig. It was about the third week of school and I can remember sitting in . . .

Unless the events of that day were salient to you for some reason, you could not rapidly retrieve them as you would the name of a good friend or your home address. Instead, you had to begin to fill in the gaps in your memory by searching for the missing pieces of information. This search process is not unlike attempting to solve a problem by breaking it into several smaller, more manageable parts and working on each in turn. In the example above, students start with the problem of where they were two years ago. Having solved that problem, they proceed to the more specific problem of what they were doing. This process continues in a cyclical fashion until the final solution is reached. In most cases, it is extremely difficult to verify the accuracy of reconstructed memories. They represent a combination of people's recall of actual events and people's reconstructions of those events.

haps more if you "chunked" or grouped the digits into meaningful units. For example, the sequence 1-9-6-7-8-0-4-3-6-5 might be easier to remember if you combine the individual digits into meaningful numerical chunks as follows: 1967 (your birth year), 804 (your license number), 365 (the number of days in a year). On a task like this, 2-year-olds will generally be able to recall about two digits, 5-year-olds about four digits, 7-year-olds about five digits, and 9-year-olds about six digits (see Figure 6.1). Adults past age 60 can remember about as many digits as adolescents and younger adults (around seven) unless they are asked to recall the digits in reverse order. We will talk about backward memory-span tasks later.

Although the memory-span task discussed above reveals some interesting developmental trends, the important question is, Why can adults remember more information than children? Is it because adults have larger memory "receptacles" or "containers" in which to store memory—that is, larger capacity? Are there differences in the efficiency of strategies adults use on memory tasks such as chunking information? Or do developmental changes in one area (such as processing capacity) lead to developments in other areas (such as strategy usage)? Little work was done on these questions until quite recently. The advent of infor-

Figure 6.1 A summary of age differences in digit-span performance (solid line). Individual differences at various ages are expressed as ranges (dashed lines).

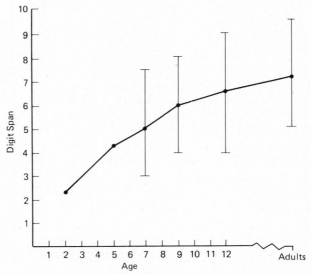

mation-processing theories of memory in the late 1960s represented a breakthrough in studying such questions because they provide a very exact and detailed model for studying individual memory processes. Many developmental researchers borrowed concepts from information processing and applied them to studies of memory development in children and adults. What emerged from these studies was a much more complex picture of developing memory, one that encompassed a variety of different competencies and explanatory mechanisms.

MODELS OF MEMORY

Information-processing models probably represent the leading approach to the study of memory at the present time. Over the past two decades information-processing theorists have introduced many terms into the literature such as *sensory register, short-term* and *long-term memory, primary* and *secondary memory, storage structures, operative structures, episodic* and *semantic memory,* and *memory code* (Klatzky, 1984). These terms will become more meaningful to you if we compare the information-processing approach with other approaches. Accordingly, three other theoretical frameworks for studying memory—organismic, behavioristic, and contextualistic—will be introduced. For consistency, the above theoretical models are presented in the order in which they were originally presented in Chapter 2, beginning with Piaget's organismic model of memory.

Organismic Models

The most fully elaborated organismic model of memory belongs to Piaget. For Piaget (see Piaget & Inhelder, 1973), the major developmental features of memory can be found in developmental changes in cognitive operations. In his theory, the operations involved in memory are structured like all other cognitive operations, that is, in sensorimotor, preoperational, concrete operational, and formal operational schemes (Reese, 1973b). The emergence of new operations should therefore lead to memory improvements. This viewpoint led Piaget to make a startling prediction: memory should improve with a longer retention interval (the interval between the presentation of the material and its recall). This prediction runs directly counter to the prevailing notion that memory declines over time. According to the latter position, the longer the retention interval, the poorer memory should be.

In explaining his position, Piaget distinguished between memory in the wider sense and memory in the strict sense (Piaget & Inhelder, 1973). "Memory in the wider sense" refers to the operation of intellectual schemes and to the retention of all the knowledge produced by the actions of these schemes during cognitive development. This type of memory is the *operative* aspect of memory. It can be distinguished from other mental operations only insofar as it refers to understanding of events and actions that have occurred in the past. "Memory in the strict sense" refers to the more ordinary use of the term for the product of mnemonic activity or what is remembered about a specific event at a particular place and time in the past. This aspect of memory is called the *figurative* aspect and represents what is usually regarded as the memory trace. The figurative component of memory is closely tied to the operative component in that retention of specific events or objects will depend on the child's operative level of development.

To test his prediction of the long-term improvement of memory, Piaget focused on a cognitive operation called **seriation**. Seriation, which will be discussed more fully in Chapter 7, is the ability to order objects in a series along some abstract dimension (number, height, brightness, loudness). Piaget (1952) investigated children's understanding of serial relationships by showing them a set of sticks of varying lengths (see Figure 6.2a). Piaget asked children to select the smallest stick first, then the next larger stick, and so on until all 10 sticks had been ordered (see Figure 6.2b). Preoperational children (4–5 years old) were unable to order the sticks serially in terms of size. Children in transition between preoperations and concrete operations (5–6 years old) ordered the sticks correctly, but only after much effort and error. By the time of concrete operations (more than 7 years old), children had no difficulty with the seriation task.

To examine directly his prediction about memory, Piaget and Inhelder (1973) conducted the following experiment. They first showed 3–8-year-old children an array of 10 sticks ordered from smallest to

Figure 6.2 Seriation task. The child is presented with (*a*) an array of unordered sticks that must be arranged in (*b*) serial order.

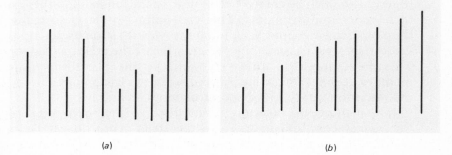

(a)   (b)

tallest. A week later, they asked the children to draw the sticks from memory. In general, the results paralleled the findings of Piaget's (1952) study. The 3- and 4-year-olds drew sticks nearly equal in length. The 5- and 6-year-olds drew various types of drawings. Some drew both tall and short sticks, while others drew sticks in seriated order, but included only a few sticks. By 7 years of age, children reproduced the sticks correctly. This study revealed that children's memory depends on their operative understanding of seriation.

Although these results were impressive, Piaget obtained more dramatic results from a longitudinal follow-up of the same children. Six to eight months later Piaget invited the children back to his laboratory and asked them to draw the sticks again as they remembered seeing them. Almost 75 percent of the children drew pictures that reflected more cognitively advanced operations than those they drew several months earlier. For example, children in transition from preoperations to concrete operations reproduced pictures that were more seriated than their first attempts. What explains these apparent improvements in memory? Piaget theorized that during the six-month interval the cognitive structures underwent modifications which in turn affected how information was organized and retrieved from memory.

Although Piaget's initial findings have been replicated (Liben, 1975a, 1975b), such replication attempts have not been uniformly successful. One team of investigators (Maurer et al., 1979) reported that only 15 percent of 6-year-olds in their study had more cognitively advanced drawings over a six-month retention interval. Other investigators (Altemeyer, Fulton, & Berney, 1969) reported that 43 percent of the children tested had more advanced drawings over a period of several months. These figures, while not as high as Piaget's, lend some support to his position.

There are two important points to bear in mind in regard to interpreting Piaget's results (Kail & Hagen, 1982). First, the typical finding in these replication studies was for children to draw operatively similar drawings regardless of the time interval since the stimulus array was presented. Thus, changes in cognitive structures probably are more influential than time in determining memory changes. Piaget himself would not predict memory improvement over intervals where no cognitive reorganizations occurred. Second, the number of children with improved drawings was generally matched by the number of children who regressed (became less advanced operatively) over time (Kail & Hagen, 1982). This latter result directly contradicts Piaget's theory and merits further empirical scrutiny.

The Piagetian approach to memory is provocative because it attempts to link memory processes closely to cognitive operations. By studying changes in memory, we may enlarge our understanding of more general changes in children's cognitive functioning. Today most investigators seem to agree that memory cannot be studied apart from other cognitive processes. Perception, imagery, problem solving, language, and intelligence all involve memory components to a significant degree. Flavell (1971b) stated this point well when he remarked: "I believe there is a growing consensus that memory is in good part just applied cognition. That is, what we call 'memory processes' seem largely to be just the same old, familiar, cognitive processes, but as they are applied to a particular class of problems" (p. 273).

Despite the implications of Piaget's model for studying memory processes, his approach is limited in several important ways. For example, cognitive operations may be necessary but not sufficient for the development of certain memory activities. Do children have to be at a certain cognitive level before they can employ memory strategies such as chunking or rehearsal? Furthermore, memory improvement over time—or *hypermnesia* as it is called in the memory literature—is found in subjects (for example, college undergraduates) who are not undergoing cognitive reorganization, at least not in the Piagetian sense (Brainerd, 1983). This phenomenon appears to be related to the consolidation of the memory trace over time or simply to the practice of retrieving information from memory. Thus, improvements in memory during adulthood may be due to nonoperative cognitive factors rather than operative advances. Finally, the Piagetian approach gives little insight into the nature of memory changes in older persons. How do cognitive operations relate to memory strategies in later adulthood? How do we account for observed memory loss in certain aspects of memory during old age? To answer these questions, we need to focus on the memory processes themselves, processes which have been peripheral features of Piaget's theory. This is exactly what the next approach to memory—information processing—purports to do.

Information-Processing Models

In information-processing models, memory is represented in terms of an active cognitive system (Reese, 1973b). How the active organism acquires, codes, and stores incoming information determines, to a large extent, how much and how well information is remembered. Information-processing models of memory (Atkinson & Shiffrin, 1968; Waugh & Norman, 1965) generally include three kinds of *storage structures* (see Figure 6.3). Figure 6.3 shows how the information-processing system works when information from a sensory stimulus passes through it. Information is passed from one storage structure to the next by means of *control operations* such as rehearsal, organization, and elaboration, which transform the information into meaningful units for recall.

Figure 6.3   Stages of a multistore information-processing model of memory.

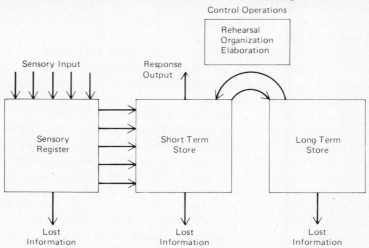

In the first stage of processing, incoming sensory information enters a **sensory register.** We call this the sensory register because information from any of the five senses remains there for a very brief period of time (about ¼–½ second) in veridical form before being passed on to the next structure. The longer information remains in the sensory register without being attended to and transformed, the more likely the information is to simply vanish. This weakening process is known as **memory decay,** or trace decay.

When information is attended to consciously, it passes into the next storage structure—the **short-term store,** or *primary* memory. In short-term store, items remain for only a brief time (about 30 seconds) and only a few items (about seven) can be held simultaneously. A familiar example of short-term memory involves trying to recall a phone number you have just heard but have not written down. If you can dial the number immediately, you will have no recall problems, but if you have to wait, or if you are given another number to remember, some information will be lost. This example demonstrates one form of *forgetting*, a process which can occur at any point in the cognitive system.

If the information in short-term store has been acted upon (rehearsed, organized, elaborated) to make it *semantically* meaningful, or more memorable, then it passes into the third storage structure—**long-term store,** or *permanent* memory. The long-term store, for all practical purposes, has virtually limitless storage capacity and contains memories that are very old (remote) in addition to more recent ones. Memories in long-term store are relatively permanent, though some may be lost. During retrieval memories are taken out of the long-term store and placed back into short-term store. The ease of retrieving representations from long-term memory, as you will see, depends upon the organization and elaboration of information as well as the availability of retrieval cues.

The control operations shown in Figure 6.3 direct the flow of information from one stage to the next and ensure that the entire memory system functions smoothly. Many of these control operations appear to be under the conscious and voluntary control of the individual. For example, to better remember a telephone number, I may actively *rehearse* the information by repeating it aloud or silently to myself. Or I may choose to *chunk* the information into a meaningful numerical code. As will be discussed shortly, developmental changes in memory are frequently due to changes in these control processes.

In summary, information-processing models see the organism as an active participator in the transformation of information into a meaningful unit for recall. Reese (1973b, 1976) argues that they are, therefore, consistent with organismic developmental views (see Chapter 2). However, information-processing models were designed to study memory in early adulthood and are not inherently developmental; in fact, much memory research within the information-processing framework is nondevelopmental. The next models we turn to—behavioristic models—are not developmental either. But as in the case of information-processing models, researchers have borrowed concepts from behavioristic approaches and applied them to developmental problems of memory.

OTHER MODELS OF MEMORY

Behavioristic approaches are no longer as popular with memory researchers as they were in the late 1950s and early 1960s. Thus, we will not deal with them extensively. For excellent overviews of the behavioral approach to memory, the reader is referred to Kausler's (1974) *Psychology of Verbal Learning and Memory* as well as Horton and Turnage's (1976) *Human Learning*. Later in this section we will also look at contextualistic models of memory, which are rapidly gaining popularity. We will examine the reasons for this increasing popularity and the implications of using contextualistic approaches for studying life-span changes in memory.

Behavioristic Models

Behavioristic models view memory in terms of a chain of *stimulus-response* (S-R) *associations.* To remember something means to emit an appropriate response under stimulus conditions that existed when the response was originally acquired (Reese, 1973b). Changes in memory can result from repeated associations of stimuli and responses or an increase in the number of associations. Failure to emit a response, or forgetting, is caused by a weakening of these associations by *interfering* associations or simply through *decay* or disuse. The associationistic process is highly mechanical, so that Reese (1973b) saw behavioristic models as consistent with a mechanistic world view.

To give you a better idea of the behavioristic approach, we will consider a procedure that has been used frequently: **paired-associate learning.** In the paired-associate procedure, subjects are first presented with a list of paired stimulus items (usually words, digits, or nonsense syllables) and then asked to respond to the second item of the pair when the first item is presented alone. For example, look at the study pairs in Table 6.1. After you study these pairs for a few seconds, cover them with a piece of paper and try to supply the missing words for the stimulus words in Table 6.1. Normally, the experimenter provides feedback after each response (e.g, "yes, that's correct"), but you will have to check the answers yourself. Did you get all the words correct on the first attempt? If not, go back and study them some more. Typically, in paired-associate learning studies, the experimenter repeats the stimulus items several times in different orders to some specified criterion such as one perfect trial.

One way to improve your learning performance on a paired-associate task is to elaborate the stimulus items by forming a visual image of them or by creating a sentence to link them (see Chapter 4). For exam-

Table 6.1
An Example of a Paired-Associate Task

Study Pairs	Stimulus Words
dime—flower	line—?
train—sink	moon—?
frog—iron	train—?
paper—clock	inch—?
inch—noise	snow—?
snow—neck	string—?
string—tent	frog—?
arrow—gift	dime—?
line—band	paper—?
moon—cork	arrow—?

ple, the paired associates *comb-cup* may be more easily remembered if you visualize a comb inside a cup. Or you may choose to use a verbal mediator such as a word phrase or a sentence ("The comb belongs inside the cup"). The main point is that the items to be recalled are linked in an image or a sentence so that remembering one will enhance memory of the other (Rohwer, 1973).

Young children and elderly adults generally find paired-associate tasks more difficult than do older children and younger adults. One possible explanation is that the young and elderly do not spontaneously employ imagery as a memory strategy for learning paired-associate items (Hulicka & Grossman, 1967; Paivio, 1969). If this is the case, then we must ask whether these two groups are incapable of using imaginal skills, or whether they have such skills but simply fail to use them unless trained or instructed. If the failure to use imaginal skills is due to cognitive immaturity (in young children) or cognitive losses (in elderly adults), then training such skills should be quite difficult. However, if the skills are intact but unused, training efforts aimed at enhancing performance of these skills should be relatively easy. (This distinction between underlying competence and actual performance is important and will be discussed in Chapter 10.)

Several investigators have reported that both young children (Levin, McCabe, & Bender, 1975; Reese, 1972) and elderly adults (Hulicka & Grossman, 1967; Treat & Reese, 1976) can enhance their performance on paired-associate tasks by using imagery when instructed. However, the use of imagery and other mediational techniques does not completely eliminate age differences in paired-associate learning. These results suggest that factors other than imaginal ability may be responsible for the age differences.

One possible factor might be the meaningfulness of the task to subjects. Subjects often regard paired-associate tasks as meaningless tasks encountered only in a laboratory situation. Hulicka (1967) reported that many older adults in her paired-associate study simply refused to complete the task because subjects did not want to learn "such nonsense"; but when the nature of the task was changed by having older subjects associate names with occupations (e.g., banker-Sloan), the subjects were more willing to cooperate.

The paired-associate task has often been employed to study learning and memory processes, but psychologists have also used it to test the *interference theory* of forgetting. Interference theory, once the most widely accepted account of forgetting, falls squarely within behavioristic or associationistic approaches to memory. According to the theory, age differences in forgetting can be explained on the basis of differences in the effects of interference across various age groups (A. Smith, 1980).

Proactive interference results from previously learned material, ret-

roactive interference from recently learned material. In a paired-associate task proactive interference is said to occur if a previously learned association *(north-south)* interferes with the memorization of a new association *(north-chair)*. Retroactive interference can be demonstrated more easily in paired-associate learning. The standard procedure is to have half the subjects learn a list of paired associates (the A-B list, where A and B represent stimulus and response items, respectively), then another list (the A-C list, where A items are identical to those in the first list but the C items are new), and finally a recall test of the A-B list. The control subjects receive the A-B list and test, but not the interfering A-C list.

The results of studies employing retroactive and proactive interference procedures have been summarized by Kausler (1970). There is only equivocal evidence to support the view that susceptibility to interference explains age-related differences in forgetting (Craik, 1977). Many of the studies using these procedures did not employ appropriate controls. More important, the age groups were not equated on their learning of the initial task (the A-B list). Although interference theory is a plausible explanation of forgetting, it has not received strong empirical support.

Contextualistic Models

Contextualistic models emphasize the use of more meaningful or ecologically valid stimulus materials in memory experiments. Perhaps this is why they have become more popular with many memory researchers than behavioristic models. For example, suppose I read you the following sentences:

> Tom went to a restaurant. He ordered spaghetti. Later, he paid and left.

Later, I ask you to recall the sentences as you remember them. You might reply as follows:

> Tom went to eat at a restaurant. He ordered spaghetti from the waitress. He then paid the bill and left.

Notice that several discrepancies exist between the original material and the material recalled. Note especially the words *eat, waitress,* and *bill.* None of them appeared in the sentences I read to you. Rather, you inferred from what you heard that I was talking about the activity of eating. Based on your knowledge of restaurant situations, you constructed an interpretation from the original material by mentally filling in the gaps.

This example illustrates the effect of *context* on memory. One's prior knowledge and current situation determine the information one recalls. People do not simply condense or omit material they hear or read. In fact, when asked to recall sentences such as the examples above, people often give you more information than you requested. Individuals actively transform and elaborate material to be consistent with their personal and social knowledge.

Contextualistic memory researchers frequently employ sentence or text materials like those in our example because they feel such materials are more ecologically or contextually valid than digit or word lists. This emphasis is reflected in a famous series of experiments by Sir Frederick Bartlett (1932). In one experiment, Bartlett (1932) presented subjects with a strange-sounding legend called "The War of the Ghosts" about a Native American tribe. Bartlett reported that his subjects (who were not Native Americans) had difficulty reproducing the exact words and made systematic errors in recall. These errors tended to be consistent with the subjects' cultural and social context. For example, subjects replaced elements in the story with terms that were more familiar to them: *canoe* became *boat*, and *hunting seals* became *fishing*. Bartlett (1932) proposed that subjects remembered the story this way because they formed an abstract representation of the story called a **schema** (the plural is *schemata*) when they first read it. In effect, subjects tried to fit the story into their existing long-term memory store.

Bartlett's work is now considered classic, but was ignored for almost 40 years. Beginning in the early 1970s, psychological investigators began to rediscover many of the issues originally raised by Bartlett (Jenkins, 1974; Meacham, 1977; Shaw & Bransford, 1977). For example, in an influential article outlining the major tenets of the contextual position on memory, Jenkins stated: "In place of the traditional [associationistic] analysis, I suggest a *contextualist* approach. This means not only that the analysis of memory must deal with contextual variables but also, and this is my point today, that *what memory is depends on context*" (p. 786). Thus, Jenkins claimed that the total context of the situation (prior knowledge states, current cognitive levels, social environment) determines what will be remembered.

The contextual view of memory fits nicely into a life-span approach because contextualists emphasize that individuals are not static organisms, but are always changing in a constantly fluctuating social-cultural environment. At an empirical level, the influence of context on memory has been most often studied in cross-cultural developmental research. Cross-cultural research enables the investigator to study population variables that would be difficult or impossible to manipulate in a laboratory setting (Wagner & Paris, 1981). For example, investigators have reported that formal schooling and urban living rather than age predict the use of rehearsal strategies in laboratory memory tasks (M. Cole & Scribner, 1977; Wagner, 1978).

In an experiment conducted in Morocco, Wagner (1978) studied schooled and unschooled individuals in both rural and urban areas. Among the individuals who attended school, rehearsal skills developed gradually between ages 7–19 in both rural and urban settings. In contrast, for individuals with no schooling, rehearsal was infrequent at all ages. By conducting research in a culture where formal schooling was not widespread, Wagner (1978) was able to separate the effects of age and education on memory abilities, something that would have been more difficult in a North American or Western European setting.

Cross-cultural research also allows us to study long-term cultural-historical changes that would be difficult to examine longitudinally. For example, researchers have compared societies with strong oral traditions to those with written languages in order to examine differences in the use of internal memory resources (Greenfield, 1972; Wagner, 1981). They found that as societies move away from oral traditions, demands on memory decline. We might also look at changes within our own culture. What effect will the increasing use of electronic calculators and high-speed computers have on our ability to remember things such as mathematical formulas?

SOME STRUCTURAL FEATURES OF MEMORY

Empirical research on the various structural features (i.e., sensory register, short-term store, long-term store) of the information-processing system will now be reviewed. Some important recent advances in conceptualizing long-term memory processes including episodic and semantic memory, the levels-of-processing approach, and automatic versus effortful processing will also be examined.

Sensory Register

Most empirical studies of sensory memory focus on either **iconic** (visual) or **echoic** (auditory) memory (Neisser, 1967). Less research has been done on memory for touch, smell, and taste, and almost no developmental research exists on memory for these sensory modalities. Therefore, they will not be discussed here. Typically, sensory memory is considered more perceptual than cognitive because the former involves the earliest stages of information processing.

Iconic Memory

Research on iconic memory often involves the use of the *partial report* technique proposed by Sperling (1960). This technique is a modified version of the memory-span task which we discussed earlier. In a typical partial report procedure, the experimenter presents subjects with three rows of three stimulus items each (numbers, letters) for a very brief time (about 50 milliseconds) on an apparatus known as a *tachistoscope*. The subject's task is to report the items in a particular row immediately after the tachistoscopic exposure. An auditory signal tone of high, low, or medium frequency occurs either simultaneously with or immediately after the disappearance of the items, indicating which row to report. Because the arrays are selected randomly, subjects have no way of knowing which row is to be reported until the letters disappear. Under these partial report conditions, subjects generally are able to report on a row of letters with few errors. Their near-errorless performance suggests that they retain most of the nine letters in sensory memory, even though the array is no longer physically present. However, under full report conditions, in which subjects are asked to report all the items in the array, they can generally report only about four or five of the nine items correctly.

Sperling (1960) explained these findings in terms of the rapid decay of the icon or iconic trace, which has a relatively large storage capacity but a duration of not more than a few tenths of a second. As a subject tries to report all nine items, the icon continues to decay, so that by the time four or five items are reported, the icon is so faint that subjects can no longer report any more letters. Thus, subjects are able to perceive more information than they can typically identify and report. This limit on the number of items reported suggests a memory limit, which has been called **span of immediate memory** (G. Miller, 1956).

Haith and associates performed a series of experiments on early visual information processing and memory in children and adults (Haith, 1971; Morrison, Holmes, & Haith, 1974; Sheingold, 1973). Using the partial report technique, they presented adults and 5-, 8-, and 11-year-old children with an array of seven geometric figures for 100 milliseconds. After a delay interval of 50–1000 milliseconds, they showed the subjects a marker where the figure had been presented and asked them to name the figure. They found no age differences in the amount of information initially available in visual storage. As the delay interval increased to about 200 milliseconds, all age groups rapidly declined in iconic memory; but beyond 450 milliseconds, adults' retention stabilized, whereas children's retention declined further. Apparently, adults used this extra time to rehearse items in order to transfer them to short-term memory, but children did not.

Researchers who study iconic memory of young and old adults also report age differences. In a study employing the partial report technique, Walsh and Thompson (reported in Walsh and Prasse, 1980) found that the iconic memory of young adults (18–31 years) was significantly better than that of old adults (60–72 years). However, the use of the Sperling technique with older subjects is problematic because the results may be due to attentional problems, not to an absence of iconic memory (Salthouse, 1976). For example, when presented with rows of letters, elderly subjects tended to concentrate only on the top letters in the row, whereas younger adults displayed more flexible attentional strategies. The partial report technique also demands a rapid refocusing of attention on a segment of information stored in iconic memory (Walsh & Prasse, 1980). As you learned in Chapter 3, rapid shifting of attention becomes increasingly difficult in old age. Similar types of attentional problems may hamper interpretation of iconic memory experiments with children.

An alternative method developed by Eriksen and Collins (1967) circumvents some attentional demand problems. In this method, the experimenter briefly presents subjects with successive visual stimuli separated by a certain time interval. The experimenter then determines the maximum interstimulus interval (ISI) during which the temporally separated stimuli appear as one continuous event. Theoretically, the ability to link information from the second stimulus with information from the first depends on iconic representation. Studies employing this procedure with younger and older adults have reported few consistent age differences in the *duration* of iconic memory (Kline & Orme-Rogers, 1978; Kline & Schieber, 1981). Our conclusion is that iconic memory ability shows no major age-related changes across the life span.

Echoic Memory

The auditory analog of iconic memory is echoic memory. In contrast to the rapid decay rate in iconic memory (⅛–1 second), auditory information shows a much slower rate of decay (about 2 seconds). The utility of this slower decay rate should be apparent; for example, in order to understand what people are saying to us, we must preserve the echoic traces long enough to provide a context for subsequent speech sounds.

Psychologists use various methods to measure echoic memory. In an auditory version of Sperling's partial report technique (see Darwin, Turvey, & Crowder, 1972), auditory stimuli such as digit or letter lists are presented simultaneously from different spatial locations, and the subject must report on one of these locations after receiving a visual cue. In a newer procedure, subjects hear a list of items such as digits or letters from several locations and are asked to recall as many items as possible from all locations immediately after hearing them. This task is quite similar to the memory-span task except that the number of items presented usually exceeds the number that can normally be spanned without error (Kausler, 1982).

Studies on developmental changes in echoic memory are few, but the pattern of results is consistent. In one study, Engle, Fidler, and Reynolds (1981) employed a stimulus suffix paradigm to assess differences in echoic memory in 7- and 11-year-old children as well as adults. They presented subjects with lists of four to nine digits at different rates, followed by the suffix -go which was not to be recalled. The suffix was expected to decrease recall of the digits by displacing items in echoic memory compared to a control condition in which no suffix was presented. Although the suffix effect was larger for young children at a slow presentation rate (they recalled more digits incorrectly), no differences were observed across age groups at a faster presentation rate. These results suggest that the capacity of echoic memory is the same for all ages. The differences in the slow presentation condition were probably due to the fact that older children and adults are more likely than younger children to encode and rehearse the items in short-term memory if given sufficient time. Thus, the differences resulted from strategic factors, not from fundamental structural change in echoic memory size. In an earlier study, A. Siegel and Allik (1973) used a series of pictures presented in a visual and an auditory way to assess sensory memory in children and adults. They found no age differences in retention of the stimulus items, but reported a "modality" effect for the last items—with the auditory items being recalled better than the visual items. This effect was the same across every age group.

Arenberg (1976) reported a modality effect in a study of young and elderly adults. Arenberg presented a series of recall lists of 16 words in either a visual or auditory way. He found that even though young and old adults differed in the total number of words recalled, the modality effect was equally pronounced for both age groups, with recall for the auditory items near the end of the list exceeding recall for the visual items. The appearance of a modality effect for older subjects provides evidence for the continuation of echoic memory into later life.

Studies attempting to assess echoic memory differences between young and old adults encounter several methodological difficulties. The most obvious is that adults past age 65 are about 15 times more likely to suffer from some type of hearing loss as young adults. Nevertheless, studies that have been performed (see Crowder, 1980; Parkinson & Perey, 1980) offer no convincing evidence for age differences in the duration of echoic memory. Thus far these studies have not looked directly at the capacity of echoic memory.

In summary, investigations of iconic and echoic memory in children and adults show few overall age differences, at least for subjects without serious sensory impairments. Estimates of the capacity of iconic and echoic memory for children and adults are similar. Adult age differences in iconic but not echoic memory have been reported, but must be interpreted cautiously because of methodological problems.

Short-Term Store and Long-Term Store

Similar to the findings on sensory memory, researchers have reported only slight age changes in short-term store. As discussed, the number of items that can be remembered in short-term memory increases steadily with age through childhood. However, this change is probably not due to changes in the overall capacity of short-term store, but in the control operations (such as rehearsal, chunking, elaboration) that people use to remember the information. For example, in order to carry out a mathematical operation such as $(3 \times 7) + (8 \times 4)$ in your head, you must be able to remember the number 21 before computing the rest of the problem. Repeating or rehearsing the number to yourself is one way to hold it in memory.

Because of the cognitive activity involved in keeping information in consciousness, some theorists prefer to view the short-term store as **working memory** (Brainerd, 1981; Case, Kurland, & Goldberg, 1982; Schneider & Shiffrin, 1977; Shiffrin & Schneider, 1977). "Working memory" refers to the amount of processing or mental work that can be carried out in short-term memory, rather than just the amount of information that can be stored. To the extent that performing a memory task requires storage of information, the amount of available working memory for operating on new information is assumed to be diminished. Baddeley and Hitch (1974) tested this assumption in a series of experiments in which subjects had to store items from a memory-span task while simultaneously working on a reasoning problem. As expected, remembering the items from the memory-span task had a pronounced adverse effect on subjects' reasoning performance. This result parallels those discussed in Chapter 3 on the allocation of attentional resources.

Many studies of short-term, or working, memory employ the forward span task with lists of digits or letters varying in length. The task is usually administered as a *free recall* task with subjects being able to recall the items in any order they desire. One consistent finding of these memory-span studies is that age differences exist at the beginning or middle of the list, but not for the last items. Older children and adults recall initial and middle items better than young children, presumably because the first two groups employ memory strategies to retain them. Recall of the last three or four items in the list is called the **recency effect.** These items are the first to be reported by all age groups and are likely to come from short-term memory store.

In a slight modification of the list-learning procedure, Myers and Perlmutter (1978) presented 2–4-year-old children with nine small toy objects. They named and then placed the toys in a box and asked each child to tell them about all the things seen. As Figure 6.4*a* shows, neither age group performed particularly well, but older children recalled on the average significantly more objects than younger children. Figure 6.4*b* presents a **serial position curve,** which plots recall scores as a function of when the object appeared in the series of objects recalled. In both age groups, level of recall for the last toys presented (the recency effect) was significantly greater than for any of the other serial positions. These results indicate a very short-term limited capacity store for the age range studied. However, there was no evidence for a **primacy effect,** in which initial items would have had been recalled better than items in the middle of the series. With adults and older children, a pri-

Figure 6.4 Children's recall of toy objects. (*a*) Mean number of objects recalled by younger and older children, and (*b*) mean percentage of objects recalled as a function of serial order of presentation.

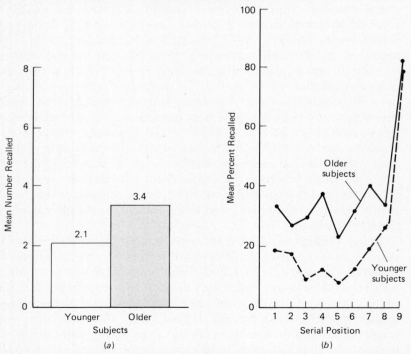

macy effect is generally associated with the use of active rehearsal strategies, so the lack of such an effect for the young age groups studied here
is not surprising.

In the Myers and Perlmutter (1978) study, recall for the early items
probably depended more on long-term than short-term store processes.
This probability highlights a major difficulty with the short-term versus
long-term distinction. Waugh and Norman (1965) drew attention to
this difficulty when they argued for defining memory in terms of **primary memory** and **secondary memory,** rather than short-term and long-
term memory. Primary memory leads to perfect retention so long as
memory capacity is not exceeded and the items to be remembered are
kept in mind (for example, by active rehearsal). When either of these
conditions is not satisfied, then secondary memory is involved, regardless of the length of the retention interval.

Short-term or primary memory difficulties in young children may
reflect not only capacity limitations and lack of processing strategies
but also deficits in processing speed. An abundance of evidence suggests
that adults encode information faster than children (Boswell, 1974;
Chi, 1976; Salthouse & Kail, 1983). For example, Boswell (1974) found
that at very short exposures with 16 letters to encode (to store in short-
term memory), adults recalled a significantly greater number of letters
than 8-year-olds. Rehearsal or organizational strategies could not have
played a role here because of the short exposure times. In another study,
Chi (1976) found that adults encoded familiar faces and retrieved the
name of a face over twice as fast as children did. The results of both
these studies suggest that children's recall is limited not only by the
lack of processing strategies but also by speed of encoding. Because
adults are faster at encoding information, they have more space in
working memory to store information.

In his recent review of memory, Poon (1985) concluded that adult
age differences in short-term or primary memory are minimal. Where
age differences are found (see Botwinick & Storandt, 1974a; Bromley,
1958; Parkinson, Lindholm, & Urell, 1980), secondary memory appears
to be involved. For example, if elderly adults are asked to repeat a list
of digits or letters in reverse order, their performance suffers relative to
that of young adults. In this backward memory-span task, individuals
must manipulate or reorganize material already in primary memory,
which requires long-term or secondary memory. Box 6.2 presents some
recent research on the development of skilled memory-span performance in young and elderly adults.

Items in short-term memory are elaborated and rehearsed as a means
of consolidating them for storage in secondary memory. Failure to
engage in these cognitive control operations results in loss of information or forgetting because short-term memory has limited structural

Box 6.2   The Development of Skilled Memory

Normally people's memory span falls within the narrow range of 7 items plus or minus 2, and this range holds across a wide assortment of memory tasks. Psychologists interpret the relative stability of memory-span performance as evidence of a most fundamental and enduring property of the human memory system— the limited capacity of short-term memory. This limit places severe restrictions on our ability to process information and to solve problems.

Recent evidence (Chase & Ericsson, 1981) now suggests that the normal memory span of 7 items may be increased more than tenfold. In an intriguing study an undergraduate (SF) with average memory abilities and average intelligence was able to increase his memory span from 7 digits to about 80 digits over a period of 20 months (see Figure 6.5). Further, SF progressed from being unable to recall any digits at the end of an hour's testing session to being able to recall over 90 percent of the digits presented to him during the session. This is one of the most impressive demonstrations of memory skill in the psychological literature. How did SF do it?

First, let us analyze SF's mnemonic skills. He was a very good long-distance runner and used his knowledge of various running times to categorize groups of digits. He coded the digits 3492 as "three forty-nine point two, near world-record mile time." When digit groups could not be converted to running times, SF invented additional mnemonics such as ages (the 3-digit sequence 896 was coded as "eighty-nine point six years old, very old man") and years (the 4-digit sequence 1943 was coded as "near the end of World War II"). If we assume that SF's original memory span was around 7, and he learned to recode single digits into groups of 3 and 4 digits, then his memory span should be about 7 groups, or a maximum of 28 digits (Chase & Ericsson, 1981). But his memory span increased steadily to about 80 digits, so a mechanism besides mnemonic skill had to be involved.

This other mechanism was SF's use of hierarchical retrieval structures. He hierarchically organized the digit groups into 4-digit groups, followed by 3-digit groups, followed by a rehearsal group (the digits he was rehearsing in immediate memory). Once SF devised a retrieval structure he could use each position in the hierarchy as a retrieval cue to activate the digit groups and recall them in proper order. This retrieval structure effectively allowed SF to bypass the capacity limitations of short-term memory by

Figure 6.5 Average digit span for SF as a function of practice. During the 20-month period which represented about 215 hours of practice, SF's digit span improved from 7 to almost 80 digits.

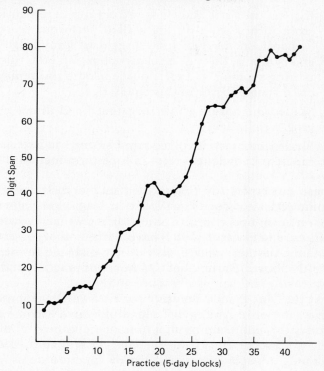

From "Skilled Memory" by W. G. Chase and K. A. Ericsson, 1981, in *Cognitive Skills and Their Acquisition* (p. 144) edited by J. R. Anderson, Hillsdale, NJ: Erlbaum. Copyright 1981 by Lawrence Erlbaum Associates, Inc. Reprinted by permission.

placing digits temporarily in a directly accessible long-term memory store.

Does this mean that *SF* increased his short-term memory capacity? Chase and Ericsson (1981) cite several reasons to think not. First, *SF*'s mnemonically coded digit groups were almost always 3 and 4 digits, and they never exceeded 5 digits. Second, his rehearsal group never included more than 6 digits, and the 6 digits were always segmented into two groups of 3 digits. Finally, after three months of practice on the digit-span task, *SF*'s memory for consonants was tested, and his consonant span was only average. Thus, he showed little transfer from one memory-span task to another. These findings suggest that the most reliable estimate of working short-term memory is around 3 or 4 digits.

Using these data, Chase and Ericsson (1981) formulated the following three characteristics of skilled memory:

1. Experts use their knowledge structures in semantic memory to store information during skilled performance of some task. Semantic memory includes organized knowledge about words and symbols, their interrelationships, and the rules for manipulating symbols and relations (episodic and semantic memory are discussed later in this chapter).
2. Skilled memory involves organized and direct retrieval from long-term memory.
3. Skilled memory involves rapid storage and retrieval of intermediate knowledge states in long-term memory.

These principles say that skilled memorizers can employ mnemonic codes to store knowledge in long-term memory and then use retrieval operations to access directly that knowledge.

Chase and Ericsson (1981) have trained other subjects to use *SF*'s system. Another subject, also a long-distance runner, performed slightly above *SF* after about 75 hours of practice, and he appeared to be using the same techniques as *SF*.

At the Max Planck Institute for Human Development and Education in Berlin, young and old adults have become expert memorizers through training in a mnemonic known as the *method of loci* (J. Smith, Heckhausen, Kliegel, & Baltes, 1984). In this method, subjects associate a list of concrete items with a set of distinct locations such as the rooms in their houses. Each item is paired with a familiar object in one of the locations. At recall subjects mentally image each location and use the object in the location as a retrieval cue. So far several younger and older adults have dramatically improved their digit recall by using 30 familiar Berlin street scenes as loci. This strategy of "testing the limits" of maximum memory performance in different-aged individuals may give us important new insights into how the cognitive system operates across the life span.

capacity. As far as we know, long-term store does not have any capacity restrictions. Long-term memory can span from a minute to days and weeks, although in laboratory situations it usually refers to a retention interval not exceeding a half-hour. Memory across very long time periods is referred to as *remote* memory, or tertiary memory.

If there are minimal age differences in sensory and short-term memory, then major developmental changes must occur in long-term, or secondary, memory. Because long-term memory is thought to have unlimited capacity, most research on the mechanisms underlying developmental changes has focused on control processes rather than capacity limitations. Indeed, considerable empirical evidence suggests that developmental differences exist in the control operations of transferring information to and from long-term memory. These include *mnemonic* (from the Greek work *mneme* for "memory") strategies such as rehearsal, chunking, and elaboration of material to be remembered.

Developmental Changes in Memory Strategies

We can only briefly review the large developmental literature on memory strategies. In an early study of verbal rehearsal strategies, Flavell, Beach, and Chinsky (1966) presented seven pictures of common objects to a group of children (aged 5, 7, and 10) and asked them to remember several pictures in serial order. Before a delayed recall task, the experimenter covered the children's eyes with a translucent visor and recorded lip movements as a measure of spontaneous labeling and rehearsal. Flavell and colleagues found that only 10 percent of the 5-year-olds used spontaneous verbal rehearsal, whereas 85 percent of the 10-year-olds did. Thus, the study provided clear evidence for a developmental increase in the use of spontaneous verbal rehearsal as a memory strategy.

Older children not only rehearse more but also rehearse information in larger and more varied units, or "chunks." Chunks reflect the use of an underlying organizational or grouping strategy, with greater chunking usually leading to better recall. Ornstein and Naus (1978) suggested that the active rehearsal employed by older children leads to the development of an organizational "plan" to consolidate information which then serves as a means for later retrieval. Numerous studies have shown that younger children can capitalize on existing groupings of stimulus objects to aid memory, but they do not organize stimulus information spontaneously (Huttenlocher & Burke, 1976; Neimark, Slotnick, & Ulrich, 1971; Samuel, 1978). Similarly, investigators of aging report that older adults fail to employ organizational strategies as extensively as young adults (Craik, 1977; Hultsch, 1969, 1971). However, when stimulus objects are first organized into groups or categories, old adults as well as young children use organizational strategies.

While we could continue to catalog the strategy failures of young children and older adults on memory tasks, a more germane issue is whether such deficits can be remediated through instructions (or training). Even though both age groups exhibit little or no spontaneous deployment of mnemonic strategies, the evidence reviewed here suggests that they have the ability to generate strategies, and certain strategies (such as rehearsal) can be readily elicited by the experimenter. This evidence has led developmental memory researchers to distinguish between **production deficiencies** and **mediation deficiencies** (Flavell, 1970). Individuals have a production deficiency if, for reasons other than ability or skill, they do not spontaneously generate mnemonic activities, such as rehearsal, which would benefit their recall. A mediational deficiency occurs when the strategy produced—whether spontaneous or experimentally elicited—fails to benefit recall performance. Flavell (1970) also referred to a **production inefficiency,** which is an actual inability to carry out a strategy skillfully and effectively.

Developmentally, (1) a stage of mediational deficiency in early childhood, in which training has no effect, appears to be followed by (2) a stage of production inefficiency, in which some improvement is produced by appropriate training; then (3) a stage of production deficiency, in which full benefit is produced; and, finally, (4) a stage in which training produces no benefit because the child already spontaneously uses the appropriate strategy (Reese, 1976). Why do children fail to employ strategies that would benefit their recall performance, given that they have the ability to use such strategies on their own? The many possible reasons for this failure include a failure to grasp the memory demands of a task, not realizing certain strategies are beneficial to memory, and the fact that the mnemonic skill is not well established. Regardless of the cause, developmental differences in memory during childhood seem not to reflect differences in memory capacity, but in the control operations governing strategy usage (Reese, 1976).

As in childhood, adult age differences in memory seem to result from changes in control operations, not absolute capacity changes. But older adults, unlike young children, have an intention to remember and presumably had appropriate mnemonic strategies in their repertoire sometime during their lives. Still, like young children, they exhibit production inefficiencies and deficiencies (Hultsch, 1971). It is tempting to relate old people's deficiencies to the causes found in childhood, but the developmental reality is probably far more complicated. First, older people often suffer a decline in self-confidence about memory, which could reflect an awareness of memory decline or a concern over what they expect to happen in their memory with age. Young children are very unlikely to possess a similar awareness or concern about memory. In addition, cohort changes may influence the types of memory strategies used by various age groups. The main point is that we cannot automatically assume that similar memory performances by children and older adults reflect the same causal mechanisms.

Although memory strategies play an important role in age-related improvements and declines in memory, the strategies alone may not account for all the developmental differences observed. Rather, the growth of a general knowledge base—an interconnected network of meanings and concepts—may influence mnemonic activities, such as chunking, which in turn can lead to memory improvements. To illustrate how this might work, consider a clever experiment conducted by Chi (1978). Children (mean age 10.5 years) and adults were administered two kinds of memory tasks. In one condition, a typical digit-span test was given, and adults' digit recall was superior as usual. In the second condition, memory for different configurations of chess positions was assessed, and the results were reversed—children's recall exceeded adults' by over 50 percent!

Why did children excel on this second task? The children were skilled chess players, whereas the adults, though knowledgeable about chess, lacked the children's expert knowledge. Because of their greater familiarity with the game, children were able to chunk the chess positions into larger units, whereas adults saw them as random arrangements of pieces. The children's general knowledge base allowed them to encode meaningful configurations, which facilitated their recall. Adults, on the other hand, had more separate pieces of information to remember than children and their recall suffered.

Encoding, Storage, and Retrieval

The studies reviewed above show that young children and old adults are less proficient in using mnemonic strategies than other individuals. But the question of *where* in the memory system difficulties arise remains unanswered. Theoretically, poor memory performance could reflect difficulties in *encoding, storage, retrieval,* or some *interaction* among these processes as well as age-related differences in the motivation to remember. If the problem is one of encoding, then individuals may fail to encode or enter material into long-term memory. A storage problem would imply that the memory trace has either decayed through disuse (by not recalling the information frequently) or has been interfered with by other incoming information. If the problem is neither in encoding or storage, then inaccessibility of the information at retrieval is probably the culprit. However, more than one process could be involved; for example, poorly encoded information would be hard to retrieve.

How can psychologists begin to isolate the locus of age-related memory difficulties? One way is to compare memory performance on tasks utilizing **recall** versus **recognition.** In recall, subjects retrieve information from their memory stores in the absence of stimulus information. A fill-in-the-blank item on a test is a recall task. Another example is the forward and backward memory-span tasks we discussed earlier. Recognition, on the other hand, requires only that subjects match information in storage with the presence of certain stimulus information. Choosing the correct answer on a multiple choice test is a recognition task. In laboratory recognition tasks, subjects are typically presented with a list of items and then a new list which contains new as well as previously presented items. Their job is to correctly identify the old items.

The developmental trends on recall and recognition memory tasks are clear-cut across numerous studies, so that some conclusions can be drawn. Generally speaking, recognition performance at every age level exceeds recall performance, perhaps because recall tasks require more active rehearsal and elaboration at the time of encoding (Myers & Perlmutter, 1978).

Recall performance shows considerable improvement with age during childhood. The youngest children tested on recall tasks (which usually require verbal responses) have been about 2 years old (Myers & Perlmutter, 1978). Children at this age have great difficulty recalling objects, which suggests a retrieval problem. From age 2 until about age 10, children gradually increase the number of items they can recall. In old age, larger declines have been observed in recall performance than in recognition performance (Botwinick & Storandt, 1974a; Erber, 1974; Perlmutter, 1979; Schonfield & Robertson, 1966). These results have led many investigators to conclude that old adults suffer from retrieval difficulties.

Recognition performance has less pronounced developmental trends. Recognition memory appears to be remarkably good even among very young children and old adults (A. Brown & Scott, 1971; Craik, 1971; Perlmutter & Myers, 1974; Schonfield & Robertson, 1966). And in a series of studies using nonverbal assessment techniques, Fagan (1982) reported that infants as young as 5 months of age have excellent visual recognition memory. (Recall memory tasks are not used in infant memory research because of their verbal nature.) Although some studies of younger children and older adults have reported recognition difficulties as well as recall difficulties (Erber, 1974; C. Hoffman & Dick, 1976; Mandler & Robinson, 1978; Rankin & Kausler, 1979), recognition performance still surpasses recall performance under most task conditions. Developmental differences on recognition tasks are often found when the stimuli employed are exceedingly complex. For example, C. Hoffman and Dick (1976) reported age-related improvements in recognition from ages 3–7 and from age 7 to adulthood for a series of very complex and detailed pictures.

Several recent lines of evidence suggest that developmental differences in memory performance may also be found at the encoding stage. In the childhood literature, investigators have reported greater age differences in recognition and recall when complex stimuli or stimuli that are not easily discriminated are employed (see Dirks & Neisser, 1977; C. Hoffman & Dick, 1976; Mandler & Robinson, 1978; Mandler & Stein, 1974). These results suggest that younger children may be less efficient at encoding more complex and detailed stimulus information than older children and adults. Recent work by A. Smith (1980) on recognition and recall in old adults also suggests that age-related differences on these tasks are a result of different encoding strategies. Older adults do not spontaneously organize information to facilitate encoding to the same extent as young adults. According to the *encoding specificity* hypothesis (Tulving & Thomson, 1973), only when information has been organized effectively during encoding will retrieval cues be effective.

The influence of encoding on retrieval highlights the conceptual difficulties with the encoding-storage-retrieval trichotomy. This point was clearly illustrated in a study by A. Smith (1977) in which memory cues were varied at the input (encoding) and output (retrieval) stages of a word recall task. The memory cues consisted of either the first letter of the word or a category label (e.g., *bird*). The main finding was that the category cues provided at input or at both input and output reduced age differences in recall between younger adult and older adult subjects. However, when no category cues were given at either input or output, or only output cues were given, age differences remained and younger adults recalled more words than older adults. Thus, the recall deficits of older adults were only overcome by giving them cues at encoding, even in the absence of cueing at retrieval.

A. Smith's (1977) study is generally viewed as supporting the existence of encoding deficits in later adulthood, but conflicting findings have been reported in which retrieval deficits account for much of the age difference commonly observed on free recall tasks (see Burke & Light, 1981; Kausler, 1982). It remains difficult to decide whether differences between the young and the old are due to retrieval problems or to processing differences at the stage of encoding.

Episodic and Semantic Memory

The topic of memory may already seem complex, but now we are going to make it more complex by drawing further distinctions. One of the most important distinctions in the memory field in recent years is between **semantic memory** and **episodic memory** (Tulving, 1972, 1983), a distinction which is roughly equivalent to Piaget's differentiation of memory in the strict sense and memory in the wider sense (Piaget &

Inhelder, 1973). In his original formulation, Tulving (1972) defines *semantic memory* as "a mental thesaurus, organized knowledge a person possesses about *words* and other verbal symbols, their *meaning* and referents, about relations among them, and about rules, formulas, and algorithms for the manipulation of these symbols, concepts, and relations" (p. 386).

In effect, semantic memory consists of knowledge of the facts of the world, meanings of words, and symbol systems, such as English grammar or mathematical formulas. In contrast, *episodic memory* is concerned with "memory for personal experiences and their temporal relations" (Tulving, 1972, pp. 401–402); it includes some reference to the self and to a particular temporal and spatial context. An example of episodic memory might be your sixteenth birthday party or your appointment at the dentist's last Friday. Some additional distinguishing characteristics of episodic and semantic memory are shown in Table 6.2.

Considerable controversy exists over the distinction between episodic and semantic memory as separate, nonoverlapping systems. In his recent book Tulving (1983) has pointed out many of the similarities between the two types of memory and proposed "that episodic and semantic memory should be regarded as separate, albeit closely interacting systems" (p. 32). For example, in many real-life situations, both episodic and semantic memory can be accessed to solve problems. Think of trying to locate a set of missing keys. You might try to reconstruct where you last saw them or what happened between the time you lost them and now (episodic memory); or you might use your general world knowledge of where missing keys are most often found, such as in a trunk lock or coat pockets (semantic memory). Thus, these two types of memory can be conceptualized as interactive, rather than as mutually exclusive.

Another problem with the episodic-semantic distinction is that the terms apply not only to memory but to the memory tasks themselves (K. Nelson & Brown, 1978). "Episodic memory" refers to a class of laboratory tasks involving deliberate learning of lists of materials, the types of tasks most often employed in memory experiments. In order to perform well on these tasks, individuals must use memory or mnemonic strategies. Because children and old adults do poorly on such tasks, investigators have claimed erroneously that these subjects have bad episodic memories.

Semantic memory has been a relatively neglected topic in the developmental literature on memory. In the cognitive literature, numerous models have been proposed to describe the contents and organization of semantic memory. *Network* models represent semantic memory as a netlike arrangement of meanings and concepts with many associations between them. The *spreading activation* model of memory, developed

Table 6.2
Differences between Episodic and Semantic Memory

Episodic	Semantic
Types of Information	
1. Occurrence of a sensory event, even if not meaningful, is sufficient for registering information in episodic memory.	For information to be stored in semantic memory, the content of the episode must be understood and comprehended.
2. Organization of knowledge is temporal. Organization is also "loose" in the sense that precisely recorded information about an event can be easily changed or lost.	Organization of knowledge is conceptual. Knowledge is tightly structured into an overall semantic organization.
3. Each event in the episodic system is defined by the rememberer's personally experienced sense of time and, at retrieval, by his or her personal past.	Knowledge in the semantic system is not connected to the knower's personal identity. Knowledge an individual possesses is connected to the external world only indirectly.
Differences in Operations	
1. Relatively limited in its inferential ability. Knowledge about the contents and temporal dates of one event is not deducible from knowledge about another.	Possesses a rich inferential capability. Highly organized conceptual knowledge structure and availability of implicit and explicit rules for making inferences.
2. Information stored in the episodic system is more vulnerable; it can be changed, modified, and lost more readily.	Information is less vulnerable because it is tightly organized. A great deal of information is overlearned rather than based on single episodes.
3. Access to or actualization of information in the episodic system tends to be deliberate and usually requires conscious effort.	Access to information in the semantic system tends to be automatic.
4. Retrieval changes the information that was stored about an episode.	Retrieval of information from semantic memory produces less readily detectable consequences.
5. Appears late in the developmental sequence (around age 3).	Appears quite early in the developmental sequence (before age 3).

Note: From *Elements of Episodic Memory* (p. 35) by E. Tulving, 1983, New York: Oxford University Press. Copyright 1983 by Oxford University Press. Adapted by permission.

by Collins and Loftus (1975), is one of the most widely accepted network models. In their model each concept is represented by a node, or particular location, in the network. The nodes are connected by a series of links, or connectors, with the length of each link reflecting the degree of semantic association. When the name of a concept is processed, the node representing the concept is activated, and the activation spreads to other nodes. The farther the concept from the original node, the weaker the activation. Figure 6.6 presents a portion of a network that involves knowledge about animals and closely conforms to the original model proposed by Collins and Loftus (1975).

Several other well-known models of semantic memory exist. The ACT model of John R. Anderson (1983) is a complex extension of the network model involving language understanding and problem solving as well as semantic memory. A very different approach can be seen in the *features comparison* model of E. Smith, Shoben, and Rips (1974). They propose that concepts are stored in memory in terms of a list of

Figure 6.6   An example of a network model of semantic memory. The length of the line represents the strength of association between concepts.

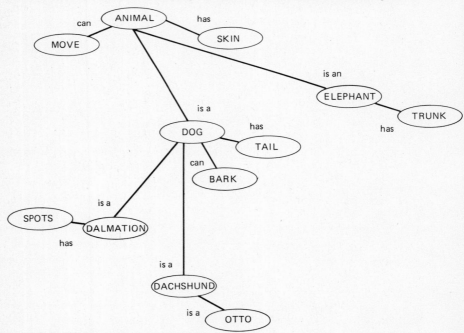

From "Information Processing and Cognitive Development" by R. Kail and J. Bisanz, 1982, in *Advances in Child Development and Behavior* (Vol. 17, p. 58), edited by H. W. Reese, New York: Academic Press. Copyright 1982 by Academic Press. Reprinted by permission.

features or attributes. For example, the concept *bird* has a set of relevant features such as *has wings and feathers, breathes, flies, nests in trees,* and *has a beak.* We do not have time to spell out all the technical details of these semantic models for you (see Johnson-Laird, Hermann, & Chaffin, 1984, for a critical review). More important for our purpose is to describe how the structure of semantic memory changes developmentally.

Very few attempts have been made to map developmental changes in semantic knowledge. In one recent study, Chi and Koeske (1983) constructed network models of a 4½-year-old boy's knowledge of dinosaurs based on how frequently dinosaurs were mentioned in the child's books as well as on information provided by his mother. Two network models were constructed from lists of better-known and lesser-known dinosaurs. The well-known network was characterized by a greater number of links between specific dinosaurs, greater strength of the links, and more direct linkings within certain related groups than between unrelated groups. This study is unique in that the semantic network was constructed from the child's verbal protocols, not from the experimenter's intuitions. In another recent study, Siegler and Richards (1983) attempted to characterize children's (aged 4–11) and adults' knowledge of life and the attributes they ascribe to living things. In Siegler and Richards' (1983) model, as in J. R. Anderson's (1983) ACT model, information is represented in terms of nodes and links connected to form propositions. They found that almost all of the subjects' responses could be categorized into one of five groups: *people, other animals, trees, other plants,* and *parts of living things.* Older children and adults included more animals and significantly more plants and trees in their representations than the younger children, with the greatest increase occurring between ages 7 and 9. In addition, older children and adults listed over twice as many attributes of living things (e.g., *eats, reproduces, dies, grows, moves*) as did the younger children. This research, like Chi and Koeske's (1983), shows developmental changes in semantic networks in the direction of increasing complexity and interconnectedness.

In recent years a growing number of studies on age differences in semantic memory have used connected verbal materials such as sentences, paragraphs, and stories. These materials are believed to be more contextually valid than the digit and word lists used in episodic memory studies.

Recall that Bartlett (1932) used a Native American folktale to assess contextualistic aspects of memory. Since his original work, several *story grammars* have been proposed to describe how people comprehend and remember the structure of a story (Kintsch & van Dijk, 1978; Mandler & Johnson, 1977; B. Meyer, 1975). The assumption underlying all of these approaches is that memory for story materials is a joint result of input information and preexisting schematic knowledge about stories.

Mandler's (1978) story grammar will be used here because it is one of the simplest. In Mandler's system a story consists of a series of basic elements or nodes which represent the syntactical structure of the story. The first node of an episode is the *setting*, which establishes the time and place of the story. The *beginning* then describes an event which starts the plot. Next is a *reaction* to the initial event, followed by a formulation of a *goal* to deal with it. Finally, there occurs an *attempt* to attain the goal through an action and then an *outcome* of success or failure. Using this set of grammatical rules, Mandler (1978) developed a set of stories such as the one presented in Box 6.3.

Box 6.3   Farmer Story (Shortened Version)

1. Once there was an old farmer
2. who owned a very stubborn donkey.
3. One evening, the farmer wanted to put his donkey into the barn.
4. First he pushed him,
5. but the donkey would not move.
6. Then he pulled him,
7. but the donkey still would not move.
8. Next the farmer thought he could frighten the donkey into the barn.
9. So he asked his dog to bark at the donkey,
10. but the lazy animal refused.
11. Then the farmer thought that his cat could get the dog to bark.
12. So he asked the cat to scratch the dog.
13. The cooperative cat scratched the dog.
14. The dog immediately began to bark.
15. The barking so frightened the donkey
16. that he jumped into the barn.

Note: From ''Remembrance of Things Parsed: Story Structure and Recall'' by J. M. Mandler and N. S. Johnson, 1977, *Cognitive Psychology, 9*, p. 127. Copyright 1977 by Academic Press. Reprinted by permission.

In a critical review of various story grammars, including Mandler's, Black and Wilensky (1979) concluded that it is more useful to focus on the semantic content of stories rather than their grammatical structure. They emphasized the importance of specific kinds of semantic knowledge needed to understand story content and how people use that knowledge during story comprehension. In their view, the major question is how individuals distinguish between stories that are "understandable" and those that are not.

In the developmental literature on children's memory, studies using different story grammars have produced fairly consistent results. Story recall generally increases with age through childhood, and violations of story structure interfere with recall (Mandler & DeForest, 1979; Mandler & Johnson, 1977; N. Stein & Glenn, 1979). Furthermore, children will typically rearrange disorganized or "nonunderstandable" (i.e., nonsemantic) stories into a more conventional story structure during recall. In the aging literature, mixed results have been obtained for developmental trends in story recall (Hultsch & Dixon, 1984). Some researchers have reported that old adults recall as much information as young adults, but recall fewer details and more "gist" information (B. Meyer & Rice, 1981; Spilich, 1983). Other investigators (G. Cohen, 1979; Dixon, Simon, Nowak, & Hultsch, 1982) have reported greater age differences for recall of gist information than for the details of a text.

In a recent study, S. Smith, Rebok, Smith, Hall, and Alvin (1983) attempted to resolve the conflicting findings by comparing well-educated young and old adults under three story structure conditions: (1) standard, (2) interleaved, and (3) scrambled. The standard version followed Mandler's (1978) structure, whereas the scrambled version violated this structure by having randomly ordered sentences. The interleaved version consisted of two story episodes woven together to form an atypical but structured story. The results revealed that both age groups recalled the standard stories equally well and the scrambled stories equally poorly, but old adults experienced recall problems on the interleaved stories and young adults did not. The investigators attributed the latter result to the demands placed on old subjects' memory by dividing attention between two story episodes.

Most investigations of age differences in story memory have been limited to either childhood or adulthood comparisons, but recently a few life-span investigations have appeared. In one study, Harker, Hartley, and Walsh (1982) assessed story recall among sixth graders, young adults, and old adults. They found age differences in overall recall scores between children and adults, but no differences between the two adult groups. One important life-span implication of the Harker et al. (1982) study is that caution must be exercised in interpreting age differences in semantic memory performance. Typically, differences in story recall between young and old adults are explained in terms of memory processing deficits, whereas those between children and adults are attributed to differences in organizational strategies or comprehension skills. Before such conclusions can be drawn, the capabilities of different aged subjects must be examined in great detail using various task materials and experimental conditions.

Levels of Processing

Memory *processing* is a key feature of the **levels-of-processing model** proposed by Fergus Craik and colleagues (Craik & Lockart, 1972; Craik & Tulving, 1975) as an alternative to multistore information-processing models of memory. Instead of viewing information as passing through a series of separate memory stores, Craik and colleagues speak of memory as a *continuous* process. In their model, incoming information can be processed in a hierarchical fashion at many different *levels* of analysis. At the "shallow" level, only physical or sensory features of stimuli are processed, and the resulting memory trace is highly fleeting. At the "deeper" level, individuals recognize patterns in the stimuli and extract meaning from stimuli, and the resulting memory trace is more durable. At the deepest, semantic level, people do some cognitive analysis of the to-be-remembered material. Thus, memory is viewed as a continuum of processing ranging from memory traces resulting from shallow, less permanent encoding to more permanent encoding of semantic features. The deeper the level at which material is processed, the better the retention.

A typical levels-of-processing study asks subjects to encode a series of words by processing them to various levels. As each word is presented, the experimenter asks subjects questions about it to which they must respond "yes" or "no." The questions may refer to nonsemantic, orthographic features of the word ("Is it printed in small letters?"), or may ask about semantic features involving category membership ("Is the word a type of vehicle?") or sentence completion ("Would the word fit into the sentence 'I saw a _____ in the pond'?"). These are called *orienting* questions because they are designed to induce a certain level of encoding. After the questions are presented, subjects are given an *incidental* or unexpected test of recall or recognition memory for the list of words (see Table 6.3).

Initial work (Craik & Tulving, 1975; Till & Jenkins, 1973; Walsh & Jenkins, 1973) has supported the levels-of-processing notion: words about which semantic questions were asked were retained far better than words preceded by nonsemantic questions. Why does semantic encoding lead to superior retention compared to other types of encod-

Table 6.3
Examples of Typical Orienting Questions and Answers in the Craik and Tulving (1975) Experiment

Processing Level	Question	Answer	
		Yes	*No*
Orthographic	Is the word in capital letters?	TABLE	table
Rhyming	Does the work rhyme with WEIGHT?	crate	MARKET
Category	Is the word a type of fish?	SHARK	heaven
Sentence	Would the word fit in the sentence "He met a _____ in the street"?	FRIEND	cloud

Note: From "Depth of Processing and the Retention of Words in Episodic Memory" by F. I. M. Craik and E. Tulving, 1975, *Journal of Experimental Psychology: General, 104,* p. 272. Copyright 1975 by the American Psychological Association. Reprinted by permission.

ing? M. W. Eysenck and Eysenck (1979) suggested that, unlike semantic encoding, nonsemantic encoding directs the learner's attention to selected parts of a word (such as the first letter or the last syllable), thereby interfering with the encoding of the entire stimulus. Fisher and Craik (1977) explained the superiority of semantic encoding in terms of the larger number of features that can be encoded uniquely at the semantic level than at shallower levels.

Like the multistore model of memory, the levels-of-processing model was initially developed and tested on adult college samples. And most of the subsequent developmental studies using the model have been conducted with adult subjects of various ages. In an influential study, Eysenck (1974) compared young adults (aged 18–30 years) and old adults (aged 55–65 years) under different orienting conditions. He found that old subjects remembered significantly fewer words on a recall task than young subjects and did not benefit from an orienting task designed to induce deep processing. There was no evidence for any age differences in recall with shallow processing orienting tasks. These results led M. W. Eysenck (1974) to conclude that older adults have a "processing deficit" at deeper semantic levels. In a more recent test of the processing deficit hypothesis, Mason (1979) compared young, middle-aged, and old adults under various orienting conditions (orthographic, rhyming, category orienting) and found that semantic orienting tasks increased adult age differences in memory performance. Not all studies agree with these results, however. Perlmutter (1979) eliminated adult age differences in free recall by using a semantic orienting task followed by cued recall, suggesting that old adults suffer from a production deficiency, not a processing deficiency.

Little research on depth of processing has used childhood samples. In one study, M. Murphy and Brown (1975) presented preschoolers with lists of pictures and gave them (1) explicit instructions to remember the items, (2) an orienting task focused on physical features such as the color of the pictures, or (3) a task requiring them to categorize the pictures. M. Murphy and Brown (1975) found that the categorization task induced a deeper level of processing and led to better recall scores than the other two conditions. S. Weiss, Robinson, and Hastie (1977) gave second and fourth graders a 40-word list under various task conditions designed to deepen processing. They discovered that the depth-of-processing manipulation aided the fourth graders' performance more than the second graders' performance. Results of both these studies provide added support for the levels-of-processing position.

Various explanations have been offered as to why young children and old adults benefit less than other age groups from conditions designed to induce deeper processing. One possibility is that young children and old adults engage in less *elaborative* rehearsal, that is, rehearsal which involves the generation of images of items and semantic associations between these images. This type of rehearsal has been called **Type II processing** and is expected to produce durable memory traces. In contrast, **Type I processing,** or *maintenance* rehearsal, is characterized by the rote repetition of material in working memory (such as simply repeating a list of items to yourself over and over again). Maintenance rehearsal is important to momentarily keep information in working memory, but it yields very transient memory traces. Maintenance rehearsal involves shallow processing and limited cognitive effort in contrast to elaborative rehearsal, which occurs at a deeper processing level and is more cognitively demanding. If the processing resources of young children and older adults are more limited than those of other age groups, the first two groups would be expected to engage in maintenance rehearsal and to show low long-term retention.

Although the levels-of-processing framework has stimulated a great deal of research, especially on adult samples, it has also come under heavy criticism. Baddeley (1978) has argued that the definition of processing *depth* is inadequate because no independent, objective measure of depth is used. Without such a measure, we are left with intuitive concepts and circular reasoning. Intuitively, shallow processing should lead to poor retention and deep processing to better retention, but how can one tell if information has been deeply processed? The only way to make this determination at the moment is to look at how well the information is remembered in the first place. Moreover, some studies have produced results inconsistent with the notion that deeper processing always leads to superior recall. In an influential series of experiments, Morris, Bransford, and Franks (1977) reported that shallower levels of processing led to better retrieval on memory tasks calling for nonsemantic encoding of stimuli (e.g., the spelling or rhyming of words). These results emphasize the importance of the learning context in considerations of the appropriateness of any memory activity.

Automatic and Effortful Processing

Another important distinction has recently been made in the memory literature between automatic and effortful processing (Hasher & Zacks, 1979). As discussed in Chapter 3, automatic processing occurs spontaneously without attentional demands, whereas effortful processing demands deliberate activation of attention. For example, someone learning to drive a car must pay attention to many aspects of driving (e.g., shifting gears, turning on directional signals) that experienced drivers perform automatically. But even experienced drivers activate attention to deal with difficult driving situations (sudden stops, heavy traffic). Thus, effortful processes can occur at the same time as automatic processes without interfering with them. When attentional demands exceed our attentional capacity, performance may suffer.

In order to study automatic and effortful processing, researchers have developed several research procedures. For example, Schneider and Shiffrin (1977) used a combined memory search and visual search procedure. Their results showed that subjects who developed automatic detection strategies were not affected by the amount of information to be remembered, but subjects who relied on effortful (which they termed *controlled*) processing that involved attentional and perceptual scanning showed reduced performance under increased load conditions.

As we discussed earlier in this chapter, the developmental literature on changes in control strategies over the childhood years is substantial. Strategies such as rehearsal and organization are used more frequently by older children than younger children, and these strategies demand most attention or effortful processing. On the other hand, strategies that rely on automatic processing show minimal developmental changes during childhood; such strategies include encoding basic temporal and spatial information as well as recognition information. Thus, remembering temporal durations, the spatial layout of one's neighborhood, and the identity of a frequent visitor require little effortful processing.

Aging has been frequently associated with reductions in the use of effortful or controlled processing strategies. Elderly adults, like young children, often fail to use deliberate mnemonic strategies on memory tasks. In a direct test of the automatic-effortful distinction, Plude and Hoyer (1981) gave a card-sorting task to groups of young (mean age 23.6 years) and elderly (mean age 75 years) adults. The task involved either an unchanging memory set (consistent mapping) or a changing memory set (varied mapping) with zero, three, or eight distractor items. In the consistent mapping condition, subjects searched for the same target over several experimental sessions. For example, the letters A and Y served as target letters printed on an index card. Each card in a stack of cards contained either A or Y, plus a number of distractors. Cards containing the letter A were supposed to be placed in one pile and those containing the letter Y were to be placed in the other pile. In the varied mapping condition, different target letters were designated for each experimental session (A and Y for the first session, L and J for the second session, and so on) with varying numbers of distractor items across sessions. The latter condition introduced a heavy memory load, which required more effortful, attention-demanding processing. When the target stimuli remained consistent from session to session, less cognitive effort was required, and processing became more automatic.

Plude and Hoyer (1981) found that under the varied mapping conditions (requiring effortful processing), the young adults performed better than the elderly adults; but no age differences were found in the consistent mapping condition (requiring automatic processing). This result suggests that age differences can be minimized when effortful processing requirements are decreased. The Plude and Hoyer study must be interpreted cautiously, however, because recent studies using other stimulus materials and task conditions have reported age differences in automatic and effortful processing components (Kausler & Hakami, 1982; Park, Puglisi, & Lutz, 1982).

REMOTE MEMORY

The observation that older adults can accurately remember *remote* events in their lives, but often fail to recall events of the recent past has been based mostly on clinical impressions and on elderly persons' observations of their own memory processes. Why should old or remote (tertiary) memories be recalled better than recent ones? Psychologists offer many explanations to account for this phenomenon. Perhaps old events are more meaningful to older adults, especially if their present situation lacks meaning and purpose. Certainly, memory of personal events may be more meaningful to elderly individuals than memory of laboratory materials used in experiments. Another possibility is that old memories have been rehearsed more often and therefore are recalled more easily.

The experimental controls needed to evaluate explanations of the purported superiority of remote memory are lacking. There is no way to determine how often a memory has been retrieved over the years or how relevant this memory is to the individual. Moreover, the quantity of information originally stored in memory is unknown. The remote memories observed may represent only a small fraction of an old adult's storehouse of old memories, many of which may not be retrievable.

Some research has focused on contrasting age differences in old versus new memories (Botwinick & Storandt, 1974a; Poon, Fozard, Paulshock, & Thomas, 1979). These studies employed an old adult group and a young adult group and compared them in terms of old and more recent recall. In addition, investigators have frequently used a questionnaire technique covering major news events from different time periods. For example, Botwinick and Storandt (1974a) employed a questionnaire to assess young and old subjects' recall on material from the 1890s to the 1960s (see Table 6.4 for sample questions). They found no significant age effects in recall of remote past events, but subjects tended to recall more material from the time when they were young (15–25 years) than for their later years. Botwinick and Storandt (1974a) also reported a sex difference in remote memory, with males showing superior memory to females at all age levels and historical periods. However, the authors acknowledged that the items may have been unintentionally biased in favor of men. In a replication study, Perlmutter (1978) used Botwinick and Storandt's questionnaire and found the same sex difference. In contrast to Botwinick and Storandt's (1974a)

Table 6.4
Sample Questions from Botwinick and Storandt's (1974a) Long-Term Memory Questionnaire

1950–1969	1. What was the name of the first man to set foot on the moon? (Neil Armstrong)
	2. In what year did the Russians orbit the first satellite? (1957)
1930–1949	3. What was the name of the only President of the United States to be elected to four terms of office? (Franklin Roosevelt)
	4. Where (in what state) did the German dirigible, the *Von Hindenburg,* crash and burn? (New Jersey)
1910–1929	5. What was the name of the ship which hit an iceberg and sank on its maiden voyage in 1912? (*Titanic*)
	6. What do the initials *WCTU* stand for? (Women's Christian Temperance Union)
1890–1909	7. Where did the Wright brothers make their first successful flight? (Kitty Hawk)
	8. In what year did Henry Ford introduce the Model T? (1908)

Note: From *Memory, Related Functions, and Age* (pp. 189–191) by J. Botwinick and M. Storandt, 1974, Springfield, IL: Charles C Thomas. Copyright 1974 by Charles C. Thomas, Publisher. Adapted by permission.

findings, recall and recognition memory for remote events improved with age.

In a study designed to clarify the conflicting results on remote memory, Poon and associates (1979) administered a memory questionnaire to a group of males aged 26–69. Their results supported Botwinick and Storandt's (1974a) findings of minimal age differences in memory for recent events. However, consistent with Perlmutter (1978), Poon et al. (1979) found that elderly adults outperformed young adults on remote recall items.

In order to study age effects on very long-term memory, it is desirable to keep the age of the person and the age of the memory separate. For example, memory of the United States moon landing dates from the same year—1969—for everyone who experienced the event. However, some studies have confounded the person's age and the date of the event. Bahrick, Bahrick, and Wittlinger (1975) tested male and female high school graduates (aged 17–74) for memory of the names and faces of their classmates from their high school yearbooks. They reported that recall and recognition memory performance declined with time (and therefore age) since graduation. Nevertheless, over 90 percent of the information about names and faces remained for at least 15 years after graduation and declined only to 60 percent 40 years after graduation. Note here that age of subjects (17–74) and age of memory are confounded, which complicates conclusions from this study. However, memory for long-term events appears critical in maintaining a sense of psychological continuity and personal identity over time.

METAMEMORY

Think about your high school graduation class. Can you recall the names and faces of most of your high school classmates, as subjects did in the Bahrick et al. (1975) study? Is it easier for you to remember names or faces? If you cannot recall a classmate, what strategies would you use to retrieve the student from memory? Answers to these questions reveal your awareness and knowledge of your own memory processes and how they operate. Flavell (1971b) referred to this awareness as **metamemory** and argued that it influences our ability to store, retain, and retrieve information from memory.

In the past 15 years, developmental psychologists have shown increased interest in studying metamemory processes and the more general process of *metacognition*, or knowledge about knowing and understanding (A. Brown, 1975; A. Brown, Bransford, Ferrara, & Campione, 1983; Flavell & Wellman, 1977; Paris, 1978). Metamemory covers a broad constellation of abilities important for remembering. One such ability is *memory monitoring*, or the ability to keep track of items currently in your memory. This type of metamemory involves knowledge about whether an item is stored in memory and whether you think you can recall it if asked. Another type of metamemory is *memory knowledge*, which includes knowledge about the number of items that can be held in memory at one time and the factors that facilitate or inhibit recall.

Because it involves abilities which are useful in grade school settings, metamemory has most often been examined by developmental psychologists studying children. However, there is increasing recognition of the role of metamemory abilities in using accumulated knowledge about the world. Whether people should spend time searching their knowledge base for an item, attempt to reconstruct the item by drawing inferences, or use an external mnemonic device (such as lists, notebooks, other people) depends to a large extent on an efficiently functioning metamemory (Flavell, 1985). In addition, in the face of declines in retrieval processes with increasing age and the accumulation of an internal store of information, metamemory may serve to maintain memory functioning. Thus, metamemory skills may be especially important in studies of life-span cognition (J. Lachman, Lachman, & Thronesbery, 1979).

Studies of metamemory in children show less accurate memory monitoring and memory knowledge in young than in old children. Two similar experiments presented children and adults with sequences of pictures beginning with 1 item and ranging to a maximum of 10 items and asked the subjects to predict the number of pictures they would be able to recall (Flavell, Friedrichs, & Hoyt, 1970; Yussen & Levy, 1975). The experimenters also tested the subjects' actual memory spans. The combined results from both experiments are displayed in Figure 6.7, which shows that through kindergarten, the discrepancy between predicted and actual recall is quite large. From second to fourth grade, the gap narrows somewhat, so that children become more realistic in their predictions. From fourth grade on, children estimate their recall just about as well as adults do. The striking discrepancy between the actual and predicted memory spans of kindergarten and nursery school children may have significant implications. If young children erroneously believe they can recall 8 items in order, they may be less likely to perceive the need to use mnemonic devices or strategies.

Such results are frequently used to explain the difficulties children experience in remembering. Young children probably have numerous gaps in their memory knowledge. First, children appear to have a much more limited understanding than adults of the need to employ deliberately mnemonic strategies. They must learn to discriminate situations which demand deliberate memorization. Children also do not

Figure 6.7   Predicted and actual memory spans by grade level. Based on data from Flavell et al. (1970) and Yussen and Levy (1975). N = nursery school, K = kindergarten.

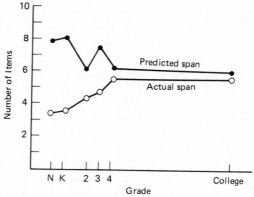

From *The Development of Memory in Children* (2nd ed., p. 51) by R. Kail, 1984, San Francisco: Freeman. Copyright 1984 by W. H. Freeman and Company. Reprinted by permission.

realize the impact the quantity of information can have on the difficulty of a memory task, as shown in the studies cited on predicted memory span. Finally, young children seem less capable of monitoring and evaluating their recall readiness. In the study by Flavell et al. (1970), preschoolers were less accurate than second and fourth graders in assessing when a set of stimulus items had been memorized.

Like other aspects of memory, children's knowledge of metamemory functioning shows age-associated improvements. What developmental factors account for these improvements? One factor may involve the sorts of memory tasks children are routinely exposed to in home and school environments. For example, children see parents writing items on a grocery list or birth dates on a calendar to help the latter remember. And children are frequently asked questions about their memory for the locations of objects ("Where is your bicycle?") or social routines ("What should you say when you answer the phone?"). When children enter grade school, the importance of memory abilities becomes even more apparent. Children must learn to judge the length of time allotted to study material, the best strategy to use for remembering, the relative difficulty level of various types of tests, and so on. Although their knowledge of these individual aspects of metamemory improves with age, children only gradually learn the impact of *combinations* of memory variables and often do not show such knowledge until adolescence or young adulthood (Kail, 1984).

Though a fair amount is known about children's metamemory knowledge, much less is known about how children *monitor* the extent to which they have stored something in memory (A. Brown et al., 1983). Much-needed information on this issue has been provided in two studies by Henry Wellman and colleagues (Cultice, Somerville, & Wellman, 1983; Wellman, 1977). Wellman (1977) investigated the memory-monitoring abilities of kindergarten, first-, and third-grade children on a name recognition task. Children were shown pictures of 30 objects and asked to name them. The objects differed in ease of naming. Some were easily named *(clown, fish)*, some were of medium difficulty *(goggles, pliers)*, and others were difficult to name *(caduceus, metronome)*. Subjects who failed to name the picture were asked to judge whether they would recognize the name if they heard it. Such judgments are called "feeling-of-knowing" judgments because they involve the subjective prediction of whether one will be able to retrieve an item from a set of items (Hart, 1965, 1967). Finally, children were given a recognition test in which they were shown a set of 9 objects and required to pick a designated object from the set. Although able to make the feel-of-knowing judgments about recognition, children's accuracy improved considerably between ages 6–9. Thus, all the children appeared to have the relevant information in their long-term memories and could make judgments about it. This result is significant for the development of optimal memory search routines. If information is not in long-term store, a search for it is inefficient and such a decision must be based on accurate memory monitoring.

In a subsequent study, Cultice et al. (1983) presented a modified naming task to 4–5-year-old children. The stimuli were photographs, some of which were easy to name (classmates, teachers), some moderately difficult to name (children attending another preschool class in the same building, researchers conducting studies in the school), and some totally unlikely to be named (children and adults who never visited the preschool). As before, the focus was on the correspondence of feeling-of-knowing judgments to actual recognition performance. The results showed that both 4- and 5-year-olds were able to monitor their memories accurately; they could distinguish names they would recognize from those they would not. Noteworthy is the fact that children in this study were substantially more accurate in their monitoring assessments than were 6-year-olds in Wellman's (1977) study, perhaps because the task in the former study involved background knowledge of personal names.

Can metamemory differences account for poor memory performance in older adults on memory tasks? Bruce, Coyne, and Botwinick (1982) addressed this question in a study comparing the accuracy of metamemory abilities in three groups aged 18–31, 60–69, and 70–79 years. Bruce et al. found that elderly adults, like young children, tended to overestimate their recall abilities, but young adults made accurate recall

Box 6.4   Complaints of Poor Memory in the Elderly

Elderly adults frequently express concern about poor memory. Surveys have shown that about 50 percent of community-living elderly report serious memory problems, and the percentage is even higher among elderly referred to a geriatric clinic (see Zarit, Cole, & Guider, 1981). These complaints usually are assumed to reflect negative age changes in actual memory ability, but evidence suggests that such complaints may reflect depressed mood. In a study comparing older adults with or without signs of organic brain dysfunction, Kahn, Zarit, Hilbert, and Niederehe (1975) found that depressed individuals had a greater number of memory complaints than those who were not depressed, even though the subjects' actual memory performance did not differ. Furthermore, even among organically impaired older adults who had performed poorly on standardized memory tasks, complaints were made only if the person was also depressed. This research suggests that memory complaints among the elderly may be related to depressed affect, rather than declining memory.

In a series of studies, Zarit et al. (1981) examined the effects of memory training on subjective complaints about memory among the elderly. In one study, subjects aged 50–88 years (mean age 72.2) were taught four different memory strategies for remembering lists of related and unrelated items, names and faces, and a long prose passage. The strategies included clustering the items into groups, constructing a meaningful connection between the items, forming a visual image of the to-be-remembered material, and making personal associations to the material. Significant improvements in memory performance occurred among subjects using clustering and visual imaging strategies, but improved performance did not lead to fewer memory complaints. And, in contrast to previous studies, depressed mood showed no significant relation to memory complaints. This lack of relationship suggests that other factors should be considered in determining the extent of concern about poor memory in the elderly (Zarit et al., 1981). Perhaps the pervasive stereotype that memory declines naturally with age causes many older adults to complain about their memory, regardless of whether they are depressed and experience actual memory deficits.

predictions. Bruce et al. (1982) interpreted these results as evidence that young adults possess more accurate metamemory knowledge than old adults. Paradoxically, many old adults in the study also expressed concern about their memory declines. Box 6.4 considers memory complaints among the elderly. In contrast to the Bruce et al. (1982) study, Perlmutter (1978) and M. Murphy, Sanders, Gabriesheski, and Schmitt (1981) reported that young adults and old adults were equally accurate in predicting their memory span on a subsequent recall task.

Although metamemory research continues to grow rapidly, serious concerns have been raised. In a comprehensive critical review, Cavanaugh and Perlmutter (1982) have argued that we still lack a clear definition of *metamemory* as well as reliable and valid measures for assessing it. They also pointed out that the relationships between metamemory and memory ability are not well understood because improvements in metamemory do not always result in better memory performances. Most researchers simply correlate the two abilities without concern for the theoretical meaning of the correlations.

In addition to these concerns, several aspects of metamemory remain inadequately studied. One area deals with **prospective memory,** or memory for future events, such as reminding ourselves to stop by the bank to cash a check before we go home. Traditionally, the bulk of memory development research has been devoted to **retrospective memory,** or memory for past experiences and events, but little research on age differences in prospective memory exists (J. Harris, 1984; Meacham, 1977). Perhaps as one's time perspective shifts from future events to past experiences with age, the importance of prospective memory also shifts.

MEMORY, THE INDIVIDUAL, AND SOCIETY

The memory models and approaches described in this chapter are based, in large measure, on studies of different-aged individuals' performances on laboratory tasks. These models fail to consider the role of social, cultural, and historical changes in developmental memory changes across the life span. As Reese (1976) has pointed out, notions of a durable memory trace or permanent long-term storage system are inconsistent with a dynamic conception of memory.

One model of memory that considers individual changes in memory abilities within the context of a changing society is the *dialectical* model, which fits nicely into the contextualistic approach to psychology described in Chapter 2. Two major features characterize the dialectical approach to memory—an emphasis on context and a focus on change.

As the context changes, changes occur in both episodic and semantic memory (Tulving, 1972, 1983). Since life-span approaches also emphasize these features, such approaches seem quite compatible with the dialectical model of memory.

In a paper on memory development in the individual and society, Meacham (1972) summarized the major dimensions of the dialectical model as exemplified by Soviet research. The Soviet approach to memory emphasizes the importance of embedding material to be remembered within the ongoing activity of the organism. For example, when you are trying to recall someone's phone number, think of all the mnemonic activities you engage in—repeating the numbers to yourself, searching through an address book for the number, using visual imagery to picture the number in your mind.

Several steps are involved in the development of memory competence, according to the Soviet model. First, a person learns an activity (action) such as rehearsing, classifying, or verbal labeling for its own sake. Later, this activity can be subordinated to reach a new goal, such as the goal of remembering. Then the new goal can be embedded within even more complex activities, such as problem solving, as a way of reaching a higher goal (Reese, 1976). In order for an activity to be subordinated to a new goal, it must be "well formed," or practiced. Once fully formed, it becomes part of a hierarchy of progressively more complex memory strategies. These hierarchical and subordination processes bring the individual into closer interaction with the material to be remembered.

One of the most striking examples of the importance of incorporating material to be remembered within an activity is found in a study by the Soviet psychologist Istomina (1975), who gave 3–7-year-old children a list of five words to remember under two different experimental conditions. In one condition, she set up a grocery store and had children remember the items so that they could buy them. In the other condition, she simply told the children to learn and remember the list of words. Istomina found that children in the grocery store condition recalled almost twice as many items as children in the list-learning condition. She attributed this finding to the "naturalness" of the shopping situation as opposed to the artificial nature of the list condition.

From Istomina's (1975) results, we can conclude that knowing about memory or its significance is not sufficient; people must see memory as a goal worth pursuing. As Hultsch and Pentz (1980) have stated, "Learning and remembering are means to ends as well as ends in themselves" (p. 85). It is likely that the goal of remembering changes across different ages. For example, there has been considerable work in gerontology on **reminiscence,** or the calling to mind of a past life experience or event. Reminiscing processes appear to become more important to individuals over 45–50 years of age, and these processes seem to help older people integrate their experiences and personality (Boylin, Gordon, & Nehrke, 1976; Butler, 1963).

The importance of memory as a goal also changes as society changes. Over 70 years ago Robinson (1912) recommended that we cultivate memory skills because, in his opinion, a good memory was the single most important factor in having a successful career. Today, most career experts emphasize good problem-solving and decision-making skills as the primary key to career advancement. Because our complex technological society changes rapidly, storing large amounts of information which may soon be outdated is less important than the ability to analyze and integrate information. In the next two chapters, you will read about problem-solving, decision-making, intelligence, and other complex thinking skills.

SUMMARY

1. Memory abilities are critical for recalling past experiences as well as for planning future actions. Because of the importance of memory in everyday functioning, psychologists have long been interested in studying it.

2. Most empirical work on memory up until 1970 was descriptive and did not deal extensively with theoretical issues. Recently, memory researchers have borrowed theoretical concepts from information-processing models and applied them to developmental problems.

3. In addition to information-processing models, three other theoretical frameworks for studying memory development are organismic, behavioristic, and contextualistic.

4. Information-processing models of memory can be represented in terms of an active cognitive system with storage structures and control operations. Storage structures include a sensory register, short-term store, and long-term store. Control operations such as rehearsal, elaboration, and organization direct the flow of information from one storage structure to the next.

5. Paired-associate tasks are often used in behavioristic studies to assess learning and memory. Failure to use mediators spontaneously is one reason why young children and old adults do poorly on such tasks.

6. From a contextualistic perspective, subjects actively construct their memories by transforming and elaborating the to-be-remembered material. Contextualistic studies of memory frequently employ meaningful sentence and text materials.

7. Developmental research on sensory memory focuses on either iconic (visual) or echoic (auditory) memory. Researchers report only slight changes in iconic and echoic memory over the life span.

8. Greater age changes are found in long-term (secondary) memory than in short-term (primary) memory. Investigators usually attribute these findings to age-related differences in the use of mnemonic strategies.

9. A major issue in memory research is whether memory difficulties represent problems in encoding, storage, or retrieval. Studies comparing recall and recognition memory locate the major difficulty in the retrieval stage, but there is also evidence for age-related differences in encoding.

10. Several important distinctions have recently been made in regard to long-term memory, including episodic and semantic memory, levels of processing, and automatic versus effortful processing. These distinctions have substantial implications for studying memory development, but they also have been frequently criticized.

11. Memory for very long-term events is referred to as "remote memory." Little empirical support can be found for the supposition that older adults can remember remote events in their lives better than recent ones.

12. "Metamemory" refers to our awareness and understanding of our own memory processes. Metamemory abilities play an increasingly influential role in memory with age, although their relationship to memory performance is not well understood.

13. The dialectical model of memory considers individual changes in memory within the context of a changing society. Soviet research on memory exemplifies a dialectical approach. Soviet researchers emphasize the importance of incorporating material to be remembered within an individual's ongoing activity.

Key Terms

seriation	paired-associate learning
sensory register	proactive interference
memory decay	retroactive interference
short-term store	schema
long-term store	iconic

echoic

span of immediate memory

working memory

recency effect

serial position curve

primacy effect

primary memory

secondary memory

production deficiencies

mediation deficiencies

production inefficiency

recall

recognition

semantic memory

episodic memory

levels-of-processing model

Type II processing

Type I processing

metamemory

prospective memory

retrospective memory

reminiscence

Suggested Readings

Baddeley, A. D. (1976). *The psychology of memory.* New York: Basic Books. An excellent comprehensive overview of memory research. Some of the material is slightly dated now, but still worth reading.

Chi, M. T. H. (Ed.). (1983). *Trends in memory development research.* Basel, Switzerland: Karger. A summary of major trends in memory development research over the past 10 years and of the unresolved problems likely to dominate future work. This book should interest students who want a brief but expert review of current issues in the memory development literature.

Kail, R. (1984). *The development of memory in children* (2nd ed.). San Francisco: Freeman. Written for individuals with limited backgrounds in psychology, this book describes current knowledge of memory development and the possible mechanisms underlying developmental changes in memory.

Kail, R., & Spear, N. E. (Eds.). (1984). *Comparative perspectives on the development of memory.* Hillsdale, NJ: Erlbaum. This volume attempts to bridge the gap between researchers studying the development of human memory and those studying memory in infrahuman organisms. Chapters by developmental psychologists and developmental psychobiologists discuss constraints on memory as well as development of various components of memory.

Luria, A. R. (1968). *The mind of a mnemonist.* New York: Basic Books. This remarkable little book describes the clinical case of a Russian mnemonist known only by his initial, *S,* and his extraordinary memory ability. Luria relates *S*'s memory expertise to various aspects of personality development.

Moscovitch, M. (Ed.). (1984). *Infant memory: Its relation to normal and pathological memory in humans and other animals.* New York: Plenum Press. This collection of articles attempts to integrate the literature on infant memory and mainstream memory development research; it should appeal to both beginning and advanced readers.

Neisser, U. (1982). *Memory observed: Remembering in natural contexts.* San Francisco: Freeman. This book emphasizes observations of memory in natural contexts rather than in the psychological laboratory. This fascinating book discusses the kinds of memory that psychologists often ignore—childhood recollections, eyewitness testimony, special memory feats, and memories of famous individuals.

Poon, L. W. (1985). Differences in human memory with aging: Nature, causes, and clinical implications. In J. E. Birren & K. W. Schaie (Eds.), *Handbook of the psychology of aging* (2nd ed., pp. 427–462). New York: Van Nostrand Reinhold. This comprehensive and scholarly presentation of the available experimental evidence on human memory and aging emphasizes the interactional effects of environmental influences and individual differences on memory performance.

Poon, L. W., Fozard, J. L., Cermak, L., Arenberg, D., & Thompson, L. (Eds.). (1980). *New directions in memory and aging: Proceedings of the George Talland Memorial Conference.* Hillsdale, NJ: Erlbaum. This book identifies the most promising areas in memory research as they relate to aging. It includes contributions by both experimental and clinical psychologists and should appeal to anyone who has active interests in research on aging or is concerned about applying research findings to the diagnosis and treatment of memory problems in the elderly.

CHAPTER 7

Problem Solving and Creativity

OUTLINE

OVERVIEW

Problem solving includes any sequence of cognitive operations which are directed toward a goal. Problems having clear goals can usually be solved with routine operations, but those with vague goals often require creative solutions.

In this chapter we present one of the oldest theories of problem solving, Gestalt theory, as well as more recent information-processing approaches. Gestalt theorists emphasize restructuring the elements of a problem to form a solution, whereas information-processing approaches focus on the search for a solution through a problem space. Neither perspective is based explicitly on developmental considerations.

Piaget's work most clearly illustrates a developmental approach to the study of problem solving. Developmental trends on several Piagetian tasks will be considered, including the famous conservation problem. Attempts to extend Piagetian research across the life span are also discussed. In addition to the large body of work on Piagetian problem solving, the developmental literature on more traditional problem-solving tasks such as concept learning will be reviewed.

Next, the topic of creativity is introduced. We will argue that creativity is not limited to the artistic or scientific genius but can be found, in varying degrees, in each of us. Researchers who study creativity distinguish among creative persons, creative products, and creative processes. Although these are not mutually exclusive categories, they help us organize and evaluate the literature on creativity.

The final sections emphasize the importance of studying creativity from a life-span perspective. Some problems related to equating creativity measures for different age groups will be examined. We also will look at empirical findings from developmental studies of creative behavior and a preliminary attempt to construct a developmental theory of creativity.

A SAMPLE PROBLEM

Suppose someone gives you the following problem to solve: Here are two decks of standard playing cards, 52 cards per deck. The backs of all the cards are identical. I am going to shuffle the two decks together into one large pile. What I would like you to do is sort the pile into two complete decks as quickly as you can and with as few errors as possible.

At this point you might be tempted to get two decks of cards and try the problem yourself. Before you do, stop for a moment and think about the ways you might proceed. You could start by sorting all the red cards into one pile and all the black cards into another. Or you might choose to divide the cards first into four piles by suit—hearts, diamonds, clubs, spades. You could also begin by sorting the deck into 13 separate piles according to the face value of the cards—aces, twos, threes, fours, and so on.

When my colleague Jerome Meyer and I gave this task to four different age groups (third graders, eighth graders, young adults, old adults), we were surprised by the variety of strategies that subjects used (J. Meyer & Rebok, 1985). You might be thinking, "Come on, there can't be *that* many ways to sort cards." (Why not try the task now and find out for yourself!) In our research on this problem, we identified at least eight different characteristic sorting strategies, which ranged from sorting the cards first by suit and then by face value, to laying all 104 cards out on the table in a matrixlike arrangement. Some of our younger subjects sorted through the entire deck and picked out all the aces first, and then went back through the deck again and picked out all the twos, threes, and so on. Older subjects tended to use more efficient strategies such as laying the cards into 13 piles by face value with a single duplicate value pile, a strategy which appeared to limit the amount of visual scanning and remembering required and involved only a single sort. Thus, problem-solving strategies can vary greatly in their effectiveness. Later in this chapter we will examine why some strategies are better than others and why strategies show changes with development.

DEFINITIONS AND DISTINCTIONS

What makes the card-sorting task a problem-solving task? The next section examines various criteria proposed to define problem solving. The topic of creativity will be introduced, and distinctions will be drawn between problem-solving processes and creative thinking processes. Contrary to what many people think, the two types of processes are not dramatically different from one another.

Problem Solving

A well-known cognitive psychologist, John R. Anderson (1985), has identified three criteria that characterize problem solving: (1) goal-directedness, (2) subgoal decomposition, (3) operator selection. By *goal-directedness*, he means that problem solving is oriented toward a desired goal or solution. On the card-sorting problem described above, there is substantial agreement about the goal or solution—divide one deck of cards into two separate and complete decks. Hence, the problem can be called a *well-defined* problem (Reitman, 1965). However, as some psychologists have pointed out (Greeno, 1976), there can be uncertainties about the exact goal of a problem and the steps to its solution, even on relatively well-defined problems. Consider again the card-sorting problem. Although the final goal of the problem seems clear enough, the intermediate goals subjects generate and use in the process of working on the problem are not ("Should I first sort the cards into face value or suit?"). Moreover, the goals may vary from one problem solver to another and may not be the same as those the experimenter had in mind. For example, in the card-sorting experiment (J. Meyer & Rebok, 1985), many subjects' behaviors, particularly those of the youngest subjects, seemed directed toward the goal of sorting the cards as quickly as possible without too much concern about separating them into two decks.

Most problems employed by psychologists in the laboratory are well defined and have clearly stated goals. However, problems encountered in everyday life tend to be *ill defined;* they lack clearly defined goals and procedures for reaching them. Consider the problem of trying to plan a dinner party. Imagine you can invite as many guests as you wish, serve whatever you like, and schedule the dinner on any day of the week. In this example, there are no obvious or direct ways of deciding which procedure to use or which solutions are correct. In making party arrangements, you need to *decompose* the problem into a series of subtasks or subgoals—J. R. Anderson's second criterion feature of problem solving. You might first decide whether to plan a small gathering with a few close friends or a large dinner party with 25 or 30 people. The next subgoal might involve decisions about the time of the party, followed by the choice of a main course.

Finally, you need to select your **operators.** Operators in problem solving are the actions or steps taken to reach a goal. In the card-sorting problem, for example, *planning* and *deciding* whether to sort first by suit or by face value, *remembering* which cards have been dealt and which remain in the pile, and *learning* that one discard pile is more efficient than several piles are operators involving a cognitive component. To achieve a problem solution, the known operators must be selected and sequenced appropriately.

No single homogeneous set of cognitive operators or actions is involved in solving a problem. Nevertheless, we can identify some cognitive processes that are common across various kinds of problems, including planning and decision-making processes, memory, attention, and learning. What about creativity? Although some problems require creative solutions, others apparently can be solved more or less automatically.

Creativity

In solving problems with clear goals or ones successfully solved on a previous occasion, people often perform a well-practiced or routine series of operations. Greeno (1980) has referred to this type of problem solving as *routine problem solving*. When the goals and procedures for reaching them are not so clear-cut, however, as in the ill-defined party planning problem discussed earlier, we frequently invent novel solutions and new procedures. The latter type of problem solving comes closer to what psychologists usually refer to as *creativity*. In creative problem solving, there is no one correct solution or standard way of achieving it.

A good illustration of the difference between routine and creative problem solving can be seen in Wolfgang Köhler's (1927) classic experiments with apes. Köhler, a German psychologist, was trapped on the Isle of Tenerife in the Canary Islands during World War I. There he began to study a local chimpanzee colony and became interested in the problem-solving behavior of animals. In one problem, Köhler placed a bunch of bananas outside the cage of his most prized ape, Sultan. He then gave Sultan a stick, and the ape had no trouble using the stick to pull the bananas into the cage. The real problem came when Köhler gave Sultan two sticks, neither of which was long enough to reach the bananas. After several frustrated attempts to reach the bananas, Sultan suddenly hit upon the idea of joining the sticks together to form a longer stick. This is clearly an example of *creative* or *insightful* problem solving by the ape. **Insight** means to suddenly grasp how the elements of a problem fit together to form a solution. Once Sultan solved the problem, he repeated his strategy on subsequent versions of the same problem. These later solution attempts are examples of *routine* problem solving because they involve the application of already established procedures.

In the following sections, problem solving and creativity will be discussed separately. In reality, however, these two concepts lie along a continuum and are not true dichotomies.

THEORIES OF PROBLEM SOLVING

There seem to be as many theories of problem solving as there are problems to solve. Rather than attempt to review each one, we will concentrate on two of the most well known—Gestalt theory and information-processing theory. By now, you should have some familiarity with both approaches.

Gestalt Theory

One of the oldest theories of problem solving is called Gestalt theory. As you may recall from Chapter 3, Gestalt psychologists dealt with organized wholes or structures in perception, and they subsequently applied these concepts to the study of problem solving. According to Gestalt theory, the process of problem solving deals with *understanding* the structural relationships between various elements of a problem and seeing how they can be *restructured* to form a solution. Köhler's studies on chimpanzees, about which you just read, are a good example of the application of a Gestalt approach to problem solving. Although Gestalt theory no longer exists in its original form, many of its concepts still influence our thinking about the nature of problem solving.

One of the most significant contributions of Gestalt psychology is the notion that people have difficulty in solving problems because they develop a **problem-solving set,** a habitual way of solving a problem based on familiar or routine solutions. In a classic experiment, Abraham Luchins (1942) demonstrated this effect by using the "water jar" problem. Luchins gave his subjects a hypothetical problem of measuring a given amount of water with three water jars varying in volume (see Table 7.1). In problem 1, you fill jar B (127 quarts) and pour out enough to fill jar A (21 quarts). Then you pour off enough to fill jar C (3 quarts) twice. Thus, the solution is Goal = B − A − 2C. The majority of subjects applied this solution to problems 2–5, but got stuck on problem 6. That is, they grew accustomed to the formula B − A − 2C

Table 7.1
Luchin's Water-Jar Problem

Problem	Volume of Jars			Goal (in quarts of water)
	A	B	C	
1	21	127	3	100
2	14	163	25	99
3	18	43	10	5
4	9	42	6	21
5	20	59	4	31
6	23	49	3	20

Note: From *Rigidity of Behavior: A Variational Approach to the Effect of Einstellung* (p. 109) by A. S. Luchins and E. H. Luchins, 1959, Eugene, OR: University of Oregon Books. Copyright 1959 by A. S. Luchins. Reprinted by permission.

on the first five problems and failed to realize that problem 6 can be solved using a new and even simpler rule: Goal = A — C. Luchins administered his task to over 900 elementary school and college-aged subjects and found that problem-solving set, or *mechanization* as he called it, was a major source of difficulty in problem solving. Rather than consider each problem on its own merits, subjects tended to mechanically apply the previous solution.

In an often cited developmental study of problem-solving sets, Heglin (1956) gave a variation of the water-jar task and a maze problem to three age groups: adolescent (mean age 16.0 years), younger adult (mean age 31.7 years), and older adult (mean age 66.0 years). On both the water jar and maze measures, the older adult group showed most susceptibility to problem-solving set and the adolescent group the least. However, after training designed to help overcome this set, younger adults showed the least susceptibility, whereas old adults continued to be the most set-prone. These results could be interpreted as evidence that older adults are less flexible than adolescents and younger adults in solving problems and that they tend to use only one solution. But this conclusion rests on the results of a single experiment and must be viewed with caution (Salthouse, 1982).

Another factor that interferes with successful problem solving is **functional fixedness,** or the tendency to view an object in terms of its characteristic function rather than to envision novel uses. For example, paper money is generally used to purchase things, but a person stranded in the middle of a desert on a cold night might use it to start a fire.

Karl Duncker (1945) illustrated the fixation effect with a "candle" problem. He gave subjects a candle, a book of matches, and a box of thumbtacks. The goal was to mount the candle on the wall in such a way that no wax drippings would fall on the floor. The solution involved emptying the box of thumbtacks, tacking the box to the wall, and using the box as a platform to hold the candle. Most subjects (between 80–90 percent) failed to solve the problem because they could not restructure the situation in such a way to see a new use for the box. However, when Duncker (1945) presented an empty box to other subjects, over 80 percent of them used it as a platform or holder.

Duncker concluded that subjects' failure to solve the candle problem was due to perceptual factors. Because of functional fixedness, they could not see how the separate elements of the problem fit together to form a new structural "whole," or "Gestalt." They failed to achieve insight.

Several investigators have challenged Duncker's conclusions and offered alternative interpretations (Weisberg & Alba, 1981; Weisberg & Suls, 1973). In a theoretical analysis of the candle problem, Weisberg and Suls (1973) argued that functional fixedness was not caused by perceptual difficulties or lack of insight, as Duncker believed, but by a variety of factors in the task environment such as not labeling the box as a separate object; unclear instructions; and the presentation of other objects. They arrived at their conclusions by applying an information-processing analysis to the candle problem.

Gestalt psychologists made substantial contributions to our understanding of problem solving. They presented many excellent, detailed discussions of complex thinking processes and proposed mechanisms to account for inflexibility in problem-solving behavior. On the other hand, their theoretical notions were often conceptually vague and difficult to test. Perhaps that is why Gestalt theory no longer motivates much research. Increasingly, researchers have turned to more experimental approaches such as information processing to answer questions about the nature and developmental course of problem solving.

Information Processing

The information-processing system has been outlined in Chapter 2. At the beginning of this chapter, we said that the defining features of problem solving are goal-directedness, subgoal decomposition, and operator selection (J. R. Anderson, 1985). Information-processing theorists treat problem solving as a search for a goal or solution through a **problem space** (Newell & Simon, 1972), which is the problem solver's mental representation of the various states of the problem. In problem-solving terminology, the given or starting situation of the problem is called the *initial state*, the situations on the way to the goal the *intermediate state*, and the final goal situation the *goal state* (J. R. Anderson, 1985). *Operators* are the moves the problem solver can make to change one state to another.

Think about these terms in relation to a situation that might be familiar—locking yourself out of the house. The initial state of the problem might be "I have forgotten to take my keys with me, so I can't open the locked door and no one is home to let me in." The goal state would be "I want to get inside my house." The following are some possible intermediate states to the problem: "The front door may be locked, but maybe the back door is open." "The neighbors are home and they have a key." "The windows may be big enough for me to crawl through." The operators are the various moves you take to bring about the goal—for example, trying the back door, contacting the neighbors, or attempting to crawl through the window. In this conception of problem solving, you *search* your problem space until you find a sequence of moves that transforms the initial state into the goal state.

The conception of problem solving as a search through the problem space was developed by Newell and Simon (1972) at Carnegie-Mellon

University. As they have pointed out, on well-defined problems, the problem space is likely to be similar from individual to individual. Thus, individuals will take similar paths in their search for a solution. But on ill-defined problems, there is greater interindividual (between-person) variability in problem-solving search.

Information-processing investigators frequently employ well-defined puzzle-type problems because their structure can be analyzed very precisely in terms of given states, goal states, and operators. One of the most widely used problems is the "tower of Hanoi" problem. The standard version of the problem consists of three pegs and a set of three doughnut-like disks of decreasing size. The goal is to get the three disks off peg 1 and onto peg 3. However, only one disk can be moved at a time, and a larger disk can never be placed on a smaller disk. The standard three-disk tower of Hanoi problem and its solution is shown in Figure 7.1. Notice that even this simple version of the problem may tax our reasoning, quantitative ordering, and short-term memory abilities. In a three-disk problem, the problem space comprising all possible arrangements of disks on the pegs contains 3^3, or 27 *nodes* or locations in the decision tree. A four-disk problem contains 3^4, or 81 nodes, and a five-disk problem has 3^5, or 243 arrangements.

Klahr (1978) used the tower of Hanoi problem as part of an information-processing analysis of young children's problem-solving strategies. To make the task more appropriate for young children, Klahr changed the Hanoi problem into the "monkey-cans" problem shown in Figure 7.2. He presented the problem as a story in which the cans are monkeys (large = daddy, medium size = mommy, small = baby) who jump from tree to tree (peg to peg). The experimenter's monkeys are "copycat" monkeys that want to look like the child's monkeys. The child's task is to tell the experimenter what to do to get his or her cans to look just like the child's. The initial state and the goal state of the problem were varied so that from one to seven moves were required for solution.

Klahr (1978) tested three groups of children on the monkey-cans problem: 3-, 4-, and 5-year-olds. He found rather striking developmental differences. Most of the 4-year-olds could reliably solve up to the four-move problem before they began to make mistakes. Only some of the 3-year-olds were able to solve the four-move problem, and many were unable to get beyond the two-move problem. Five-year-olds were about evenly split between five- and six-move problems, and one of them could solve the seven-move problem. From these results it can be concluded that the length of the solution path through the problem space increases with development.

What developmental changes enable older children to outperform younger children on this and similar types of problems? Klahr (1978)

Figure 7.1 The three-disk tower of Hanoi problem and its solution.

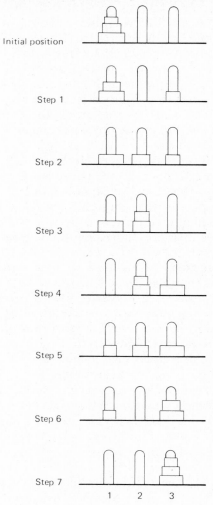

suggested a number of possibilities. With regard to general cognitive characteristics, what develops are abilities such as planning a strategy, keeping track of goals and subgoals in working memory, ignoring distracting information, and focusing on a solution. Children also develop, among other abilities, specific knowledge about procedures or *strategies* for reaching the desired goal state. Youngest children's strategies contain no plans; they want to get directly to the goal. Older children make plans before they move, but still have a tendency to move directly, rather than generate a series of subgoals. Subgoals are states of

Figure 7.2 Child trying to solve a one-move version of the monkey-cans problem.

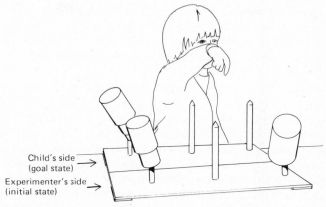

Child's side
(goal state)

Experimenter's side
(initial state)

From "Goal Formation, Planning, and Learning by Pre-School Problem Solvers or: 'My Socks Are in the Dryer,'" by D. Klahr, 1978, in *Children's Thinking: What Develops?* (p. 185) edited by R. S. Siegler, Hillsdale, NJ: Erlbaum. Copyright 1978 by Lawrence Erlbaum Associates, Inc. Reprinted by permission.

a problem that are intermediate between an initial state and the final goal state. The oldest children can postpone immediate action and have the ability to generate subgoals. As Klahr and Robinson (1981) have suggested, difficulties in mental representation may account for some of these differences in problem-solving strategies. Although investigators often cannot tell how children mentally represent and encode problem information, young children may fail to encode the problem correctly, so that their problem-solving strategies do not get a chance to operate effectively. In the next two sections we continue our discussion of problem-solving strategies and internal representation of problems.

Strategies for Solving Problems

Simon (1975) has shown that even with a relatively simple problem such as the tower of Hanoi puzzle, several distinct solution strategies are available. These different strategies place various demands on attention and short-term memory. For example, in a **random search** strategy, the problem solver randomly applies operators in a trial-and-error fashion until a solution is generated. Thus, if the problem solver is in a certain problem state, he or she randomly chooses any permissible move as the next move. For example, in the tower of Hanoi problem shown in Figure 7.1, if you are at step 3, you could randomly choose among three possible moves: step 2, step 4, or some unnumbered step (Mayer, 1983). The greater the complexity of the problem, the more extensive the search through the problem space becomes, and the less efficient random search becomes.

Random search strategies, whether efficient or inefficient, rely on the use of **algorithms,** which are methods guaranteed to generate a solution to a problem sooner or later. To solve the three-disk tower of Hanoi problem, you could systematically generate the complete problem space consisting of 27 different nodes and randomly search for moves leading to the goal state. This would be a time-consuming process but would eventually lead you to a solution.

Algorithmic methods generally contrast with **heuristic search** strategies. In heuristic searches, problem solvers limit themselves to the portion of the problem space most likely to produce a solution. Unlike algorithmic methods, heuristic methods may never lead to a successful solution, but they are often much more efficient. For example, suppose you play a game of chess. You could decide to test each possible move, which would involve approximately 10^{120} possible combinations (Moates & Schumacher, 1980). When the problem space becomes this large, or when no algorithm exists, heuristic methods are preferable.

Many problems such as the tower of Hanoi problem consist of an initial state, a well-defined goal state, and a set of operators (steps) for moving from the initial state to the goal state. In solving such problems, people often employ a heuristic called **means-ends analysis.** This strategy entails comparing the differences between the initial state and the goal state, and then identifying the operators and subgoals that will reduce those differences. For example, on the three-disk tower of Hanoi problem, the stated goal is to move all the disks from peg 1 to peg 3. The most conspicuous subgoal is to move the large disk onto peg 3 (step 4 in Figure 7.1). This subgoal consists of various other subgoals such as moving the small disk to peg 3, moving the medium disk to peg 2, and then moving the small disk back to peg 2, thereby freeing peg 3 for the large disk.

Another useful heuristic for solving problems is to *work backwards* from the goal. This strategy is useful in cases where many paths in the problem space lead from the initial state, but few paths lead to the goal state. For example, on maze problems, people often first identify the goal and then work backwards to the starting point. Rather than try to draw a line from the beginning point of the problem, they might draw a line from the goal leading back to the starting point.

Both means-ends analysis and working backwards are simple yet powerful heuristics for solving laboratory-type problems as well as problems in everyday life. Both strategies involve considering the goal state of the problem and choosing operators that will lead to problem solution. Nevertheless, there is a major difference between the two strategies. Means-ends analysis takes into account the differences between the goal state of the problem and the current problem state, whereas working backwards does not (J. R. Anderson, 1985). Therefore, means-ends analysis provides a more constrained or focused way of searching the problem space. For example, means-ends analysis would be more useful than working backwards on a problem such as the tower of Hanoi, where as many paths lead from the goal state back to the initial state as lead from the initial state to the goal state.

Prior Knowledge and Problem Solving

What determines which of several alternative strategies will be used in a problem situation? One major factor is a person's prior knowledge of the problem or similar set of problems. Perhaps a child who has a toy peg-and-disk set would perform differently on the tower of Hanoi problem than a child who has never seen such a toy.

The effects of prior knowledge on problem solving show up very clearly in the game of chess. Expert chess players approach the game differently than unskilled beginners. Chase and Simon (1973), and later Chi (1978), proposed that chess expertise depends on chunking the information for recall into larger units. Simon (1979) defined *chunking* as any perceptual configuration (visual, auditory, and so on) that is familiar and recognizable. Expert chess players are estimated to have about 50,000 such configurations stored in long-term memory.

In an interesting demonstration of the chunking hypothesis, Chi (1978) gave a memory-for-chess-positions test to children (mean age 10.5 years) and college-aged adults. As you may recall from our discussion of this study in Chapter 6, the children were chess experts, whereas the young adults could only play chess to a limited degree. Chi found that children's immediate recall for structured (or meaningful) chess positions was far superior to adults', despite the fact that adults' digit-span memory (which Chi also assessed) was higher than that of children. These results strongly suggest that subjects with more prior knowledge about a particular domain will perform better than those without such knowledge.

In a life-span investigation of chess skill, Charness (1981) proposed that factors other than chunking may account for developmental differences in chess performance. Charness equated chess players aged 16–64 years on overall chess skill. He then examined the component cognitive processes (such as memory) that distinguished between the younger and older players. The results showed that even though chunking was negatively related to age, older players matched the performance of younger ones. Charness speculated that older players compensated for declines in chunking ability with increased efficiency in searching through the problem space. Specifically, they took less time than younger players to select an equally good move. Although the reasons for increased search efficiency are unclear, this increase could be due to the older players' greater number of years of playing chess compared to younger players' experience.

In an earlier study, Charness (1979) reported similar relationships between age and performance in the game of bridge. Subjects aged 19–68 were first matched on skill level and were subsequently given various bridge-related tasks such as planning a play and recalling a bridge hand. Charness found that skilled problem solving in bridge depended on factors related to prior knowledge and experience rather than age.

Charness's (1979, 1981) research is important because it suggests that present information-processing models may need to be modified to account for performance changes over the life span. Indeed, most information-processing analyses have been based on narrow age ranges; and despite their detailed descriptions of problem solving, they do not form a coherent framework for explaining age changes in performance across a variety of tasks. In the next section, we turn to developmental studies of problem solving and focus our attention on various Piagetian problem-solving tasks.

PIAGETIAN RESEARCH

Up to this point we have concentrated on two theoretical frameworks—Gestalt and information processing—for describing problem-solving processes. Neither framework is based explicitly on developmental considerations. To examine an approach to problem solving that is grounded in developmental theory, we need to look at Piaget's research. The Piagetian problems described below have most often been used to assess the onset of concrete operations in school-aged children (see Chapter 2).

Conservation

In what is probably the most famous experiment in developmental psychology, Piaget assessed children's understanding in a series of conservation problems. In the broadest sense, "conservation" refers to a person's ability to understand that the essential properties of objects (such as number, weight, length, area, volume) do not change despite superficial changes in their external appearance. In a typical conservation-of-liquid-quantity task, the experimenter presents a person with two equivalent sets of objects, such as two identical glasses with the same quantity of a liquid such as water (see Figure 7.3, glasses A and B). The experimenter then changes the external perceptual appearance or form of the objects (in Figure 7.3, glass B's contents are poured into glass C, a taller and thinner glass). The conserver is able to state not only that

Figure 7.3   Piaget's conservation-of-liquid task.

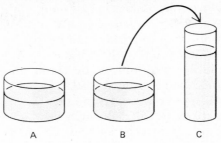

A   B   C

the amount of water in the two containers has remained the same, but also to state *reasons* why the quantities are equivalent.

The developmental trends in conservation-of-liquid performance have been relatively clear-cut across hundreds of studies. Before age 4 or 5 children fail to conserve. They frequently focus on the most salient, or noticeable, characteristics of the object (such as the height of the glass) and fail to simultaneously consider other important dimensions (such as width). For example, they will say "There's more in this glass because it looks higher" or "There's more because that glass is bigger." During a transitional stage (somewhere around age 5 or 6) children give intermediate answers to the problem. They may conserve when there has been minimal change in the external form of the objects, but fail to conserve when the change becomes more striking. For example, if the experimenter pours the liquid from one glass into four or five small flat bowls, the children may be misled by the perceptual appearance of the display and give nonconserving responses.

Only during the third stage, concrete operations, when children are 7 or 8, does full-blown conservation normally appear. At this stage children are certain that the liquid in the two containers has not changed, and generally they can offer one or more of the following reasons:

1. *compensation*—"The water in one glass is higher but that glass is also thinner, so one thing [height] makes up for the other [width]."
2. *identity*—"You [experimenter] didn't add any water or take any water away, so the amount of liquid is the same as it was originally."
3. *reversibility*—"You could pour the liquid back into its first glass and that would show they were the same all along."

Thus, concrete operational children can go beyond misleading superficial appearances by using logical operations to *infer* that the two quantities are equivalent. Moreover, when children fully master concrete operations, they can understand the logical interconnections of the factors of compensation, identity, and reversibility (H. Gardner, 1978).

On the basis of the information given so far, you may be wondering why the conservation problem has intrigued psychologists since Piaget first described it around 1940. Piaget candidly admitted that after 30 years of studying the problem, he could not satisfactorily explain it. The importance of the problem certainly does not lie in the child's ability to physically pour water from one glass to another or to notice the perceptual features of the task (such as color of the liquid, shape of the glass). Piaget referred to the latter as **figurative knowledge** because it is based on static perception of objects or events in the world. This type of knowledge contrasts with **operative knowledge,** which derives from the ability to think about transformations from one state to another. A good example of the ability to envision transformations comes from an experiment in which Piaget asked children to draw a picture of a vertical stick as it fell to a horizontal position. Older (concrete operational) children were able to draw the intermediate positions of the stick shown in Figure 7.4. In contrast, younger (preoperational) children focused on the static beginning and end states of the problem and had great difficulty integrating the intermediate states into a sequence of events. In the conservation-of-liquid problem, the transformation is the event of pouring liquid from one glass into another. This event transforms one static state into another static state.

The conservation task is significant because it signals a shift away from childhood egocentricity and an increasing capacity to engage in operative thought. In Piaget's words, a child learns to *decenter*, or focus attention simultaneously on two or more relevant dimensions. Initially, children *center* on only one dimension (height), then height and width (but not at the same time), and finally they attend to both dimensions. This ability to focus on both dimensions and organize experience into a conceptual unit is similar in many respects to the process of chunking.

Conservation ability may also have important implications for a

Figure 7.4   A falling stick. Children who understand the notion of transformation should be able to draw the stick as it undergoes a sequence of changes from a vertical to a horizontal position.

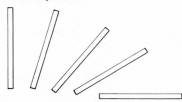

child's understanding of others in social situations. In social encounters, children often face changes in the physical appearance of other people. For example, children may run into a teacher in a grocery store wearing jeans and old sneakers. To what extent do children realize that the teacher remains the same person despite changes in outward appearance? Not much evidence exists on this question. However, some studies of character constancy have indicated by age 8 children understand that personality characteristics (e.g., kindness) do not change, despite changes in facial expression or physical appearance (Rotenberg, 1980, 1982). More will be said about children's conceptions of self and others as part of our discussion of social cognition in Chapter 9.

So far only one conservation skill—conservation of liquid quantity—has been discussed. Other forms of conservation such as number, substance, length, area, weight, and volume, and their approximate ages of acquisition, are illustrated in Figure 7.5. These conservation skills, like conservation of liquid quantity, involve children's reactions to transformations of the visual display, and the results are in many respects similar to those for liquid conservation. For example, in a conservation-of-number problem, children are shown two parallel rows of pennies (see Figure 7.5). Each row contains an equal number of pennies arranged in one-to-one visual correspondence. The experimenter then transforms the arrangement, usually by spacing the pennies in one of the rows farther apart. Nonconservers insist that more pennies are now in the second row because "they are more spread out" (Piaget, 1952). From the age of 7 or 8 on, children recognize that the pennies in each row are numerically equal.

Rochel Gelman and colleagues have done many studies on number conservation in preschool and elementary school children (Gelman, 1972; Gelman & Baillargeon, 1983; Gelman & Gallistel, 1978). Their research indicates that children can conserve number at an earlier age than Piaget's (1952) findings suggested. To test children's understanding of number conservation, Gelman developed an ingenious experimental paradigm involving a "magic" task. In one experiment using this task (Gelman, 1972), 3- and 4-year-old children were shown two plates, one with a row of three toy mice and the other with a row of two toy mice. Without mentioning number, the experimenter pointed to the three-mouse plate and declared it to be the "winner." The experimenter and the child then took turns playing a game in which one of them hid the plates under a cover and shuffled them. As in the old shell game, the child was asked to guess the winning plate after the covering and shuffling.

After several trials on which the child responded correctly, the experimenter covertly changed the "winner" either by lengthening or short-

Figure 7.5 Types of conservation skills and approximate ages of acquisition.

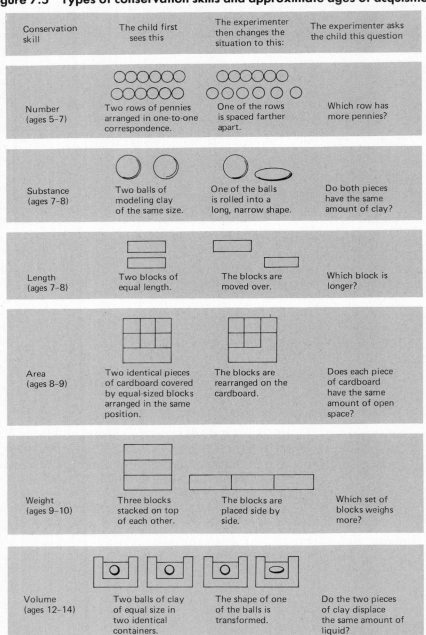

Conservation skill	The child first sees this	The experimenter then changes the situation to this:	The experimenter asks the child this question
Number (ages 5–7)	Two rows of pennies arranged in one-to-one correspondence.	One of the rows is spaced farther apart.	Which row has more pennies?
Substance (ages 7–8)	Two balls of modeling clay of the same size.	One of the balls is rolled into a long, narrow shape.	Do both pieces have the same amount of clay?
Length (ages 7–8)	Two blocks of equal length.	The blocks are moved over.	Which block is longer?
Area (ages 8–9)	Two identical pieces of cardboard covered by equal-sized blocks arranged in the same position.	The blocks are rearranged on the cardboard.	Does each piece of cardboard have the same amount of open space?
Weight (ages 9–10)	Three blocks stacked on top of each other.	The blocks are placed side by side.	Which set of blocks weighs more?
Volume (ages 12–14)	Two balls of clay of equal size in two identical containers.	The shape of one of the balls is transformed.	Do the two pieces of clay displace the same amount of liquid?

298

ening the row or by increasing or reducing the number of mice. On subsequent trials the child was asked after uncovering the altered plate whether it was the winner. Gelman was interested in children's surprise reaction. Would children notice the alteration and, if so, would they think the change mattered? Gelman found that the majority of children showed surprise when there was an extra mouse or when one of the mice was missing. In contrast, few children expressed surprise when confronted with the rearrangement of the mice into a shorter or longer row. For example, a child might say, "They moved out. It still wins. It's three now and it was three before" (Gelman & Gallistel, 1978, p. 162). These results strongly suggest that preschool children know more about number conservation than originally supposed.

Gelman and Gallistel (1978) were quick to point out that the numerical abilities of young children who pass the magic task are not necessarily as complex as those of older children. Young children seem to conserve only when the set size of the number display does not exceed four or five items; on larger sets, they often give nonconservation responses. Moreover, young children have considerable difficulty using the one-to-one correspondence principle to make judgments about numerical equivalencies. They tend to count the number of items in the display rather than make judgments based on logical operations such as reversibility (e.g., putting a missing item back into a display will return it to its original state). Despite these limitations, young children apparently know more about number conservation than psychologists have realized. Yet young children have a long way to go before they have a complete understanding of number; and even concrete operational children show gaps in their knowledge of numerical principles (Gelman & Baillargeon, 1983).

As is true for other cognitive abilities, not all conservation skills emerge simultaneously. Conservation of number usually appears first, followed by substance, length, area, weight, and volume, as shown in Figure 7.5. Some cross-cultural variation occurs in this sequence of acquisition; for example, Australian Aboriginal children appear to conserve weight before they conserve substance (de Lemos, 1969).

Regardless of the precise sequence, cognitive developmentalists agree that different conservation abilities emerge at different ages within the same developmental stage (such as concrete operations). At first glance, this seems to violate Piaget's theory. Shouldn't a child who can conserve on one problem be able to conserve on all other conservation problems, assuming the others involve the same cognitive skills? Piaget called these lags or gaps in the developmental sequence **horizontal décalages,** a term that refers to situations in which the attainment of the structure to solve one problem precedes the attainment of structures to solve another problem (D. Kuhn & Angelev, 1976). Piaget believed that area, weight, and volume problems require more abstract cognitive structures than number, substance, and length problems. He also believed that the later forms of conservation build on the earlier forms and that repetition of earlier conservation skills allows more advanced skills to emerge.

Currently, the major controversy surrounding the various conservations is not the sequence of conservation behaviors, but determining how to explain this sequence and how much it can be altered by training. The issue of training for conservation is discussed with intervention studies in Chapter 10. The explanatory issue centers on whether developmental changes in conservation can be accounted for on the basis of a single, overarching process such as equilibration or whether several subprocesses are involved. Piaget invoked the process of equilibration (see Chapter 2) as the principal mechanism for the acquisition of various cognitive behaviors, including conservation. Other psychologists believe that various attentional, memory, and linguistic subprocesses underlie the development of conservation. For example, Klahr (1984) recently proposed an information-processing account of how children acquire knowledge about conservation of number.

Class Inclusion and Multiple Classification

According to Piaget (1952; Inhelder & Piaget, 1964), during the concrete operations stage children develop the ability to classify objects hierarchically. One measure of children's understanding of hierarchic classification is **class inclusion.** In a class inclusion task, children are typically shown two subclasses that form a superordinate class and are asked to compare the two subclasses with the more inclusive superordinate class. For example, an experimenter shows the child five dogs and two cats and asks, "Are there more dogs or more animals?" Younger children often focus on the two subclasses and choose the larger of the two (i.e., dogs). Older children can simultaneously compare the subclasses with the superordinate class and produce the correct answer (i.e., animals). In Piagetian terms, class inclusion involves the child's ability to conserve the whole (*superordinate class*) while maintaining the identity of the separate parts (*subclasses*).

Inhelder and Piaget (1964) showed that children who can group objects into hierarchical classes often fail the test of class inclusion. According to their studies, class inclusion is generally exhibited between ages 8–13 during the development of logical operations. Winer (1980) has suggested that failure on a class inclusion task may depend on logical reasoning deficits, but could also be a function of linguistic difficulties. Children and even some adults may misinterpret the linguistic content of class inclusion questions. By changing the language of the questions, investigators have been able to obtain class inclusion at earlier ages (Winer, 1980). To return to our example, substituting the comparison word *than* for the word *or* in the question "Are there more dogs or more animals?" makes the question less difficult. Other factors such as the nature of the objects being classified (animals are more difficult to classify than flowers) also affect class inclusion performance. Some information-processing analyses of the class inclusion problem have been conducted in order to identify the factors and processes involved (see Wilkinson, 1976). Thus far most of this work has focused on class inclusion in a single age group (nursery schoolers) rather than on inclusion skills at different age levels, so that its relevance for understanding developmental changes in class inclusion is questionable.

Another important aspect of classification ability is known as **multiple classification.** Like class inclusion, this ability requires the capacity to reason simultaneously about two separate classes. In multiple classification, the attributes or dimensions common to both subclasses define the multiple class. To illustrate, suppose I gave you a set of red squares and triangles and a set of red and blue squares. The multiple class would be the set of red squares because redness and squareness are the common properties across both subclasses.

Researchers have found that multiple classification ability generally appears at about 7–9 years of age (Inhelder & Piaget, 1964; P. Jacobs & Vandeventer, 1971). However, according to Inhelder and Piaget (1964), even 4-year-old children can solve multiple classification tasks if they use a preoperational perceptual strategy relying on a symmetrical arrangement of a matrix into rows and columns (see Figure 7.6). Older children, on the other hand, tend to use logical operations to solve such problems.

Seriation and Transitive Inference

Another cognitive achievement during the concrete operational stage is *seriation*, which was introduced in Chapter 6. Recall that in seriation, objects are organized in a series along some abstract dimension such as size, weight, or brightness. In several studies, Inhelder and Piaget (1964) reported that children of different ages vary in their ability to seriate. In one seriation task they gave children sticks of varying lengths and asked them to arrange the sticks from shortest to longest (see Figure 6.2). In studies using this task and similar seriation tasks, Inhelder and Piaget found consistent developmental trends. Children younger than age 6 (preoperational) rarely ordered the sticks in correct sequence. Children around age 6 (transitional) sometimes arranged the

Figure 7.6   Examples of multiple classification tasks. The subject must find the correct small picture to complete the large pattern.

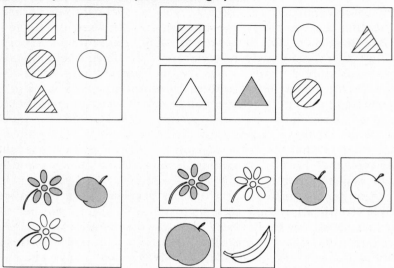

From *The Early Growth of Logic in the Child* (p. 160) by B. Inhelder and J. Piaget, 1969, New York: Norton. Translated by E. A. Lunzer and D. Papert. English Language translation copyright 1964 by Routledge & Kegan Paul Ltd. Reprinted by permission of Harper and Row Publishers, Inc.

sticks in their correct arrangement, but this took time and considerable trial and error. Children older than 6 (concrete operational) approached the task in a systematic way, first choosing the shortest stick, then the next shortest stick, and so on until all the sticks had been seriated. Many of the older children seemed surprised that Piaget would even ask them to perform such an "easy" task.

As in his other problem tasks, Piaget was not simply concerned with children's ability to produce a solution, but with the mental processes that enable children to reach the goal. On the seriation task, children older than 6 appear to use a relational rule (i.e., stick B is larger than stick A, but smaller than stick C) in order to solve the problem. On the other hand, children around age 6 who use a trial-and-error procedure seem to rely on perceptual processes, such as making the sticks look like a "staircase." These developmental trends are similar to those discussed for the multiple classification problem.

In an effort to identify the type of strategies used on seriation tasks, Piaget conducted the following experiment. He first had children seriate a set of 10 sticks of varying lengths. He then gave the children a second set of nine sticks, and asked them to add the set to the already seriated one to create a single series of 19 sticks. Younger children experienced great difficulty in performing the task and made comments such as "My staircase is finished," and "No, that's not right, it's too difficult." They succeeded in making only several short series which they placed side by side without regard for the order of the whole series. Or they succeeded in building the staircase, but only took the tops of the sticks into account and disregarded the bottoms. In contrast, older children had no difficulty with the task and did not hesitate to create a seriated set of 19 sticks. Thus, younger children were more bound to the figurative, or perceptual, aspects of the task, whereas older children showed evidence of operative strategies by generalizing a rule from one task to the next.

As is true for other Piagetian tasks, research on the seriation problem shows that children younger than age 6 have the ability to seriate. For example, Koslowski (1980) tested 3- and 4-year-olds on a seriation task consisting of four easily discriminable sticks. Children given the simplified version of the task seriated the sticks, although these children were not able to seriate a set of 10 sticks. These findings, while impressive, do not necessarily constitute evidence that the children used operational reasoning to solve the problem.

Another task that involves the ability to order an array of objects is called **transitive inference.** In fact, seriation and transitive inference may be thought of as two versions of the same problem; only the manner in which the problem is presented differs.

If I told you that Ron is older than Jane, and Jane is older than Larry, you would probably infer that Ron is older than Larry. This type of inference is usually referred to as a transitive inference because it involves logical reasoning about the comparative relations among a seriated set of objects. The relationships among two pairs of objects are directly stated, whereas the relationship among the other two objects in the series must be inferred from the first pairs. This particular type of transitive inference problem is called a **linear syllogism** because subjects are presented with two *premises* (the first two sentences), each describing a relation between two terms; subjects must order the terms in the premises in a linear sequence.

What kind of cognitive operations are involved in solving transitive inference problems? According to Piaget's theory, concrete operational structures for dealing with logical relations are necessary for transitive inferences to develop. Piaget, therefore, maintained that transitive inferences are beyond children's ability until about age 6 or 7. In contrast, information-processing theorists maintain that children as young as 4 or 5, who are presumed to be preoperational, have the basic logical skills to solve a transitive inference problem (Bryant & Trabasso, 1971; Trabasso, 1975, 1977). Failure to solve transitive inference problems is due, in large part, to memory difficulties that hide children's true reasoning competencies. Bryant and Trabasso (1971) have shown that young children can solve transitive inference problems when retention factors are controlled. To control for children's memory of the premises, children are first taught the premise relations. For example, to solve the problem "the blue stick is longer than the red stick and the red stick is longer than the green stick," children learn the premise relations (i.e., blue > red, red > green). During the testing phase of the procedure, children are questioned on all possible comparisons—both premise comparisons and inference comparisons (i.e., blue > green). By including the premise comparisons, the experimenter can determine whether children continue to remember the premises while they are solving inferences.

Trabasso (1975) described results of studies for almost 30 groups of children, adolescents, and adults who were trained and tested using these procedures. The correlation between the mean percentage correct in retrieval of the premise comparisons and the mean number of correct answers on the inference questions was positive and very high. Thus, strengthening people's retention of the premises led to corresponding increases in inferential performance, even among young children. From these results Trabasso (1975) concluded that memory plays a major role in transitive reasoning performance at all ages.

Trabasso's conclusion has not gone unchallenged. In an extensive review of the transitive reasoning literature, Breslow (1981) offered an alternative explanation of children's performance on transitive inference problems. Breslow (1981) proposed that after extensive training children may simply form a mental image of the array and then read off the correct comparison without combining the premises in a logical fashion. Breslow's proposal has received some support from a recent study by Kallio (1982), which employed a five-term transitive inference task developed by Bryant and Trabasso (1971). In Kallio's study preschoolers, second graders, fourth graders, and college students were tested on a series of inference problems involving seriated sticks A–E. To assess the effect of memory on transitive reasoning, Kallio used a serial presentation order (i.e., A > B, B > C, C > D, D > E) and a nonserial presentation order (i.e., B > C, D > E, A > B, C > D) during training. Under the serial order condition, preschoolers were able to respond with the correct inferences, as Trabasso would predict. However, nonserial ordering of the premises made it almost impossible for preschool subjects to form an internal linear ordering and to solve the transitive inference. And, transitive inferences did not appear until after 8 years of age under the nonserial presentation condition, which is consistent with Piaget's theory. After age 8, developmental increases in the ability to correctly solve inference problems with nonserial order cues were observed. Kallio (1982) attributed his results to developmental changes in subjects' linguistic ability and mental representation.

Whether some combination of these factors or those related to logical ability better explain age-related changes in transitive reasoning will continue to be a controversial issue.

EXTENDING PIAGETIAN RESEARCH ACROSS THE LIFE SPAN

Several investigators have attempted to give Piagetian tasks to adult subjects (Papalia, 1972; K. Rubin, Attewell, Tierney, & Tumolo, 1973; Storck, Looft, & Hooper, 1972). Papalia (1972) tested subjects aged 6–82 on standard measures of conservation of number, substance, weight, and volume. She found that while number conservation held up well with age, quantity conservation performance generally declined in subjects past age 65. Moreover, the last-developed and most complex type of quantity conservation, volume, showed the earliest decline. Storck et al. (1972) presented subjects aged 55–79 with a multiple classification task in addition to other Piagetian tasks (seriation, conservation) and found no significant relationship between age and performance. However, a later study by N. Denney and Cornelius (1975) reported that middle-aged subjects performed better on multiple classification and class inclusion tasks than older adults and that noninstitutionalized older adults did better than their institutionalized age-mates. Thus, some studies indicate age differences among adults in performance on Piagetian tasks, while others report no differences.

When declines are found in Piagetian studies of adults, they are usually attributed to age-related cognitive regression and deterioration. Neurophysiological degeneration and lack of environmental stimulation are thought to lead to declines in logical operations abilities. However, the regression explanation of cognitive aging has several major drawbacks (Bearison, 1974). Foremost is the problem that regression is inconsistent with Piagetian theory. As you recall, Piaget proposed an invariant sequence of stages which allows for no sliding backward in a structural sense during adulthood. Furthermore, most of the Piagetian research on adult samples has been cross-sectional, so that one cannot entirely rule out the possibility of an age-by-cohort confounding effect. For example, in several cross-sectional studies of conservation (Papalia, Kennedy, & Sheehan, 1973; Papalia, Salverson, & True, 1973; Selzer & Denney, 1980), education and conservation performance were significantly related, but age and conservation were related only when educational differences had not been controlled for statistically. Perhaps the more educated subjects continued to be active in their adult years, thereby preventing deterioration.

TRADITIONAL PROBLEM-SOLVING TASKS

In addition to the voluminous research on Piagetian problem solving, there exists a substantial developmental literature on more traditional, non-Piagetian problem-solving tasks. Numerous reviews (Giambra & Arenberg, 1980; N. Denney, 1979, 1982; Klahr & Wallace, 1976; Weir, 1964) of this literature are available, and we will summarize only the studies related to two types of problems: (1) concept learning and (2) verbal search. Studies using these problems reflect a wide range of theoretical orientations.

Concept Learning

Suppose I were to present you with a series of cards, with each card having three dimensions of variation: color, shape, and size. I then select a rule to define a concept (e.g., "large triangle"), and your job is to discover this rule by learning which patterns describe the concept. Such a concept-learning task is given in Box 7.1. After reading the instructions, see if you can solve the problem.

The problem in Box 7.1 is an instance of concept learning because you had to learn the rule for classifying the sets of items into mutually exclusive *categories.* When all the dimensions and values (or attributes) are described in advance and the subject must identify the rule, concept learning is called **concept identification** (Mayer, 1983). Box 7.1 presented you with the dimensions of color, shape, size, and their respective attribute values. When a subject must identify the dimensions and values in addition to learning the relevant concept, the problem is called **concept formation.**

In what is perhaps the best-known and most frequently cited study in the concept-learning literature, Bruner, Goodnow, and Austin (1956) presented college students with cards such as those in Figure 7.7. Bruner and colleagues used 81 stimulus items, each of which varied along four dimensions. There were three values per dimension: shape (circle, square, cross), color (red, green, black), number of borders (1, 2, 3), and number of objects (1, 2, 3).

Bruner et al. (1956) used three main classification rules to define their concepts:

1. A *conjunctive concept* has one value on one dimension and another value on another dimension (e.g., red circles).

2. A *disjunctive concept* has one value on one dimension or a different value on another dimension (e.g., red or circle).

3. A *single-value concept* has a particular value on one dimension (e.g., red) while all other dimensions and values are ignored.

Box 7.1   An Example of a Concept-Learning Problem

You will be shown a set of three different stimulus items on each trial with each item varying along the dimensions of color (red, green, blue), shape (triangle, square, circle), and size (large, medium, small). For each trial you will be informed whether the set of items is a positive (+) or negative (−) instance of the concept. For example, any trial having items with the attribute values "large" and "triangle" is a positive instance of the concept "large triangle." Before you begin the problem, cover the right-hand column with a piece of paper. Then for each of the set of items presented on the left, try to predict if it is or is not an instance of the concept. Move your paper down a notch each time to see if your prediction is correct. Continue the problem until you think you know what the concept is.

	Trial	*Type of Instance*
1.	large blue circle	+
2.	small red circle	+
3.	small blue square	−
4.	medium blue triangle	−
5.	large blue square	+
6.	large green circle	+
7.	medium red circle	+
8.	medium green triangle	−
9.	large green square	+
10.	large blue triangle	+
11.	small green square	−
12.	small blue circle	+
13.	large red triangle	+
14.	medium red triangle	−
15.	small red triangle	−
16.	medium green circle	+
17.	medium green square	−
18.	small red square	−

The concept is "large" or "circle."

Figure 7.7 Sample stimulus cards used in the Bruner et al. (1956) study.

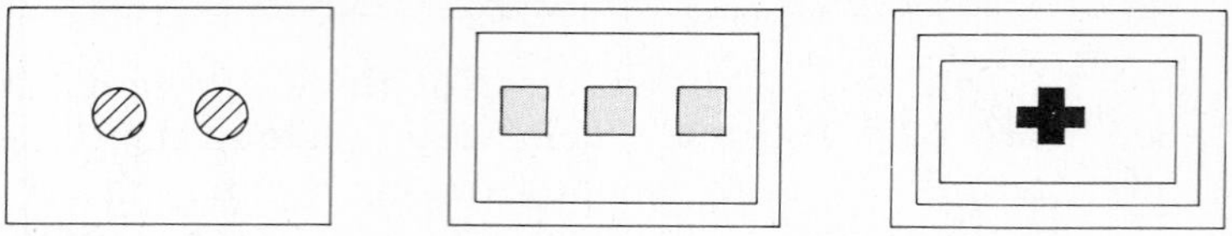

Shape	circle	square	cross
Color	red	green	black
Number of borders	1	2	3
Number of objects	2	3	1

From *A Study of Thinking* (p. 42) by J. S. Bruner, J. J. Goodnow, and G. A. Austin, 1956, New York: Wiley. Copyright 1956 by J. S. Bruner. Adapted by permission.

Bruner et al. (1956) used two different methods for presenting positive instances (*exemplars*) and negative instances (*nonexemplars*) of the concept. Concept learning was said to occur when the subject could categorize the stimuli as exemplars or nonexemplars of the concept. The two methods used were the **reception method** and the **selection method.** In the reception method, the experimenter picked the stimulus cards one at a time and the subject decided if each card was a positive or negative instance of the concept; then the experimenter told the subject whether the chosen instance was correct (Mayer, 1983). In the selection method, the subject picked cards from the array of 81 stimulus items one at a time and identified each as a positive or negative instance, and the experimenter indicated whether the card exemplified the rule.

In studying people's performance on concept-learning problems, Bruner et al. (1956) found that solutions could be understood in terms of different types of learning strategies. For example, for problems using the selection method, three major strategies were identified: (1) *simultaneous scanning,* in which subjects attempted to evaluate all possible hypotheses at once, and eliminated the incorrect hypotheses after each instance; (2) *successive scanning,* in which subjects concentrated on a single hypothesis and evaluated subsequent instances only in terms of that hypothesis; and (3) *focusing,* in which the subjects chose a positive instance and then selected cards that changed one or more attribute values at a time.

Of these three strategies, focusing is the most efficient because it limits the demands placed on memory by eliminating the need to keep track of many hypotheses at once. Do these strategies change with development? A study by Olson (1966) of problem solving in 3–9-year-old children suggested that these strategies do change with age. One of the most striking changes occurs around 5 years of age when children begin to use successive scanning approaches. From age 7 on, children use more systematic information-selection strategies such as focusing. Olson (1966) suggested that strategies change because of the more advanced modes of representation available to children as they grow older.

The results of research by Olson (1966), Bruner et al. (1956), and other investigators provided early evidence that subjects use an active hypothesis-testing approach to concept learning. In other words, subjects sample and test hypotheses until a correct solution is reached. This hypothesis-testing explanation of concept learning contrasts sharply with conditioning theory. According to conditioning theory, concept learning can be explained in terms of the reinforcement and extinction of specific stimulus-response associations. Learning occurs as a gradual, incremental process in which increases in associative strength accumulate over positively reinforced trials (Tumblin & Gholson, 1981). In contrast, hypothesis-testing theories characterize concept learning as a discrete all-or-nothing process in which performance operates at a chance level until the correct hypothesis is selected. Once subjects choose the correct hypothesis, they continue to use it because it is positively associated with reinforcement. Thus, learning shifts from knowing "nothing" about the hypothesis to knowing it perfectly.

Blank-Trials Procedure

One procedure for identifying hypotheses that subjects use on concept-learning tasks is the **blank-trials procedure** (Levine, 1963, 1975). In this procedure subjects are provided with either feedback or no feedback (blank) on a series of learning trials. For example, turn back to Box 7.1. Let's assume that I do not inform you whether each item set represents a positive or negative instance of the concept. If you have a specific hypothesis (e.g., "green"), you should respond with positive instances on trials 6, 8, 9, 11, 16, and 17 and negative instances on the remainder of the trials. A different pattern of responding would be evident if "red" were your hypothesis. In this case, trials 2, 7, 13, 14, 15, and 18 would be identified as positive instances and the rest would be identified as negative instances. The response patterns subjects display across a series of no-feedback or blank trials can be used to predict the hypotheses or rules they are using.

The blank-trials procedure has been widely employed in research with children as well as adults (Tumblin & Gholson, 1981). This research indicates that individuals aged 5–80 base their response choices on specific hypotheses. They do not respond randomly or haphazardly from trial to trial. Using a blank-trials procedure similar to the one described above, Eimas (1969) tested children in grades 2, 4, 6, 8, and college students on a series of four-dimensional concept-learning problems. He found that even the youngest age group exhibited a hypothesis-testing response pattern on over 70 percent of the blank trials, and this percentage increased steadily with increasing age.

Types of Hypotheses in Concept Learning

Although subjects do not respond haphazardly to concept-learning and problem-solving tasks, their strategies are not always directed toward reaching a solution (Tumblin & Gholson, 1981). Infrahuman organisms and children younger than approximately 6 years of age exhibit a type of hypothesis called a *response set*. Response-set hypotheses are not sensitive to feedback and are maintained over many trials despite repeatedly being disconfirmed. In contrast, older children and adults exhibit mostly *prediction hypotheses*, which are sensitive to feedback consequences and which are rejected if not confirmed.

Researchers have assumed that both types of hypotheses—response-set and prediction—emerge in their complete form in the problem-solving repertoire of the child. However, considerable controversy surrounds the question of whether young children really exhibit hypothesis-testing behavior or whether their behavior can be explained in other ways. For example, T. Kendler (1979) proposed a two-stage model of development in which two modes of learning, or *levels of functioning*, may exist side by side in the individual. One level is a cognitive, all-or-nothing type of learning, which is similar to learning through testing hypotheses. The other level is incremental or associationistic learning, which results from conditioning and extinction of stimulus-response connections. In T. Kendler's (1979) view, children younger than age 6 function primarily at the associationistic level; older children and adults may function at either level, but the cognitive mode becomes dominant with increasing age. Adults almost always function at the cognitive level.

To support her levels-of-functioning theory of problem solving, T. Kendler applied her assumptions to data derived from an earlier series of experiments involving shifts in rules (see H. Kendler & Kendler, 1975, for a historical review of this work). Subjects initially learn to discriminate between stimuli that differ on two dimensions such as size and shape (see Figure 7.8). Reinforcement is always administered if a response is made to either of the large stimuli (designated +) and is never given if it is made to either of the small stimuli (designated −). After the subject "successfully" learns the discrimination (usually by achieving a preestablished number of errorless trials), the second phase of the problem, called the shift discrimination or optional shift, begins. In this phase, "large" is no longer reinforced and subjects have to learn the correct (reinforced) value. As the test series in Figure 7.8 shows, the shift problem allows either (1) a **reversal shift,** which requires a response

Figure 7.8 The different stimulus settings presented over trials in each phase of the optional shift procedure.

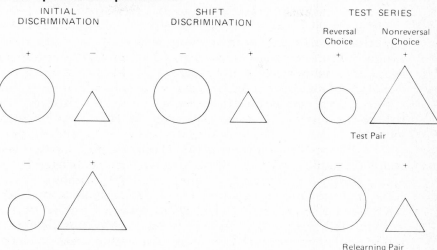

Adapted from "Toward a Theory of Mediational Development" by T. S. Kendler, 1979, in *Advances in Child Development and Behavior* (Vol. 13, p. 85) edited by H. W. Reese and L. P. Lipsitt, New York: Academic Press. Copyright 1979 by Academic Press. Reprinted by permission.

in the presence of "small" and no response in the presence of "large," or (2) a **nonreversal shift,** which requires a response to "triangle" and no response to "circle." Notice that in the reversal shift, the same dimension continues to be reinforced (i.e., size) but the individual "reverses" on this dimension by selecting the alternate value. The nonreversal shift involves switching to a completely different dimension (i.e., shape) to solve the problem.

If concept learning involves primarily the strengthening of S-R associations, as conditioning theory predicts, then the nonreversal shift should be easier to master because it requires relearning only two associations, whereas the reversal shift requires relearning four associations (see the test series in Figure 7.8). However, if concept learning involves a cognitive rule which mediates between the stimulus and the response, then the reversal shift should be easier to relearn than the nonreversal shift. T. Kendler defines mediators as covert internal responses which control overt responses to the test stimuli. For example, a subject may say to herself, "Oh, I see, shape is what is important, not size." This covert response, or mediator, guides the overt response of responding to the triangles and not responding to the circles. Assuming that individuals made mediating responses during the testing phase, we would predict reversal shifts would be easier to learn than nonreversal shifts. In the reversal shift, only the overt response must be relearned (for example, respond to triangles and not to circles). However, in the non-reversal shift, the covert mediating response (e.g., shape rather than size) as well as the overt response must be relearned.

Using this ingenious method, T. Kendler and Kendler (1959) discovered that animals and children younger than age 6 are more likely to exhibit nonreversal shifts than reversal shifts. Children beyond age 6 and adults are more likely to show reversal shifts. These findings led T. Kendler and Kendler to conclude that infrahuman organisms and young children use associationistic learning to solve problems, whereas hypothesis testing becomes important to cognitively mature individuals.

T. Kendler's (1979) conclusions about the findings derived from studies of discrimination-shift tasks have been challenged by Gholson and colleagues (Gholson & Schuepfer, 1979; Tumblin & Gholson, 1981). Gholson points out that children's responding is sometimes controlled by position cues (e.g., always respond to the object on the right) rather than by reinforcement contingencies. Moreover, children often fail to exhibit the expected *win-stay, lose-shift* patterns of responding on shift problems. Normally we expect children to stay with a hypothesis after receiving positive reinforcement for a correct choice. Similarly, following no reinforcement or negative feedback, a new hypothesis is selected and the child is said to lose-shift. However, developmental studies show that children younger than age 6 rarely display win-stay behavior, whereas older children and college students almost always do.

Kendler has argued that win-stay behavior implies operating in a cognitive mode, and the absence of such behavior implies operating in an associationistic mode. Thus, she claims that young children, who fail to display win-stay responding, do not operate in a hypothesis-testing cognitive mode. Gholson has disputed the claim on the basis of the position preference data discussed above. If young children show position preference (e.g., left, right, left), then their behavior can be classified as win-shift, lose-shift, with respect to position (Tumblin & Gholson, 1981). That is, they shift to their preferred position regardless of whether the response is reinforced or not. According to Gholson, this preferential pattern of responding among young children reflects a primitive form of hypothesis-testing behavior, which eventually must be coordinated with feedback and other stimulus cues to become more sophisticated. Contrary to T. Kendler's view, this pattern does not require a separate level of functioning for its explanation.

What can we conclude about conceptual learning in children and adults? It seems that from about age 6 on, individuals are capable of approaching concept-learning problems as active information processors and hypothesis testers. The evidence is less conclusive regarding whether the behavior of young children conforms to a hypothesis-testing model or can be better understood within a conditioning theory framework. The available research on position preferences and other types of preferences (such as consistent responding to an object of a certain shape) as well as research on stereotypic response patterns is interpreted by some psychologists as evidence for hypothesis-testing behavior in young children. With increasing age, children become more responsive to positive and negative feedback cues during concept learning.

Adult Age Differences in Concept Learning

Not all cognitive psychologists are satisfied with the concept-learning tasks described here. Because these tasks typically involve abstract, geometric figures, some psychologists have criticized them as being highly artificial. For example, Arenberg (1968) worked with older adults using problems modeled after those of Bruner and colleagues (see Figure 7.7). Arenberg's pilot research found that older subjects with less education had difficulty understanding the dimensions of these problems and the problem instructions. However, when he converted the task to a "poisoned food" problem, older subjects were better able to understand it. On the poisoned food problem, older and younger adult subjects were presented with nine foods and told that one of the foods had been poisoned. Arenberg then informed subjects that they would either "live" or "die" after eating certain food combinations. Their task was to identify the poisoned food. The results showed that younger adults solved significantly more of the problems correctly than older adults. Thus, making concept-learning problems more naturalistic and easier to understand does not automatically eliminate developmental differences in performance.

Arenberg's work perhaps represents the most comprehensive and systematic research program on adult developmental differences on concept-learning problems. Recently, Arenberg (1982) reported the results of an ongoing 13-year longitudinal study of concept problem solving using various versions of the poisoned food task. He began data collection in 1967 on a well-educated group of 20–80-year-old men as part of the Baltimore Longitudinal Study of Aging. In analyzing his data, Arenberg examined cross-sectional means for subjects in each decade from the 20s to the 80s as well as longitudinal means for all subjects who returned to be retested following a six-year interval. As you will read in Chapter 8, cross-sectional and longitudinal comparisons do not always yield equivalent results, so it is important to include both types of comparisons in developmental studies of problem solving.

The results of Arenberg's (1982) analysis are displayed in Table 7.2.

Table 7.2
Cross-Sectional and Longitudinal Results from Arenberg's (1982)
Study of Concept Problem Solving

Age	Mean Number of Problems Correct[a]		
	Cross-Sectional Means	Longitudinal Time 1	Means Time 2
20s	10.4	10.3	10.8
30s	9.7	10.1	10.2
40s	9.0	8.9	9.2
50s	8.2	8.4	8.5
60s	8.0	8.5	8.1
70s	6.6	6.9	6.7
80s	5.4	3.5	4.5

Note: Adapted from "Changes with Age in Problem Solving" by D. Arenberg, 1982, in *Advances in the Study of Communication and Affect: Vol. 8. Aging and Cognitive Processes* (pp. 226–227) edited by F. I. M. Craik and S. Trehub, New York: Plenum Press. Copyright 1982 by Plenum Publishing Corporation. Adapted by permission.
[a]Maximum number of problems correct = 12.

Note that the cross-sectional age comparisons reveal clear age differences in problem-solving performance, with systematic decreases in the mean number of problems solved correctly across each decade after the 20s. The longitudinal data, however, show that problem solving improved from the first to the second time of measurement for every age group except men in their 60s and 70s. These results indicate not only that the concept problem-solving performance of older men is poorer than that of younger men but also that older men's performance declines with age over a testing period of six years.

Verbal Search

A fundamental aspect of problem solving is knowing how to search for information. One way to obtain information is to ask questions, and question asking begins at a very early age. Children as young as 2 or 3 often bombard their parents with an endless stream of questions: how come? why? where? Although adults may tire of hearing this barrage of questions, question asking forms an important part of children's comprehension of the world.

The nature of children's questions and their strategies for seeking information change with age. One of the most common tasks for studying question-asking strategies at different ages is the old parlor game of "twenty questions" (Mosher & Hornsby, 1966). In this procedure, the subject is presented with an array of everyday objects such as pieces of furniture, articles of clothing, and methods of transportation. The subject's task is to discover the object the experimenter has in mind by asking questions. The idea is to try to narrow the range of possibilities and arrive at a solution using the fewest number of questions possible. The experimenter answers only "yes" or "no" to subjects' questions and does not provide any other information.

Mosher and Hornsby (1966) presented the twenty-questions task to children aged 6–11. They found that the youngest children asked **hypothesis-scanning** questions, which eliminated only one item from the array at a time; for example, "Are you thinking of the chair? the frying pan? the airplane?" These questions relied on "lucky guesses" and had very little relationship to one another. The oldest children used **constraint-seeking** strategies, which are more general than hypothesis-scanning questions and eliminate many items with a single question; for example, "Is it something you use to cook with?" Eight-year-old children tended to begin by asking constraint-seeking questions, but if they received an affirmative reply, they quickly jumped to hypothesis-scanning questions. Older children followed up positive replies by asking questions that further "constrained" the range of possibilities. The investigators also reported that children recognized the superiority of constraint-seeking questions over hypothesis-scanning questions before they could generate such questions on their own.

In another version of the twenty-questions problem, Mosher and Hornsby (1966) asked the same children to listen to the following brief story and then to ask questions of the storyteller to find out what had happened: "A man was driving along the road, the car goes off the road and hits a tree. Why?" This version of the problem differs from the first in that children have no concrete visual array to scan while trying to ask questions. Thus, it probably taps more formal operational as opposed to concrete operational thinking processes. Not unexpectedly, 6-year-olds continued to ask hypothesis-scanning questions on the task, but so did the 8-year-olds. They asked specific, inefficient questions such as "Did the driver get stung on the eye by a bee and lose control and go off the road into the tree?" followed by a question about a wasp sting. Eleven-year-olds, however, continued to use constraint-seeking questions, such as "Did it have anything to do with weather?" "with the car?"

Question asking is also an important cognitive activity for adults, and various versions of the twenty-questions task have been used with adult samples. In one study N. Denney and Denney (1974) compared middle-aged women (mean age 38.3 years) and elderly women (mean age 82.5 years) on an array of problems. They found that elderly women asked far fewer constraint-seeking questions, required more questions to arrive at a solution, and asked more redundant (noninformative) questions than middle-aged women. N. Denney and Denney's findings are similar to those of other investigators who investigated question-asking strategies among the elderly (Jerome, 1962; Young, 1966).

Why do younger children and older adults ask fewer constraint-seeking questions than older children and younger adults? Several investigators have suggested that the difficulties the former groups experience on the twenty-questions problem may be due to memory factors.

One way to study the effect of memory on question asking is to vary the *size* of the array. Eimas (1970) compared the frequency of constraint seeking among children aged 7–13 and young adults on two different-sized arrays of 8 items and 16 items. He found no significant differences in question strategies as a function of array size. In a more recent study, Hartley and Anderson (1983) compared question-asking strategies among younger and older adults on arrays of squares varying in size and complexity. Like Eimas (1970), Hartley and Anderson (1983) found no evidence that task size or complexity affects question strategies, which suggests that memory may not play a major role in question asking.

When the experimenter models the use of constraint-seeking strategies, children over age 6 and elderly adults quickly adopt the more efficient strategy. This finding suggests that both groups have the necessary cognitive skills, but prefer to use less efficient strategies. Perhaps there is less environmental demand for a young child and an elderly person to organize their worlds in highly abstract, logical ways. Or younger children and older adults may simply lack exposure to twenty-questions tasks, perhaps because of their educational backgrounds. When given this exposure through modeling, however, they can quickly shift to more sophisticated strategies. Children under age 6 do not appear to benefit from such exposure and probably lack the component cognitive skills (such as planning a strategy, remembering questions) needed to solve the problem.

CREATIVITY

When you hear the word *creativity*, you may think of famous people such as Shakespeare, Beethoven, da Vinci, or Einstein (see Figure 7.9). However, in the opinion of many writers, creativity is not limited to the great writer, musician, artist, or scientist. Indeed, each of us in our unique way expresses creativity in everyday life. Cooking a special dish using a personal "secret" recipe, wearing novel color combinations of clothing, and interacting with others in our own inimitable style are examples of how we express ourselves creatively on a daily basis. Chil-

Figure 7.9 Albert Einstein's penetrating mind formulated a creative theory about the nature of space and time.

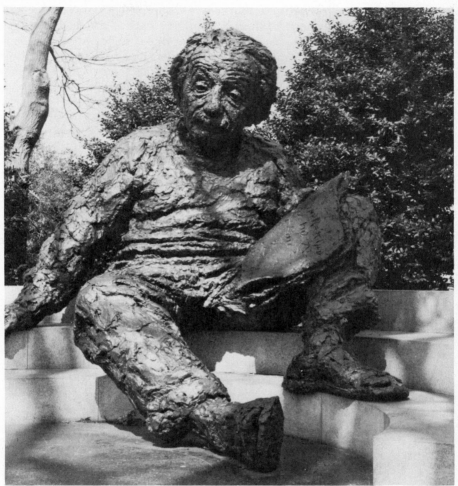

Photograph courtesy of Dr. Lynn R. Offerman. Reproduced by permission.

dren too show creativity in their day-to-day activities, as when they draw a picture for class, use language in novel ways, or play house.

We will not limit our discussion of creativity to the highly gifted person and the creative adult. Even these individuals have dry spells during which inspiration does not readily express itself. And a person who is creative is not necessarily creative in every endeavor. For example, a great poet probably will not be a great musician or talented painter. The extraordinarily creative genius may be ordinary in most everyday activities and functions.

These observations highlight an important point about creativity. Unlike intelligence, which can be characterized by a general factor cutting across many ability domains (see Chapter 8), creativity seems to be more limited to specific talents or abilities such as music, dancing, writing, and painting. This is not to say that one cannot be talented in many areas. Leonardo da Vinci, for instance, was not only a great painter but also a superb sculptor, architect, musician, and scientist. However, cultural pressures and time limitations often force a person to specialize in one creative endeavor.

Scientific interest in the study of creativity began roughly 30 years ago. A main reason for the increased interest is that a highly technologically advanced society such as ours depends on creative ingenuity. As David Wechsler (1958), the developer of several successful intelligence tests, expressed it, "Wisdom and experience are necessary to make the world go round; creative ability to make it go forward" (p.143). Box 7.2 presents two methods of stimulating creativity.

During the three decades since serious research on creativity began, a huge body of data has been collected. However, the literature on creativity—much like the literature on problem solving—is fragmented and disjointed and has no consistent pattern of results. One of the problems that besets research in this area is the difficulty of defining *creativity.* Many terms such as *insight, discovery, intuition, imagination,* and even *intelligence* have been used to describe creativity and creative thought processes.

"Creativity" is most often defined in terms of a process or a product but can also be defined in terms of persons and their individual characteristics. One leading researcher in the creativity field, E. Paul Torrance (1966), has described creative thinking as

> a process of becoming sensitive to problems, deficiencies, gaps in knowledge, missing elements, disharmonies, and so on; identifying the difficulty, searching for solutions, making guesses, or formulating hypotheses about the deficiencies, testing and retesting these hypotheses, and possibly modifying and retesting them; and finally communicating the results. (p. 6)

The process Torrance described may lead to a variety of creative products or outcomes, ranging from concrete to very abstract. In the next sections we will look at three lines of research on creative persons, creative products, and creative processes and examine the major areas of investigation in each.

Creative Persons

The first line of research focuses on the qualities or characteristics of the creative personality. This work is based primarily on a **trait** concep-

Box 7.2 Stimulating Creative Thinking: Two Techniques

Can people be taught to be creative? Can a creative individual who is currently experiencing blocks overcome these difficulties? Are certain training procedures better than others in stimulating people to think more creatively? These are some of the questions Morris Stein (1974) explored in his influential two-volume series *Stimulating Creativity*. Although Stein presented evidence that creativity can be trained, he cautioned that there is no easy short-cut to the development of creativity. The creative process requires time and a motivation to learn.

Probably the most common approach to stimulating creativity in a group setting is called *brainstorming* (Osborn, 1957). One of the most important rules for a brainstorming session is that the participants must suspend their criticisms of others' ideas and adopt an openness to all suggestions. The wilder the idea is, the better. Session members also are encouraged to produce as many ideas as possible. There is some empirical evidence that brainstorming can increase the quantity and quality of ideas produced.

Another method used to improve creativity is called *synectics.* Synectics was developed by W. Gordon (1961) to encourage the use of analogies in creative thinking. In mathematics, the word *analogy* indicates a correspondence of ratios or proportions; for example, the ratio 2:4 is the same as the ratio 4:8. In general, "analogy" refers to any relationship between two concepts or things that helps us explain the relationship between two other concepts or things. An analogy is usually stated in the form "A is to B as C is to _____?" (A:B::C:?). For example, apple:eat::milk:? The answer is *drink.*

The synectic method employs several types of analogies including *personal analogy* (imagining yourself directly in the situation), *direct analogy* (finding something else that solves the problem you are investigating), *symbolic analogy* (using an objective, impersonal, or poetic image to solve a problem), and *fantasy analogy* (freeing yourself of the boundaries of the normal world). For example, Gutenberg invented the printing press in part from the direct analogies he saw in the wine press and punches used for making coins. As W. Gordon (1961) observed, analogies make the strange familiar and the familiar strange. Despite many anecdotes about the role of analogies in scientific and artistic activities, there is only mixed support for the effectiveness of the synectic method for improving creative thinking (M. Stein, 1974). Furthermore, the synectic method, like the brainstorming technique, has been used mainly with adults, so its usefulness for improving children's creativity is unknown.

tion of personality. Traits are aspects of one's personality (such as shyness, anxiety, trust) that show themselves regardless of situations or circumstances. For example, from the trait perspective, a shy person would be expected to be shy whether in a classroom, home, or job situation. This view of personality contrasts with the **situationist** view, which sees personality as more situationally dependent (Mischel, 1968, 1977). For example, from a situational viewpoint, an individual might be shy around strangers, but outgoing when interacting with friends.

The major question in trait conceptions is whether creative persons differ in systematic ways from their noncreative counterparts. In other words, do creative people have different personalities or personality traits than people who are not consistently creative? Research on this question effectively began with Frank Barron's finding in the early 1950s that art students described as creative by their professors tended to prefer drawings and block arrangements of greater complexity than did students seen as noncreative (Feldman, 1980). This observation led Barron to hypothesize that creative persons prefer more complex and ambiguous stimuli than do noncreative persons. Using the Barron-Welsh Art Scale, which assesses people's preferences for simple or complex figures, Barron (1969) performed a series of studies comparing individuals from various professions and groups including artists, architects, physicists, and others. In general, these studies showed that, as hypothesized, persons designated by their peers or superiors as creative tended to prefer more complex patterns of stimuli than noncreative persons.

A colleague of Barron's, Donald MacKinnon (1962), carried out a related series of studies on personality differences among groups of creative architects using a wide range of measurement techniques, including a battery of psychological instruments and intensive interviews. MacKinnon found that the creative architects had a greater preference for complexity, were more flexible and open-minded, and had a wider range of interests than noncreative architects. Both Barron's and MacKinnon's studies focused on the occupational achievements of mature adults. These studies tell us little about developmental changes in various aspects of creativity over the life span. A useful review of the person-centered approach to creativity and some recent investigations of the creative personality can be found in Barron and Harrington (1981).

Creative Products

The second line of research on creativity, creative products, overlaps considerably with the research on creative persons. However, it differs in terms of the degree to which investigators are concerned about the creative works rather than the individuals who produced them (Wallach, 1970). Here again, investigators have frequently focused on the creative output of mature adults rather than of children or adolescents. Nonetheless, much of the developmental work on creativity has creative products as a focus, as we will discuss later in this chapter.

By a "creative product" do we mean the dinner we cooked last night, the clothes we are wearing today, or the outcomes of our daily interactions? While these products may qualify as creative by some standards, researchers tend to look more at the creative output of research scientists like themselves (S. Cole, 1979). Studies include such diverse criteria for creativity as occupational status; number of publications; number of patented inventions; and ratings by peers, supervisors, and trained judges. At this point, you may be thinking, can the term *creativity* apply to all of these examples? The answer is probably "no." As Wallach (1970) has indicated, the product-centered criteria are not correlated highly among themselves, and there is no strong evidence for a general factor of creativity.

One of the principal difficulties with the product-centered approach to creativity involves choosing the criteria by which to judge creative products. In measuring intelligence, psychologists can categorize items on an intelligence test as right or wrong, true or false. That is, they can use an objective criterion to decide on the adequacy of the response. In contrast, creative responses or products are not usually seen as correct or incorrect. Rather they are evaluated on the basis of subjective criteria, such as how good they are. But what determines goodness?

Jackson and Messick (1965) suggested four different criteria or standards that can be used to evaluate the worth, or "goodness," of creative products: (1) unusualness, (2) appropriateness, (3) transformational power, and (4) condensation of meaning. Let us examine each of these criteria in turn.

Unusualness can be defined as the infrequency of a response relative to some norm or standard. For example, a person who judges a painting to be unusual typically uses a chosen class of paintings as a norm of comparison (Jackson & Messick, 1965). If people evaluate a child's painting as containing an unusual color scheme, they most often use other children's paintings as a standard of comparison. To use adult paintings as the standard would certainly be unfair to the child.

Although the unusualness of a product is an important factor in evaluating its creativeness, we must also consider how *appropriate* the product is to its context. Bizarre or strange responses may be unusual, but not creative. For example, a creativity measure called the "unusual-uses" task asks subjects to think of as many different uses as they can for a common object (e.g., a brick). The response "use a brick as a pillow" would be unusual but not especially creative because it is obviously inappropriate. On the other hand, the response "use a brick as a doorstop" would be uncommon or unusual and also appropriate to the demands of the situation.

In judgments of more complex products such as paintings, the criterion of appropriateness is more difficult to apply. What makes one color scheme in a painting unusual and creative but another merely bizarre? Contemporary artist Jackson Pollock painted by dripping, flicking, and dribbling different colors onto a canvas laid on the floor. To some his paintings represent a complex and elegant intermingling of line and color, but to others they look like nonsensical splatter. Such differences of opinion reflect a great deal of subjectivity.

In interpreting the appropriateness of any creative product, the intentions of the creator must be taken into account along with the product's suitability to its context. A child who splatters paint on a piece of paper without much awareness of the outcome of these actions is different in many ways from an artist who intentionally or planfully produces a painting. Although the child's painting might be considered creative by some, it may be more of a serendipitous outcome than a carefully planned construction. Arlin (1984) has summarized the difference between a Pollock and a young child in the following manner: "Both splash paint on paper. The child does so because he/she is constrained by his/her limited competencies and skills to do so. A Pollock does so because he *chooses to* out of his universe of possibilities" (p. 262, italics added).

Jackson and Messick's (1965) third criterion, *transformational power*, involves the creation of products that irreversibly change or transform one's view of the world. Once transformed, they invite further thought and speculation. A good example is the Copernican revolution in science (see Chapter 1), which dramatically altered our conception of the earth's position in the universe. Another example is the Piagetian conception of cognitive structures, which changed our view of children's thinking and led to further empirical research. Transformations are not simply quantitative shifts in our thinking, but qualitative reorganizations. You might think of them as the ability to overcome problem-solving sets and engage in flexible thought.

Jackson and Messick's (1965) fourth and final criterion is *condensation of meaning*. Creative condensation reflects the interconnection between apparent simplicity and complexity in any great creative work. That is, something that appears quite simple turns out to be highly complex, and complexity often masks an underlying simplicity. Consider the painting by artist Paul Klee in Figure 7.10. At first glance, it seems simplistic, almost child-like, but if one looks longer, an intricate pattern of line and form can be seen. Or consider the case of the DNA

Figure 7.10 *Group of Masks* by Paul Klee, 1939.

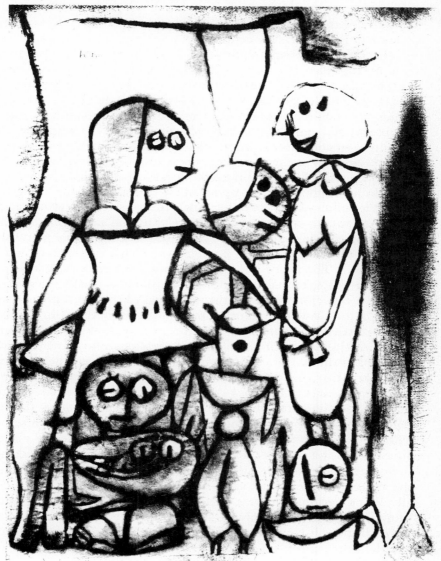

molecule. Its molecular structure at first appeared almost incomprehensible to scientists, but research revealed a simple and understandable patterning of sugar and phosphate bases. To date, very little empirical work has operationalized Jackson and Messick's (1965) four response criteria (see Feldman, 1980).

Creative Processes

Unlike research on the creative products of mature adults, research on creative processes has concentrated on children, adolescents, and young adults. Two major issues in this line of study are (1) the degree to which creative thought processes are similar to other cognitive processes such as intelligence and (2) the identification of the processes believed necessary for creative productivity (Wallach, 1970). Before reviewing these issues, we should emphasize that research on creative processes cannot occur entirely apart from the context of creativity. To understand creative thinking, one must take into account the goal or outcome and the appropriateness of the thought process in relationship to the goal. For some individuals, the joy of creating may be the goal; for others, the end product may be more important.

Early studies of creative thinking processes tended to use concepts drawn from the study of problem solving and intelligence (Wallach, 1970). But psychologists soon began to doubt that creativity involves the same thinking processes involved in general intelligence and problem solving. The major impetus for studying creativity as a skill separate from intelligence came from J. P. Guilford and associates. Guilford devised a model of how humans think, called the structure-of-intellect model, which you will learn more about in Chapter 8. In this model, Guilford tried to identify (1) the *processes* or thinking operations carried out, (2) the *content* to which the operations apply, and (3) the *products* that result. Guilford distinguished between **divergent thinking** and **convergent thinking.** Divergent thinking involves the ability to produce many novel associations to a stimulus. It is scored in terms of number of responses (fluency), number of categories (spontaneous flexibility), uniqueness of responses (unusualness), and quality of responses (originality). Generating many unusual and unique responses to a question about uses for a paper clip would demonstrate divergent thinking. On the other hand, convergent thinking is indicated by an ability to give the appropriate or correct answer to a question such as $8 \times 6 = ?$ Usually we associate divergent thinking with creativity and convergent thinking with problem solving and intelligence.

As intuitively appealing as Guilford's approach sounds, psychologists have had considerable trouble devising creativity tests that do not correlate highly with intelligence. Most of the tests that claim to measure fluency, unusualness, or originality of thinking also tend to correlate highly with standardized intelligence tests. In an effort to separate empirically the constructs of intelligence and creativity, Getzels and Jackson (1962) undertook a massive study of students ranging from sixth grade to senior year in high school. Using an IQ measure and five measures of creativity (including one devised by Guilford), Getzels and

Jackson attempted to identify individuals who were high in intelligence but not as high in creativity, and those who were high in creativity but not as high in intelligence. Although Getzels and Jackson partially succeeded in empirically separating the two groups, the high-creativity group also tended to score well on the standardized test of intelligence. Thus, the results did not provide solid evidence that intelligence is distinguishable from creativity.

Not long after Getzels and Jackson's inconclusive study, Wallach and Kogan (1965) investigated creativity-intelligence relationships among 151 fifth-grade children enrolled in a New England public school. Using a narrower criterion of creativity, they defined *creative process* in terms of the following two considerations: "first, the production of associative content that is unique; second, the presence in the associator of a playful, permissive task attitude" (Wallach & Kogan, 1965, p. 289). In their view, the creative scientist or artist should be able to generate many hypotheses, some quite unusual, and should be able to entertain many ideas without rushing to evaluate them. Applying these two criteria for creativity, the investigators devised five measures of *associative fluency,* the ability to generate many unusual and original responses.

Three of these measures involved verbal procedures. In the *instances* test, children were asked to generate as many examples as they could for a category of objects such as round things or things that move on wheels. The *alternate uses* test required children to think of as many uses as possible for an object such as a newspaper, a cork, or a shoe. The *similarities* test asked for all possible similarities between pairs of objects such as a cat and a mouse, or milk and meat. The final two measures used visual procedures, although a verbal response was required. In *pattern meanings,* abstract designs were presented and subjects were asked to think of as many meanings or interpretations as they could. In *line meanings,* the subjects received the same instructions, but the stimuli consisted of nonobjective line forms. On each of these five creativity measures, the number and uniqueness of responses were recorded.

In addition to the creativity tests, Wallach and Kogan (1965) administered a standardized intelligence test, but they did not follow the normal procedure for its administration. Typically, intelligence tests are given under timed conditions in a controlled group setting, as in the Getzels and Jackson (1962) study. Assuming that creativity occurs primarily under playful circumstances, Wallach and Kogan administered their tests individually without time limitations in a comfortable, unpressured environment.

The results of their study showed that creativity and intelligence could be validly distinguished. Wallach and Kogan (1965) were able to identify four distinct subgroups: (1) high intelligence–high creativity; (2) high intelligence–low creativity; (3) low intelligence–high creativity; and (4) low intelligence–low creativity. These groups could be differentiated in terms of psychological characteristics. Children who were highly intelligent and highly creative were self-confident in school, excelled academically, and were well liked by peers. In contrast, children who scored low in both creativity and intelligence lacked self-esteem, performed poorly in school, and were not as popular. The psychological profiles of the children in the other two groups were more complex and more interesting. The high creativity–low intelligence children were the least confident of all the groups and least sought after by their peers. They deprecated their academic accomplishments and did poorly in the classroom. These children seemed worse off than their low creativity–low intelligence peers. The low creativity–high intelligence children devoted themselves to academic achievement and seemed aloof in their social behavior, though they were well regarded by their peers. These results underscore the need to consider children's joint standing on measures of creativity and intelligence if we are to generalize about either construct.

To evaluate Wallach and Kogan's research, let us reconsider their definition of creativity. They viewed creativity as an associational process involving the generation of many unique and original ideas. But is this ability the major one underlying the creative activities of the master artist, the creative writer, or the ingenious inventor? After all, a young child or a psychotic person may produce many unusual associations without ordinarily being considered creative (H. Gardner, 1978).

Associational fluency may be necessary, but not sufficient, for creativity. Equally significant is the possession of expert knowledge in a content domain such as music, poetry, mathematics, or painting. Possibly, the difficulty many people experience in being creative results from a failure to generate appropriate internal representations (i.e., a knowledge base) upon which creative thought processes can operate. Future research on creativity needs a more balanced focus on creative processes as they interact with domain-specific knowledge. Both process and knowledge are important.

MEASUREMENT OF CREATIVITY

Some problems in selecting measures for assessing creativity across the life span will now be examined. We will then review results of developmental studies of creativity that have employed either real-life or laboratory-based measures.

Problems in Measuring Creativity

Although the tests used by Wallach and Kogan (1965) appear to be face valid (they appear to measure what they are designed to measure), can we be certain that they assess the same creative processes in different age or cohort groups? In an excellent review of creativity across the life span, Romaniuk and Romaniuk (1981) have pointed out the problem in attempting to equate creativity measures for different age groups. For instance, on the unusual-uses task, sizable differences in experience with a particular object (such as a brick) may exist across different age or cohort levels. A young child with limited experience may respond quite differently than a retired homebuilder when asked to think about various ways to use a brick.

Another problem in measuring creativity is the meaningfulness of the task to individuals. How do we know that tasks which are novel or challenging to children are not boring or even trivial to adults? Furthermore, it would be helpful to know if persons had solved the task before and how they went about solving it (Treffinger, Runzulli, & Feldhusen, 1971). We also need to know if laboratory tests of creativity mirror creative processes in real life. Is giving a set of discrete answers to an unusual-uses item under timed conditions with a group of subjects the same as working alone on a new invention over a period of many years? Although the problem of relating laboratory and real-life types of creativity is formidable, this issue deserves greater attention.

Changes in Creativity across the Life Span

Keeping in mind the measurement problems involved in assessing life-span changes in creativity, let us examine some of the developmental studies that have been conducted. From a developmental perspective the major question is, How do creative thinking processes and products change with advancing age? A nineteenth-century life-span study by Quetelet, discussed in Chapter 1, indicated that creativity peaks between ages 25–35 among playwrights and declines gradually after age 55. How generalizable are Quetelet's findings?

In a widely cited study, Lehman (1953) investigated the age of peak creative achievement among professionals in different fields. Using data on the number of contributions and expert ratings of the contributions, Lehman (1953) concluded that superior creativity generally rises to its highest point in the 20s and 30s and declines thereafter. However, the peak varies by profession. Among chemists, the period of greatest contribution is from ages 26–30 (see Figure 7.11), whereas musicians and mathematicians reach their highest creativity between ages 30–40. Lehman (1956) subsequently pointed out that age is not the

Figure 7.11   Contributions to chemistry as a function of age. Based on 222 men who lived to age 70 or beyond and who made 653 total contributions. Average number of contributions = 2.94.

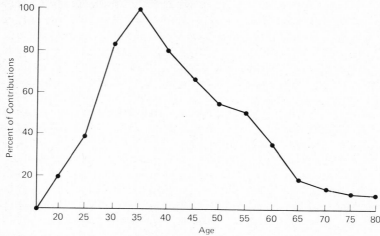

only determinant of creativity trends. Other factors such as declines in physical energy, loss of sensory capacity, and increased personal and social responsibilities also play a role.

Dennis (1966) published a similar study on the creative productivity of people from ages 20–80. He reported that the peak period of creativity occurred later in life. For example, historians produce most of their creative work in their 60s, and novelists in their 50s. More recently, Simonton (1975, 1977) has published a series of studies on literary creativity in well-known creative persons across the life span. Simonton (1977) looked at the creative works of 10 classical composers born before 1870. Productivity peaks occurred in the composers' early 30s for musical-theme compositions and the middle 40s for musical works.

The studies of Lehman, Dennis, and Simonton all attempted to measure creativity in a real-world environment. Alpaugh and Birren (1977) took a different approach by testing a cross-sectional sample of 111 teachers aged 20–83 years in a laboratory situation. They administered standardized measures of creativity (several Guilford tasks and the Barron-Welsh Art Scale) and intelligence (Wechsler Adult Intelligence Scale). The authors reported age-related declines on the creativity measures, but no significant decline on the intelligence measure. They concluded that age differences in divergent thinking and preference for complexity are more compelling explanations for the observed decrease in creativity over the life span than age-related declines in intelligence.

DEVELOPMENTAL THEORY OF CREATIVITY

As mentioned, there is no single accepted theory of creativity, and much of the creativity research is limited to one age group or cross-sectional age comparisons. Moreover, studies on creativity often are not based on theoretical considerations. What we badly need is a theory of creativity framed within a developmental context, preferably a life-span context. A preliminary step has been taken in this direction, and we will outline it for you.

J. Meyer (1983) has proposed a structural theory of creativity based on the organismic developmental position of Piaget. Although Piaget did not discuss creativity per se, he labeled newly formed thought structures as "novelties" or "creations" (Feldman, 1980). In J. Meyer's proposal, cognitive structures are seen as inherently creative because they can be characterized by developmental *transformations*, rather than by specific content. However, structures must be applied to content for creativity to become manifest. Meyer discusses four qualitatively distinct stages of creative development which parallel the cognitive stages of Piaget. Sensorimotor creativity is linked to the infant's failure to differentiate self from the world resulting in novel forms of behavior (e.g., creative sucking). Preoperational forms of creativity can be found in a child's novel use of symbolism such as language. The degree to which these activities are truly creative or are primarily simple expressions of spontaneity is unclear.

What about the concrete operational child who is often seen as less creative because of the orientation to the concrete "here-and-now" (Dudek, 1974)? J. Meyer argued that the concrete structures which emerge in middle childhood (e.g., seriation, reversibility, causality) result in greater flexibility in thought and enable the child to apply alternative mental schemes to the same content. Concrete operational children may express their new ability through more differentiated, more realistic drawings and paintings (Dudek, 1974). For example, they may draw a person to look like a person rather than a circle and four sticks. Although this concern with realism may represent a loss of the child's earlier imagination and creativity, it does prepare the child for more complex cognitive activity and creative expression.

Finally, in formal operations, reality becomes subordinated to the hypothetical, and the adolescent can go beyond immediate experience to create novel mental products. Having acquired formal operations, the child can begin to hypothesize, to perform combinatorial analyses, and to imagine a greater range of possibilities. Creativity at the formal operations stage is more congruent with many adults' conceptions of mature creativity.

J. Meyer's proposal is promising because it is based on a theory of cognitive development and because it broadens adult-centered notions of creativity to include the childhood years. To be considered creative, one usually must produce a product that is unique and socially useful according to adult standards; by this definition, children are seldom seen as creative. Meyer's ideas give us a new means of conceptualizing creativity, at least across the earlier portion of the life span. The task that remains is to link such ideas with the current theorizing on adulthood changes in creative thought. Some of these changes will be considered in Chapter 8.

SUMMARY

1. Problem solving involves a sequence of cognitive operations directed to a goal.
2. Problems with clear goals are called well-defined problems and can usually be solved with routine mental operations. Ill-defined problems, which lack clear goals, often require the use of creative problem solving.
3. Gestalt theorists emphasize understanding the structural elements of a problem and restructuring them to form a solution. According to Gestalt theory, people have difficulty solving problems because of problem-solving sets and functional fixedness.
4. Information-processing perspectives view problem solving as a search for a solution through a problem space.
5. Two search strategies for solving problems are algorithms and heuristics. Algorithms will always lead to a solution; heuristics, though more efficient, do not guarantee a solution.
6. Piaget's work is the clearest example of a developmental approach to problem solving. Five widely used Piagetian problems are conservation, class inclusion, multiple classification, seriation, and transitive inference.
7. "Conservation" refers to the ability to understand that the essential properties of objects (e.g., quantity) do not change despite changes in their surface appearance.
8. In addition to Piaget's work, there exists a large developmental literature on more traditional problems such as concept learning. Concept learning involves learning a rule for classifying instances of the concept into different categories.

9. Older children and adults use an active hypothesis-testing approach to concept learning. The evidence for hypothesis-testing behavior in young children's concept learning is less conclusive.
10. Creativity is not limited to the genius or gifted adult, but can be found in varying degrees in everyone.
11. Researchers who study creativity distinguish among creative persons, creative products, and creative processes.
12. A major problem in measuring creativity across the life span is equating the meaningfulness and difficulty level of creativity tasks for various age groups.
13. There is no single accepted theory of creativity, and we badly need a developmental theory of creativity.

Key Terms

operators	**linear syllogism**
insight	**concept identification**
problem-solving set	**concept formation**
functional fixedness	**reception method**
problem space	**selection method**
random search	**blank-trials procedure**
algorithms	**reversal shift**
heuristic search	**nonreversal shift**
means-ends analysis	**hypothesis scanning**
figurative knowledge	**constraint seeking**
operative knowledge	**trait**
horizontal décalages	**situationist**
class inclusion	**divergent thinking**
multiple classification	**convergent thinking**
transitive inference	

Suggested Readings

Bransford, J. D., & Stein, B. S. (1984). *The IDEAL problem solver: A guide to improving thinking, learning, and creativity.* San Francisco: Freeman. This practical how-to guide for solving brain teasers, puzzles, and everyday problems suggests strategies for improving memory, learning new knowledge, and enhancing creative solutions to problems. Challenging and fun.

Kuhn, D., & Phelps, E. (1982). The development of problem-solving strategies. In H. W. Reese (Ed.), *Advances in child development and behavior* (Vol. 17, pp. 1–44). New

York: Academic Press. This article describes an innovative method for studying patterns of changes in problem-solving strategies over repeated encounters with the same problem. This method's use with preadolescents is discussed, and implications of the results for developmental theories of problem solving are considered.

Newell, A., & Simon, H. A. (1972). *Human problem solving.* Englewood Cliffs, NJ: Prentice-Hall. One of the most influential volumes on problem solving ever written, this book describes an information-processing theory of problem solving and computer simulation of problems in cryptarithmetic, logic, and chess.

Perkins, D. N. (1981). *The mind's best work.* Cambridge, MA: Harvard University Press. A fascinating look at the creative process in the arts and the sciences. Also includes some "personal experiments" in creativity which the reader can attempt.

Reese, H. W., & Rodeheaver, D. (1985). Problem solving and complex decision making. In J. E. Birren & K. W. Schaie (Eds.), *Handbook of the psychology of aging* (2nd ed., pp. 474–499). New York: Van Nostrand Reinhold. This scholarly review of the experimental literature on problem solving and decision making from young adulthood through old age includes a section on age changes in problem solving of real-life tasks.

Tuma, D. T., & Reif, F. (Eds.). (1980). *Problem solving and education: Issues in teaching and research.* Hillsdale, NJ: Erlbaum. This collection of papers by top scholars on basic research in problem solving and its relevance to education emphasizes the need to teach students improved problem-solving skills.

CHAPTER 8

Intellectual Development and Complex Thinking Processes

OVERVIEW

Because of its significance for psychological theory and everyday functioning, human intelligence has been studied intensively for many years. Psychologists differ, however, in how they describe and measure intelligence. Some psychologists focus on intelligence as a general, global ability, whereas others concentrate on specific intellectual skills.

This chapter examines various intellectual abilities as they change across the life span. We will attempt to explain the nature of intellectual change by looking at individual, societal, and cultural factors affecting IQ. We will also examine attempts to produce culture-fair and age-fair measures of intelligence.

We will discuss complex thinking processes such as formal operations and wisdom. Two Piagetian tasks used to assess formal operations in adolescents and adults will be described, and some stage models of adult thought that go beyond the Piagetian end stage of formal thinking will be considered. Finally, the notion of wisdom as a positive developmental outcome of later-life cognition will be discussed.

DEFINITIONS OF INTELLIGENCE

The concept of human intelligence occupies a central position in psychological theory and measurement as well as in everyday life. Because intellectual competence is so highly valued in Western culture, intelligence has been one of the most heavily researched psychological constructs for the past 75 years. Despite the lack of precise operational definitions, work on the study of intelligence has proceeded at a rapid rate, particularly over the last decade.

What is meant by the concept of intelligence? Does the concept developed by so-called experts on the subject match our intuitive everyday notions of intellectual ability? Although the word *intelligence* is an old one—coming from Latin words meaning "to choose between" and "the ability to make wise choices"—the term did not find its way into psychological literature until well into the twentieth century (Wechsler, 1958). This is not to say that psychologists had no interest in what we now describe as intelligence. James Baldwin (1906), an influential early psychologist, defined *intellect* (a synonym for intelligence) as "the faculty or capacity of knowing." Since Baldwin's time our definitions of the concept have expanded considerably. We will examine various definitions to give a basis for understanding the material to follow.

Psychologists have defined intelligence in a myriad of different ways.

More than a half-century ago, Boring (1923) pragmatically defined *intelligence* as the behaviors which an intelligence test measures. This definition is unsatisfactory, because of its circularity and vagueness. How can one be certain intelligence tests measure intelligence in the same way, say, a ruler measures inches? The lack of consensus about what intelligence tests measure led to a famous symposium in the *Journal of Educational Psychology* in 1921. Seventeen leading experts of the day responded to the question "What do you conceive intelligence to be and by what means can it best be measured?" Their responses yielded little agreement, as is shown by the following sample of definitions:

the ability to carry on abstract thinking (Terman)
the power of good response from the point of view of truth or fact (Thorndike)
learning or the ability to learn to adjust oneself to the environment (Colvin)
general modifiability of the nervous system (Pintner)

More recently, Neisser (1979) has suggested that intelligence has no defining attributes, but should be viewed in terms of various *prototypes.* To understand the idea of prototypes, consider the concept of games. We are all familiar with games such as chess, Monopoly, hearts, baseball, and tennis; yet if asked to describe common properties that apply to all games, we might be hard pressed to produce a definition. We have in our minds a prototype, or "best instance," of what a game is like as well as more marginal instances. Each game is compared to this ideal model or prototype. Neisser (1979) suggested that we do much the same thing with the concept of intelligent person and, by extension, intelligence. We mentally imagine a protypically intelligent person and compare everyone to the imagined prototype.

What does a prototypically intelligent person look like? To answer this question, Siegler and Richards (1982) asked introductory psychology students at Carnegie Mellon University to list the five traits most characteristic of a 6-month-old, a 2-year-old, a 10-year-old, and "an intelligent adult," and then to weight these characteristics according to their relative importance. As Table 8.1 shows, the students viewed an intelligent adult quite differently than intelligent infants and children. For example, at 6 months of age, recognition ability, motor coordination, and alertness were listed as the most important characteristics of intelligence; none of these characteristics was mentioned in describing intelligent adults or 10-year-olds. Reasoning, verbal ability, and problem solving were mentioned with increasing frequency with age, whereas perceptual and motor abilities were mentioned less frequently. Learning ability was considered an important characteristic from age 2

Table 8.1
Five Traits Most Frequently Mentioned as Characterizing
Intelligence at Different Ages

6-Month-Olds	2-Year-Olds	10-Year-Olds	Adults
Recognition of people and objects	Verbal ability	Verbal ability	Reasoning
Motor coordination	Learning ability	Learning ability; problem solving; reasoning (all three tied)	Verbal ability
Alertness	Awareness of people and environment		Problem solving
Awareness of environment	Motor coordination		Learning ability
Verbalization	Curiosity	Creativity	Creativity

Note: From "The Development of Intelligence" by R. S. Siegler and D. D. Richards, 1982, *Handbook of Human Intelligence* (p. 899) edited by R. J. Sternberg, 1982, New York: Cambridge University Press. Copyright 1982 by Cambridge University Press. Reprinted by permission.

onward. Thus, two people can be perceived as intelligent, but share few of the same traits (Neisser, 1979).

Siegler and Richards (1982) also asked the students to estimate the relationship between traits by indicating correlations (1.00 = perfect relationship, .50 = moderate relationship, .00 = no relationship). They found that students perceived some overlap between traits (e.g., the average estimated correlation between problem solving and verbal ability was .65), but there was also a good deal of distinctiveness (e.g., the estimated correlation between motor ability and verbal ability was only .28). Thus, the students seemed to think that a common core of intellectual abilities exists, although these abilities need not be highly related.

The view of intelligence as comprised of overlapping but distinctive abilities has been the subject of intense debate for decades. This view is nicely illustrated by Howard Gardner (1983) in *Frames of Mind: The Theory of Multiple Intelligences.* Gardner proposes a theory which goes well beyond existing theories in the kinds of human abilities it considers "intelligent." Based on various sources of evidence, Gardner concludes that there are six distinct intelligences: *linguistic intelligence, logical-mathematical intelligence, spatial intelligence, musical intelligence, bodily kinesthetic intelligence,* and *personal intelligence.* The first three are typically included in traditional models of intelligence, but the latter three are not usually seen as evidence of intelligence or, at best, are seen as secondary in importance to the other abilities. On what basis does Gardner label musical ability, bodily motor skill, and social-interpersonal skills as intelligent?

H. Gardner (1983) has proposed a set of signs that can be used to identify distinctive intelligences. Not every form of intelligence exhibits all the signs, nor do behaviors that exhibit one or two signs automatically qualify as intelligent. Therefore, you should think of these signs as guidelines for identifying intelligent behaviors, rather than as exact, hard-and-fast criteria.

1. *Potential isolation by brain damage*
Damage to the brain often results in impairment of a specific intellectual ability while other skills are spared. Such selective impairment (and sparing) indicates that the ability is at least partially autonomous of other skills.

2. *The existence of exceptional individuals*
Some individuals exhibit extraordinary talent and skill in one domain, but are mediocre or retarded in other domains. This selective competence, like selective impairment, indicates the autonomy of the particular intellectual competence. A good example is an *idiot savant*, a retarded person who shows exceptional numerical or musical ability.

3. *A distinctive developmental history*
Each distinct intelligence should have its own sequence of development through which normal as well as exceptional individuals pass.

4. *An evolutionary history*
Intellectual skills emerge as individuals develop, just as they have emerged as the human species has evolved. A well-defined phylogenetic sequence suggests the autonomy of an intellectual competence in the same way that a reliable ontogenetic (developmental) sequence does (Kail & Pellegrino, 1985).

5. *A set of core operations*
If an intelligence is truly distinct, a set of basic information-processing operations should comprise the core of the intelligence. An example might be a sensitivity to pitch relations as a core of musical intelligence.

6. *Experimental evidence from laboratory tasks*
The autonomy of intelligence is implicated in laboratory demonstrations where subjects are asked to perform two tasks concurrently. If there is minimal interference between the tasks, then the abilities are

separate. Where two tasks are difficult to perform concurrently—as in cases of trying to type and listen to speech—then it can be said that the two tasks require an overlapping set of intellectual skills. The autonomy of intellectual abilities can also be established statistically via a procedure known as factor analysis, which will be discussed in the next section.

7. *Encoding in a symbol system*
The intelligence has its own distinct symbol system such as language and pictures.

H. Gardner has used the above signs to support his view of six distinct types of intelligence. As an illustration of his argument, let's examine musical intelligence, something not typically measured by standardized intelligence tests. H. Gardner believes that musical intelligence forms a central part of our intellectual competence. He cites composers who were afflicted with Wernicke's aphasia; their speech was impaired, but their ability to comprehend and compose music remained intact. There are also many famous cases of exceptionality in musical talent at very young ages, perhaps none more celebrated than the Austrian composer Wolfgang Amadeus Mozart. In addition, laboratory studies of memory for musical tones and for verbal materials consistently support the hypothesis that they are separate intellectual abilities. Thus, several signs point toward music as a distinct form of intelligence.

H. Gardner's proposal is certain to spark lively debate concerning the nature and distinctiveness of human intellectual skills. It is one of the most ambitious efforts yet to integrate the more traditional approaches to intelligence, including psychometric models, information processing, and Piagetian theory. Because H. Gardner's proposal is too new to have been substantiated by empirical research, it is best thought of as a heuristic framework rather than a full-blown theory.

PSYCHOMETRIC MODELS OF INTELLIGENCE

Psychometric models of intelligence are concerned with such practical issues as the construction of intelligence tests and the prediction of future performance. Of greatest concern is the development of intelligence tests that are valid (or measure what they are supposed to measure) and reliable (or measure performance consistently). Despite an interest in practical matters of testing, there has also been considerable concern for the underlying nature of intelligence. As Carroll (1976) has stated:

However great their interest in practical matters, all the leading figures in psychometrics—Binet, Spearman, Thurstone, and Guilford (to name but a few)—have had an abiding concern for the nature of intelligence; all of them have realized that to construct a theory of intelligence is to construct a theory of cognition. (p. 27)

It can be said, therefore, that the first cognitive psychologists were the psychometricians (Carroll, 1976).

Binet and the First Intelligence Test

The developer of the first successful IQ test, Alfred Binet, a French psychologist, believed that intelligence is a multifaceted construct consisting of many different abilities and skills. He demonstrated this conviction by developing an intelligence measure that combined several different types of tests into a composite scale. Although Binet did not know exactly what abilities were being measured by his scale, he felt that judgment, comprehension, and reasoning were very important. Binet developed his test in response to a request by school administrators in Paris, France, for an instrument that would distinguish children who lacked the capacity for schoolwork from children who had the capacity but lacked the interest and motivation. Because the immediate goal was a practical one—to predict success in school—Binet followed others' suggestion to use only a single overall score, although he believed in multiple intelligences (Guilford, 1979).

Binet began his development of the intelligence test by observing his own children's activities. He assumed that intelligence increased with age, so that older children and adolescents should outperform younger children. Accordingly, he and his colleague, Théophile Simon, devised a test consisting of a series of age-graded questions (see Table 8.2). Binet ordered the test items according to their level of difficulty, from simple to complex. As Table 8.2 indicates, 3-year-olds were expected to be able to point to their nose, eyes, and mouth and to name objects in a picture (e.g., a picture of a man and boy pulling a cart loaded with furniture). An 11-year-old was expected to be able to point out absurdities and contradictory statements (e.g., "I have three brothers, Paul, Ernest, and myself.") and to rearrange randomly ordered words (such as "A defends dog good his bravely master") into a sentence. A "successful" item was one that approximately 60 percent of children at a given age level could answer correctly and that significantly fewer children one year below and significantly more children one year above the level got correct. Thus, item selection was guided by how well the items discriminated among children of consecutive ages.

Binet and Simon administered their test to hundreds of children aged

Table 8.2
Sample Items from the 1908 Binet-Simon Scale

Level (years)	Item
Age 3	1. Points to nose, eyes, mouth. 2. Names objects in a picture.
Age 4	1. Knows sex. 2. Repeats three digits.
Age 5	1. Indicates the heavier of two cubes (of 3 and 12 grams and also of 6 and 15 grams). 2. Copies a square, using pen and ink.
Age 6	1. Knows morning and afternoon. 2. Defines familiar objects in terms of use.
Age 7	1. Describes pictures as scenes. 2. Tells what is missing in an unfinished picture.
Age 8	1. Gives differences between two objects from memory. 2. Counts backward from 20 to 0.
Age 9	1. Makes change on 4¢ out of 20¢ in simple play-store transactions. 2. Arranges five blocks in order of weight.
Age 10	1. Answers easy comprehension items. 2. Constructs a sentence to include three given words—*Paris, fortune, gutter.*
Age 11	1. Points out absurdities in contradictory statements. 2. Puts words, arranged in a random order, into a sentence.
Age 12	1. Repeats seven digits. 2. Answers problem question—a commonsense test.
Age 13	1. Rearranges in imagination the relationship of two triangles and draws the results as they would appear. 2. Gives differences between pairs of abstract terms such as *pride* and *pretension.*

Note: From *Intelligence: Nature, Determinants, and Consequences* (pp. 6–7) by E. B. Brody and N. Brody, 1976, New York: Academic Press. Copyright 1976 by Academic Press. Reprinted by permission.

3–13 years and compared each child's performance to the *norm* (or average) for his or her age group. This comparison procedure enabled the testers to establish a **mental age** for each child based on the number of items the child got correct relative to the number of items the average child of the same chronological age would get correct. For example, a 6-year-old child who passes all the items that the average child of 8 passes is said to have a mental age of 8.

The mental age concept proved extremely useful for measuring children's absolute levels of intellectual performance, but was of limited value in comparing the relative intelligences of children. For example, two children with mental ages of 8 but different chronological ages will not be equally intelligent for their age. A 6-year-old with a mental age of 8 would be considered quite bright, but a 10-year-old with the same mental age would be considered quite dull.

In 1912 William Stern, a German psychologist, proposed the concept of the **intelligence quotient,** or IQ, to deal with this problem. To find the IQ, a child's mental age (MA) was first divided by his or her chronological age (CA) and then multiplied by 100 to eliminate the decimal:

$$IQ = \frac{MA}{CA} \times 100$$

If a child passed all the items typically passed by his age group, the child's IQ score would be 100, or average IQ. Scores greater than 100 indicate above-average intellectual ability, and those less than 100 below-average intellectual ability.

The use of mental age for deriving a person's IQ score proved problematical for a variety of reasons. First, change in intelligence across one age range (e.g., 10–12 years) is not always equivalent to change across an equivalent age range (e.g., 5–7 years). Furthermore, the highest mental age a person can achieve on the revised Binet-Simon test (discussed below) is 16 years. Thus, when psychologists tried to apply the IQ formula to adults, the calculations became rather meaningless. A 50-year-old, regardless of true ability, would appear to be quite unintelligent with an IQ score of 32. For this reason, the ratio IQs derived from the MA/CA formula have been replaced by **deviation IQs.** Deviation IQs are computed on the basis of an individual's performance relative to the performance of others within the same age group. Although they have been used in much the same way as the original ratio IQs, they are in principle quite different (Sternberg & Powell, 1983).

Today psychologists continue to follow many of the same procedures originated by Binet. For example, they use varied tests to measure intelligence and base their selection of items on a person's ability to pass the items. A Stanford University psychologist, Lewis Terman, imported Binet's test into the United States in 1916. Terman made extensive modifications in Binet's test, and this verson became known as the Stanford-Binet Intelligence Scale. The Stanford-Binet included more items than the original Binet-Simon scale and could be used for children aged 2–16. Terman subsequently employed this scale in his landmark longitudinal studies of highly gifted individuals. Though subjected to much criticism, these studies provide a fascinating glimpse of life-span changes in intelligence among an unusually intelligent group of individuals. The background of the Terman research program and some recently reported findings from that program are described in Box 8.1.

The Binet-Simon and its successor, the Stanford-Binet, are both heavily loaded with items that tap verbal skills. In contrast, a series of intelligence tests developed by David Wechsler emphasizes nonverbal as

Box 8.1   Terman's Longitudinal Study of Gifted Men and Women

In what has been called the classic life-span research project, Lewis Terman and colleagues traced the life histories of more than 1500 men and women who had IQs of 135 or higher (the average IQ was 150). Scores at or above 135 are usually considered gifted IQs and place a person in the top 1 percent of the population. To find his gifted subjects, Terman sifted through the records of over a quarter-million California public school children. Most of the children in the final subject pool were in grades 3–8, and their average age was 11 when they were originally selected in 1922. The original sample had 857 boys and 671 girls and was not necessarily representative of the national population. There were only 2 Blacks, 1 Native American, and no Chinese; Latin American, Italian, and Portuguese groups were also underrepresented. Almost one-third of the children were from professional households, and few were children of unskilled laborers.

The sample was administered questionnaires and rating scales and interviewed in 1922 and in 1928, 1940, 1950, 1955, 1960, and 1972. Parents and teachers of these children were also surveyed periodically during the early years of the study. The amount of data gathered was enormous. The first reports from the study are contained in the five-volume *Genetic Studies of Genius* (Terman, 1959). Later reports have been published (Oden, 1968; Sears, 1977), and the data from the last data collection are still being analyzed.

Although all the subjects in Terman's study had high IQs, they were far from a homogeneous group. As adults, the subjects varied widely in their occupational achievements. To determine what accounted for these differences, Terman and his associate Melita Oden compared the 100 most successful individuals (the A group) and the 100 least successful individuals (the C group). Success was determined by occupational income and the status accorded to the job by society as measured by a standard scale. Several significant differences between groups A and C were found in childhood, and these differences became more exaggerated in adulthood. Although both groups had scored the same on intelligence tests, group A members graduated earlier from high school and received more graduate training. As children, group A members had many more collections and took part in more extracurricular activities, and as adults, they belonged to more professional societies and were more physically active. In addition, group A members came from more educationally and economically advantaged families than group C. Group A also seemed to become more intelligent with age. In both the 1940 and 1950 follow-up, groups A and C were given the Concept Mastery Test (CMT), an adult intelligence test that is heavily weighted with verbal items (such as synonyms, antonyms, analogies). In 1922, the initial time of measurement, the average IQ was 157 for group A and 150 for group C. On the follow-up tests, group A continued to do well relative to group C, and group A's advantage actually increased—group A's average CMT score was 147 and group C's was 130. A score of 130 is a superior score but not generally considered in the "gifted" range.

Why did group A excel? The answer appears to lie in motivation and attitude, not intellect. Group A seemed to possess greater perseverance, self-confidence, and goal orientation from an earlier age than group C. In short, the former group showed greater ambition and a special drive to succeed, which made a major difference in their lives.

In spite of their great career success, the men in group A put greater emphasis on a satisfactory family life than satisfaction in their work. From their earliest years, these men had most wanted a happy, rewarding family life, and most had found it. The gifted women in Terman's study valued family life to an even greater degree than the men. They also reported deriving more satisfaction from friends and cultural activities and less satisfaction from work than gifted men. Apparently, even gifted people find more satisfaction in their personal relationships than they do in work or intellectual pursuits.

Terman's study highlights the intellectual, emotional, occupational, and physical diversity of a group of exceptionally gifted individuals. By any standard their accomplishments have been remarkable. They have published almost 2000 scientific reports; 100 books; 375 plays and short stories; and more than 300 magazine articles, essays, and critiques. These achievements far surpass those expected from a group of 1500 people chosen randomly from the population. The gifted group as a whole also ranked far below the national average in number of cases of ill health, mental illness, suicide, and delinquent behavior (Terman, 1959). These data reveal that giftedness may lead to a healthier, happier, and more productive life, although within any gifted group there are wide individual differences in achievement and life satisfaction.

well as verbal abilities. Two of Wechsler's most widely used tests are the Wechsler Adult Intelligence Scale (WAIS; Wechsler, 1955) and a downward extension of the WAIS for children called the Wechsler Intelligence Scale for Children (WISC; Wechsler, 1974). Each test consists of subtests, approximately half of which deal with verbal content and the other half with nonverbal (performance) content. The WAIS and the WISC yield separate verbal and performance IQs as well as a full-scale (composite) IQ. Like later versions of the Binet tests, IQs on the Wechsler tests are based on deviation scores, not mental ages.

Spearman's "G"

Both Binet and Terman were less concerned with the theoretical aspects of intelligence than with the pragmatic concerns of test construction and human assessment. However, a prominent English psychologist of the era, Charles Spearman, was concerned with articulating a basic psychological theory of intelligence. Spearman believed that a single, unitary intellectual ability called "G" (for "general capacity") cut across many seemingly unrelated intellectual tasks. Thus, a person who does well on, say, a test of mathematical reasoning should also tend to do well on other types of intelligence items, such as verbal reasoning items. But Spearman thought that intelligence also consisted of a variety of specific, largely unrelated abilities required for particular cognitive tasks.

To test his theory, Spearman developed a highly sophisticated statistical procedure called **factor analysis.** Factor analysis is a correlational technique for observing *clusters* of relationships among a large number of items (e.g., the items found on an intelligence test). This procedure can determine whether certain items tend to cluster or correlate together. If they do, they are said to constitute a *factor.* Spearman was unable to support his theory completely employing factor analysis methods. While he did identify test-specific factors, called "S" factors (for "specific capacity"), there was only limited evidence for a G factor. For example, on his tests of verbal, numerical, and spatial reasoning, the items correlated more highly within each type of ability than they did across abilities.

Spearman described the G factor as a kind of mental energy which can appear in different forms. Some later theorists, including Thurstone, Guilford, and Cattell, followed Spearman's lead in explaining the existence of one general or central factor as a property of the faculties and abilities of the organism. Other theorists explained the existence of G quite differently. For example, G. Thomson (1939) tried to explain G on the basis of a large number of interconnected bonds including reflexes, habits, stimulus-response associations, and the like. Related psychological tests would activate overlapping sets of bonds. Although a factor analysis might yield an apparent general factor, the stimulus bonds actually are common to the various tests.

Many factor theorists conceded that regardless of its exact nature, G was exceedingly hard to find using a factor analysis approach (Guilford, 1979). Hence, they turned to a search for group factors. One of the major theories was proposed by Thurstone (1938), whose initial studies reported the existence of nine psychologically meaningful factors, which he termed *primary mental abilities*. Thurstone tested abilities that he identified as visual, perceptual, inductive, deductive, numerical, spatial, verbal, rote memory, and word fluency. In subsequent studies, Thurstone and his students identified additional primary abilities. A current version of the Primary Mental Abilities Test (PMA) consists of five different abilities: number, word fluency, verbal meaning, reasoning, and space (Thurstone, 1958).

The Structure-of-Intellect Model

Other theorists have gone further than Thurstone in identifying distinct abilities. Probably the most well-known psychologist to use this approach has been J. P. Guilford. Through factor analysis and logical analysis, Guilford identified 120 different factors in intelligence. According to Guilford, the differences among abilities can be indicated in three ways: (1) operations (the kinds of cognitive processing involved), (2) content (the type of information processed), and (3) product (the form that the information takes). Representing these required a multidimensional model, which Guilford called the **structure-of-intellect model,** or SOI model. The original model (Guilford, 1959) had five categories of operations, four of content, and six of product (see Figure 8.1).

To give you some idea of how the SOI model works, consider the following test item:

a. Name as many objects as you can that are both white and edible.

This is a test of "ideational fluency"; the greater the number of appropriate words produced in a limited time, the better the person's score. Instead of producing single words, item b asks a person to generate a list of short sentences:

b. Give as many sentences as you can that would fit into the form:
    W_____   c_____   s_____
    d _____.
    [e.g., Workers could seldom deviate.]

Figure 8.1   Guilford's structure-of-intellect model.

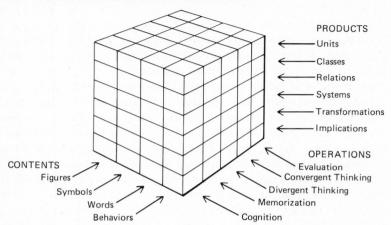

From *The Nature of Human Intelligence* (p. 63) by J. P. Guilford, 1967, New York: McGraw-Hill. Copyright 1967 by McGraw-Hill. Reprinted by permission.

Guilford calls item b a test of "expressional fluency." In both items a and b, the *operation* is divergent thinking. (As Chapter 7 noted, divergent thinking is a key ability in creativity.) The *content* in both items is also similar, consisting of conceptual material (words). The difference between the two items is in the *product* generated. In item a, the information is in the form of single objects or ideas, and the product is a *unit.* In item b, the product consists of an organized sequence of words or units called a *system.*

Guilford and colleagues are still trying to devise different items to fit the SOI model, the most recent version of which contains 150 factors (Guilford, 1982). So far, they have designed items to measure 105 of the 150 separate factors. Although the search for different factors of intelligence is likely to continue, the crucial question for developmentalists is how the various factors change with age. The next model we are going to discuss was designed with this question in mind.

The Fluid-Crystallized Model of Intelligence

Although the factor analytic methods discussed above are useful for identifying clusters of various intellectual abilities, they can be employed more effectively if guided by a theory of intelligence. And, as Guilford recognizes, the search for more separate ability factors seems to be reaching a stage of diminishing returns. McNemar (1964) pointed out the subjectivity in identifying and interpreting factors, many of which overlap considerably. If there can be 150 factors, why not 200,

500, or 1000? At this stage of our knowledge, a simpler approach seems best.

The problem of fractionalizing the intellect into progressively greater numbers of factors is avoided in the *hierarchical* approach (Cattell, 1963, 1971). This approach recognizes relatively independent primary abilities, but also includes broader, higher-order mental abilities which can be identified by factor analyzing relationships of the primary ability components. By examining correlated factors, hierarchies of intellectual abilities can be constructed from very specific primary factors of intelligence to more general second-, third-, and even fourth-order factors. The products of these higher-order factor analyses are referred to as *dimensions* or *components* of intelligence. A fully hierarchical model consists of several levels of mental abilities with a general factor at the top of the hierarchy.

The theory of **crystallized intelligence** (Gc) and **fluid intelligence** (Gf) proposed by Cattell (1971) and extended by Horn (1972, 1978) is a hierarchical approach to intelligence. This theory is based on the factor analytic study of the correlational structure among primary mental abilities, but also deals with the development of these abilities over the life span and proposed causal influences. The theory distinguishes between two independent second-order factors: crystallized intelligence and fluid intelligence. ("Independence" does not mean that the factors are correlated zero, only that they represent independent scientific constructs.) Crystallized intelligence is said to reflect the systematic influence of variables such as schooling, acculturation, and learning experiences. It can be measured by means of primary abilities such as verbal comprehension, concept formation, logical reasoning, and general reasoning. For example, a vocabulary test ("Define the word *impale*") and an untimed test of information recall ("How far is it from New York to Los Angeles?") measure crystallized knowledge.

Fluid intelligence is said to reflect intelligence that is relatively independent of systematic educational or acculturation experiences and can be described as incidental learning or *casual learning* (Horn, 1982). A good example of casual learning can be seen in the child who acquires ideas about conservation without being exposed to systematic efforts by parents or teachers to teach this concept. Fluid ability is believed to operate through a different pattern of neural and biological organization than crystallized intelligence. It can be seen in primary abilities such as inductive reasoning, figural flexibility, and integration. For example, a letter series task in which one has to find the letter that completes a sequence of several letters is a measure of the primary ability of induction:

  d   f   i   m   r   x   e   _____

Other primary abilities which show a consistent relationship to fluid intelligence are associative memory and spatial orientation. Because fluid intelligence and crystallized intelligence are indexed by many primary abilities, no single measure of either intelligence exists. Thus, any given measure may reflect both fluid and crystallized abilities, although some tests are purer measures of one or the other.

In their theory of crystallized and fluid intelligence, Horn and Cattell (1967) proposed a specific life-span developmental sequence. Because crystallized intelligence is held to reflect accumulated knowledge and experience, it is expected to continue to increase throughout most of adulthood, at least from people's 20s to their 60s. Fluid intelligence is expected to increase with age through adolescence, level off in young adulthood, and decline in middle and old age. When measures of crystallized and fluid ability are combined into a composite *omnibus* score, these discrepant developmental trends are obscured, and no systematic age-related increases or declines can be observed (see Figure 8.2).

We noted that incidental learning produces fluid intelligence; according to Horn (1982), this type of learning is particularly susceptible to neurological and physiological alterations in the body with age. As Fig-

Figure 8.2 Intellectual performance as a function of age.

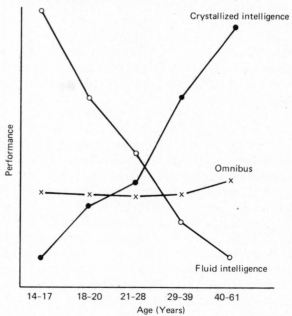

From "Organization of Data on Life-Span Development of Human Abilities" by J. L. Horn, 1970, in *Life-Span Developmental Psychology: Research and Theory* (p. 463) edited by L. R. Goulet and P. B. Baltes, New York: Academic Press. Copyright 1970 by Academic Press. Reprinted by permission.

Figure 8.3 Life-span development of fluid intelligence (Gf) and crystallized intelligence (Gc) and their relation to maturational growth and decline of neural structures (M), accumulation of injury to neural structures (I), accumulation of educational exposures (E), and overall ability (G).

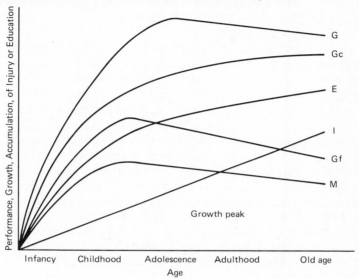

From "Organization of Data on Life-Span Development of Human Abilities" by J. L. Horn, 1970; in *Life-Span Developmental Psychology: Research and Theory* (p. 465) edited by L. R. Goulet and P. B. Baltes, New York: Academic Press. Copyright 1970 by Academic Press. Reprinted by permission.

ure 8.3 shows, the physiological base which supports fluid functioning deteriorates from birth until death as a result of the accumulation of injuries to the neural structures. For example, in later adulthood the number of active neurons in the central nervous system decrease; blood flow and oxygen use, especially in the limbic area of the brain, decrease; and waste by-products build up in the neural cells. Maturational growth offsets injuries to the biological base during childhood and adolescence, leading to a gain in fluid intelligence. But after biological maturity is attained, maturational declines heighten the effect of such injuries, and fluid intelligence decreases.

Crystallized abilities appear less vulnerable to the damaging effects of biological deterioration and injury. For example, many of the crystallized abilities immediately affected by a stroke recuperate over time or with some cognitive retraining (Horn, 1982). In contrast, fluid abilities affected by brain damage are less responsive to the recuperative effects of time or rehabilitation. As Figure 8.3 shows, educational learning experiences, which accumulate over time, increase crystallized ability. Much of this learning occurs through systematic exposure to the knowledge and skills of the culture at home, school, or work. Although some crystallized knowledge is forgotten over time, a surprisingly large amount of what people learn intentionally tends to be maintained. Moreover, with repeated use, crystallized knowledge may be reorganized into new knowledge structures as new associations are learned and old ones reevaluated.

As support for their theory, Horn and Cattell (1967) presented data based on a cross-sectional study of 279 adolescents and adults. The findings of their study were consistent with the proposed model, though one must interpret the data cautiously (see Guilford, 1980). Very few subjects in their study were over age 50. Further, the use of cross-sectional methodology introduces the potential confounding of age and cohort variables. When cohort variables were controlled for by using sequential developmental studies, results failed to corroborate the large fluid decrement in adulthood (Schaie, 1979; Schaie & Labouvie-Vief, 1974). However, there is consistent support for the finding of increased crystallized ability in cross-sectional as well as longitudinal and sequential studies. Indeed, crystallized abilities may be more relevant to the types of tasks individuals perform in everyday life and may form the basis of what we commonly call the "wisdom" of older people. These notions will be discussed fully in a later section.

The Age Differentiation–Dedifferentiation Hypothesis

For a life-span cognitive psychologist, the concept of factors of intelligence raises a whole set of important issues. Chief among these is whether intelligence factors remain the same across the life span or whether they change. Do children have the same number and type of factors as adults? Which factors go together and which remain independent?

Interest in these questions grew out of work in the childhood literature on the **age differentiation hypothesis,** which states that abstract intelligence changes in organization with age from a general ability, or G factor, to a more loosely organized group of special abilities, or S factors (Garrett, 1946). To support the hypothesis of differentiation, various intellectual abilities should have a lower correlation within different age levels later in childhood than earlier in childhood. Although these abilities might still depend on a general G factor, they should do so to a lesser degree. The evidence for the differentiation hypothesis has been mixed, with just about as many empirical studies supporting the hypothesis as failing to support it (see Reinert, 1970, for a review).

From a life-span perspective, we can ask whether abilities continue to differentiate or whether they show evidence of **dedifferentiation.** That is, do individuals return to the general, global structure character-

istic of childhood intelligence, or do the abilities grow more specialized? Once again, the empirical data yield conflicting findings. Some
studies show factor variability (or differentiation); others support factor
stability (or dedifferentiation). These findings must be interpreted cautiously because of statistical difficulties and an overreliance on cross-
sectional comparisons of age groups. In a study that overcame many of
these problems, Cunningham (1981) reported that the number of factors remained fairly stable across the adult years, but the pattern of
interrelationships was not the same across different factors and age
groups. The factors of Cognitive Flexibility and Perceptual Speed were
more high related to the other cognitive factors in an older age group
(51–83 years) than in a younger age group (15–32 years). On the basis
of his results, Cunningham (1981) suggested that the dedifferentiation
hypothesis should not be thought of as a simplification of the structure
of abilities with age, but as "an increasing *interdependence* of different
aspects of intellectual functioning" (p. 19). He also suggested that intellectual speed and health factors may account for these increased inter-
dependencies. Cunningham's results provide fruitful avenues for further theoretical and empirical study on the age differentiation-
dedifferentiation hypothesis.

In conclusion, the factor analytic approach has been a major tool for
answering questions about the nature of human intelligence. While this
approach has told us a great deal about how intelligence is structured,
serious questions have been raised about its usefulness for analyzing
the cognitive processes underlying intellectual ability (see Sternberg,
1977). Such questions have arisen because factor analytic methods
focus on the answers to intelligence test items, rather than on the cognitive processes used to arrive at the answers. And depending upon the
type of factor analysis used, different factors of intelligence may
emerge, making comparison of various theories of intelligence difficult.
A recent theory that overcomes many of these limitations is described
in Box 8.2. This theory, known as *triarchic theory,* is grounded in the
information-processing tradition but also incorporates elements of contextualistic approaches to intelligence.

Box 8.2   A Triarchic Theory of Human Intelligence

   Robert Sternberg (1985) has recently proposed a triarchic theory
of intelligence that goes well beyond existing theories in its
breadth and conceptual scope. The theory is composed of three
subtheories: (1) *contextual subtheory,* which emphasizes the role
that intelligent behaviors play in successful adaptation to the environment; (2) *componential subtheory,* which specifies the mental
structures and mechanisms underlying intelligent behavior; and

(3) *experiential subtheory,* which indicates that intelligence is best demonstrated in situations requiring the ability to deal with novelty or to automatize information processing. Collectively, these three subtheories can be used to understand individual differences in intelligence or to identify who is intelligent (Sternberg, 1985).

In discussing contextual subtheory, Sternberg claims that individuals strive for an optimal fit to their environment. If the degree of fit falls below what is considered satisfactory, then adaptation to the environment at one level may be perceived as maladaptation at another. For example, an employee's attitudes and values may be so discrepant from the employer's that a satisfactory fit does not seem possible (Sternberg, 1985). When adaptation is impossible or undesirable, individuals may attempt to *reshape* the environment to achieve a better contextual fit or *select* an alternative environment. Thus, the employee might seek another job or try to get the employer to view matters differently. One implication of this contextual view is that intelligence will vary across individuals and cultures as well as across age levels. For example, spatial representation skills (see Chapter 4) may be one of the most important indices of adaptive intelligence in an environment in which people must navigate through unfamiliar terrain, but may be largely irrelevant in a context in which people spend most of their time in familiar surroundings. Similarly, the operational definition of what is intelligent will differ between children and adults, and between adults at different age levels. Does this mean that intelligence is entirely age- or culture-specific?

Sternberg (1985) avoids the problem of a relativistic point of view by positing a set of mental components that underlie adaptive, intelligent behavior, regardless of behavioral contexts. A *component* is an elementary information process that operates on internal representations of objects or symbols (Sternberg, 1977). Sternberg distinguishes three broad classes of components: *performance components, metacomponents,* and *knowledge acquisition components.* Performance components are the basic mental operations used to execute various cognitive tasks, such as encoding information, combining and comparing information, and responding with a solution. Sternberg believes that performance components are potentially important as sources of individual and developmental differences in intelligence.

An even more fundamental source of such differences are the control processes or executive routines known as metacomponents. Metacomponents are used in deciding what problem is to be solved, selecting appropriate performance components, selecting the representation or organization for the information, and choosing the appropriate strategy for combining the performance components. Metacomponents are also used to allocate attentional resources, monitor the solution to the problem, and modify performance in light of external feedback. Changes in metacomponents lead to critical changes in the functioning of the performance components.

The last major components are knowledge acquisition components, which are used to gain new knowledge. These components, like the other two, have several aspects, including selectively encoding relevant information, combining this information into a structured whole, and selectively comparing newly acquired information with information acquired in the past.

The third part of triarchic theory is experiential subtheory. Sternberg contends that intelligence is best demonstrated when individuals are confronted by relatively novel tasks or are in the process of automatizing their performance on a given task. These two facets of the subtheory—novelty and automatization—interact. For example, automatization of information processing frees more processing resources to deal with novelty in the task. Conversely, adaptation to novelty enables people to automatize a task early in their experience with it. The idea that intelligent actions involve adaptation to novel circumstances is not altogether new. Experts and lay persons believe that more intelligence is revealed in rapidly adapting to unfamiliar and challenging situations than in carrying out daily routines (Sternberg, Conway, Ketron, & Bernstein, 1981). Later in the situation, automatization comes into play. People who can perform a task automatically are generally seen as more intelligent than people with the same amount of experience with the task who can only perform it haltingly and with considerable conscious effort (Sternberg, 1985). Experiential subtheory has important implications for selecting items to assess intelligence across different age groups. Similar tasks presented to children and adults may measure the former's ability to deal with novelty and the latter's level of automatization. In addition, the tasks should not be so unfamiliar that an individual cannot apply past knowledge to their solution. Asking a 5-year-old to solve a calculus problem would be a meaningless measure of intellectual ability.

Sternberg's (1985) triarchic theory is an ambitious attempt to provide a more complete view of human intelligence than previous theories can offer. Although in need of further empirical validation, the theory gives a conceptually integrated framework for studying the nature of human intelligence. And it may offer us additional insights on the course of intellectual development across the adult life span (see Berg & Sternberg, 1985).

INTELLECTUAL DEVELOPMENT OVER THE LIFE SPAN

Since their inception intelligence tests have been administered to thousands of people of varying ages. Though certain age groups (e.g., schoolchildren) are more likely to be tested than other age groups (e.g., infants, old adults), enough data are available to draw some conclusions about the course of intellectual development over the life span. From a life-span perspective, many important questions can be asked. Does an infant's intelligence predict its intellectual performance in the school years? Which intellectual abilities develop fastest? Does intelligence "peak" at a certain age? Do declines in intelligence occur in old age?

Intelligence in Infancy

Earlier in the chapter we noted that undergraduates in Siegler and Richards's (1982) study characterized an "intelligent" infant by traits such as perceptual recognition ability, motor ability, and alertness. This characterization is remarkably similar to the way in which psychologists describe infants' intellectual capacity. To measure this capacity, psychologists have devised tests that rely heavily on sensorimotor content. One of the best standardized and widely used measures of infant intelligence is the Bayley Scales of Infant Development (Bayley, 1969), which consists of a 163-item mental scale and an 81-item motor scale (see Chapter 4). Table 8.3 shows sample items from each scale and the approximate ages at which 50 percent of the babies tested passed the items. As Table 8.3 shows, most of the items from the scales measure sensorimotor and perceptual abilities, but a few tap beginning language skills.

Testing an infant's intelligence can be highly problematical. Psychologists must judge many novel or unusual responses and decide whether the infant is attending or not attending to stimuli. Moreover, the scales used to measure an infant's mental ability must be administered individually by a very patient tester. Why then do psychologists insist on measuring infant intelligence? One reason is that such tests can distinguish between normal and handicapped babies. A well-trained and sensitive examiner may detect early sensory or neurological difficulties that call for intervention. Several new tests designed to detect mental deficiencies among infants have been developed, including the Denver Developmental Screening Test and Brazelton's Neonatal Behavioral Assessment Scale (Brooks-Gunn & Weinraub, 1983).

A broader use of infant intelligence tests is to make developmental predictions. For many years psychologists hoped to be able to predict children's future mental status by their performance on IQ tests during

Table 8.3
Examples of Items on the Bayley Scales

Age	Mental Scale Items	Motor Scale Items
Newborn	Baby quiets when picked up.	Baby makes a postural adjustment when examiner puts her to his shoulder.
2 months	When examiner presents two objects above infant in crib, she glances back and forth from one to the other.	Baby holds her head steady when being carried about in vertical position.
5 months	Baby is observed to transfer object from one hand to the other during play.	When seated at a feeding-type table and presented with a sugar pill out of reach, baby attempts to pick it up.
8 months	When object in plain view of baby (on table) is covered by a tissue, baby removes tissue to recover toy.	Baby raises herself to a sitting position.
12 months	Baby imitates words when examiner says them.	When asked by the examiner, baby stands up from a position lying on her back on the floor.
16 months	Baby builds a tower with three small cubes after demonstration by examiner.	Baby stands on her left foot alone.

Note: From *Bayley Scales of Infant Development* by N. Bayley, 1969, New York: Psychological Corporation. Copyright 1969 by The Psychological Corporation. Reproduced by permission. All rights reserved.

the first few months of life. For the most part, this hope has been unrealized. In Bayley's (1943) longitudinal studies, assessments of infants at several times of measurement failed to correlate with their performance on the Stanford-Binet at age 6 and 7. J. E. Anderson (1939) conducted a longitudinal study of predictive validity at about the same time as Bayley. He tested over 100 infants on a composite intelligence scale during the first 2 years of life and the Stanford-Binet at age 5. J. E. Anderson (1939) found low or no correlations between the 5-year-olds' IQ scores and the earlier scores. Few items predicted later intelligence; the only exceptions were alertness to the external environment in the first few months of life and language ability in the second year of life. More recent studies also failed to find a systematic relationship between infant tests and later IQ score or scholastic achievement (Honzik, 1976; R. Rubin & Balow, 1979). As Brooks-Gunn and Weinraub (1983) pointed out, results like this supported arguments that intelligence varies not only quantitatively across the life span but qualitatively as well.

Why do infant intelligence tests fail to predict preschool or school-aged IQ? For one thing, an infant's intelligence may change so rapidly that measurement is impossible (Birren, Kinney, Schaie, & Woodruff, 1981). In addition, the sensorimotor content tapped by infant measures may not have much to do with the verbal and symbolic activities measured by later IQ tests. Finally, even within the infancy period, there is little consistency in IQ performance (M. Lewis, 1983). Some attempts have been made to increase the predictive validity of infant intelligence tests by collecting additional measures (e.g., category ratings, clinical appraisals) and by conducting more sophisticated statistical analyses. Thus far such attempts have not succeeded in significantly improving the predictive accuracy of these tests.

Intelligence in Childhood and Adolescence

The first intelligence tests were used to predict scholastic performance, and their greatest success was in this area. For example, correlations between a child's IQ score and current grades in school average about .50 (Minton & Schneider, 1980). Because success in our culture is so intimately connected to success in school, intelligence tests also seem to be a good yardstick of a broad range of human activity in everyday life. However, much less attention has been paid to the relationship between intellectual abilities and real-life activities. We are not saying that a high IQ causes success in school or in other situations, only that the two go together.

During the childhood years, individuals make their most rapid strides in intelligence. But children show wide individual differences in intellectual development as they do in physical development. Children seem to go through two spurts in intellectual growth: first around 6 years of age and then around age 10 or 11. The age 6 spurt may be associated with entry into a school system or may be connected with the shift from preoperational to concrete operational development which occurs around this time. The reasons for the age 10–11 spurt are less clear. Perhaps it is associated with a general set of physical and psychological changes occurring around the time of puberty or with the transition from concrete to formal operational thinking.

Although intelligence undergoes occasional rapid spurts, it begins to stabilize during middle childhood. For example, Honzik, Macfarlane, and Allen (1948) found a strong relationship between IQ scores at ages 8 and 9 and those at age 10. The correlation between the IQs was .88 for ages 8 and 10, and .90 for ages 9 and 10. Both are very high correlations and show a strong degree of relationship across ages and IQ. Furthermore, by age 10, predictions of adolescent and adult IQs can begin to be made with considerable accuracy. For example, the correlation between IQ at age 10 and IQ at age 18 was .76, a statistically significant correlation. Despite the stabilization of IQ scores during childhood, IQ can show considerable variability. Honzik et al. (1948) reported that 60 percent of the children tested had IQ scores that changed 15 points or more in the period from ages 6–8.

More recently, McCall, Applebaum, and Hogarty (1973) looked at the consistency of scores among children who had been given intelligence tests at regular intervals from age 2½–17. Because they were concerned with individual differences in IQ, the investigators identified five distinct groups of children with different patterns of IQ change over age. As Figure 8.4 shows, group 1 evidenced little systematic change in IQ, while groups 2–5 displayed considerable year-by-year fluctuation. Notice that groups 2 and 3 showed predominately decreasing scores during the preschool years, while groups 4 and 5 showed primarily increasing scores. When individual scores were averaged across all groups, the range of IQ scores shifted an average of 28.5 points from 2½–17 years of age. More than one out of every three children displayed performance shifts of 30 points, and approximately one out of seven increased or decreased by as much as 40 points. One child increased 74

Figure 8.4 Change in IQ scores over age for five IQ groups. The data are from the Fels Longitudinal Study.

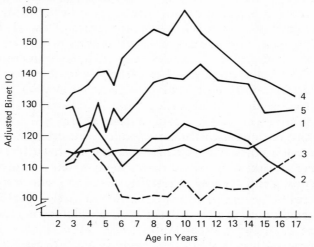

From "Developmental Changes in Mental Performance" by R. B. McCall, M. I. Applebaum, and P. S. Hogarty, 1973, *Monographs of the Society for Research in Child Development, 38* (Serial No. 150, No. 3), p. 48. Copyright 1973 by The Society for Research in Child Development, Inc. Reprinted by permission.

points! Since the standard error of measurement (an alternative way of expressing reliability) for most intelligence tests is only 3 or 4 points, these results indicate that IQ is influenced by other factors such as testing conditions or characteristics of the home or school. Thus, caution must be exercised in drawing conclusions about later-life IQ from early performance data because intelligence is not as fixed as the original theories assumed.

Testing Biases and IQ

One factor that markedly affects children's performance on intellectual measures is the nature of the testing conditions (Scarr-Salapatek, 1975). For example, cross-cultural research shows that children's performance may not be optimal under unfamiliar or threatening testing conditions (Cole, Gay, Glick, & Sharp, 1971). As noted in Chapter 5, many Black children use simplified speech registers when interacting with authority figures (such as IQ testers), but complex speech forms with peers.

Items on intelligence tests also may be inappropriate for various ethnic cultures and social class groups. Critics charge that IQ tests have not been standardized on minority groups and that the content of the tests is based heavily on White middle-class children's school and home experience. Intelligence tests are considered biased to the extent that they depend on middle-class language, values, and experience.

Attempts to deal with culture bias in standardized IQ tests have taken several different directions. One attempt involves the development of tests that draw on the special knowledge, language, and skills of minority children. For example, the Dove Counterbalance General Intelligence Test, sometimes referred to as the "chitling test," was facetiously developed by Black sociologist Adrian Dove (1968) to show that testing biases can operate both ways. Dove's test includes many vocabulary items from Black street slang such as "handkerchief head" (an Uncle Tom). Although Black children would doubtless score higher on this test than most White children, many educators might question its value for predicting academic performance and grades in school systems dominated by White middle-class values and norms.

Attempts to develop culturally unbiased tests or to modify existing test items involve "renorming" the standardized tests and compiling separate statistical profiles for minority group children. Probably the best-known and successful attempt at cultural adjustment is Jane Mercer's (1971) System of Multicultural Pluralistic Assessment (SOMPA). This scale consists of a battery of interrelated measures for children aged 5–11 years. The battery includes a Wechsler IQ test; a one-hour interview with parents on the child's health history and family background; an adaptive behavior inventory of the child's nonacademic functioning in school, home, and neighborhood; and a complete medical exam. According to Mercer (1971), SOMPA is better able than standardized IQ tests to identify children who do not perform well academically, but who are capable of taking care of themselves and functioning effectively in the community. In her opinion these children should not be labeled retarded, but should be placed in a regular classroom environment that takes into account their unique cultural background and learning history. This is especially important in that minority children are more likely to be diagnosed as retarded than White children based on standard criteria (usually an IQ of 84 or below on the Stanford-Binet and impaired adaptive behavior).

Proponents hail SOMPA as the first nondiscriminatory, culture-free assessment battery. Many states such as California and Louisiana have already adopted it for use in determining student placement in special education programs. On the other hand, opponents claim that SOMPA creates unrealistically high expectations about a child's ability among parents and teachers and pressures children to measure up to these expectations. Some psychologists point out that the battery contains a Wechsler IQ test, so that it is not a totally unbiased measure.

Other psychologists argue that not only are IQ tests biased against minority children, but they are also unfair to White middle-class children. Consider the following question from a well-known standardized test:

> Which of these four sports—field hockey, pool, football, or baseball— doesn't belong on the list?

The "right" answer is *pool* because it is not a team sport. But one could also make a case for any of the other three sports. For example, field hockey is played mostly by females, football is not played with a bat or stick, and baseball does not involve putting the ball into a goal ("Ban on IQ Tests," 1976).

Responding to pressure from parent and teacher organizations, California, New York City, and Washington, D.C., have banned standardized group intelligence tests from their schools because of concerns about fairness and reliability. Moreover, several states have passed legislation mandating that questions and answers on standardized tests be made available to students who have taken the tests. Despite the controversy, more tests are being mass-produced and administered. The reasons behind this phenomenon, other than obvious economic ones, are subtle and complex. Many educators are alarmed by the sharp drop in scores on tests such as the Scholastic Aptitude Test (SAT) over the last decade and insist that tests measuring basic verbal and quantitative abilities be given. Others fear that reliance on teachers' or employers' judgments about intellectual proficiency will invite even more abuse and unfairness than the tests create.

Serious efforts are being made at universities and research centers across the country to develop fairer, more reliable, and more contextually valid intelligence tests (B. Rice, 1979). Several of these tests have a futuristic quality. For example, computerized audiovisual tests are now being used by some psychologists to assess intellectual skills such as listening and perception, which are not easily measured with traditional paper-and-pencil tests. Other psychologists are measuring *evoked potentials* of the brain by monitoring electroencephalographic (EEG) recordings of brain-wave activity in response to sensory stimuli such as sounds or light flashes. Brain diagnoses may prove particularly useful for testing nonverbal children and those with language and neurological problems. Finally, following the tradition of Soviet psychologists such as Vygotsky (see Chapter 5), psychologists in the United States are developing tests that measure "learning potential" or modifiability rather than what the child already knows. According to Vygotsky's (1978) notion of the "zone of proximal development," we should examine the difference between a child's existing intellectual performance and the competence he or she could achieve with proper instruction and training. Children with greater potential should require fewer prompts or less coaching to do well than children with less potential. Such innovative approaches promise to change dramatically the way intelligence is conceptualized and assessed in the future.

Social Class, Racial, and Ethnic Differences in IQ

Individual differences in performance among children on standardized IQ tests have been attributed not only to testing biases but also to social class, racial, and ethnic differences. Lower-class children reliably score 10–15 IQ points below middle- and upper-class children, and Black children on the average score 15–20 IQ points below their White agemates (Hall & Kaye, 1980; Jensen, 1969; Kennedy, 1969; Loehlin, Lindzey, & Spuhler, 1975). Hispanic and Native American children also score well below the White norm on standardized intelligence tests. These differences do not become apparent until the early school years, and they increase with age through childhood.

Many studies on intellectual performance have confounded the factors of social class and racial group because Blacks, Hispanics, and Native Americans are found disproportionately in the lower social classes. When these factors are controlled, social class differences occur within racial groups; for example, middle-class Blacks have higher IQs than lower-class Blacks. Similarly, middle-class Whites have higher IQs than lower-class Whites. How can these differences be explained?

One environmental explanation is that the combined effects of poverty, ill health, poor nutrition, inadequate living environment, and limited education are responsible for the poor cognitive performance of children from ethnic groups and lower social classes. These factors may in turn lower achievement motivation, self-esteem, and feelings of personal efficacy, which negatively influence performance on IQ tests.

Another environmental suggestion is that differences in parenting behaviors may play an important role in explaining the relationship between social class and IQ. The largest differences between middle-class and lower-class parents are seen in their use of language toward children. Middle-class mothers are more likely than lower-class mothers to respond quickly to infant vocalizations, to continue vocalizing to infants when they cease to speak, and to play language games with their children (Golden & Birns, 1976; M. Lewis & Freedle, 1973). Significant differences also exist in parenting styles and control techniques. Middle-class parents tend to use child-centered disciplinary methods. They explain the reasons behind their actions, emphasize the child's feelings, and make the child aware of the complexities of physical and social surroundings. Lower-class parents tend to use parent-centered child-rearing methods, which emphasize the adults' superior power and status. For example, they stress conformity and obedience to parental demands (e.g., "Do it because *I* told you to"). This style of communication is less likely to equip the child with the complex problem-solving and thinking skills required in everyday and academic life. Because of the importance of parent-child relationships for later intellectual development, many psychologists have tried to develop intervention programs to improve the communication and teaching skills of parents (see Chapter 10).

In contrast to the preceding explanations is the argument that social class and racial differences in intelligence involve differences in hereditary background. The most outspoken exponent of this genetic position is Berkeley psychologist Arthur Jensen. In a controversial article in the *Harvard Educational Review,* Jensen (1969) concluded that compensatory educational programs for culturally disadvantaged children had failed dismally because the environment contributes to only a small portion of the variance (about 20 percent) in IQ scores. The remaining variance (about 80 percent) is due to hereditary factors. Jensen based his conclusions on data from twin studies which show that identical twins (with identical heredity) reared in different environments have highly similar IQs. Jensen also argued that there are two different levels of genetically determined abilities. Level I learning, or **associative learning,** involves abilities such as short-term memory, rote learning, attention, and simple associative thinking. This type of learning, which does not predict school performance well, is equally distributed among different racial, ethnic, and social class groups. In contrast, Level II learning, or **cognitive learning,** is predictive of school performance because it involves abstract reasoning, symbolic thinking, and problem-solving skills. The cognitive learning skills measured by standardized IQ tests are concentrated more in middle-class and Anglo-American populations than in lower-class and ethnic groups.

Jensen's arguments provoked a storm of protest in 1969 and are still the subject of heated debate. In fact, at a recent meeting of the American Psychological Association in Anaheim, California, scattered protests erupted outside where Jensen was speaking. Why are his ideas so controversial? First, critics charge that Jensen seriously overestimates the influence of genetic factors on intelligence. Even if his estimate of 80 percent heritability were correct, all efforts to modify or improve intelligence would not be fruitless. Intelligence may or may not be difficult to change. For example, Scarr and Weinberg (1976, 1977, 1983) reported a series of studies of disadvantaged Black children who were adopted early in their lives by White middle-class families. The researchers discovered that as schoolchildren, the Black adoptees averaged 10 points above the average IQ of the population as a whole and about 20 points above age-mates raised in the Black community. These findings indicate that the home and school environment can play a significant role in boosting IQ performance.

Jensen's critics also argue that even though individual IQ differences within a group have a large hereditary component, one cannot automatically conclude that IQ differences between two groups are genetically based. Consider an example described by H. Gardner (1978). Suppose you measure the average heights of children in a rural Mexican village and find a strong positive correlation between the heights of children and those of their parents: taller parents have taller children. Since all the children grew up in the same environmental setting, you might conclude that height is based on the hereditary makeup of the family. Suppose that you measure children in Mexico City and find the same strong positive relationship between children's and parents' heights, but you notice that urban children are taller on the average than rural children. These between-group urban-rural differences might be due to environmental factors such as nutrition, medical care, and living conditions. Thus, within-group (individual) variations in height might be primarily due to genetic differences, but between-group variations might be due to environmental conditions. The same logic applies to conclusions about social class, racial, and ethnic group differences in intellectual performance. Even though IQ may be equally heritable within a sample of Black and White children, the 15–20 point average IQ difference between groups may reflect differences in the environmental conditions under which the two groups live.

Jensen has been roundly criticized for downplaying the impact of the environment on intelligence during the early years. Leon Kamin (1974, 1981a, 1981b), a Princeton University psychologist, claimed that the experimental designs and statistical procedures for analyzing the results of the twin studies on which Jensen based his argument are flawed. The most serious shortcoming is that identical twins reared apart are often placed in very similar home circumstances, and identical twins reared together are treated more similarly by parents than nonidentical twins or siblings. The implication is that similar environments, not similar hereditary backgrounds, may explain the high correlation of IQ scores among identical twins.

Kamin (1981a, 1981b) also cited evidence from adoption studies which compared IQs of adopted and natural children raised in the same household. Studies done in Texas and Minnesota did not find the intellectual resemblance between pairs of biological siblings to be appreciably greater than between biological and adopted siblings. Apparently, children growing up in identical environments will be similar to each other in IQ, whether or not they share the same genetic heritage.

Kamin's arguments have been welcomed by those favoring an environmental position, but many psychologists remain unconvinced that the heritability of intelligence is negligible. Although he is probably correct in stating that the heritability of intelligence has been overestimated, Kamin overstated the lack of evidence for genetic factors in IQ. Moreover, his argument about the greater similarity of the environments of identical twins reared apart compared to nonidentical twins reared together is debatable. Finally, Kamin ignored recent evidence from adoption studies showing that the correlations between the IQ scores of children and their biological parents (after controlling for family placements) were significantly higher than between children and their adoptive parents. The only definite conclusion we can draw from this IQ controversy is that the environment plays an influential role in intellectual development, but genetics sets limits on the nature and extent of environmental influence.

Intelligence in Adulthood

Most early work on intelligence focused on the acquisition of intellectual abilities during the childhood years. Terman's standardization of the Binet-Simon intelligence test for use in the United States assumed that intellectual development peaked at age 16 and remained constant thereafter (Schaie, 1979). However, when intelligence tests were administered to large numbers of adults, some puzzling findings emerged. Nearly all the initial studies suggested that intellectual abilities peaked sometime in early adulthood and then declined systematically with age (H. Jones & Conrad, 1933; Wechsler, 1939). In the H. Jones and Conrad (1933) study, a cross-section of persons aged 10–60 was tested on an early group intelligence test, the Army Alpha. The

Army Alpha was designed to classify men for various military activities during World War I and was subsequently put to civilian use. It consists of eight timed subtests, many of which are similar to the verbal subtests on the WAIS. H. Jones and Conrad (1933) showed that younger adults performed better than older adults, but the peak of intellectual performance varied considerably with the specific ability tested. For example, the numerical and reasoning abilities showed the greatest decline; the verbal abilities declined least. Wechsler (1939) reported similar findings using the Wechsler-Bellevue Intelligence Scale (W-B), the forerunner of the WAIS. Verbal abilities "held up" well with age, whereas performance abilities failed to hold. Indeed, the data compelled Wechsler to include an age adjustment in his scoring system. If we were to administer the WAIS to different age groups, we would find that the average IQ for any group is around 100. However, a 20-year-old must achieve a higher raw score on the test than a 50-year-old to be given a normal IQ score. For example, a 20-year-old with a raw score of 80 would have an IQ of only 87, a subnormal IQ, whereas a 50-year-old with this same raw score would have an IQ of 101, an average IQ.

The above findings and interpretations were all based on cross-sectional studies. When data from longitudinal studies became available, a different picture emerged. Early longitudinal investigations by Bayley and colleagues (Bayley, 1968; Bayley & Oden, 1955) and Owens (1953, 1959) reported that intellectual ability is maintained into middle age. Bayley tested individuals who participated in the longitudinal Berkeley Growth Study. She found that IQ scores, as measured by the W-B at ages 16, 18, 21, and 26, and by the WAIS at age 36 increased through age 26, after which they leveled off and remained unchanged for the next 10 years. Using these data, Bayley developed a "theoretical curve" of intellectual growth, extending through age 36 (see Figure 8.5). Owens (1953) tested 127 50-year-olds on the Army Alpha Test, which they had taken as 19-year-old freshmen at Iowa State College. Their overall total IQ scores at age 50 were significantly higher than their scores at age 19. A later follow-up of these same subjects showed that they maintained their abilities well into their 60s (Cunningham & Owens, 1983).

Why do we find a discrepancy between cross-sectional and longitudinal findings? As you may recall from Chapter 2, cross-sectional studies confound the developmental variables of subject age and cohort membership. The older people tested in these studies differ from younger people not only in their age but also in average educational level, familiarity with the tests, and health care. In the early longitudinal investigations, the subjects were highly educated, intellectually gifted, and in cognitively demanding occupations. Typically, the brightest and healthiest subjects remained in the studies; the less bright

Figure 8.5 Theoretical curve of the growth of intelligence, based on repeated testing of the same individuals. The data are from the Berkeley Growth Study.

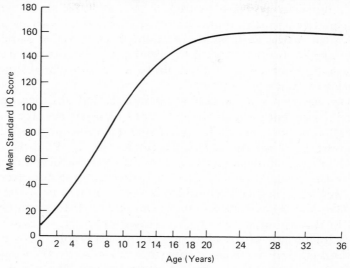

From "Development of Mental Abilities" by N. Bayley, 1970, in *Carmichael's Manual of Child Psychology* (3rd ed., Vol. 1, p. 1176), edited by P. Mussen, New York: Wiley. Copyright 1970 by John Wiley & Sons, Inc. Adapted by permission.

or less healthy ones dropped out. So longitudinal studies probably underestimate the amount of age-related decline in intelligence, whereas cross-sectional studies probably overestimate it (Horn & Donaldson, 1976).

In one of the most comprehensive and well-known studies of adult intelligence, K. Warner Schaie and associates used a combined cross-sectional and longitudinal approach (Schaie, 1979, 1983; Schaie & Labouvie-Vief, 1974). In 1956 Schaie administered the Primary Mental Abilities Test to a group of 500 subjects aged 20–70 years of age, all of whom were part of a group health plan in Seattle, Washington. These subjects were retested at seven-year intervals in 1963, 1970, and 1977. Thus, the study consisted of four cross-sectional comparisons and a longitudinal comparison covering 21 years.

The cross-sectional comparisons showed the usual pattern of age-related decline across all abilities. However, three variables—verbal meaning, space, and reasoning—showed an increment across successive cohorts (Schaie, 1979). This means that 60-year-olds of the 1910 cohort performed better on these variables than 60-year-olds of the 1903 or 1896 cohorts. The longitudinal findings do not support a conclusion of age-related decline in intelligence. The results for the five primary mental abilities—verbal meaning, reasoning, space, number, word fluency—at the 1970 testing showed little, if any, reliable age decrement until age 60 (see Figure 8.6). As Figure 8.6 shows, some abilities, especially verbal and number abilities, improved with age in adulthood. For most of the abilities represented, declines were rather small until after age 74. But we are talking about *average* performance curves here, which does not negate the possibility of an individual improving his or her IQ beyond age 74.

Despite the finding that most intellectual abilities do not decline until the seventh or eighth decade of life, some average decline occurs. What accounts for such decline? Several investigators (Kleemeier, 1962; Palmore & Cleveland, 1976; Riegel & Riegel, 1972) have argued that little or no decline occurs across the life span until the months or years preceding natural death, when terminal drop occurs (see Chapter 2). Because each successively older cohort contains proportionately more people who are within five years of death, greater numbers of subjects are in the terminal drop phase. However, those in this phase may be uncharacteristic of the older age group as a whole. They may represent individuals whose physical functioning is also declining at a rapid rate.

How do researchers study terminal drop? The usual way is to go backward in age starting at the time of death. For example, in a longitudinal study in north Germany during the 1950s and 1960s, Riegel and Riegel (1972) gave a variety of cognitive tests to men and women over age 55. They then compared the initial scores of the survivors with those who had died in the interim between times of testing and those who refused to be retested. Riegel and Riegel used the first testing as the point of comparison because data for all three groups were available then. Their retrospective analysis showed that nonsurvivors and retest refusers had significantly lower scores than survivors. Riegel and Riegel suggested that there may be small or no changes in performance and behavior among survivors. Among nonsurvivors, the causes of terminal drops remain unclear, but most investigators assume a connection between biological factors and behaviors predictive of survival. This does not rule out the influence of environmental determinants of survival on intelligence. In the next section we will take a closer look at biological and environmental variables affecting intellectual performance in adulthood.

Individual Differences in Intelligence in Adulthood

There are tremendous individual differences among adults, both within and across cohorts. And in regard to IQ test performance, these differences tend to become larger with increasing age (Matarazzo, 1972). The correlation between age and IQ rarely exceeds −.50, which means that

Figure 8.6 Comparison of cross-sectional with longitudinal findings (dotted lines) by age for subjects initially tested in 1963 and retested in 1970.

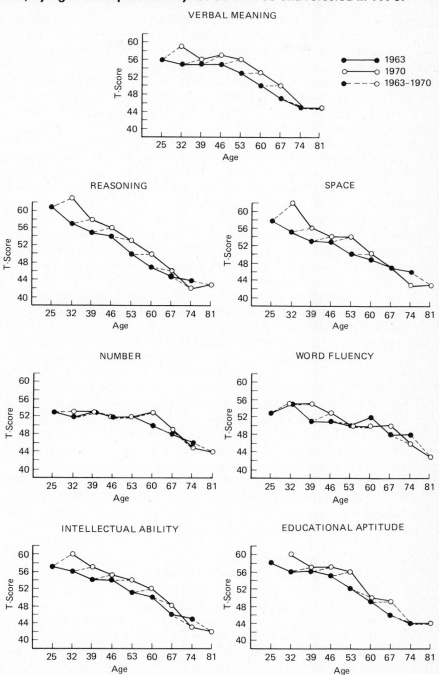

From "Generational versus Ontogenetic Components of Change in Adult Cognitive Behavior: A Fourteen-Year Cross-Sequential Study" by K. W. Schaie and G. Labouvie-Vief, 1974, *Developmental Psychology, 10*, pp. 309–312. Copyright 1974 by the American Psychological Association. Reprinted by permission.

age accounts at most for only about 25 percent of the variability in intelligence scores. The remaining variability (about 75 percent) must be explained by a broad range of biological and environmental variables that influence the age-intelligence relationship. These variables include health status, education, personality, social class, occupation, and the nature of the tests and testing conditions. These factors are not thought to affect intellectual competence or underlying capacity, but the level of intellectual performance.

This competence-performance distinction is critical for studying individual differences in intellectual development. Someone taking an IQ test may be fatigued, ill, unmotivated to perform well, or unfamiliar with the test. Therefore, one's observed performance may not accurately reflect what one is capable of doing in principle (i.e., true competence). However, there is little agreement among psychologists about how to best estimate actual competency level. Should it be estimated by an individual's single best performance in a given situation, by individuals' performance across comparable conditions among individuals, or by averaging performance across many situations (Scarr, 1983)?

Willis and Baltes (1980) have recommended "testing the limits" as a means of obtaining information on the range of intellectual performance. By examining variability in performance within an individual subjected to different testing conditions—which Willis and Baltes refer to as "intraindividual variability," or "plasticity"—one can gain a better picture of the person's capacity or competence. (The most direct way of doing this is to provide performance-enhancing treatments or interventions; see Chapter 10.) Traditional psychometric testing procedures, which yield an average score on a variety of tests at a single time of measurement, yield little information about the possible range or limits of intellectual performance. Thus, people's performance on an intelligence test does not reveal how they could potentially perform under different testing conditions. Studies examining intraindividual variability in performance can provide valuable additional data on the factors affecting intellectual development across the adult life span. Let us now examine some of these factors.

Health Status and Intelligence

The relationship of intellectual functioning to physical and mental health status is an important one in adult developmental studies. As Birren (1973) remarked, "It has become apparent that if one is to study seriously the nature of intellectual change in the adult years, he must consider health a dynamic factor of greater importance than it is in childhood" (p. 151). Too many developmental investigators fail to adequately describe the health status of their subject samples (W. Hoyer, Raskind, & Abrahams, 1984), thereby limiting our ability to draw inferences about the relationship of health and intelligence.

Several writers have suggested the potential importance of cardio-vascular diseases in intellectual impairment (see Thompson & Marsh, 1973). It is now well documented that cardiovascular problems such as coronary artery disease and hypertension may play significant roles in the development of intellectual deficits (Abrahams, 1976; Elias & Stree-ten, 1980). The usual explanation for such findings involves circulatory insufficiency as the most significant factor in age-related declines in cross-sectional studies. Failure of the brain cells to receive an adequate oxygen supply may result in oxygen starvation and tissue death. Lon-gitudinal studies of health disorders and intelligence confirm the cross-sectional findings.

One major longitudinal study (Wilkie & Eisdorfer, 1971) investi-gated the relationship between intellectual decline and elevated blood pressure. Two age groups (60–69 and 70–79 years at initial testing) were tested on the WAIS over a 10-year period. In the 60–69 age group, subjects' diastolic hypertension was related to significant intellectual loss over the 10-year period. (Diastolic pressure is the maximal pressure during the diastole, or dilation phase of the cardiac cycle.) Losses were not seen in the nonhypertensive or mildly elevated blood pressure sub-jects in the 60–69 age group. In the 70–79-year-old subjects at initial test, none with hypertension returned to be retested. Subjects with nor-mal and mildly elevated blood pressure showed some intellectual de-cline over the 10-year period. These results indicate that only beyond some critical level are there consistent intelligence–blood pressure rela-tionships among older adults.

In a more recent longitudinal study, Schultz, Elias, Robbins, Streeten, and Blakeman (1986) tested nonhypertensives (mean age 42 at first test-ing) and medically treated hypertensives (mean age 46 at first testing) on the WAIS over a 5–6 year test interval. Nonhypertensive subjects improved significantly over time on the verbal tests but not on the per-formance tests, while hypertensive subjects showed no significant improvement or decline. The latter result contrasts with the findings reported by Wilkie and Eisdorfer (1971) and may be due to the younger sample employed and the shorter test-retest interval.

There is more to age-related disease processes than cardiovascular pathology. Brain disorders such as Alzheimer's disease have an enor-mously negative impact on intellectual functioning in later life. The effects of Alzheimer's disease on intellectual changes are detailed in Box 8.3. Whether these changes are simply the extreme of normal aging pro-cesses or represent a qualitatively different disease state is a matter of controversy (Labouvie-Vief, 1985). One thing is certain: senile pro-cesses contribute to a breakdown of normal intellectual functioning by producing massive and diffuse brain cell loss. Today, a great deal of research is being done to identify the cause of dementia and possible cures.

Box 8.3 Intellectual Changes in Alzheimer's Disease

Over the past decade a senile brain disorder known as Alzheimer's disease has emerged as one of the leading mental health concerns in the United States. Alzheimer's disease is a chronic, relentlessly progressive, degenerative brain disease characterized by profound changes in cognition, memory, perception, personality, and ability for self-care (Hughes, 1978). Traditionally, dementias of the Alzheimer's type were seen as a normal part of growing older, but recent research suggests that this untreatable and invariably fatal condition is not part of the normal aging process. In fact, the vast majority of older people do not develop any type of senile dementia, and only an estimated 5–7 percent of the population at age 65 show any signs of Alzheimer's disease. However, Alzheimer's disease is strongly age correlated, and the risk of developing the disease increases markedly as one becomes older. Because the elderly are the fastest growing segment of the population, Alzheimer's disease is attracting considerable attention from mental health professionals.

The term *dementia* implies a disturbance of intellectual functioning (E. Miller, 1981). Demented individuals perform lower on all types of cognitive tasks, including standardized tests of intelligence, with average IQs falling below the statistical mean for the population of 100. But the nature of these changes is far from simple. Among studies employing the Wechsler scales (the W-B and the WAIS), the typical finding is that verbal IQ is decreased, and performance IQ is even lower. Tests that require new mental habits and unfamiliar ways of thinking show the greatest decline. Thus, individuals with dementia appear to have lost much of their verbal, crystallized intelligence as well as their nonverbal, fluid intelligence. Whether these declines are the same as those observed at a slower rate in normal individuals is an open question. Many writers have pointed out the similarities between this pattern of differential decline and that found among normal old people, but the patterns of change on individual subtests of intelligence may not be identical (E. Miller, 1981).

Although declines in the intellectual abilities are central to the concept of dementia, they have rarely been examined. One of the main reasons for this inattention involves the practical difficulties in measuring the amount of intellectual decline in a person with a progressive disorder such as Alzheimer's disease. The ideal would be to compare predisease levels of intellectual functioning with current levels, but this is only occasionally possible because most people have not had previous psychometric assessments. In addition, psychometric measurement is restricted by the limited availability of valid tests that yield information on specific intellectual skills. Alternative approaches such as studying thought processes of demented persons by information-processing analyses have not yet been widely applied. The information-processing approach appears to offer an excellent means of isolating specific intellectual, linguistic, spatial, and memory difficulties in cases of Alzheimer's disease.

Education and Intelligence

It is not surprising that the more education one has, the more likely one is to do well on standardized tests of intelligence. What is surprising is that education may be more significant than age in determining test performance. Birren and Morrison (1961) found a higher correlation between intelligence test scores and educational level than between these scores and age. Similarly, Granick and Friedman (1967) administered a battery of more than 60 cognitive, perceptual, and psychomotor tests to a group of noninstitutionalized older adults. When the educational differences were statistically controlled for, the number of tests showing significant age decline fell from 27 to 19 (a 30-percent decrease). Results such as these converge with results from longitudinal studies of intelligence in showing little or no decline among well-educated adults.

Education may function in various ways to improve performance and to reduce age-related declines in intelligence. For instance, those with more education are more likely to develop scholastic abilities related to vocabulary, mathematical reasoning, and memory, which are assessed by IQ tests. In addition, these people are more likely to have been exposed to intelligence tests during their school years. Finally, those with more education probably perceive the benefits of scholastic achievement and remain involved in activities that maintain intellectual effectiveness.

Involvement in higher education activities among adults of all ages has been increasing. It is estimated that by the late 1980s 40 percent of all collegians will be above the age of 25. In addition, many colleges and universities now offer special programs for older adults that make courses available on a low-cost space-available basis (Birren & Woodruff, 1973; Schaie & Willis, 1978). As the number of older adults with previous higher education experience increases, more of them will return to college to renew their education.

Personality and Intelligence

It is commonly believed that highly intelligent individuals differ in their personality from less intelligent people. Research on this issue suggests that a link may indeed exist between personality and intelligence. Schaie (1958) showed that one dimension of personality, rigidity, correlated with scores on the PMA test at every adult age level tested; the higher the rigidity scores, the lower the PMA performance. Whether rigidity caused poor performance or vice versa was unclear because this was a correlational study.

In a longitudinal study of personality development and intellectual functioning from childhood to 40 years of age, Honzik and Macfarlane (1973) reported several interesting relationships. Ten different personality characteristics measured during the subjects' first 18 years and at age 30 years were correlated significantly with the 40-year-old IQs of both males and females on the WAIS. These characteristics included such aspects of intellectual functioning as (1) a high degree of intellectual capacity, (2) verbal fluency, (3) concern with philosophical problems, (4) ability to see to the heart of important problems, and (5) high aspiration level for oneself. Some highly significant sex differences in personality characteristics also were related to IQ. High-IQ females at age 40 had the following personality characteristics at age 30: "has a wide range of interests" and "does not create or exploit dependency in people." For high-IQ males at age 40, the most salient personality characteristics were "is introspective," "is not satisfied with physical appearance," and "not responsive to humor." Thus, the links between personality and intelligence appear to be moderated by sex.

Other Factors

A host of other factors can affect age-intelligence relationships, and only a few can be mentioned here. Individual differences in socioeconomic status and occupational background are known to be linked to intellectual ability (Fozard & Nuttall, 1971; Pressey & Kuhlen, 1957). During both world wars, tests of general ability given to individuals of different occupational backgrounds revealed marked differences in intelligence (Stewart, 1947). In general, professionals tended to score highest on these tests and unskilled workers the lowest, as Figure 8.7 shows. But notice the overlap in general ability scores between the different occupations in Figure 8.7. The upper 10 percent of machine operators scored above the median for lawyers. Thus, IQ alone cannot be used to predict the occupational level of which an individual is capable (Pressey & Kuhlen, 1957).

Fozard and Nuttall (1971) examined the significance of age-related changes in intelligence by administering the General Aptitude Test Battery (GATB) to a group of more than 1000 employed and retired men (age range 28–83 years). The GATB consists of 12 manual, perceptual, and verbal tests used to match aptitude to jobs. Fozard and Nuttall (1971) found significant declines among the oldest age groups and those from the lowest social class, but no significant interactions occurred

Figure 8.7   General ability in relation to occupation during World War II. Data are from Stewart (1947). The bars show the 10th, 25th, 50th, 75th, and 90th percentiles.

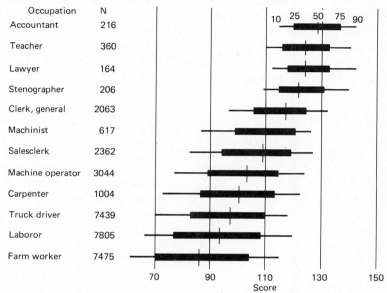

From *Psychological Development through the Life-Span* (p. 97) by S. L. Pressey and R. G. Kuhlen, 1957, New York: Harper & Row. Copyright 1957 by Harper & Row Publishers, Inc. Reprinted by permission.

between age and social class. Interestingly, the abilities most affected by age were least affected by socioeconomic status, and vice versa.

Another set of factors influencing the age-intelligence function includes the test content and procedures used to measure intelligence. As noted, intelligence tests for children and adolescents predict scholastic performance accurately because they mirror the content taught in schools. Such predictive accuracy was not found for adult intelligence tests when they were used to forecast success in adult occupations. This result is not surprising because the abilities required for job success (persistence, interpersonal skill, creativity, inventiveness) vary tremendously and are not typically measured by standardized intelligence tests. We may say that most intelligence tests lack contextual validity for assessing the abilities of adults.

Some investigators have attempted to deal with the validity problem by constructing intelligence measures applicable to the problems of everyday life. For example, Schaie (1978) argued that fresh approaches are needed to assess intellectual competencies at various stages in the adult life span. In one study, Scheidt and Schaie (1978) identified several real-life situations that require intellectual competence. They then asked more than 300 older adults to classify these situations in terms of four molar dimensions—whether the situations involve (1) high or low activity, (2) social or nonsocial activity, and whether they are (3) common or uncommon and (4) supportive or depriving. These four dimensions and examples of their manifestations in specific situations are shown in Table 8.4. Scheidt and Schaie (1978) recommended that the next step in this type of research should determine the intellectual abilities needed for each category.

Table 8.4
Four Dimensions of Intellectual Competence and Examples of Their Manifestation in Real-Life Situations

Situational Attributes	Social	Nonsocial
High Activity		
Common-Supportive	Being visited by son or daughter and their children.	Gardening in yard, planting seeds, and weeding.
Common-Depriving	Pressured by salesperson to buy merchandise.	Cleaning apartment or household.
Uncommon-Supportive	Traveling around city looking for a new residence.	Exercising for a few moments each day.
Uncommon-Depriving	Waiting at the end of a long line for tickets to entertainment.	Driving auto during rush-hour traffic.
Low Activity		
Common-Supportive	Offering money to son or daughter who needs it.	Making plans for future.
Common-Depriving	Hearing that close friend has recently died.	Worrying about ability to pay a debt.
Uncommon-Supportive	Attending art exhibit.	Recording day's events in diary.
Uncommon-Depriving	While talking with someone, you feel you have unintentionally hurt their feelings.	Discovering you locked keys in car while shopping.

Note: From "A Taxonomy of Situations for an Elderly Population: Generating Situational Criteria" by R. J. Scheidt and K. W. Schaie, 1978, *Journal of Gerontology, 33*, p. 851. Copyright 1978 by the Gerontological Society of America. Reprinted by permission.

It is generally acknowledged that tests such as the WAIS and PMA provide only limited information about behavior in real-life situations. Several investigators have tried to construct more contextually valid versions of IQ tests for adults (Demming & Pressey, 1957; Monge & Gardner, 1976). These attempts to develop "age-fair" tests parallel the numerous attempts to devise culture-fair intelligence tests for children. Demming and Pressey (1957) developed an intelligence test with items that they felt would be more meaningful and less threatening to older adults. A sample item on their test deals with the use of the yellow pages of a telephone directory.

> Where in the yellow pages of the telephone directory would you look if you wanted to buy an Airedale? Under heating equipment, kennels, shoe stores, real estate, dairy equipment?

On items like this one, adults in their 40s and 50s scored higher than did younger adults. In an extensive study, Monge and Gardner (1976) developed a battery of tests to measure knowledge of real-life domains such as disease and death, finances, sports, art, transportation, and religion as well as items employed in more traditional IQ measures. They administered these tests to a large sample of men and women aged 20–79. In general, the results showed that performance increased with age through the 40s and 50s and then declined to a level similar to that of the 20s and 30s. Thus, adults in their middle years exhibited greater everyday knowledge than younger adults, even in cases where the former showed declines on the more traditional IQ items.

Many psychologists would not agree that the tests described above are true measures of intellectual ability. One reason is that the tests assess informational and comprehension items, which normally show little decline on standardized intelligence measures for healthy persons. Moreover, the questions included in the tests have been deliberately chosen for older adult samples, so it is not surprising that older adults do well on such questions compared to younger adults. Finally, psychologists still do not know how well knowledge of this crystallized information relates to everyday behaviors. Despite these problems, efforts to develop age-fair tests are likely to continue, and such tests may prove useful for predicting performance in real-life situations and settings.

One other major problem with intelligence tests for older adults is that many of the items are timed. For example, on the WAIS, performance tests such as the block design and digit symbol are timed, and bonuses are given for rapid solutions. Another scoring procedure only credits performance within some allotted time limit. What would happen if the time restrictions were removed? Klodin (1976) compared young men (mean age 22 years) and old men (mean age 73 years) on the object assembly subtest of the WAIS under timed and untimed conditions. The object assembly task requires that subjects assemble an object such as a person's head into a familiar configuration. Klodin (1976) reported that the scores of the young adults were not affected by the untimed conditions, and the old adults' scores improved only slightly. This result was probably due to the fact that the young adults' scores were near ceiling levels without the treatment, whereas the older adults had more room for improvement. Elimination of timed testing conditions thus reduces but does not totally erase age differences in intelligence.

In summary, intelligence can be influenced by a variety of factors not related to intellectual competence, such as health status, education, personality, occupation, socioeconomic status, and testing procedures. Thus, conclusions about whether intelligence does (or does not) decline with age in adulthood must be qualified in several ways. Perhaps the best we can do at present is to state which specific abilities and skills change most rapidly and under what circumstances. This task will require a complex multicausal multidirectional conception of adult intellectual development.

COMPLEX THINKING PROCESSES

In contrast to approaches that emphasize the number of test items an individual can answer correctly at a given age, some psychologists have been interested in the individual's underlying thought processes. Psychologists such as Piaget have focused on thought processes in childhood and adolescence and how these processes differ qualitatively at different times in development. Other psychologists such as Klaus Riegel and Gisela Labouvie-Vief have focused their attention on adult thinking processes as qualitatively different from those of preadulthood. Few theorists have dealt with developmental changes in cognition for the entire life span. In this section we will concentrate on cognitive processes in adolescence and adulthood.

Formal Operations

Chapter 2 introduced the major tenets of Piagetian theory. From his work on the sensorimotor period, you learned that children gain knowledge about their world by their immediate actions on the world. In the preoperational and concrete operational stages, children use symbols to represent the world. By age 10 or 11, the transition to formal operational thinking occurs; but research suggests that formal operations may occur much later in adolescence than originally believed (Ashton, 1975; Dulit, 1972).

Piaget characterized the qualitative shift in thinking from concrete to formal operations as a shift in reasoning from the actual to the possible (Flavell, 1963; Neimark, 1975a, 1975b, 1982). In this stage of thinking, the individual is able to reason with logical propositions as well as with concrete physical objects. "Possibility no longer appears merely as an extension of an empirical situation or of actions actually performed. Instead it is *reality* that is now secondary to possibility" (Inhelder & Piaget, 1958, p. 251). In other words, instead of focusing on tangible objects and events, children must begin to consider a whole set of hypothetical possibilities. This ability enables adolescents to differentiate the form of an argument from the content and to evaluate the logical validity of any proposition from a purely hypothetical standpoint. In contrast, concrete operational children are incapable of disregarding the content of an argument and are limited to the empirically knowable world.

To illustrate the difference between concrete and formal reasoning, consider the following situation in which a concrete operational thinker is asked to reason in a manner contrary to empirical fact. Given the propositions "all mice are bigger than dogs" and "all dogs are bigger than elephants," the subject would have difficulty reaching the logically correct conclusion that "all mice are bigger than elephants" because both propositions violate empirical fact (Neimark, 1982). Concrete thinkers are unable to focus on the form of the argument regardless of content. In contrast, formal thinkers can manipulate the logic of the propositions without regard to their content. They are much more likely than concrete thinkers to approach a problem from the standpoint of all possible solutions and then to narrow the problem to the solution that exists in reality. Concrete operational children, on the other hand, begin with tangible reality and reluctantly, if at all, venture into the realm of possibility (Flavell, 1985).

Combinatorial Reasoning

One of the hallmarks of formal operational thinking is the ability to operate on symbolic propositions or variables through a higher-order combinatorial scheme. A formal thinker can use an efficient method to generate and test all possible combinations and permutations of a set of elements. This aspect of formal thinking has been extensively investigated by Piaget and can be illustrated by one of his most famous problems, the "colorless-liquids" task.

In this problem Inhelder and Piaget (1958) presented children of varying ages with four similar beakers of colorless, odorless liquids numbered 1, 2, 3, 4, and a fifth bottle labeled g. Each child was asked to produce a yellow color by dropping g into any one of the combinations of beakers (the correct answer was 1, 3, and g). Inhelder and Piaget (1958) identified three different performance strategies for solving the task corresponding to the preoperational, concrete operational, and formal operational stages, respectively. The youngest children approached the task in a haphazard, unplanned manner. At the preoperational stage their attention was attracted by figurative aspects of the task (e.g., the color of the liquid in the beakers), and they rarely solved the problem. At the concrete operational stage, the beginning of a systematic strategy was discernible. Children began by combining the liquids two at a time, but when that failed they were lost. Only when prompted did concrete operators combine more than two liquids, and, even then, they could not envision all possible combinations. Finally, formal operations children could systematically test all possible combinations involving two, three, and four beakers according to a rational plan. Not only did they reach the correct solution, but having done so, they continued to carry out tests to see if there were any other possible solutions.

By calling these mental operations *formal* operations, Piaget tried to emphasize the adolescent's concern with the formal or logical aspects of the problem (H. Gardner, 1982). No longer do children attend to the perceptible, figurative properties of the problem. Instead, they try to envision all the possible combinations of a given problem, hypothesize about which possibility may be correct, deduce the consequences of each hypothesis, and carry out tests to determine which one is correct. We term this characteristic approach to problem solving *hypothetico-deductive*, in contract to the reality-based and nontheoretical *empirico-inductive* reasoning of concrete operational children. This is not to say that adolescent and adult approaches to a problem are always as systematic and efficient as described. Rather, a good deal of trial and error may occur before a systematic hypothetico-deductive approach to the problem develops. The major difference between the haphazard solution attempts by children and those of adolescents and adults lies in the two latter groups' ability to reflect on their own mental processes—an ability called *reflective*, or *recursive*, thinking. They can think about their own thinking and operate on ideas as well as concrete objects and events to solve a problem. The formal operational thinker is not necessarily consciously aware of all the possible combinations to a problem, but engages in various forms of thought which would be impossible without some sort of combinatorial thinking (Neimark, 1975a, 1975b, 1982).

Isolation of Variables

One more example should help to clarify the concept of formal operations. The ability to isolate and manipulate a single variable in an experiment while holding all the others constant is presented as an indication of formal operations by Inhelder and Piaget (1958). D. Kuhn and Brannock (1977) assessed this ability among 80 fourth, fifth, and sixth graders and college students using a "natural experiment" situation as well as three traditional Piagetian problems. The naturalistic task was the "plant problem" shown in Figure 8.8. Two of the plants appeared quite healthy and two were in poor condition. The subjects' task was to figure out which of the variables presented (large or small glass of water, dark- or light-colored plant food, and leaf lotion) was responsible for each plant's health. As Figure 8.8 shows, the problem was constructed so that the plant food was effective in influencing a plant's health and the other two variables were ineffective. The subjects' performance on the plant problem is presented in Table 8.5. Notice that the ability to isolate the effective variable develops only gradually. Level 0 subjects have no concept of variable isolation. For example, many subjects incorrectly

Figure 8.8 The plant problem.

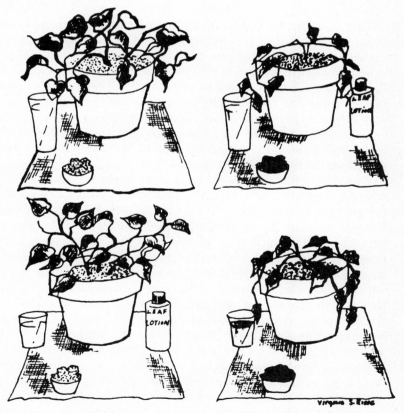

From "Development of the Isolation of Variables Scheme in Experimental and 'Natural Experimental' Contexts" by D. Kuhn and J. Brannock, 1977, *Developmental Psychology, 13,* p. 10. Copyright 1977 by the American Psychological Association. Reprinted by permission.

Table 8.5
Subjects' Performance on the Plant Problem

	Grade 4	Grade 5	Grade 6	College
Level 0 (concrete)	7	8	3	1
Level 1 (emergent formal)	3	2	2	1
Levels 2 and 3 (transitional)	7	6	7	5
Level 4 (formal)	3	4	8	13

Note: From "Development of the Isolation of Variables Scheme in Experimental and 'Natural Experiment' Contexts" by D. Kuhn and J. Brannock, 1977, *Developmental Psychology, 13,* p. 13. Copyright 1977 by the American Psychological Association. Reprinted by permission.

assumed that because the leaf lotion was next to one healthy plant, the lotion must have played a key role in the experimental outcome. At level 1 some concept of variable isolation exists, but the correct variable is not isolated. Levels 2 and 3 represent a transitional phase in which subjects isolate variables and perform valid experiments part of the time, but at other times perform invalid, confounded experiments and draw erroneous conclusions. Only at level 4, in formal operations, can subjects isolate the effective variable and logically exclude all of the ineffective variables. Competence on the plant problem was not closely related to ability to solve the Piagetian-type problems, which suggests that different formal abilities may be involved in the different tasks.

Inhelder and Piaget (1958) emphasized the interdependence of the isolation-of-variables scheme and combinatorial thinking. Both forms of thought reflect the existence of what they called *structured wholes* having properties similar to a coherent logical system. These structured wholes integrate a group of transformational rules into a single higher-order system that can be used to manipulate operations. This system of rules is referred to as the **INRC group** (for "identity, negation, reciprocity, and correlation"). Consider the balance-scale problem discussed in Chapter 2, in which subjects must alter the balance by moving unequal quantities of weights at specific distances along the arms of the balance. An identity rule would simply indicate to the subject that the transformation had no effect, as when more weight was added to the side of the scale that was already tipped down. The operation could be negated by simply subtracting the additional weight. If the subject moved the weight a certain distance from the fulcrum of the balance scale, a reciprocal transformation would be effected by moving an equal weight an equivalent distance on the opposite side of the scale. A correlational transformation would involve learning a mathematical rule for computing the relation between the weight (W) and distance (D): $W_1/W_2 = D_2/D_1$. By using the concept of proportionality, the formal operational thinker can accurately predict which side of the scale will lower. In addition to the INRC group, the hypothetical structured wholes include other operational schemes, such as the concept of probability and some advanced forms of conservation (Neimark, 1975a).

Age and Formal Operations

Nearly every study using Piagetian tasks such as the colorless-liquids task or the balance-scale problem has found a significant age effect (D. Kuhn & Angelev, 1976; Neimark, 1975a, 1975b). Piaget (1972) assumed that formal thinking begins around age 11 and is completed no later than ages 15–20 in normal subjects. However, research has shown that the proportion of adolescents who function at the formal operational stage may only be found predictably among 30–40 percent (Arlin, 1975; Neimark, 1975a; Tomlinson-Keasey, 1972). The reasons for such low percentages are the subject of intense debate. Furthermore, in some cultures, formal thinking skills altogether seem to be absent (Berry & Dasen, 1974; Neimark, 1975a).

Two explanations have been offered for the nonuniversality of formal operations across age and culture. One explanation concerns the nature of the tasks. Inhelder and Piaget (1958) used 15 different tasks, most involving problems in physics, chemistry, and mathematics. On several of these tasks, children have more difficulty than on others (Keating, 1978; Neimark, 1975a). Piaget (1972) conceded that some formal problems are more difficult than others, and he used the concept of horizontal décalage to account for this (see Chapter 7). Piaget (1972) also acknowledged that experience with a task has an effect on the tendency to engage in formal thinking. Individuals may use formal thinking according to their aptitude, cultural membership, and professional specialization. For example, a carpenter may employ formal thought to solve a problem in building a house, but use concrete operations in solving a physics problem. Similarly, a theoretical physicist may be formal operational in thinking about a physics problem, but use concrete operational thought to build a tool shed.

A second explanation for why everyone does not engage in formal thinking at the same time in development has to do with neurological maturity. Epstein (1974) has shown that the brain undergoes different "spurts" in development at approximately ages 2–4, 6–8, 10–12, and 14–16. During the intervening periods, growth is more gradual. Epstein (1974) argued that the age period between the last two spurts does not include the new neurological development that may be necessary for the more advanced stages of formal thinking to develop. Thus, adolescents of this age (e.g., 13) may be neurologically unprepared to handle the more advanced material they are given (see Kohen-Raz, 1974; Petersen, 1976). The search for the neurological concomitants of formal thought is difficult but exciting.

Despite the problems associated with the concepts of formal operations, almost everyone agrees that adolescents think about or "cognize" the world differently than their younger counterparts. Although adolescents may engage in considerable trial-and-error learning, they also approach problems systematically, keep a record of all the possibilities, and modify hypotheses in light of new evidence. Furthermore, formal operational reasoning brings other changes into adolescents' lives. Adolescents begin to be interested in political, religious, and moral systems, and a code of values to live by. They are able to consider the forms different arguments may take and imagine the way things "ought to be" rather than the way they "are." Their view of themselves also becomes more highly differentiated and abstract and less tied to immediately perceptible characteristics. Adolescents strike most of us as a group highly dissimilar in thought and behavior from younger children.

Beyond Formal Operations

Piaget considered formal operations to be essentially complete by late adolescence, with no further qualitatively distinct levels of development emerging in adulthood. Though quantitative change within the stage of formal operations is possible—for example, an individual may acquire more vocabulary knowledge—formal operations represent the final and most mature stage of cognitive development in Piaget's theory. This assumption has been questioned recently by adult developmental psychologists who argue for the possibility of progressive developmental changes in thought structures beyond the formal operational stage (Dittmann-Kohli & Baltes, in press; D. Kramer, 1983; Labouvie-Vief, 1985; Riegel, 1973a).

Another assumption made by Piaget is that once formal operations are achieved, there can be no "sliding back" to an earlier period. Although one may occasionally use earlier forms of thinking, one never loses the ability to think formally. In Piaget's view, cognitive development is always progressive and cumulative. This assumption has been challenged by studies showing age-related declines on formal operational tasks (Botwinick, 1977; N. Denney & Wright, 1976).

The formal operational tasks described earlier all involve finding the correct solution to an abstract problem. Though different strategies, which vary in their effectiveness, may be used, only one solution is possible. Thus, formal operational problems qualify as convergent thinking tasks (see Chapter 7). However, many situations call for a range of possible solutions and divergent thinking.

Arlin (1975) has suggested a fifth stage of cognitive development, a **problem-finding stage,** which may reflect an ability to think divergently. The characteristics of this hypothetical stage include an ability to think creatively, to "discover" new problems, to raise general questions about ill-defined problems, and to demonstrate cognitive abilities like those represented in the most significant scientific thought (Arlin, 1975). Arlin tested her hypothesis by giving 60 female college seniors a set of formal operations tasks used by Inhelder and Piaget (1958) as well as a problem-finding task consisting of a problematic situation. This problematic situation involved examining an array of 12 common objects (e.g., a wooden cube, a scissors, a quarter, a piece of red cardboard) and raising questions about them. Arlin reported that formal operations are a necessary but not sufficient condition for high problem finding. Arlin's results imply a two-stage sequence: a formal problem-solving stage (traditional Piagetian formal operations stage) followed by a separate problem-finding stage (possible postformal stage). However, other investigators (e.g., Fakouri, 1976) have pointed out that elements of Arlin's problem-finding stage are likely to be found in the Piagetian stages of concrete and formal operations. Thus, one cannot regard formal operations as a necessary but insufficient condition for the problem-finding stage.

Riegel (1973a) proposed a position similar to Arlin's. He suggested that adult thinking can be characterized by dialectic maturity, not formal thought. According to Riegel, dialectical maturity involves the ability to live with and accept contradictory evidence. For example, a general principle in physics is that light can be both a wave and a particle. A psychological example might involve the observation that two objects can be very different (a small light object and a large heavy one), but they both can act in the same way (i.e., they can float). Or think of answering an ambiguous multiple choice item where two answers appear to be correct.

Unlike Riegel, Piaget argued that organisms tend toward equilibrated states. They try to overcome contradictions and conflict through their actions and cognitions. Before an organism progresses to a new stage of cognitive development, a marked disequilibrium occurs and is eventually resolved. In contrast, Riegel's theory sees contradiction and conflict as a fundamental property of thought and creativity. Though Riegel's ideas are provocative, the dialectical stage cannot be taken as evidence for a fifth cognitive stage because dialectical operations are potentially found in some form at every Piagetian stage (Commons, Richards, & Kuhn, 1982; Riegel, 1973a).

Some theorists postulate only a single postformal stage, whereas others propose multiple stage models (Labouvie-Vief, 1982; Schaie, 1977–1978). Schaie has offered the five-stage model depicted in Figure 8.9. Of the five stages proposed, four (*achieving, responsible, executive,* and *reintegrative*) apply to adulthood. Schaie (1977–1978) contends that much of the traditional work on intellectual development, whether in the psychometric or Piagetian tradition, focuses on intellectual skills

Figure 8.9   A five-stage model of adult cognitive development.

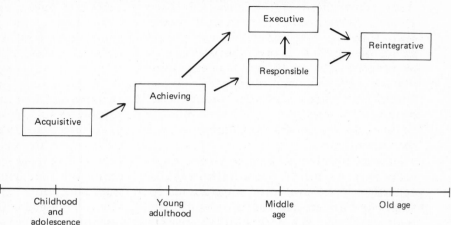

From "Toward a Stage Theory of Adult Cognitive Development" by K. W. Schaie, 1977–1978, *International Journal of Aging and Human Development, 8,* p. 133. Copyright 1977 by Baywood Publishing Company, Inc. Reprinted by permission.

acquisition. In adulthood, however, the individual must learn to creatively apply these skills. Young adults' major concern is achieving. Formal operations thinking acquired in adolescence is used in the service of personal and career goals. The next stage, responsibility, occurs when the middle-aged individual has achieved role independence and cognitive competence and must take responsibility for other people such as a spouse or children. This stage requires that the person integrate long-term goals and consequences within the context of real-life problems. The executive stage is parallel to the responsibility stage, except that responsibility for others now extends beyond one's immediate social system to encompass wider systems such as work groups, communities, and even nations. In the final stage of reintegration, cognitive development is influenced to a greater degree by motivational and attitudinal variables. When faced with role constrictions such as retirement or the relinquishment of family responsibilities, older individuals must attend to the problems that have the most meaning for them. This last stage comes close to what is meant by the "wisdom of old age."

The notion of embedding intelligence within the practical and social responsibilities of the adult thinker can be seen in Labouvie-Vief's (1982) theory, which discusses a broad restructuring of adult thought in terms of self-regulated social and personal goals. Three adult stages of logic are proposed: (1) *intrasystemic,* or formal, realism; (2) *intersystemic,* or contextual, realism; and (3) *autonomy.* In the intrasystemic stage, reality is ordered according to logical and universal truths. At the intersystemic level, the basic duality of logical truth and logical relativism is acknowledged. For example, a college student comes to accept the inherent relativity of multiple intellectual perspectives (Perry, 1970). But the search for logical certainty eventually must end, and the student must make a responsible commitment to a course of action. Thus, to paraphrase Piaget, possibility once again is subjected to reality. During the autonomous stage, truth acquires meaning by reference to a matrix of social and personal goals (Labouvie-Vief, 1982). The logic of truth is widened to encompass the self and the other and their interactivity.

The theoretical proposals of Schaie and Labouvie-Vief raise crucial questions about complex thinking processes in adulthood. We are faced with the possibility that adult thought, perhaps more than children's thought, can assume multiple forms, depending upon an individual's personal and social context. Within this multiplicity of developmental forms lies a broad-stage framework that captures the intellectual changes in adulthood.

Wisdom and Development

Traditional psychometric models and Piagetian models of adult intellectual development emphasize the decline or regressive features of cognition later in life. But the aged years have been valued for centuries as a time of wisdom and superior knowledge. In their thoughtful review of the wisdom literature, Clayton and Birren (1980) state that "Wisdom has always had an association of a positive nature with the later years of life. Those older individuals who possessed wisdom often held positions of social consequence and were given respect in their communities" (p. 104). Today, greater numbers of researchers are analyzing the psychological nature of wisdom (Clayton, 1975, 1982; Dittmann-Kohli & Baltes, in press.

The term *wisdom* has been used for centuries in philosophical and religious literature to describe a person with special insight and understanding. Trying to define *wisdom*, however, is no easier than trying to define *intelligence*. Recently, Dittmann-Kohli and Baltes (in press) characterized wisdom as "an individual's ability to exercise superior judgment about *important* but *uncertain* matters of life". In addition, Dittmann-Kohli and Baltes (in press) differentiated between **practical wisdom,** which relates to one's personal life and life span, and **philosophical wisdom,** which involves the relationship of the self to human life and the world at large. Practical wisdom can be seen in the older person who accepts the losses of later life and mortality within the context of generational transmission. Philosophical wisdom might be manifested in a recognition of the limits of political systems for effecting societal change.

These theoretical formulations should help lay the foundation for the development of measurement instruments to assess the content domain of wisdom-related knowledge (Clayton, 1982). Once satisfactory measures of wisdom have been developed, empirical research on the construct can proceed. Questions for future research include: How are wisdom and crystallized intelligence related? What is the connection between wisdom and creativity? Another aspect of wisdom is social intelligence, which is an important but much neglected dimension of intelligence in need of further study.

In concluding this chapter, we encourage cognitive developmental researchers to avoid narrowly limiting their study of intellectual development to IQ or logical operational ability. Rather, studies should be geared to the whole person functioning within a complexly changing ecology over long time spans (Bronfenbrenner, 1977). Cognitive development is best understood not in isolation from, but in relation to, the total psychological and social functioning of the person. In Chapter 9, we continue this theme by examining the relationship of cognitive development to social development.

SUMMARY

1. Psychologists have defined the concept of intelligence in a wide variety of ways. Recently, Neisser proposed that intelligence should be viewed in terms of prototypical characteristics that describe an ideally intelligent person.

2. Psychometric models of intelligence deal in a practical way with the construction of intelligence tests and the prediction of performance. Alfred Binet, a French psychologist, is credited with developing the first successful IQ test; psychometricians continue to follow many procedures initially proposed by Binet.

3. English psychologist Charles Spearman theorized that intelligence consists of a single, universal ability, called G, as well as several separate abilities. Spearman used a method called factor analysis to test his theory.

4. Factor analysts such as Thurstone and Guilford focused their attention on the identification of group factors of intelligence. Thurstone identified several primary mental abilities; Guilford

proposed a structure-of-intellect model consisting of 120 different factors of intelligence.

5. The fluid-crystallized model of intelligence is one of the most important developmental theories of intelligence based on a factor analytic approach. Fluid abilities reflect the incidental learning of the organism and are thought to increase through young adulthood and then decline. Crystallized abilities reflect schooling and acculturation influences and hold up well with age.

6. The age differentiation–dedifferentiation hypothesis states that intelligence begins as a general ability, proceeds to a loosely organized set of specific abilities, and then returns to the general ability structure characteristic of its beginning. Empirical support for this hypothesis has been mixed.

7. Several major intellectual changes occur across the life span. These changes are not limited to one age group or type of intelligence.

8. Measures of infant intelligence rely heavily on sensorimotor content, and therefore are poor predictors of school performance. However, infant intelligence tests are useful for identifying early developmental problems in infants.

9. Intelligence undergoes several spurts during childhood, but begins to stabilize around age 8 or 9. Wide individual differences in intelligence exist as a result of variations in testing procedures, social class background, and ethnicity. Several attempts have been made to develop culturally unbiased tests of intelligence.

10. Cross-sectional studies of adult intelligence tend to overestimate the amount of age decline, whereas longitudinal studies underestimate it. The concept of terminal drop is used to explain intellectual decline in late life. Other key factors influencing the age-intelligence relationship are health status, education, and personality.

11. In contrast to quantitative, measurement-based approaches to intelligence, psychological models such as Piaget's focus on qualitative differences in thinking between children and adults. The qualitative shift from concrete to formal operational thinking involves a shift in reasoning from the actual to the possible. Combinatorial reasoning and the isolation of variables are two examples of formal thought.

12. Several psychologists argue the possibility of one or more cognitive stages beyond formal operations. Perhaps more than children's thought, adult thinking can take many different forms depending on a variety of personal and social variables.

13. "Wisdom" refers to an individual's ability to exercise superior judgment in the most important but uncertain matters of living. Wisdom has always had a positive association with the later years of life.

Key Terms

psychometric models	age differentiation hypothesis
mental age	dedifferentiation
intelligence quotient	associative learning
deviation IQs	cognitive learning
factor analysis	INRC group
structure-of-intellect model	problem-finding stage
crystallized intelligence	practical wisdom
fluid intelligence	philosophical wisdom

Suggested Readings

Brody, E. B., & Brody, N. (1976). *Intelligence: Nature, determinants, and consequences.* New York: Academic Press. This good source of background information on the major issues in the field of intelligence includes discussions on the history of intelligence testing, age changes in intelligence, intelligence and achievement, biological and social determinants of intelligence, and the uses of IQ tests.

Case, R. (1985). *Intellectual development: Birth to adulthood.* New York: Academic Press. This book proposes a provocative new theory of intellectual development. It focuses on how children's minds function at different stages of development, the mechanisms governing transition from one stage to the next, and the steps parents and educators can take to optimize intellectual development in children.

Gardner, H. (1983). *Frames of mind: The theory of multiple intelligences.* New York: Basic Books. This provocative book outlines a bold new theory of human intellectual competencies that goes well beyond the narrow confines of a single IQ score derived from an "intelligence" test. Research from many diverse and previously unrelated sources is integrated. Fascinating reading.

Kail, R., & Pellegrino, J. W. (1985). *Human intelligence: Perspectives and prospects.* San Francisco: Freeman. The purpose of this book is to bring together and evaluate three major theoretical perspectives on intelligence—the mental testing approach, the information-processing approach, and the cognitive developmental tradition as exemplified by Piaget's theory. Emerging perspectives on intelligence are also discussed. Very clear and comprehensive.

Kluwe, R. H., & Spada, H. (Eds.). (1980). *Developmental models of thinking.* New York: Academic Press. This volume presents a detailed overview of different theoretical models of thinking and intellectual development. Included are mathematical and psychometric models, information-processing models, and Piagetian-centered approaches. A state-of-the-art book.

Labouvie-Vief, G. (1985). Intelligence and cognition. In J. E. Birren & K. W. Schaie (Eds.), *Handbook of the psychology of aging* (2nd ed., pp. 500–530). New York: Van Nostrand Reinhold. This excellent review chapter emphasizes the structural growth and adaptive reorganization of intelligence in adulthood. Research from studies on biological aging processes and the ecology of intellectual aging is reviewed, and a model of intelligence stressing cultural evolution is proposed.

Resnick, L. B. (Ed.). (1976). *The nature of intelligence.* Hillsdale, NJ: Erlbaum. This book examines cognitive processes involved in intelligent behavior and how these processes relate to tested intelligence. The emphasis is on the constructs and methods of the information-processing approach to intelligence, although other approaches are also considered. For advanced readers.

Sternberg, R. J., & Powell, J. S. (1983). The development of intelligence. In J. H. Flavell & E. M. Markman (Eds.), *Handbook of child psychology: Vol. 3. Cognitive development* (pp. 341–419). New York: Wiley. This comprehensive review considers several alternative conceptions of intelligence and the nature of its development. Both implicit and explicit theories of intelligence are covered and the authors then propose a unified and coherent view of intelligence that transcends any one specific conception.

CHAPTER 9

Social Cognitive Development

OVERVIEW

Social cognition is rapidly emerging as a key topic in life-span developmental psychology. Social cognitive phenomena include conceptions of self, knowledge of others, social perspective taking and role taking, moral judgments, and prosocial behaviors such as empathy. Although all forms of cognition are inherently social, an important distinction can be made between knowing about people and knowing about objects. For example, both objects and people can be acted upon (pushed, hit), but people react less predictably.

This chapter presents the influential theoretical model of social cognition proposed by John Flavell. Then we examine developmental processes in various types of social cognition. Regardless of the aspect of social cognitive knowledge considered—self, others, rules and conventions of society—the same basic developmental trend appears. The infant is initially profoundly egocentric and fails to differentiate between self and others. With development in childhood and adolescence, there is progressively greater self-other differentiation and increased awareness of the psychological and social complexities of living. Beyond adolescence, individuals' logical understanding of social cognitive events becomes embedded within a complex matrix of personal and social realities.

In the final part of this chapter, the relationship between social cognitive events and social behaviors is discussed. The ability to understand and vicariously experience what others are experiencing, an ability called "empathy," will be used to illustrate that relationship. Finally, we attempt to bring together the various threads of development by considering some cognitive, social, and affective components that any comprehensive life-span model of cognition should include.

THE IMPORTANCE OF SOCIAL COGNITION

The ability to understand our thoughts, feelings, needs, and intentions as well as those of others is a developmentally important phenomenon. One might expect to find a great deal of information about the development of self-knowledge and knowledge involving the social world— how people see themselves in society; how they view social interactions between individuals or groups; and how they view the rules, roles, and conventions of society. However, most of the research in cognitive developmental psychology, at least until about 15 years ago, focused on the development of impersonal logical problem-solving and mathematical reasoning skills such as conservation of physical objects. When investigators applied the knowledge gained from this research to the developing child's knowledge of the self, social roles, and relations between people, a new field of inquiry called **social cognition** was born (Overton, 1983; Shantz, 1975, 1983; Youniss, 1975).

One reason for the past neglect of social cognitive development can be found in the paradigmatic orientations held by various psychologists (D. Kuhn, 1978). (You may wish to review the discussion of scientific paradigms in Chapters 1 and 2.) In spite of the acknowledged importance of the relationship between cognitive and social development, psychologists have chosen to study phenomena which their paradigm handles best. In cognitive developmental psychology, the traditional paradigm has been organismic, as exemplified by the work of Jean Piaget and Heinz Werner. For example, Piaget's conservation experiments were concerned with the acquisition of knowledge about the physical world. The understanding of a phenomenon such as conservation seems to require an organismic paradigm in which internal mental structures undergo a radical process of reorganization. In contrast, psychologists who study social development tended to focus on observable social behaviors (e.g., aggression, cooperation) and the external stimuli which influence them. The latter psychologists have typically operated within a behaviorist social learning theory or, more broadly, a mechanistic framework. D. Kuhn (1978) has suggested that such differences in paradigmatic preferences may have prevented researchers in the two areas from communicating, thereby limiting progress in both areas.

Increasing numbers of psychologists gradually realized that studying cognition in isolation from social behavioral processes is too narrow and limiting. As the field of social cognition emerged, researchers discovered that cognitive and social functioning are intimately linked, and this linkage is not as straightforward as once imagined. Today much of the research in this field is concerned with how people cognitively appraise and interpret social situations. Suppose that two children are trying to decide what to buy a third child for a birthday present. They finally agree to buy a dog after learning that their friend's pet dog has been missing for several weeks. Before buying the dog, however, they learn that their friend is so upset that "he never wants to look at another dog again." They set off to purchase another present, only to pass a store with a sale on puppies; only one or two are left and they will soon be sold (after Selman, 1976). In this case, the researcher might be interested in discovering how a child who hears this story would cognitively evaluate the feelings and traits of the main characters. Would the child be cognitively advanced enough to realize that the boy might feel both happy and sad if he received a puppy for a present—sad about the lost dog, but happy about the new one?

Social cognitive processes can also be looked at from the opposite direction (Light, 1983) if we ask, How do social situations and inter-actions affect cognitive development and what mechanisms are involved? For example, do verbal interactions with a peer discussion group foster one's ability to think logically, to take another's perspective, and to engage in advanced moral reasoning? In this chapter we will look at both aspects of the social cognitive picture.

SOCIAL AND NONSOCIAL COGNITION

Let us begin our discussion by drawing a distinction between social and nonsocial cognition. Is social cognition different from any other form of cognition in developmentally significant ways? This question can be answered at several different levels of analysis. At a more general level, Piaget (1963), Chandler (1977), Bearison (1982), and Damon (1979) argue that all cognition is inherently social. As Damon (1979) has stated:

> The human construction of knowledge in *all* of its manifestations entails an interaction of subject and object, and can never consist of a purely objective "discovery" of impersonal, physical reality. Further, the subject is contin-ually guided in his or her cognitive development by the social context in which all knowledge is presented and created. (p. 207)

Social cognition, from this broader perspective, is explained by recourse to the same mechanisms as cognition in general.

A good example of this viewpoint can be seen in Vygotsky's theory of mental development (see Chapter 5). Vygotsky (1962, 1978) believed that all higher mental functions originate from interpersonal interac-tions among individuals. Every cognitive function appears first on the in-terpsychological (social) plane and only later is transformed onto the intrapsychological (individual) plane.

Even if one accepts the position that all cognition is social, it may still be useful to distinguish between social and nonsocial cognition. Social cognitive knowledge may follow different principles of structure and organization than nonsocial cognitive knowledge, even though the two are fundamentally similar (Damon, 1979). The differences between these two realms of knowledge can be summarized as follows (based on Shantz, 1983):

1. Actions on physical objects are more predictable than actions on or with people.
2. The range of possible actions on objects is much less than that on people.
3. People but not objects can be understood, in part, by underlying thoughts, emotions, and intentions.
4. Affective relations between people are more intense than between objects and people.
5. Person-person relations, but not person-object relations, are characterized by shared, coordinated intentions.

The distinctions outlined here confirm our personal intuitions that people are different from objects. We feel the distinctions are important because they influence the topics chosen for social cognition research and the methods used to study them.

MODELS OF SOCIAL COGNITIVE DEVELOPMENT

Although social cognitive development is now a large and vigorous field of study, no single theory of social cognition exists. Much of the work in this area is an outgrowth of the theories of Piaget (1970) and Werner (1948). As you know, Piaget was concerned primarily with children's knowledge about basic physical concepts such as space, time, number, and causality. He emphasized that these concepts develop through a child's progressive adaptation to the environment. Because people constitute a very important part of the environment, they may play a major socializing role in a child's cognitive development. Indeed, in many of his early works, Piaget (1932) emphasized the importance of social cooperation and conflict for counteracting children's egocentric tendencies. Werner also was interested in the individual's developing ability to assume the perspective of others.

Piaget's (1932) and Werner's (1948) emphasis on the significance of social interaction and the coordination of other perspectives was virtually ignored for many years. However, their theoretical concepts have stimulated the development of promising models of social cognition. We will now look at one of these models.

Drawing on Piaget's theory as well as non-Piagetian perspectives, John Flavell and associates have proposed a general model for the study of social cognition (Flavell, Botkin, Fry, Wright, & Jarvis, 1968). This model can be used to construct inferences about the social world and to apply these inferences to social situations. According to Flavell et al. (1968), at least four sequential steps are involved in this social inference process: (1) *existence*, (2) *need*, (3) *inference*, and (4) *application*. "Existence" refers to a person's knowledge or awareness of certain social facts or events. In order to use social cognitive thinking, one must be aware that certain social phenomena exist. For example, a 4-year-old may be unaware of people's ulterior motives and may not understand why accepting candy from a stranger is not a good idea. A 10-year-old may be more wary of strangers and see through surface appearances.

A child who is unaware of the existence of a given social fact cannot perceive the need to consider it as a possibility. However, at times children may be aware of a social fact, but not see a need to consider it in a given situation. Either the child does not think about the fact or does not wish to for whatever reason (Flavell, 1985). For example, children who are offered candy by a well-dressed, friendly stranger who they have seen around before may perceive this person as safe and sense no need to refuse the candy. The term *need* here is similar to Flavell's notion of *production deficiency* (see Chapter 6) in that children may possess a strategy but fail to use it spontaneously.

"Inference," the third component of Flavell's model, refers to an ability to identify another person's feelings, thoughts, and perceptions. Children may recognize the existence of another's subjective state and even the need to consider such states; but on the basis of the information given, they may have no way of inferring what the other person is experiencing. For example, a child may realize that a parent is upset (which requires some inferential ability), but have no clear idea about the exact nature of the parent's feeling (e.g., anger, disgust, sadness) or why it has occurred.

Once the steps of existence, need, and inference have been taken, the individual is ready for the last step—application. He or she applies the knowledge gained from steps 1–3 to real-life social situations. Suppose you are aware that your instructor is upset with a piece of work you just handed in (existence). You may want to figure out why the instructor is feeling this way in order to protect your grade (need). You infer, perhaps, that the instructor is upset because you handed in the work a day late (inference). That inference may or may not be correct, and unless you talk to the instructor about your work (application), your conclusions will remain idle speculation. If you find that the instructor is upset at something totally unrelated to your work, you would be forced to *reassess* your original inference.

To summarize, Flavell's model provides a useful heuristic framework for evaluating how people process social cognitive information in everyday activities. Since cognitive processing abilities are known to change developmentally, it is expected that knowledge about and awareness of social cognitive phenomena might also change. Specifically, as a person grows older, there should be a greater awareness of the existence of social realities, a more highly developed need to draw inferences about others' experience, and an increased ability to cognitively represent and infer information from ambiguous-appearing social situations.

Flavell has presented his sequential steps (see Figure 9.1) as a way of describing developmental changes in social *role-taking* ability. Role taking will be discussed later; first, we must discuss the point at which the development of all social cognition begins, namely, the understanding of one's self.

CONCEPTIONS OF SELF

To introduce a section on social cognition with a discussion of the self may seem a bit strange. But self-conceptions and conceptions of others cannot be considered apart from one another. How we understand others' intentions, motives, and feelings depends, in part, on our current self-knowledge and the inferences we draw from past experience. Our cognitions and personalities limit our knowledge of ourselves as well as of other people. How early does a concept of self develop?

Figure 9.1 Flavell's model of social cognition. The dashed arrow represents a reassessment of the original inference.

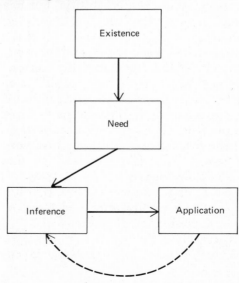

As yet, there is relatively little evidence on the development of a **self-concept** in early infancy. Self-concept is the sum total of ideas and perceptions a person has about himself or herself. As you learned, one of the major tasks infants face in the sensorimotor period of development is to differentiate themselves from other people and objects in the everyday environment. Not only must infants differentiate themselves as physical objects among a set of physical objects but they must also differentiate themselves as psychological subjects among things and other people (Flavell, 1985). By the end of the sensorimotor period, with the development of an object concept, infants have made a major step in this direction.

Michael Lewis and Jeanne Brooks (now called Brooks-Gunn) have conducted some intriguing investigations of an infant's sense of self (Brooks & Lewis, 1976; M. Lewis & Brooks, 1975). These investigators found that by age 20–24 months, infants have a rather well-developed self-concept and a concept of other people. In one experiment M. Lewis and Brooks (1975) surreptitiously dabbed a spot of rouge on babies' noses and placed each infant in front of a mirror. Babies under 1 year of age failed to recognize that the rouged nose reflected in the mirror belonged to them. Babies aged 15–18 months reacted differently: almost one-quarter of them immediately grabbed their nose. By 2 years of age, over three-quarters of the infants reached for their nose when they looked into the mirror. Is the development of self-concept related to the infant's cognitive development? The results of a similar study by Mans, Cicchetti, and Sroufe (1978) suggest that it is. Cognitively retarded Down's syndrome children tested in this study were almost 3 years of age before they reached for their rouged noses.

During early and middle childhood, the self-concept continues to develop as the child's cognitive and social worlds expand. By the time they enter elementary school, children can give a fairly accurate self-description based on concrete characteristics such as gender, age, size, possessions, and personal appearance (Livesley & Bromley, 1973; Montemayor & Eisen, 1977). In one study, Montemayor and Eisen (1977) used the "Twenty Statements Test" procedure to investigate self-concepts among children and adolescents in grades 4, 6, 8, 10, and 12. They asked subjects to write 20 different answers to the question "Who am I?" As expected, they found that 9-year-olds, still in concrete operations, used surface qualities and physical appearances to describe themselves. The following is a set of responses given by a 9-year-old boy in the fourth grade:

My name is Bruce C. I have brown eyes. I have brown hair. I have brown eyebrows. I'm nine years old. I LOVE! Sports. I have seven people in my family. I have great! eye site. I have lots! of friends. I live on 1923 Pinecrest Dr. I'm going on 10 in September. I'm a boy. I have a uncle that is almost 7 feet tall. My school is Pinecrest. My teacher is Mrs. V. I play Hockey! I'm almost the smartest boy in the class. I LOVE! food. I love freash air. I LOVE school. (Montemayor & Eisen, 1977, p. 317)

By 11–12 years of age, with the beginning of formal operational thinking skills, children give more internal, abstract, and differentiated descriptions which capture more of their personality characteristics. The following is a sample description given by an 11-year-old girl in the sixth grade:

> My name is A. I'm a human being. I'm a girl. I'm a truthful person. I'm not pretty. I do so-so in my studies. I'm a very good cellist. I'm a very good pianist. I'm a little bit tall for my age. I like several boys. I like several girls. I'm old-fashioned. I play tennis. I am a *very* good swimmer. I try to be helpful. I'm always ready to be friends with anybody. Mostly I'm good, but I lose my temper. I'm not well-liked by some girls and boys. I don't know if I'm liked by boys or not. (Montemayor & Eisen, 1977, p. 318)

As you can see, both of these children include some concrete characteristics in their self-descriptions, but the older child's contains more abstract internal characteristics.

During adolescence conceptions of self become even more complex and encompass personal values, belief systems, and ideologies. Adolescents can make inferences and formulate hypotheses about their underlying personality characteristics based on their own behavior. Montemayor and Eisen (1977) quoted a 17-year-old girl in her senior year in high school, who wrote:

> I am a human being. I am a girl. I am an individual. I don't know who I am. I am a Pisces. I am a moody person. I am an indecisive person. I am an ambitious person. I am a very curious person. I am not an individual. I am a loner. I am an American (God help me). I am a Democrat. I am a liberal person. I am a radical. I am a conservative. I am a pseudoliberal. I am an atheist. I am not a classifiable person (i.e., I don't want to be). (p. 318)

Other studies asking children and adolescents to describe themselves have reported similar trends from physical to psychological self-conceptions and from an unintegrated sense of self to a conceptual integration of the self-system. Nevertheless, it would be unwise to reduce these trends to a simple set of changes paralleling more general trends in cognitive development. As Damon and Hart (1982) have argued, many young children express self-statements that are not purely physicalistic (e.g., they describe their emotions), just as many adolescents give self-descriptions that are not purely psychological (e.g., they describe the physical self). To account for this complexity, Damon and

Hart (1982) have proposed a multidimensional model of self-understanding that describes how the aspects of the self interact in the course of development. Their model is largely speculative, but draws attention to the fact that development of self-conceptions proceeds along several dimensions simultaneously, rather than from one level of understanding (e.g., outer, physical) to another (e.g., inner, psychological).

Search for Identity

The adolescent's self-description in the Montemayor and Eisen (1977) study discussed above seems to contain a certain amount of role confusion and ambiguity. According to renowned psychoanalyst Erik Erikson (1968), adolescence is especially a time of search for an *identity*. The adolescent has many new roles and decisions involving heterosexual contacts, peer relationships, moral commitments, and educational and occupational activities as well as an increased capacity for formal, rational thought. If the adolescent succeeds in synthesizing these various roles and commitments, a (more or less) stable *ego* (self-) *identity* results. Failure to establish a meaningful synthesis leads to a sense of *identity diffusion* and a *totalistic* self-concept. **Totalism** means a conception of self characterized by arbitrary, rigid, and absolute boundaries (Erikson, 1968).

In Erikson's view, a certain amount of conflict and confusion is inevitable, and even desirable, in adolescence because of rapid physical, psychological, and social changes and because of the many decisions faced during this period. These factors can help account for some of the periods of relative instability of self-conceptions during the adolescent years. On the other hand, a growing body of empirical evidence suggests that a stable sense of identity and self emerges in adolescence (Dusek & Flaherty, 1981; Monge, 1973). This stabilization of personal identity may be related to the emergence of the equilibrated cognitive structures of formal operations. Although Erikson and others have speculated on such a link between cognitive development and identity formation, empirical research examining the two domains remains rare.

Self-Concept in Adulthood

According to Erikson, each individual faces a series of personal crises or choice points throughout the adult life span. Each of these involves some reevaluation of a person's identity, so that a complete resolution of identity status is neither possible nor desirable. Rather, the individual is expected to undergo a series of self-assessments involving some degree of change in identity. Such reevaluations are essential if a person is to achieve an integration of identity in late adulthood.

In Erikson's theory the major crisis of young adulthood is *intimacy versus isolation*. "Intimacy" means the establishment of close relationships with other people (e.g., spouse, friends, co-workers) characterized by sharing of feelings and ideas. To be intimate is to be able to identify with and relate to another person without fear of losing one's own identity. On the other hand, a failure to achieve intimacy produces a sense of isolation from others. Successful resolution of the intimacy-versus-isolation stage enables the adult to become concerned with producing and caring for a new generation. This concern for younger persons, or *generativity*, contrasts with *stagnation*, in which an individual becomes self-absorbed and self-indulgent. Energy that otherwise would be channeled toward rearing and teaching the young is focused inward toward the self. The generativity-versus-stagnation stage becomes important during the middle years of adulthood.

The final crisis of adulthood is that of *ego integrity versus despair*. Older people who can reflect on their lives and discern an integrated pattern—a feeling of having made the correct choices—experience a sense of self-integrity or wholeness and can face the end of their lives with feelings of satisfaction. If they do not perceive a meaningful pattern or carefully woven fabric in their lives, they feel a sense of despair and loss, and face death with anxiety and resentment.

In a study using an Eriksonian approach, Nehrke, Hulicka, and Morganti (1980) reported that self-conceptions become more positive during late adulthood from the 60s on. Nehrke et al. (1980) interpreted their results as showing that increasing numbers of older people successfully resolve the integrity-versus-despair conflict as they advance through their later years, but not every study has reported positive changes in self-concept during the adult years. Some studies show no changes or show self-concepts becoming more negative.

The notion of stability (no change) is critical in the developmental literature on self-conceptions. This issue was dealt with extensively in Chapter 8's discussion of intelligence and the age differentiation–dedifferentiation hypothesis, which states that intellectual development proceeds from a global, undifferentiated state to a more specific, differentiated one. In other words, intelligence is expected to develop a more complex structure as it evolves over the life span. Using this hypothesis as a point of comparison, should we similarly expect self-conceptions to become increasingly complex, multidimensional, and differentiated after adolescence?

The empirical evidence on this question suggests a great deal of stability in self-concept in adulthood, although allowing for the influences of certain life experiences and events. Some recent longitudinal research on self-concepts by Mortimer, Finch, and Kumka (1982) is germane here. Mortimer et al. (1982) studied 368 males from the University of Michigan in 1962–1963, when the subjects were freshmen; in 1966–1967, when they were seniors; and in 1976, 10 years after their college graduation. To assess self-concept, they used a **semantic differential scale,** which is a self-rating scale composed of several bipolar adjectives (e.g., *happy-unhappy, relaxed-tense, confident-anxious, social-solitary*) describing different personality dimensions. A sample scale used by Monge (1973) to assess adolescents' self-concepts is shown in Figure 9.2.

The Mortimer et al. (1982) study assessed four different personality dimensions: well-being, evaluation of interpersonal qualities, competence, and unconventionality. Subjects were asked to rate "Myself as a Person" on each adjective set at each time of testing. The most striking finding was the degree of stability in self-concepts over time. Through the multiple role transitions in the 14-year period (e.g., graduation from college, entry into an occupation, career changes, marriage, becoming a parent), most respondents' self-concepts remained fairly stable. However, life events did have an impact, as indicated by self-concept changes. For example, males who experienced prolonged periods of unemployment and less positive relationships with their parents had a decreased sense of personal competence. And the subjects' level of self-competence during the senior year of college partially predicted certain life experiences. For example, a high level of self-competence predicted high job satisfaction. These findings indicate a dynamic and reciprocal relationship between life experiences and self-concepts. They also raise the fascinating prospect of predicting adult experiences such as occu-

Figure 9.2 Sample items from a semantic differential scale used to rate the concept "My Characteristic Self." Italicized items appeared on the left-hand pole in the original scale.

smart	___	___	___	___	___	___	___ dumb
success	___	___	___	___	___	___	___ failure
leader	___	___	___	___	___	___	___ *follower*
confident	___	___	___	___	___	___	___ unsure
good	___	___	___	___	___	___	___ *bad*
happy	___	___	___	___	___	___	___ sad
refreshed	___	___	___	___	___	___	___ *tired*
stable	___	___	___	___	___	___	___ unstable
hard	___	___	___	___	___	___	___ soft
healthy	___	___	___	___	___	___	___ *sick*

From "Developmental Trends in Factors of Adolescent Self-Concept" by R. H. Monge, 1973, *Developmental Psychology, 8,* p. 388. Copyright 1973 by the American Psychological Association. Adapted by permission.

pational success from multidimensional self-concept measures, something that has been difficult to do using only cognitive measures such as IQ scores.

CONCEPTIONS OF OTHERS

Do people conceive of themselves in the same way that they conceive of others? As we observed, individual self-concepts become more differentiated and more abstract with age, at least through adolescence. Ample evidence shows that conceptions of others also show a developmental progression toward greater abstractness and complexity (Barenboim, 1981; Flapan, 1968; Livesley & Bromley, 1973; Peevers & Secord, 1973).

Person Perception

The area dealing with how people view the internal and external attributes of others is called **person perception.** Several reviews of this literature are available (Dubin & Dubin, 1965; Livesley & Bromley, 1973; Rosenberg & Sedlak, 1972; Shantz, 1975). In person perception research, the most frequent method is simply to ask people to describe either orally or in writing individuals whom they know (Shantz, 1975). Though this method of free description suffers from drawbacks such as overreliance on verbal skills, the method is less biased than having subjects rate a list of experimenter-selected adjectives. It has been pointed out that trait adjectives (e.g., *social, confident, aggressive*) account for only about 20 percent of children's descriptions of others (Peevers & Secord, 1973).

A recent series of studies by Carl Barenboim (1981) helps to illustrate the nature of research in the area of person perception. Barenboim asked 6-, 8-, and 10-year-old children to describe three different persons whom they knew well, excluding immediate family members. One year later the children were retested using the same procedure, except that they were asked to describe three new persons. Each of the children's descriptions was then scored for the use of (1) behavioral comparison—comparison of the person described to another person's behavior or to a general norm of behavior; (2) psychological constructs—personality or trait-like descriptions; and (3) psychological comparison—comparison of the person being described to another person in terms of psychological constructs or psychological dispositions.

Barenboim (1981) hypothesized that the youngest children should describe the people they know primarily in behavioral terms such as "Billy runs a lot faster than Jason" or "She draws the best in our whole class." This hypothesis was based on the finding that children around age 6 or 7 characterize other people in terms of concrete, observable characteristics such as physical appearance, social roles, habits, possessions, age, and sex, rather than deeper psychological characteristics (Livesley & Bromley, 1973). As children grow older, they begin to observe certain regularities in their friends' behavior, and therefore should endow others with traits, motives, needs, and other psychological attributes. For example, at about ages 8–10, children may describe another child with statements such as "He's really conceited, thinks he's great" or "Sarah is so kind." However, children at this age do not spontaneously produce psychological comparisons. By age 11 or 12, children should be able to compare persons on psychological dimensions (e.g., "He's much more shy than most kids would be in a situation like that" or "Billy is much more thoughtful than Ted").

The results of Barenboim's study provide strong support for his hypotheses. As Figure 9.3 shows for both cross-sectional and longitudinal methods, the descriptions of the younger children were typically couched in behavioral terms; there was a significant increase in behavioral comparisons between ages 6–8 and a significant decrease between ages 9–11. In contrast, the use of psychological constructs began to increase among the 6–8-year-olds, and increased even more dramatically among the 9–11-year-olds. The longitudinal data were also in

Figure 9.3 Mean percentage of behavioral comparisons, psychological constructs, and psychological comparisons for children aged 6–11.

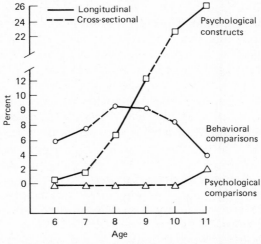

From "The Development of Person Perception in Childhood and Adolescence: From Behavioral Comparisons to Psychological Constructs to Psychological Comparisons" by C. Barenboim, 1981, *Child Development, 52*, p. 134. Copyright 1981 by The Society for Research in Child Development, Inc. Reprinted by permission.

accord with the hypothesized developmental sequence. For example, 8-year-olds' behavioral comparison scores predicted their psychological construct scores at age 9, and the psychological construct scores of 10-year-olds similarly predicted their psychological comparison scores at age 11. But even 11-year-olds used few psychological comparisons in their descriptions.

To find out when children first use psychological comparisons, Barenboim (1981) conducted a similar study with 10-, 12-, 14-, and 16-year-olds. He found that children between ages 10–12 begin to employ psychological comparisons spontaneously in describing others, with some gradual increases thereafter. The vast majority of children aged 12 or older used psychological comparisons, whereas less than 20 percent of 10-year-olds did.

What factors underlie the developmental sequence from behavioral comparisons to psychological constructs to psychological comparisons? Barenboim suggests that the transition from concrete to formal operations accounts for the changes in children's social conceptions. At the beginning of the concrete operational period, children classify others in terms of concrete, behavioral characteristics. Gradually, children begin to include covert, psychological constructs in their descriptions of other people. Shantz (1975) argued that this developmental trend from describing people's surface appearances to inner qualities corresponds to the development of conservation abilities. While surface features (e.g., height, number of possessions) may change, underlying qualities (e.g., friendliness, sociability) remain the same.

By the time of formal operations, individuals' descriptions of others increase in scope and complexity. Adolescents are aware of the existence of contradictory tendencies and traits in other people (e.g., someone is kind and cruel) and attempt to explain them. They become increasingly aware that a person's characteristics may vary as a function of family background, situational constraints, internal states, or other fluctuating events (e.g., someone is even shyer than I am when near strangers, yet is very talkative with friends). In their descriptions they explain behavior, describe how traits are manifested in particular situations, and employ qualifying terms (e.g., *sometimes, quite*). These changes are significant because they reflect adolescents' growing knowledge about other people and knowledge about causal networks involving personal and situational factors.

To review, changes in children's conceptions of others parallel changes in the way they conceive of themselves. They first employ overt, behavioral conceptions which are eventually replaced by internal, psychological conceptions. They also shift from merely describing another person's behavior to trying to explain it. The major developmental changes in person concepts have been summarized by Shantz

(1983) using the notion of differentiation. In contrast to the older child and adolescent, the younger child

1. fails to differentiate a person as a *psychological* entity from his physical context (i.e., a person is what he owns or wears);
2. fails to differentiate external, observable aspects of a person from internal, covert aspects (i.e., a person is how she looks or behaves);
3. does not differentiate his or her conceptions from the set of all possible conceptions about others (i.e., a person is what the child thinks him to be);
4. tends not to differentiate both good and bad qualities within the same person (i.e., a person is either good or bad).

Perceptions of Aging Persons

Thus far we have concentrated largely on childhood and adolescent changes in the conceptions of others. Studies of person perception in the adult developmental literature have focused on the existence of age-role stereotypes and intergenerational perceptions. However, most of the research has been conducted on perceptions of old age, and there is a lack of information on people in other age groups as perceptual targets (Nardi, 1973). In addition, the use of a wide variety of assessment methods—including semantic differentials (Kogan & Wallach, 1961), adjective checklists (Fitzgerald, 1978), and attitude scales (Tuckman & Lorge, 1953)—makes comparisons across studies difficult. Nevertheless, a perception of old age as characterized by dependency, passivity, low intelligence, poor health, and mental problems emerges as a consistently documented finding. These negative age perceptions may have a negative impact on the older generation's cognitive and social functioning.

Reno (1979) illustrated the pervasiveness of age-role stereotyping. She gave young adult subjects information about a fictitious person who had begun college after working for several years. Half of the subjects were told that the new student was 25 years old, while the other half were told the new student was 63 years old. Subjects were then informed that the student failed to graduate from college and were asked to attribute probable causes for the failure. The younger student's failure was attributed primarily to alterable temporary causes, such as not trying hard enough. In contrast, the older student's failure was attributed mainly to a permanent ability deficit, such as lacking the intellectual ability for college. Not only do young people rate older people more negatively but many older people also hold negative attitudes toward their age-mates (Nardi, 1973). This observation underscores the pervasiveness of age-role stereotyping in our culture, although the stereotyping may be less widespread than current research studies would have us believe (see Fitzgerald, 1981).

Egocentrism and Self-Other Differentiation

Developmental changes in conceptions of others can be conceived of as a shift from egocentricism to perspectivism (Piaget, 1970; Werner, 1948). **Egocentrism** can be defined broadly as an inability to differentiate between self and others, whereas **perspectivism** refers to the capacity to differentiate between one's own and others' points of view. In Piaget's view, egocentrism stands as the major obstacle to progress in both social and cognitive development (Light, 1983). In the social domain, "egocentrism" refers to the inability to take on the viewpoint of another; in the cognitive domain, it deals with fixation, or *centration*, on one aspect of a stimulus. Both uses of the term have been discussed previously—social egocentrism in Chapter 5 and cognitive egocentrism in Chapter 4.

Because egocentrism is critically important in self-other differentiation, we need to consider it in some detail. As mentioned above, egocentrism can be characterized as a lack of differentiation between the self and nonself. According to Piaget, infancy is a period of almost total egocentrism. Young infants think the world is physically *centered* on them, not realizing that objects and people have a separate existence apart from the infants' immediate actions. By gaining a concept of objects and people as separate entities in a space-time matrix, infants gradually begin to overcome this profound egocentrism. In middle childhood and toddlerhood, children show less egocentrism, but they still tend to confuse self and nonself. The onset of preoperational thinking signals the beginning of symbolic modes of thought. Though the symbolic function represents an advance in thinking, preoperational children tend to confuse their own psychological states with those of other people. For example, the child assumes others know his dreams, thoughts, and wishes.

Piaget found a decline in egocentrism among most children by age 6 or 7. Children become increasingly accurate in recognizing that other people have perspectives different than their own. For example, in the social communication problem discussed in Chapter 5, children are increasingly likely to take the listener's perspective into account as they grow older. Piaget felt that peers have an influential role in helping the child overcome egocentric thinking. In childhood games such as marbles, children make up rules and solve rule conflicts, which demand the consideration of other perspectives.

By adolescence egocentrism declines even further, although it does not disappear entirely. The beginning of formal operations ensnares the adolescent in another form of egocentrism, one in which new mental abilities are misused. Formal thinking opens up a whole range of imagined possibilities, among them an ability to engage in *recursive* thinking (e.g., "The boy is thinking that the girl is thinking of him talking to her."). In effect, adolescents can think about their own thinking, can think about themselves thinking about their thinking, and so on in a recursive fashion. According to psychologist David Elkind (1967, 1980), these changes in adolescent thought are reflected in two forms of egocentrism: (1) imaginary audience and (2) personal fable. An **imaginary audience** refers to the adolescents' belief that the concerns of others are the same as theirs. They develop a self-conscious feeling of always being "on stage" or "in the spotlight." For example, an adolescent may spend hours combing his hair in front of a mirror, imagining the impact he will make when he enters the dance hall with his friends. A **personal fable** is a story a person constructs which idealizes his or her unique feelings and experiences. Keeping a diary, as many adolescents do, in which one chronicles heroic personal adventures is a familiar example. In the imaginary audience, adolescents underdifferentiate between themselves and others; whereas in the personal fable, they overdifferentiate their experiences from those of others.

These forms of adolescent egocentrism eventually yield to more mature forms of thinking as individuals reality-test their own views against those of others. But some residual egocentric thinking may remain, even in adulthood. Flavell (1985) has speculated on this possibility:

> Unlike, say, nonconservation of number, I believe we are "at risk" (almost in the medical sense) for egocentric thinking all of our lives, just as we are for certain logical errors. The reason lies in our psychological designs in relation to the jobs to be done. We experience our own points of view more or less directly, whereas we must always attain the other person's in more indirect manners. (p. 125)

Thus, a certain amount of egocentrism appears to be inevitable, even among mature adult thinkers.

The notion of egocentrism serves as a unifying thread tying together the various strands of mental development. However, it has come under some severe criticism. Critics charge that the amount of egocentrism in early life has been seriously overestimated (Borke, 1975; Cox, 1980; Gelman, 1979; Gelman & Baillargeon, 1983). They point to instances of young children sharing toys with another child or comforting a child who is upset. Furthermore, how the social environment (i.e., peers, friends, family) counteracts egocentric tendencies is not clear, because most of the research has focused on egocentric cognitions, not on how environmental experiences affect them. In addition, differentiating between an egocentric and nonegocentric response is often difficult. For example, a person who sees a similarity between herself and another individual is not necessarily egocentric; the assumed similarity may exist. Perhaps the most damaging criticism is that research studies fail to support the view of egocentrism as a valid psychological construct (Ford, 1979, 1985). In his comprehensive review of this issue, Ford (1979) concluded that measures of egocentrism are typically as highly correlated with other constructs, such as IQ and conservation, as they are with each other. This lack of construct validity casts serious doubt on Piaget's interpretation of egocentrism as a generalized psychological trait.

ROLE TAKING

No matter how confident we are of objectively apprehending the physical and social world, individuals of all ages use a good deal of subjectivity in their perceptions of people and objects (Chandler, 1977). This observation is conveyed in such sayings as "Love is blind" and "Beauty is in the eye of the beholder." Children in particular are believed to be susceptible to subjective biases in personal judgments, whereas adults are thought to be more objective. Much of the research on subjectivity in personal judgments involves a capacity known as **role taking,** which refers to the ability to adopt the roles and perspectives of other people.

Before we discuss the developmental research on role-taking abilities, several preliminary comments are in order. First, as you may suspect, there is a close relationship between role taking and egocentrism, but the two concepts are not identical. The ability to take on the role of another requires nonegocentric thinking, but nonegocentric functioning does not require role-taking skills (Shantz, 1983). To illustrate this point, think about Flavell's concepts of existence, need, and inference (see Figure 9.1). You may be aware of the existence of another's point of view (nonegocentric thinking), but not be able to understand the other's view (role taking). On the other hand, you must recognize the existence of another social reality before you can understand that perspective.

We also need to clarify the meaning of *role* in the present context. In the social psychological literature, the term refers to a culturally specified set of expectations for appropriate behavior (e.g., the role of parent). Here the term *role* refers to the awareness that various ways of being are possible. Given this definition, whether people can be said to occupy different roles depends on the degree to which they can differentiate themselves from others. Role taking requires that people recognize both the existence of other points of view and the necessity of putting themselves in another role or vantage point.

Development of Role-Taking Skills

Several different measurement procedures have been designed and used to assess the development of role-taking skills. All of them require subjects to describe objects or events from multiple points of view. In Piaget's and Piagetian-inspired work, role taking has been assessed by visual perspective-taking tasks such as the three-mountain problem (see Figure 4.8). In contrast, other investigators have employed measurements which are more interpersonal and require subjects to retell or interpret a story about others.

Selman and Byrne (1974) used a story procedure to study stages of role taking in children. They showed 4-, 6-, 8-, and 10-year-olds filmed stories and asked them questions about the perspectives, feelings, and thoughts of the character in the story. One of these stories is about 8-year-old Holly, who likes to climb trees. One day Holly's father sees her fall off a tall tree and asks her not to climb trees anymore. Holly promises her father that she will refrain from tree climbing. Later that day, Holly and her friends meet a child whose kitten is caught in a tree. Because Holly is the only one who climbs trees well, she is confronted with the choice of trying to save the kitten or obeying her father. Children in the Selman and Byrne (1974) study were asked about how Holly felt in this situation and how they would handle the situation.

Box 9.1 presents four stages in role taking identified by Selman and Byrne (1974) on the basis of children's responses to these questions. Box 9.1 also includes a fifth stage later identified by Selman and Jaquette (1978) to describe role-taking ability in adolescents. The major developmental trend seen in Box 9.1 is the greater degree of role taking at the higher age levels. The initial two stages (Stages 0 and 1) are marked by a high level of subjectivism. In these stages the child does not have the inference skills needed to figure out the subjective state of another. For example, Stage 0 children who hear Holly's story will assume that everyone in the story recognizes how everyone else thinks and feels. Stage 1 children begin to understand that people have different perspectives and therefore realize that Holly's friends may be puzzled by her reluctance to climb the tree, because the friends are unaware of Holly's promise to her father.

By Stage 2, children can reflect on themselves from another's cognitive perspective. A Stage 2 child can also make inferences and evaluations of others' thoughts and feelings. In the sample story, Stage 2 children can understand that Holly and her father are mutually aware of

Box 9.1   A Stage Model of Children's Role Taking

1. *Egocentric or undifferentiated perspectives—Stage 0*
   (approximately ages 3–6)
Children can recognize the reality of subjective perspectives (e.g., thoughts and feelings) within the self and the other. But because children do not clearly distinguish their own perspective from that of the other, they do not recognize that another may interpret similarly perceived social experiences or courses of action differently than they do. Similarly, children still show some confusion about the subjective (or psychological) and objective (or physical) aspects of the social world (e.g., between feelings and overt acts, between intentional and unintentional acts).

2. *Subjective or differentiated perspectives—Stage 1*
   (approximately ages 6–8)
Children understand that even under similarly perceived social circumstances, the self and the other's perspective may be the same or different. Children realize that the self and the other may view similarly perceived actions as reflections of disparate or distinct individual reasons or motives. Stage 1 children are newly concerned with the uniqueness of the covert, psychological life of each person.

3. *Self-reflective or reciprocal perspectives—Stage 2*
   (approximately ages 8–10)
Children are able to reflect on their own thoughts and feelings from another's perspective, to put themselves in the other's shoes and to see themselves as a subject to the other. This new awareness of the relation between self and other's perspective allows children to consider their own conceptions and evaluations of another's thoughts and actions. Children are able to take a second-person perspective, which leads to an awareness of a new reciprocity of thoughts and feelings ("I know that he likes me; he knows that I like him"), rather than a reciprocity of action ("She does for me; I do for her").

4. *Third-person or mutual perspectives—Stage 3*
   (approximately ages 10–12)
In Stage 3, the subject moves to a qualitatively new level of awareness—the ability to abstractly step outside an interpersonal interaction and coordinate simultaneously the perspectives of each

party in the interaction. This third-person perspective leads to the subject's awareness of the mutuality of human perspectives and hence of the self-other relationship.

5. *Societal or in-depth perspectives—Stage 4*
 (approximately ages 12–15 and beyond)
The subject conceptualizes subjective perspectives of persons toward one another (mutuality) as existing not only on the plane of common expectations or awareness but also at multidimensional or deeper levels of communication. For example, perspectives between two persons can be shared at the level of superficial information, common interests, or deeper and unverbalized feelings. Also, perspectives among persons are seen as forming a network or system. These perspectives become generalized into the concept of society's perspective or a legal or moral point of view.

From "Stability and Oscillation in Interpersonal Awareness: A Clinical-Developmental Analysis" by R. L. Selman and D. Jaquette, 1978, in *Nebraska Symposium on Motivation* (Vol. 25, p. 274) edited by C. B. Keasey, Lincoln: University of Nebraska Press. Copyright 1978 by University of Nebraska Press. Reprinted by permission.

the other's perspective and this awareness will influence Holly's father's evaluation of her action of saving the kitten. This awareness goes beyond merely thinking about another person's thoughts. It includes the ability to think about another person thinking about one's own thoughts.

In the last two stages (Stages 3 and 4), children not only can think about the perspectives of other people but also can view others' perspectives from the point of view of a third person (e.g., parent, teacher, peer—Stage 3) or a group of people in general (e.g., political party, religious group—Stage 4). The development of formal operational thinking contributes to this ability to take the multiple perspectives of different individuals and groups.

Selman and Byrne's (1974) results are consistent with other research (Feffer & Gourevitch, 1960; Looft, 1972) in showing a steady decline of egocentrism in adolescence and an advance in role-taking skills. By Selman and Byrne's Stage 4, adolescents realize that another can share their third-person perspectives of a given social interaction; consequently, adolescents appear to be less egocentric about their own third-person perspectives than children (Forman & Sigel, 1979). In addition, adolescents become increasingly aware of the mutuality of human perspectives, but their thinking is still limited because they view societal and group belief systems in the context of the society in which they have been socialized. Thus, though not as egocentric as children, adolescents tend to be *sociocentric.*

Sometime in young adulthood, sociocentrism may give way to a more pluralistic and multicultural perspective. Customs, values, and beliefs that appear peculiar or threatening if viewed from a societal perspective can be comprehended more meaningfully from a nonsociocentric view. Formal operations are now applied to deduce the meaning of customs, behaviors, or beliefs within the changing context of a particular culture. This application is a somewhat idealized version of adult social inference skills. Like adolescents, adults often lapse into sociocentric errors in thinking and are less likely to adopt others' perspectives than the literature leads us to believe (Chandler, 1976). This lapse is similar to the already noted frequent failure of adults to use formal operational thought in everyday problem situations (Piaget, 1972).

The fact that chronological age is not always accurate in predicting the level of role-taking ability suggests the operation of other factors. Characteristics of the subject, especially the subject's cognitive ability, may influence the ability to role take. K. Rubin (1978) reported that the correlations between mental age and six perspective-taking tasks ranged from .43–.77 for children aged 5½–11½. However, correlations between intelligence measures and measures of social cognitive ability tell us little about the specific cognitive processes involved. Piaget (1970) suggested that conservation abilities are related to role-taking development because certain cognitive operations (e.g., decentering, reversibility) are necessary for role taking. Little research has addressed the specific cognitive skills underlying social role taking.

Sex is another subject characteristic that may be involved in role taking. The stereotype that females are more sensitive to social cues, and should therefore be in a better position to take on the perspective of another person, is not upheld by the developmental literature. The majority of studies on social perspective taking have found no significant differences between males and females (Kurdek, 1977; Rothenberg, 1970; K. Rubin, 1978). A few studies have reported superior spatial perspective-taking ability in males (e.g., Coie & Dorval, 1973), but others have not (e.g., Cutrona & Feshbach, 1979).

Characteristics of the tasks employed to measure role taking also seem to influence the results obtained. Because social cognition is a relatively new area and because of the complexity of the field, dozens of different tasks have been employed. Naturally, tasks vary widely in the degree to which the problem engages the self (observer versus participant) with others, the nature of the social inferences involved (inferring thoughts or feelings), and the type of response required (retelling a story versus selecting a picture from a set of pictures). For example, Selman and Byrne (1974) asked children to judge how they would resolve a dilemma faced by a story character, but in spatial role-taking tasks such as the three-mountain problem, children must be participants in the different perspectives. Children in the Selman and Byrne (1974) study also were asked to answer a series of questions in their own words, whereas children in the original three-mountain study (Piaget & Inhelder, 1967) pointed to a picture. Finally, subjects in the storytelling study had to infer the feelings and thoughts of another; subjects in the three-mountain study had to infer another's visual perspective. Differences in task content and procedures undoubtedly influence role-taking performance. Little empirical evidence has documented exactly which task dimensions are responsible for performance differences.

Role Taking as a Problem-Solving Skill

We have discussed role taking as an ability to take on the perspective or viewpoint of another, but such role-taking skills may not be enough to resolve many real-life conflict situations. Knowing that a problem exists and needs to be resolved is often insufficient; people need to know what to do. Several training programs have been developed to teach interpersonal problem-solving skills. In one of the most successful programs, Spivack and Shure (1974; Shure & Spivack, 1978) have identified interpersonal cognitive problem-solving (ICPS) skills important to good social adjustment. Though most of their work focuses on young children, several of their colleagues have now examined ICPS with other age groups (Platt & Spivack, 1973; Platt, Spivack, Altman, Altman, & Peizer, 1974).

Spivack and Shure (1974) began with the observation that in spite of similarities in IQ and other cognitive abilities, disturbed middle-class adolescents showed pronounced deficits in a variety of interpersonal thinking skills, compared to nondisturbed adolescents (Shure, 1982). One interpersonal thinking skill seems especially crucial in the mediation of social behavior—*means-end thinking.* As discussed in Chapter 7, means-end thinking is an ability to plan a sequence of actions to reach an anticipated goal, to consider alternatives if the solution path is blocked, and to realize that goal achievement may not occur immediately. Maladjusted adolescents seem to lack the ability of planning to reach a goal. They go impulsively toward the goal, become easily frustrated if they do not reach it immediately, and do not consider alternative paths to goal satisfaction.

The training program developed by Spivack and Shure (1974; Shure & Spivack, 1978) concentrates on helping children and adolescents identify what they would do in interpersonal situations and encouraging them to generate alternative solutions. Daily 20-minute small-group training sessions have been created which can be applied by teachers and aides in the school setting. In the following example of a teacher applying this method, one child has just pushed another child off a bike:

TEACHER: Steven, what happened?
STEVEN: He won't give me the bike.
TEACHER: What happened when you pushed Robert off?
STEVEN: He started fighting.
TEACHER: How did that make you feel?
STEVEN: Mad.
TEACHER: How do you think Robert felt when you pushed him?
STEVEN: Mad.
TEACHER: Pushing him off is *one* way to try to get to ride the bike. Can you think of a *different* way so he won't fight and so you won't both be mad? (Shure, 1982, p. 143)

In this dialogue the teacher tries to get Steven to think through the problem, see the consequences of his actions, and generate alternative ways of handling the situation. What Steven says is not as important, in Spivack and Shure's opinion, as how he thinks about the problem. They find that "thinking through" the problem is much more effective than simply having an adult tell or order the child to take a course of action. Moreover, they report that gains in a child's interpersonal solution skills occur independently of initial IQ or IQ change.

During the early phases of the training program, Spivack and Shure (1974) did not directly measure social perspective taking, or what is more commonly known as role taking. However, in recent work they have added a series of role-playing exercises. They hypothesize that children who become emotionally sensitive to others through role playing should be better able to envision a broader range of problem solutions. Though their findings are preliminary, there appears to be some empirical support for their hypothesis (Shure, 1982).

Although apparently related to interpersonal problem solving, is role-taking ability a prerequisite for it? In an important study, Marsh, Serafica, and Barenboim (1980) trained middle-class eighth graders of average ability in various perspective-taking skills. The researchers' goal was to determine if increasing children's ability to role play would lead to improvements in children's interpersonal problem solving. They found that compared to a control group, the treatment group improved on one measure of interpersonal problem solving involving analytical thinking, but not on another involving means-ends analysis. Nor did treated children improve on social and affective perspective taking (though many of the subjects had high levels of perspective taking at the start of training). Thus, perspective-taking skills may be necessary but not sufficient antecedents for effective interpersonal problem solving. A similar conclusion has been reached by Selman (1981) in his work on the development of friendship conceptions (see Box 9.2).

MORAL DEVELOPMENT AND MORAL BEHAVIOR

In this section, we will shift to a social systems level of analysis and take a critical look at children's developing conceptions of morality. We will also examine some recent evidence on changes in moral thinking during adulthood. It is hardly surprising that the topic of moral development is a very large one. Each of us has a great personal stake in the moral order of society. Without some agreed-upon code or standard of morality for deciding between "right" or "wrong," society, as we know it, would cease to exist. And each of us, regardless of age or social position, is constantly confronted with important moral questions. For adults, such questions might involve government intervention in a foreign country, access to a controversial drug such as laetrile, or whether women have a right to abortion. Children are also faced with serious moral decisions which may not encompass the wider societal and cultural sphere, but are significant in a child's day-to-day life and later moral development. Many of a child's moral decisions revolve around loyalty to friends, cheating, lying, and stealing. For example, "Should I allow my friend Billy to sneak in front of me in the cafeteria line ahead of others who are hungry and have been waiting for a long time?" Or "Should I report a suspected cheater to the teacher?"

At least four different theories of moral development have been proposed—including psychoanalytic (Erikson, 1963; Freud, 1930), social

Box 9.2 The Development of Friendship Conceptions across the Life Span

The development of friendship conceptions is a major part of social cognitive knowledge. Until recently, most of the empirical research in this area concentrated on behavioral interactions between friends rather than on individuals' ideas about friendship. Although interest in friendship interactions remains, developmental psychologists have increasingly turned their attention to studying how concepts of friendship change with age.

One of the most comprehensive and well-articulated theories of friendship conceptions has been proposed by Robert Selman (1981; Selman & Jaquette, 1978) as part of a broader research program on children's social reasoning. Using an organismic developmental framework, Selman has suggested that the development of friendship conceptions can be studied by assessing children's reflections on six key issues in the interpersonal domain: (1) friendship formation, (2) closeness and intimacy, (3) trust, (4) jealousy, (5) conflicts and their resolutions, and (6) friendship termination. To study children's as well as adolescents' and adults' understanding of these issues, Selman used an open-ended clinical interview in which he asked 93 male and female subjects (aged 3–34) to discuss and resolve a series of interpersonal dilemmas. For example, to explore thinking about conflict resolution, subjects were presented with a hypothetical dilemma in which a person around the subject's age is asked by a newcomer in town to go to a special event that conflicts with a previous engagement made with a longtime close friend. To make matters worse, the old friend does not like the new friend.

In subjects' answers to a series of probe questions concerning the dilemma, Selman (1981) identified the following developmental progression.

1. *Momentary, physicalistic playmateship —Stage 0*
   (approximately ages 3–6)
In Stage 0, friendship relations are viewed in terms of propinquity and proximity (physicalistic) to the exclusion of other parameters. A close friend is someone who lives nearby and who the child happens to be playing with at the moment. Friendship issues such as jealousy and intrusion of a third party in the play situation are seen by the Stage 0 child as fights over toys or space, rather than as conflicts involving personal feelings.

2. *One-way assistance—Stage 1 (approximately ages 7–9)*
In Stage 1, a friend is someone who performs activities to meet one's goals or expectations. In contrast to Stage 0, a friend is someone whose likes and dislikes are known, not someone with whom one simply interacts.

3. *Fair-weather cooperation—Stage 2 (approximately ages 8–12)*
By Stage 2, the child has a new awareness of the reciprocity of interpersonal relations. Friendship is viewed as a two-way affair involving each person's adjustment to the likes and dislikes of the other, rather than as one person's simply matching expectations to the other's standards. However, friendship is "fair weather" and can easily be broken by arguments.

4. *Intimate and mutually shared relationships—Stage 3 (approximately ages 11–12)*

At Stage 3, friendship is interpreted within the context of enduring affective bonds. Friends share personal problems and give each other support. Stage 3 is limited by its overemphasis on the two-person clique and the possessiveness that grows from the realization that intimate relations are difficult to form and maintain.

5. *Autonomous interdependent friendships—Stage 4 (approximately ages 12–15 and beyond)*

Finally, by Stage 4, friendship rests on each partner's ability to balance feelings of independence and dependence. Close friends rely on each partner for psychological support and gain a sense of self-identification through identification with the other. At the same time friends recognize that each partner has needs which may require other relationships for their satisfaction.

What accounts for these developmental changes in friendship conceptions? According to Selman (1981; Selman & Jaquette, 1978), social perspective-taking or role-taking structures, such as described in Box 9.1 (see Selman & Byrne, 1974), underlie friendship developmental stages. These role-taking stages are necessary but not sufficient for the development of a given friendship stage. Individuals can demonstrate a certain level of awareness about the perspective of another person without manifesting an awareness of the issues (e.g., conflict resolution, friendship termination) that define a stage of friendship concepts. Still, the stages of role taking and of friendship conceptions correlate highly with one another (Selman, 1981).

Selman's research has described developmental levels of friendship concepts in children and adolescents. His theory is much less specific about how adults conceive of their friends. As Huyck (1982) has indicated in her recent review, there is little agreement about how to define or measure friendship during the adult years. Researchers have found considerable variability in the kinds of relationships adults view as friendships. In one 1980 study by Cohen, Cook, and Raykowski (cited in Huyck, 1982), a significant number of nonfriend contacts were considered "intimate" and "important" to the adults interviewed, but many people seen as friends were not considered intimate or important. Future research needs to determine if friendships have the same psychological meaning in adulthood as they do in childhood and adolescence (see Tesch, 1983).

learning (Aronfreed, 1968; Bandura, 1977), social evolutionary (Hogan, 1973, 1975), and cognitive developmental theory (Kohlberg, 1963; Piaget, 1932)—and countless empirical studies have been performed. We will concentrate on the theory that has had the most impact on the field—the cognitive developmental theory of morality. Two of the principal theorists in the cognitive developmental tradition are Jean Piaget and Lawrence Kohlberg. Because Kohlberg's theory extends and refines Piaget's, we will first look at Piaget's theory of moral development.

Moral Judgment

Piaget (1932) wrote an important and still highly influential book on moral development called *The Moral Judgment of the Child.* In this classic text, which spawned the scientific study of moral development, Piaget contended that moral development, much like cognitive development, follows an orderly, sequential path of changes. As the child progresses from preoperational to concrete operational to formal operational thinking, a parallel set of changes occurs in his or her moral judgments. Although Piaget labeled these changes moral "stages," they are really more like opposite ends of a continuum (Rest, 1983). In fact, Piaget's moral stages are much less formalized and stage-like than his cognitive stages.

In his experiments Piaget presented children with a series of double-episode short stories dealing with a moral issue. In one story pair, a little boy named John accidentally breaks 15 cups while opening a door, and another child, Henry, accidentally breaks 1 cup while trying to get some jam out of the cupboard against his parents' wishes. After presenting the stories, Piaget asked subjects if the children were equally naughty, and, if not, which was naughtier, and why. Young children generally focus only on the *objective* consequences of the action and conclude that the child who did the most damage is naughtier. In contrast, older children consider the *intentions* of the actors and conclude that Henry was naughtier because he was violating a rule. The responses of younger children parallel their tendency to describe others in terms of outward appearance and not inner qualities.

From his observations, Piaget formulated a two-stage model of moral development. In the first stage—called the *morality of constraint*—obeying the rules consists of strict obedience to authority. Rules are considered absolute and rigid and are not to be broken, regardless of circumstances (e.g., "My mommy says it's right, so it must be right."). Any transgressions of the rules inevitably result in strict and swift punishment inflicted by nature or God. This view of punishment is known as **immanent justice.** For example, a 6-year-old child who lies to her parent and then falls off her bike may see the fall as punishment for lying. Furthermore, a 6-year-old still evaluates the rightness or wrongness of behaviors in terms of objective consequences, not underlying intentions.

The second stage—called the *morality of cooperation*—begins in late childhood, around age 10 or 11. In making moral judgments, the child realizes that intentions of the person described are more important than the outcome of the act. Rules are not always followed, nor is breaking the rules always punished. Punishment, when it does occur, should be more restitutive (restoring conditions to the way they were) or equitable than expiatory (punishing for the sake of punishment). For example, a child at this stage may decide that a boy who breaks a cup while stealing jam from a cupboard should pay for the cup out of his allowance rather than simply be spanked. In general, morality comes to be characterized by a greater degree of social consciousness, cognitive abstractness, and flexibility. Piaget emphasized that interactions with peers are critical in helping the child develop a mature sense of morality. Through peer interactions, such as game playing, children learn concepts of fairness, reciprocity, sharing, and concern for others. Piaget believed that peers may be more effective than parents in promoting moral development because peers' cognitive levels are more similar to the child's.

Although Piaget's studies of children's morality were fascinating and led to a great deal of research, recent work has revealed some shortcomings. The stories used by Piaget, like the one about John and Henry, may be unfair to young children because of their difficulty level. The stories require that children remember two separate actors and two separate outcomes, and the intent of the actors is not always clearly stated. When the stories are altered so that only one actor and one intent have to be considered simultaneously, young children may show more mature forms of reasoning (Berg-Cross, 1975; S. Nelson, 1980). When told the altered versions, not only do children distinguish between good and bad intentions in making moral judgments, but they also can take into account both the intentions and consequences of an action. In addition to problems with the stories, Piaget's theory of morality overlooks many important factors in how people arrive at moral judgments. Besides intentions and consequences, other studies have shown the influence of a multitude of variables such as whether the consequences are positive or negative, whether the effects of the action are physical or psychological, and whether social sanctions follow the act (Rest, 1983). Piaget's beliefs that children's consistency of moral understanding and peer interactions would lead to high levels of moral thinking have also been challenged (Hogan & Emler, 1978; Lickona, 1976). Despite these criticisms, Piaget's ideas have been enormously influential in shaping later work.

Kohlberg's Stage Model of Moral Reasoning

Harvard psychologist Lawrence Kohlberg has formulated what is probably the most comprehensive and appealing approach to the problem of moral thinking from a cognitive developmental perspective. Building on Piaget's work, Kohlberg has proposed that morality shows a sequence of changes paralleling the cognitive stages of development. Like Piaget, Kohlberg presented subjects with a hypothetical set of stories, in this case, stories containing a *moral dilemma*. The dilemma involves choosing obedience to the rules and regulations of authority or the well-being of individuals and society. The following is Kohlberg's (1969) most famous moral dilemma:

> In Europe a woman was near death from cancer. One drug might save her, a form of radium that a druggist in the same town had recently discovered. The druggist was charging $2,000, ten times what the drug cost him to make. The sick woman's husband, Heinz, went to everyone he knew to borrow the money, but he could only get together about half of what it cost. He told the druggist his wife was dying and asked him to sell it cheaper or let him pay later. But the druggist said "No." The husband got desperate and broke into the man's store to steal the drug for his wife. Should the husband have done that? Why? (p. 379)

After presenting subjects with a series of these dilemmas, Kohlberg asked them to choose a course of action and provide reasons for their choices. The subjects' moral reasoning, not their choices per se, ultimately determines their moral levels.

Kohlberg (1963, 1969) proposed the original six-stage model of moral reasoning shown in Table 9.1. As Table 9.1 reveals, the stages are defined not by the individual's actions, but by the individual's reasons for the actions. Kohlberg believes that these stages are developmentally universal and that people the world over pass through them in a fixed, invariant sequence. People differ only in how quickly they pass through the stages and whether they reach the higher stages. Before advancing to a higher moral stage, one must understand the reasoning characteristic of a lower stage. Each new stage is accompanied by a reorganized and more complex outlook of the self in relation to society.

The six stages can be grouped into three broad developmental levels: **preconventional**—Stages 1 and 2; **conventional**—Stages 3 and 4; and

Table 9.1
Kohlberg's Original Six Stages of Moral Judgment

Level and Stage	Content of Stage		Social Perspective of Stage
	What Is Right	*Reasons for Doing Right*	
LEVEL 1—PRECONVENTIONAL Stage 1—Heteronomous Morality	To avoid breaking rules backed by punishment, obedience for its own sake, and avoiding physical damage to persons and property.	Avoidance of punishment, and the superior power of authorities.	*Egocentric point of view.*
Stage 2—Individualism, Instrumental Purpose, and Exchange	Following rules only when it is to someone's immediate interest; acting to meet one's own interests and needs and letting others do the same. Right is also what's fair, what's an equal exchange, a deal, an agreement.	To serve one's own needs or interests in a world where you have to recognize that other people have their interests, too.	*Concrete individualistic perspective.*
LEVEL II—CONVENTIONAL Stage 3—Mutual Interpersonal Expectations, Relationships, and Interpersonal Conformity	Living up to what is expected by people close to you or what people generally expect of people in your role as son, brother, friend, etc. "Being good" is important and means having good motives, showing concern about others. It also means keeping mutual relationships, such as trust, loyalty, respect, and gratitude.	The need to be a good person in your own eyes and those of others. Your caring for others. Belief in the Golden Rule. Desire to maintain rules and authority which support stereotypical behavior.	*Perspective of the individual in relationships with other individuals. Aware of shared feelings, agreements, and expectations which take primacy over individual interests.*
Stage 4—Social System and Conscience	Fulfilling the actual duties to which you have agreed. Laws are to be upheld except in extreme cases where they conflict with other fixed social duties. Right is also contributing to society, the group, or institution.	To keep the institution going as a whole, to avoid the breakdown in the system "if everyone did it," or the imperative of conscience to meet one's defined obligations. (Easily confused with Stage 3 belief in rules and authority. . . .)	*Differentiates societal point of view from interpersonal agreement or motives.*
LEVEL III—POSTCONVENTIONAL, or PRINCIPLED Stage 5—Social Contract or Utility and Individual Rights	Being aware that people hold a variety of values and opinions, that most values and rules are relative to your group. These	A sense of obligation to law because of one's social contract to make and abide by laws for the welfare of all and for the	*Prior-to-society perspective. Perspective of a rational individual aware of values and rights prior to*

Table 9.1 (Continued)

Level and Stage	Content of Stage		Social Perspective of Stage
	What Is Right	*Reasons for Doing Right*	
	relative rules should usually be upheld, however, in the interest of impartiality and because they are the social contract. Some nonrelative values and rights like *life* and *liberty*, however, must be upheld in any society and regardless of majority opinion.	protection of all people's rights. A feeling of contractual commitment, freely entered upon, to family, friendship, trust, and work obligations. Concern that laws and duties be based on rational calculation of overall utility, "the greatest good for the greatest number."	social attachments and contracts.
Stage 6—Universal Ethical Principles	Following self-chosen ethical principles. Particular laws or social agreements are usually valid because they rest on such principles. When laws violate these principles, one acts in accordance with the principle. Principles are universal principles of justice: the equality of human rights and respect for the dignity of human beings as individual persons.	The belief as a rational person in the validity of universal moral principles, and a sense of personal commitment to them.	*Perspective of a moral point of view* from which social arrangements derive.

Note: From "Moral Stages and Moralization: The Cognitive-Developmental Approach" by L. Kohlberg, 1976, in *Moral Development and Behavior: Theory, Research, and Social Issues* (pp. 34–35) edited by T. Lickona, New York: Holt, Rinehart and Winston. Copyright 1976 by Holt, Rinehart and Winston. Reprinted by permission of CBS College Publishing.

postconventional, or principled—Stages 5 and 6 (see Table 9.1). These levels can be distinguished by the moral values considered right or true. The first two stages are called preconventional, or premoral, because the individual responds to moral prescriptions of right and wrong, but interprets them according to physical needs and hedonistic consequences (i.e., what feels good is "right" and what feels bad is "wrong"). In the next two stages, the individual is concerned with maintaining social conventions and the expectations of social groups for their own sake. This concern results in a high level of conformity to the expectations of others coupled with loyalty to their values (see Box 9.3). The final two stages comprise the principled level, where the individual tries

Box 9.3   Can Moral Thinking Be Taught?

Public concern over declining moral values and standards of behavior has led to renewed interest in introducing moral education into the curricula of the nation's schools. Among the many educational programs proposed is the "just community," started by Lawrence Kohlberg in 1970 (see Muson, 1979). The just community is conceived of as an experiment in teaching moral values through open group discussions of moral dilemmas. Kohlberg first tried the just community program in a prison setting, but it has since been extended to high school settings in Massachusetts, New York, and Pennsylvania.

Currently, the just community program is composed of a cross-section of high school students who volunteer to spend part of their day taking classes in which moral issues are discussed. The students are granted full power—within limits imposed by the law and the state penal policy—to make decisions about school-related matters ranging from student theft to elective classes. The decisions are to be based on moral principles such as fairness and justice. For example, after a rash of thefts, one school's just community met and ruled that if any member of the group was the culprit, he or she should come forward, make full restitution, and apologize to the group. In this case the thief, a friend of one of the community's members, admitted stealing the missing items and apologized in front of the group. According to Kohlberg, the members' concern with protecting the interests of the community rather than those of a friend or clique of friends represents Stage 4 thinking, which is the level of thinking the program aims to achieve.

In evaluating the effects of the just community experiment, Kohlberg has claimed that participation in the classroom discussions stimulates development of higher stages of moral thinking. While most students are at Stage 2 when they enter the program, almost all have reached Stage 3 or 4 by the time they graduate. But as Kohlberg admits, much of the data on the program has not been analyzed, so that his conclusion remains in doubt.

Kohlberg's just community approach has not been free of problems or criticisms. Some educators question whether the approach can be value free or whether it reflects a liberal Ivy League emphasis on social conscience and democracy. Other educators see the emphasis on communal values as a subtle form of peer pressure and control. Finally, student participants in the program sometimes complain that theirs is only a pseudodemocracy, with the real decision-making power remaining in the hands of teachers and school administrators. For example, students at one school who voted to cancel afternoon classes were overruled by school officials. Despite these problems, the just community is a unique experiment in participatory democracy which encourages students to change their way of thinking about moral issues.

to define moral values and principles that have universal and logical validity apart from a group or society.

In order to engage in the higher levels of moral reasoning, Kohlberg assumes that a person must have achieved a certain cognitive stage. Some evidence supports this assumption. For example, adolescents who had not reached formal operations could not understand or paraphrase reasoning more advanced than their own (Rest, Turiel, & Kohlberg, 1969). Studies have also shown that the more cognitively advanced people are, the more morally advanced they are. However, the attainment of a cognitive stage does not guarantee the attainment of an equivalent moral level. People who are highly intelligent and verbal may not always be more principled in their moral judgments (Kohlberg, 1973). The moral logic of the Watergate conspirators provides a good example.

Kohlberg's theory paints a rich and provocative picture of the course of moral growth. But, like Piaget's theory, Kohlberg's has been criticized (M. Hoffman, 1979; Kurtines & Grief, 1974). Some critics' charges are that not enough empirical support exists for the stages, the stages are difficult to distinguish using Kohlberg's scoring criteria, and the theory is culturally biased toward Western democratic ideals. Another criticism is that the theory is based on a male perspective of morality emphasizing justice and rules (Gilligan, 1977, 1982). Some reports have shown that adult females typically are at Stage 3 of Kohlberg's stage sequence, whereas adult males generally are at Stage 4 (Holstein, 1976; Parikh, 1980). According to Gilligan (1977, 1982) the interpersonal orientation that women use in reasoning about moral dilemmas is no less mature than the law-and-order reasoning adopted by men. Rather each level of reasoning reflects the primary concerns associated with the female and male roles. For example, the female role emphasizes mutuality and nurturance of others, whereas the male role stresses competition and the establishment of ground rules to manage conflict.

In view of the mounting criticisms of Kohlberg's theory, some psychologists have called for its wholesale rejection (see J. Murphy & Gilligan, 1980). Other investigators have accepted the first four stages of the theory, but presented evidence that the postconventional Stages 5 and 6 do not occur in the stage sequence that Kohlberg suggested (Gibbs, 1979; Gilligan, 1977; J. Murphy & Gilligan, 1980). Kohlberg (1976, 1978) amended his theory in light of these criticisms and also revised his scoring system to make it more objective and easier to use (Kohlberg, Colby, Gibbs, & Speicher-Dubin, 1978). Kohlberg has added new substages and transitional stages to replace Stage 6 of moral development, because he feels that almost no one reaches the principled reasoning criteria of Stage 6. Originally, he expected to find some individuals whose moral thoughts and behaviors were guided by abstract concepts involving universal justice, respect for all humanity, and true equality. But few individuals—other than perhaps great religious and political leaders such as Mahatma Gandhi, Dr. Martin Luther King, Jr., or Mother Teresa—seem to reach this lofty plateau.

Moral Reasoning beyond Adolescence

In his original theory, Kohlberg felt that the fifth stage of moral reasoning was achieved by the end of high school or, at the latest, young adulthood. The major change in moral development beyond adolescence, Kohlberg believed, was stabilization prior to reaching the highest stage (Stage 6), rather than the development of new stages. In some early work Kohlberg and Kramer (1969) reported an apparent regression in moral thinking before individuals attained the highest stage. They observed that around the sophomore year of college, individuals did not use the highest moral stages of which they were capable (Stages 4 and 5), but returned to a Stage 2 moral hedonism level. Kohlberg and Kramer (1969) interpreted these findings in terms of Erikson's concepts of identity crisis and identity *moratorium* (i.e., a person has not established an identity but is seeking commitments). Before individuals can achieve morally principled thought, they must make a commitment to do so.

Closer observation forced Kohlberg to reconsider his initial argument (Kohlberg, 1973; Turiel, 1974) and reject the notion that fully stabilized, principled thought is attained by the end of high school. Rather, he created a Stage 4½, in which individuals have rejected the conventional morality of adolescence, but have not constructed the principled reasoning of Stage 5:

> Fully-principled or Stage 5 and especially Stage 6 thinking is an adult development, typically not reached until the late twenties or later. Structural development and stabilization are not two different things. The fact that the apparently Stage 5 thinking of high school students was vulnerable to retrogression or was not yet stabilized was, in fact, evidence for the fact that such thinking was not really principled. (Kohlberg, 1973, p. 190)

To reach the highest stages of principled moral judgment, one needs to be faced with "sustained responsibility for the welfare of others" and irreversible moral choices (Kohlberg, 1973, p. 196). Only rarely do students have such experience.

Although Kohlberg's (1973) reformulation resolves the problem of regression in adult moral thought, it does not explain the unique features of the adult moral experience. Why would one expect adult experiences to lead to the type of abstract moral reasoning displayed by the bright high school students in Kohlberg's original studies? J. Murphy and Gilligan (1980) have argued that the key to understanding adult morality lies in the balancing of abstract, logical concepts of equality, justice, and reciprocity with real-life experiences of moral conflict and choice. Therefore, they propose reconceptualizing principled moral thinking within a contextualistic framework.

To illustrate the embedding of moral principles within the wider context of social reality, consider the following story told by an adult in response to the Heinz dilemma. In the story, he is responding to his own postconventional response to the same dilemma six years earlier.

> This is a very crisp little dilemma and you can latch onto that principle pretty fast and in that situation you can say that life is more important than money. But then, when you reflect back on how you really act in your own life, you don't use that principle, or I haven't yet used that principle to operate on. And none of the people who answer that dilemma that way use that principle to operate on because they were blowing $7,000 a year for their education at Harvard instead of giving it to the Children's Fund to give porridge to the kids in Botswana and to that extent answering the dilemma with that principle is not hypocritical, it's just that you don't recognize it. I hadn't recognized it at the time, and I am sure they don't recognize it either. (Gilligan & Murphy, 1979, p. 24)

After reading this dilemma, you should recognize the contextual dependency of the respondent's answer. His answer reflects an attempt to choose among alternative courses of action that are not entirely context free. What, then, is the major change in moral development in adulthood? According to Labouvie-Vief (1982), the major change is not simply a matter of perfecting logic, but consists of relating logic to other systems—action, affect, interpersonal relations—which have previously developed in a largely parallel fashion.

Perry (1970) investigated this issue in his study of Harvard University students' movement from logical reasoning to moral relativism or contextualism (see Chapter 8). As freshmen these students seemed to be searching for a single path to truth, but were profoundly troubled when they found that many of the problems confronting them (e.g., choice of a mate or occupational role) could not be solved with logical reasoning alone. Gradually they realized that no logical certainty, no single correct answer, existed. Exposed to professors and classmates with diverse viewpoints and confronting the possibility of multiple contexts for truth, the students eventually adopted a relativistic stance toward morality. This relativism was accompanied by a sense of responsibility and moral commitment. Students realized that although no single moral orientation is objectively correct, some positions are better than others and are worth caring about (J. Murphy & Gilligan, 1980).

The research reported by Perry (1970), Gilligan (1977, 1982), and others is a useful step in building a life-span theory of moral development. Whereas in the context of the absolute logic of adolescent thinking, adult morality may be interpreted as "retrogression" or decline, this reconceptualization transforms it into a higher level of development. Thus, the current work on adult moral development seems to parallel the work on higher-level concepts such as wisdom and problem finding discussed in Chapter 8.

Given that young adults' thinking shows a considerable amount of moral relativism, would we expect older people to show such relativism, perhaps even to a greater degree? Answers to this question are speculative. In one cross-sectional study, Bielby and Papalia (1975) reported that moral reasoning is at its highest level in middle age (30–49 years) and declines significantly from age 50 onward. Even in middle age, consistent with Kohlberg's theory, the majority of people are at the second, or conventional, level of development (Stages 3 and 4). After age 50, the individual's level of moral reasoning regresses to Stage 2 or 3. Whether this regression represents a true decline in moral reasoning skills or is a cohort-related phenomenon is not clear. Perhaps older adults grew up in a cultural environment which emphasized obedience to external rules and authority. Alternatively, the observed adult declines in moral reasoning can be seen as the product of the age-inappropriateness of the moral dilemmas used to assess moral thought (Rybash, Roodin, & Hoyer, 1983). Rybash et al. (1983) report that the moral dilemmas faced by older adults seldom involve abstract principles of equity and justice (i.e., postconventional level), but revolve around real-life experiences. These concerns include problems involving family members such as whether to give or take advice, caregiving and living arrangements, and financial matters. Thus, moral reasoning may take on a more pragmatic function in later life, reflecting the major developmental concerns of the age period. Or older adults simply may have less emotional energy to invest in the legalistic and philosophical problems embodied in Kohlberg's higher stages of morality (Roodin, Rybash, & Hoyer, 1984; Rybash et al., 1983). But this would not automatically mean that they use less mature forms of moral reasoning.

RELATIONS OF SOCIAL
COGNITION TO SOCIAL BEHAVIOR

Earlier in this chapter we compared the paradigmatic orientations of investigators in the cognitive and social domains of research. Cognitive theorists primarily concentrate on internal processes and operations that undergo transformations or reorganizations with development. By contrast, social behavioral theorists emphasize observable social behaviors and the causal role of external environmental stimuli in shaping social development. However, very little research has examined social cognitive–social behavioral relations. Probably the most espoused position is that social cognitive abilities should be positively related to the occurrence of **prosocial behaviors,** which are behaviors intended to benefit another person without the expectation of a personal reward. Such behaviors include cooperation, altruism, friendliness, generosity, and kindness (Feshbach, 1978; M. Hoffman, 1977b, 1983; Kohlberg, 1969).

The ability to take other people's affective perspectives, or *empathize* with them, is seen as critical in the development of prosocial behavior. Therefore, the development of **empathy** is the focus of this section. M. Hoffman (1983) has maintained that empathy reduces to two major categories: (1) *cognitive awareness* and (2) *vicarious affective responses.* The first category involves our conscious awareness of other persons' inner feelings (e.g., perceptions, thoughts, emotions, intentions); the second category concerns our affective response to other persons which is more appropriate to their situations than our own.

M. Hoffman (1977b, 1979) has formulated one of the two major theories of empathy (Feshbach's, 1978, theory is the other). M. Hoffman focuses on the vicarious affect of empathy, although he makes clear that the cognitive aspects of empathy cannot be ignored. For example, imagining oneself in another's shoes is a cognitive process that triggers an empathetic response (M. Hoffman, 1977). Hoffman believes that children pass through four social cognitive stages in developing empathetic responses. In addition to feeling what others feel, the child increasingly realizes that the source of affect (e.g., distress, pain) lies in the other's situation and not the self.

The first stage, *global empathy,* lasts for most of the first year of life. Because infants have not differentiated themselves from other people, they have trouble distinguishing who is experiencing any distress they witness. They sometimes act as if what is happening to others is happening to them and respond with a global empathic distress response. As an example, Hoffman described an 11-month-old who saw another child fall down and cry. The child responded by putting her thumb in her mouth and burying her head in her mother's lap, which were her usual responses when she was injured.

The second stage, *egocentric empathy,* occurs after the child has differentiated between self and others (around age 1 or 2). Now the child begins to experience empathetic distress, but realizes that another individual—and not the self—is the victim. But children's understanding is limited. They still experience difficulty distinguishing between their own and others' inner states and tend to confuse them. M. Hoffman (1983) cited the example of a 13-month-old who responded with a distressed look to an adult who appeared sad and then offered the adult his favorite toy. Hoffman points out that such behavior is not entirely egocentric because the child is responding with the appropriate affect, even though he fails to distinguish between what comforts himself and what comforts others.

As role-taking abilities begin to develop around age 2 or 3, a third stage of empathy, *empathy for another's feelings,* is attained. Children come to realize that other people's feelings may differ from their own and that others' perspectives are based on other interpretations, needs, and emotions. As children begin to appreciate the independence of their own and others' feelings, they become more cautious about falsely attributing certain causes to what others are feeling. Even as young as age 4, children can recognize others' affective cues (e.g., sadness, happiness, anger) and respond appropriately (Borke, 1971). Language ability is important here because the child starts to recognize verbal cues of emotion, not just physical, nonverbal ones such as facial expression.

In late childhood (8–12 years of age), as children develop a more differentiated concept of self, they become aware that other people have feelings that extend beyond the immediate situation. M. Hoffman calls this fourth and final stage *empathy for another's general plight.* Although children may respond empathically to a person's present distress, they now show even greater concern when they realize that such distress may be chronic and not transitory. At this stage, the child can empathize with the plight of an entire social group or class, such as the retarded, handicapped, poor, or oppressed. This general empathic distress may include the child's awareness that providing a meal to a group of starving people does not automatically solve their hunger problem. Hoffman sees this awareness as the highest level of empathy, which can lead adolescents and adults to political and social action to relieve the plight of disadvantaged groups.

One important factor that determines whether people actually help others is the **attribution** they make about the cause of others' plight. Attributions are the inferences we draw about the causes for others', as well as our own, behavior. The majority of attribution theories (Heider, 1958; E. Jones & Davis, 1965; Kelley, 1973) deal with the way adults infer when given only a limited amount of information about another's behavior, feelings, and situation. Although attribution theories differ widely in their concepts, they all distinguish two major causes of behavior: (1) internal causes (abilities, effort, attitude) and (2) external causes (situational circumstances, luck). For example, in Kelley's (1973) model, behavior that occurs in certain situations in most people most of the time is seen as caused by external or environmental factors. Behavior occasionally shown by a few people is thought to have an internal locus.

Let us consider these two categories of causes in relation to the development of empathetic affect. Imagine that you are observing a person who appears to be asking for money. If you believe the person is responsible for his plight, you may end up blaming him for the distress you observe. In this case, you are unlikely to respond empathetically. But suppose that the clues indicate that another person is to blame for this person's distress, say, an employer who has unjustly fired him. In this instance, you may empathize with the person and direct the blame toward the employer.

What happens when no information is available about who is responsible for the person's plight? Here, the tendency seems to be to overestimate the importance of internal, personal factors and to "blame the victim" for her distress (Nisbett, Borgida, Crandall, & Reed, 1976; L. Ross, 1977). This internal attribution is used by many individuals to support a "just world" hypothesis (i.e., people get what they deserve). Despite this tendency to blame the victim, people still show an almost universal tendency to empathize with others (M. Hoffman, 1981). How much we empathize with the plight of others is affected by different factors. If the person's distress becomes too intense, we may direct most of our attention to ourselves in order to avoid an aversive situation. Individuals will also empathize more with people who they perceive as similar to themselves in either physical (e.g., sex, race) or psychological (e.g., personality) characteristics. M. Hoffman (1979) has suggested that moral education which points out similarities between people may foster feelings of empathy.

TOWARD DEVELOPMENT OF THE WHOLE PERSON

Psychologists generally acknowledge that cognitive and social affective processes are equally significant in humans' functioning. Yet cognitive psychologists especially have tended to regard the cognitions people bring to laboratory situations as primary, and social affective phenomena as relatively unimportant. The research cited in this chapter, however, shows that children's and adults' social development and its relationship to cognition cannot be ignored. Nor should the importance of affect as a major component of social cognition be overlooked. The study of affective development has long been one of the most neglected areas of research across the life span (Malatesta, 1981).

Although it is beyond the scope of this chapter to discuss the full range of social and affective phenomena to which a life-span analysis of cognition may apply, we can suggest a few components that a developmental model of the "whole person" should include. First, the model should be bidirectional rather than unidirectional (D. Kuhn, 1978). Affective responses influence our cognitive systems, just as cognitions influence our affect. Therefore, the view of human beings as passive, information-processing computers, uninfluenced by affective evaluations, should be modified.

In a highly influential and controversial essay in the *American Psychologist*, Robert Zajonc (1980) has gone so far as to argue that affective reactions are primary (see also Zajonc, 1984). In reacting to various kinds of stimuli (e.g., voices, faces, shapes), people often form affective preferences before they engage in much cognitive activity. For example, one cannot be introduced to another individual without immediately forming some subjective impression of like or dislike. Zajonc has even proposed the existence of two relatively independent information-processing systems—one for affective information and the other for cognitive information. Figure 9.4 shows you his information-processing model of affect. You may want to compare this model to the information-processing model presented in Figure 6.2.

If valid, Zajonc's model could have major implications for developmental studies of cognition. For example, Flavell and Ross (1981) have speculated that psychologists might need to rethink the whole area of infant visual responding (see Chapter 3). Until now, psychologists have thought of infant visual preferences to patterned stimuli as reflecting cognitive judgments, but perhaps these preferences are better thought of as primary affective reactions. The recent flurry of research activity on early affective development (Izard, 1977, 1978; Oster, 1978) should be extended to other age populations and to complex, ambiguous emotions such as jealousy or chagrin.

Figure 9.4   A general information-processing model of affect.

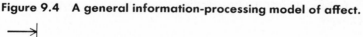

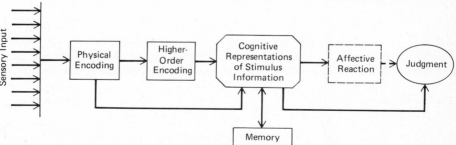

From "Feeling and Thinking: Preferences Need No Inferences" by R. B. Zajonc, 1980, *American Psychologist, 35,* p. 153. Copyright 1980 by the American Psychological Association. Reprinted by permission.

A life-span model of the whole person also needs to take into account the changing relation between the social behaviors of children and adults and their cognitive abilities. Researchers in cognitive development have typically not been concerned about how cognitive stages or sequences in development may lead to certain behaviors within particular situations. For example, current methods of assessing moral judgments rely heavily on verbal reasoning about hypothetical dilemmas. To what extent these verbal reports relate to moral behavior in realistic situations is unclear (see Blasi, 1980, for a review). In one of the few studies on this subject, Haan, Smith, and Block (1968) examined the relationship between moral reasoning and civil disobedience in students attending the University of California at the time of the sit-ins during the 1960s. Haan et al. (1968) found that 80 percent of the students who participated in the sit-ins were at a principled moral level, compared to only 10 percent who were at a conventional level. However, 60 percent of the students who were at a preconventional level also participated. As these results show, similar types of behavior can stem from different levels of moral reasoning. This suggests that both internal cognitions and external environmental events (e.g., peer influence) may be influencing behavior. A model of the whole human being would need to incorporate both of these causal factors.

Finally, psychology in general needs to know when certain cognitive judgments, inferences, or events lead to appropriate behavioral outcomes and when they do not. We do not want to risk portraying human beings as attending, remembering, creating, and problem-solving creatures who never *do* anything (Flavell & Ross, 1981). Perhaps children and adults engage in a great deal of thoughtless or mindless behavior in their everyday interactions (E. Langer, 1978; Taylor & Fiske, 1978). They may approach most routine social situations using global intuition and impression and reserve complex cognitive inferential processes for situations where routine habits and behaviors cannot be applied. The systematic relationship between thoughts, feelings, and behaviors across the life span remains uncharted territory for developmental research.

SUMMARY

1. Social cognition deals with the way one conceptualizes and reasons about the self and others. Following years of neglect, largely caused by the paradigmatic isolation of cognitive and social

researchers, social cognition has suddenly become a "hot topic" in developmental psychology.

2. All knowledge is basically social—rooted in the language, beliefs, and customs of a particular culture. However, knowing people differs from knowing objects in several important ways. The range of actions on people is greater and less predictable than on objects, and relations between people are more complex than relations between objects and people.

3. Flavell has proposed a useful model for predicting social inferences. According to Flavell, the four steps in the development of a social inference are (1) existence, (2) need, (3) inference, and (4) application.

4. Conceptions of one's self are important for understanding others. The development of a self-concept is evident as early as 1½ years of age. Children's descriptions of self focus on external, physical qualities; adolescents' descriptions are more abstract, internal, and differentiated. Self-concept appears fairly stable over the adolescent and adult years.

5. The area of research dealing with the way we describe the inner and outer qualities of other people is called person perception. People's descriptions of others seem to parallel the way they describe themselves.

6. Developmental changes in descriptions of others can be characterized as a shift from egocentric to other-oriented conceptions. Although egocentrism is most profound in early infancy, various forms of egocentric thinking persist into adolescence and adulthood.

7. Role-taking or perspective-taking ability requires nonegocentric thinking. Selman has identified five stages of role taking in childhood and adolescence, characterized initially by a high level of subjectivism and later by the ability to take the perspective of a third person or group.

8. Several training programs have been developed to teach role-taking and interpersonal problem-solving skills. These programs try to help people recognize the consequences of their actions and generate multiple solutions to problems.

9. Moral development provides an important link between the individual and society. Piaget and Kohlberg have proposed two major stage models of morality. In Piaget's model, children pass from a morality of constraint to a morality of cooperation. Kohlberg's revised model includes five developmental stages of moral reasoning.

10. The ability to empathize with others is seen as an influential factor in the development of prosocial behavior. M. Hoffman has pro-

posed one of the major developmental theories of empathy. He believes empathy contains both a cognitive and an affective component.

11. Attribution theories deal with the causes we infer about the behavior of self and others. Causes can be categorized as internal or external. How we interpret the cause of another's behavior partly determines our response to it.

12. Cognition is not exclusively important in studying development. The study of the whole person must involve changing relationships between cognitive, social, and affective factors across the life span.

Key Terms

social cognition

self-concept

totalism

semantic differential scale

person perception

egocentrism

perspectivism

imaginary audience

personal fable

role taking

immanent justice

preconventional

conventional

postconventional

prosocial behaviors

empathy

attribution

Suggested Readings

Chandler, M. J., & Boyes, M. (1982). Social-cognitive development. In B. Wolman (Ed.), *Handbook of developmental psychology* (pp. 387–402). Englewood Cliffs, NJ: Prentice-Hall. This transactional approach to social cognitive development focuses on the interaction of the structure of the organism and structure of the stimulus environment. It summarizes developmental steps in role-taking ability and moral thinking.

Izard, C. E., Kagan, J., & Zajonc, R. B. (Eds.). (1984). *Emotions, cognition, and behavior.* New York: Cambridge University Press. This book marks an attempt to bring together contributions to the study of emotions from the diverse areas of cognitive psychology, developmental psychology, psychophysiology, and personality-clinical psychology. It contains many innovative suggestions for examining the emotion-cognition interaction and relationships.

Kurtines, W. M., & Gewirtz, J. (Eds.). (1984). *Morality, moral behavior, and moral development.* New York: Wiley. This comprehensive collection of writings by leading scholars on current theory and research in the area of morality and moral development includes sections on cognitive developmental, constructivist, learning behavioral, and social personality theory approaches to moral development. Directions for future work also are described.

Lamb, M. E., & Sherrod, L. R. (Eds.). (1981). *Infant social cognition: Empirical and the-*

retical considerations. Hillsdale, NJ: Erlbaum. Each chapter in this volume deals with how infants acquire knowledge about the social environment and their role in it. Among the important issues discussed are how infants recognize and remember social objects, how they make inferences about other people's emotions and behaviors, and how they attribute meaning to their social experience. One of the best resources available on infant social cognition.

Masters, J. C., & Yarkin-Levin, K. (Eds.). (1984). *Boundary areas in social and developmental psychology.* New York: Academic Press. This book focuses on the different perspectives social and developmental psychology bring to problems in theory and research. Chapters deal with social processes in peer relationships, cognitive and social aspects of group influence processes, and developmental changes in children's understanding of the social world.

CHAPTER 10

Intervention in Cognitive Development

OVERVIEW

In the past two decades, intervention has been used increasingly to modify the course of cognitive development. This chapter examines the types, goals, levels, and strategies of intervention. Each of these aspects of intervention overlaps considerably with the others and cannot be understood in isolation. This chapter also looks at theoretical and ethical issues in planning and evaluating intervention research programs. Interventions differ in their substantive emphasis. Some are conducted primarily for theoretical reasons, others for practical reasons. However, neither is exclusive of the other. The goals of intervention also differ. Some interventions aim at removing an immediate problem behavior, whereas others seek to prevent the occurrence or recurrence of a problem or to enhance functioning beyond its normal level.

Once the goals of intervention are identified, the level of intervention must be determined. Interventions can aim at individuals, a small group of individuals, or societal institutions using an array of different strategies and training procedures. In predicting and evaluating the outcomes of intervention, psychologists need to consider important developmental issues such as the relative amount of plasticity or modifiability at different age levels and the degree of generalization of training across related and unrelated tasks. They must also consider the ethical issues involved in interfering with the natural course of development and terminating successful intervention programs.

THE CONCEPT OF INTERVENTION

The concept of **intervention** does not have a single, precise meaning. Various terms such as *education, reform, rehabilitation, remediation, training, prevention, enrichment, therapy,* and *treatment* have been used at one time or another to describe intervention (Reese & Overton, 1980). According to the dictionary, to "intervene" means to come between or interfere with the affairs of others. In the present context, "intervention" refers to the systematic attempt to modify the course of cognitive development and aging for purposes of preventing cognitive deficits and enhancing cognitive functioning and psychological well-being.

As mentioned in Chapter 1, the initial focus in developmental and gerontological research was the description of normative changes, rather than their explanation or modification. In child developmental work, pioneer researchers such as Arnold Gesell attempted to catalog descriptively children's physical and behavioral characteristics at different stages in development. Likewise, gerontological research efforts described the cognitive deficits of older people relative to younger comparison groups. In fact, Kastenbaum (1968) chided gerontological researchers for simply "counting and classifying the wrinkles of aged behavior" (p. 282). However, as Baltes and Danish (1980) wisely have noted, the descriptive phase in early developmental work was probably a valid and necessary step in establishing a preliminary knowledge base.

In the past 20 years, psychologists and educators have made numerous attempts to intervene in the normal course of cognitive development and aging. Because intervention is a relatively new and untested concept, not all psychologists understand the purposes of intervention or readily accept the need for such research. Therefore, we need to review the two major types of intervention research.

TYPES OF INTERVENTION RESEARCH

Following a proposal made by Flavell (1985), the types of intervention research can be grouped into two broad categories: theoretical-developmental and practical-educational. These two areas will be discussed separately, but the theoretical and practical sides of intervention are not easily distinguished. Traditionally, intervention was seen as the application of existing theoretical knowledge to a problem of "applied" importance such as designing a more effective educational program. However, intervention concerns not only the application of knowledge derived from theory but also the production of new theoretical knowledge (Baltes & Willis, 1977; A. Brown, Bransford, Ferrara, & Campione, 1983; Montada & Schmitt, 1982). As A. Brown et al. (1983) have pointed out, intervention is a powerful means of constructing and evaluating cognitive theory. By understanding something about the underlying cognitive processes involved and something about developmental differences, psychologists should be in a better position to intervene in cognitive development more effectively. Furthermore, the outcome of such efforts will allow psychologists to evaluate the adequacy of their theories and alter them if necessary (A. Brown et al., 1983).

Theoretical-Developmental Research

Intervention studies in cognitive development differ in their substantive emphasis. Most aim to establish the range of modifiability, or *plasticity*, in cognitive development. Such intervention studies are called "training" studies. They address the question of cognitive potential in children and adults (Baltes & Danish, 1980; A. Brown & French, 1979; Carlson & Wiedl, 1978). That is, how much can individuals of varying ages profit from a certain type of laboratory training or educational experience?

Training studies are not usually undertaken to facilitate cognitive functioning in the real world, although they may produce this effect. Rather, their objective is to identify the alternative forms of development that can emerge under varying experimental conditions. Thus, intervention studies move us beyond the descriptive phase of research to questions about why and how development occurs.

In the child development literature, the majority of training studies have focused on the Piagetian stages of cognitive development. In their most general form, these studies usually assume that a specific environmental experience is instrumental in the acquisition of some Piagetian concept (e.g., conservation). The investigator first assesses the child's preexperimental knowledge of the concept. The child who fails most or all of the items assessing the concept is selected for training. Next, a treatment (or intervention) is introduced, followed by a postexperimental assessment and follow-up. If the treatment is successful, then the child's performance in the postexperimental period should exceed that of the preexperimental period compared to a no-treatment control group. Ideally, the posttest period should extend over several weeks so that training effects can be evaluated more accurately (Brainerd, 1983).

Some examples from the training literature on the acceleration of the natural process of conservation will help you understand the basic design of these studies. Developmental psychologists have used a variety of training procedures to accelerate the acquisition of conservation skills (see Brainerd, 1974; Inhelder, Sinclair, & Bovet, 1974; Kingsley & Hall, 1967; Murray, 1978). As Chapter 7 noted, conservation reflects a general understanding about invariant relationships among objects. One group of conservation studies focuses on the use of attentional training strategies. These studies have suggested that children's failure to solve conservation problems may be due not to cognitive limitations such as a lack of reversible thinking, but to limitations in perceptual cue processes. The hypothesis is that children fail to conserve because they attend to perceptually irrelevant aspects of the problem such as shape, color, and spatial orientation.

In a frequently cited study, Gelman (1969) employed discrimination learning procedures to train 5-year-olds to attend to the relevant stimuli on number and length conservation tasks. On each learning trial children saw three rows of stimulus objects; two rows contained the identical quantity, and one row contained a different quantity. Children were asked to point out the row with the "different" objects. In some cases, the objects were arranged so that two of the three rows contained the identical number of objects (e.g., two rows of five chips and one row of three chips). In other cases, the objects were arranged so that two of the three rows were the same length (e.g., two 6-inch sticks and one 10-inch stick). Thus, in order to solve the problems, children had to learn to discriminate whether number (or length) was relevant or irrelevant. They also had to ignore irrelevant cues that changed from problem to problem (e.g., color of the chips, size and shape of the sticks, spatial orientation of the objects). Gelman found that not only did the attentional training procedures improve performance on the conservation tasks for number and length, but they also generalized to untrained concepts such as conservation of mass and liquid. In addition, children continued to conserve when they were tested two or three weeks later.

Gelman initially concluded that the attentional training provided to the children produced the improvements, but she now admits there are other interpretations (see Gelman & Baillargeon, 1983). Perhaps Gelman induced **cognitive conflict** in her subjects by presenting different perceptual and quantitative cues. Conflict procedures are frequently used by Piagetian researchers to induce contradictions in children's reasoning (Inhelder et al., 1974). According to equilibration theory (Piaget, 1971), only when children sense a conflict between two contradictory answers will they rethink their original responses. The internal disequilibrium induced by the contradiction leads children to reorganize their thoughts, thereby furthering their own cognitive development. For example, Inhelder et al. (1974) had children place 10 small clay balls into a tall, narrow glass and 10 small balls of clay into a short, wide glass. The children dropped the balls one at a time into each glass simultaneously. If children focused on the height of the beakers, they erroneously said that the tall, narrow glass contained more balls. But counting the balls contradicted the children's perception and led them to eventually conclude that height compensated for width and that both glasses contained the same number of balls.

Attempts to train conservation of number (Field, 1981; Gelman, 1969; Sigel & Hooper, 1968) have generally been more successful than efforts involving other types of conservation, suggesting that number may be an easier concept for children to grasp. In an initial series of studies, Norwegian psychologist Jan Smedslund (1961a, 1961b, 1961c) tried to train children on weight conservation using three different training techniques: training of weighing operations, teaching an addition-subtraction rule, and perceptual set training. In one of his studies, Smedslund (1961a) showed children aged 5–7 a ball of clay and asked them to judge sameness of weight after the ball had been misshapened. By using a balance scale, Smedslund showed the children that a misshapened piece of clay continues to weigh the same as a piece not deformed. After seeing this weighing demonstration several times, children began to give conserving responses (e.g., "You just changed the shape" and "You didn't add anything").

But then Smedslund altered the experiment to show how fragile the trained conservation responses were. He repeated the procedure described above, but secretly removed a small piece of clay as he was misshaping it. When asked which should weigh more, the children said both balls of clay should weigh the same. They were surprised to see that the balance scale showed the misshapened ball weighed less. Children's reactions to this event varied, however, by whether they had been nonconservers initially and received additional training or whether they had been conservers and did not receive additional training. The nonconservers who had been trained returned to their pretest performance and accepted the unequal weight without suspicion or questioning. On the other hand, the untrained conserving children reacted with surprise and attempted to explain the unusual event ("You must have taken some clay away" or "A piece fell on the floor").

Smedslund concluded that the trained children were imitating an adult-provided rule without really understanding or accepting it. When confronted with a novel situation, their trained responses extinguished. Children who had acquired conservation naturally (without training) had a deeper grasp of conservation and were able to explain the unanticipated event satisfactorily.

Developmental investigators in North America quickly challenged Smedslund's conclusions (see Beilin, 1965; Kingsley & Hall, 1967; Murray, 1978). Using an assortment of ingenious training procedures, these investigators succeeded in training most of the basic varieties of conservation. From an extensive review of such research studies, Brainerd and Allen (1971) concluded that short-term training experiences can improve conservation performance. However, their major criterion for a "successful" training study was the statistical significance of the posttest difference between the training and no-training groups on the various indices of conservation. As D. Kuhn (1974) has indicated, Piagetian researchers insist on a different set of criteria. In order to show that a trained child has truly attained conservation, three Piagetian criteria must be met. (1) The child must be able to justify the conservation response by providing an appropriate explanation. (2) The response must persist over time. (3) The response should generalize to problems not used in training. In addition, genuinely conserving children should be able to resist a cognitive challenge (i.e., apparently disconfirming evidence) from the experimenter, something that trained subjects in Smedslund's (1961a) study failed to do. Prior to the 1970s few training studies satisfied these three criteria, but recent studies have provided more definitive evidence on the trainability of conservation. As you will read later in this chapter, questions remain about the relative effectiveness of the various training techniques (e.g., Piagetian versus non-Piagetian) and the need to consider the child's stage or level of cognitive functioning in training Piagetian concepts.

In the adult development literature, training studies have focused on attempts to modify performance on standardized intelligence measures. Because fluid intelligence has been reported to show age-related decline in adulthood (Cattell, 1971; Horn, 1970, 1978), intervention efforts have been most often targeted at fluid abilities. The theoretical rationale for these studies is that evidence on the trainability or reversibility of fluid declines should provide strong support for the notion of plasticity in human intellectual functioning because such declines are thought to be based on irreversible, biological processes (Baltes & Goulet, 1971). However, the results of training studies do not allow us to ignore totally the influence of biological decrements.

Baltes, Willis, and co-workers have put together a well-designed and systematic training research program as part of the Adult Development and Enrichment Project (ADEPT) at The Pennsylvania State University (Blieszner, Willis, & Baltes, 1981; Hofland, Willis, & Baltes, 1981; Willis, Blieszner, & Baltes, 1981). One of their studies examined the degree to which a component of fluid intelligence called figural relations could be modified (Willis et al., 1981). *Figural relations,* often considered a pure primary ability of fluid intelligence (see Cattell, 1971; Horn, 1970), is defined by tasks involving the detection of relations within figural patterns (see Figure 10.1). Fifty-eight old adult subjects (mean age 69.8 years) participated in the study, with about half being assigned to a training condition and the other half to a no-training control condition. Four different training sessions were conducted, each focusing on one of four types of figural relations problems—series (see Figure 10.1*a*), classification (see Figure 10.1*b*), topology (see Figure 10.1*c*), and matrix (see Figure 10.1*d*). A fifth training session involved a review of the four types of problems. During the training sessions the trainer modeled verbal rules associated with the problems and gave subjects practice in using the rules. Subjects also received feedback about their performance and participated in group discussion.

The effects of training were assessed across three different posttests (at one week, one month, and six months). A broad array of fluid and crystallized measures was used to assess the training outcomes. To evaluate the generalizability of the training, transfer effects were examined using the pattern of transfer predicted from the fluid-crystallized theory of intelligence and the level of similarity of the transfer measures to the training program content. The transfer measures were of two types: **near transfer** (measures containing content similar to the training measures) and **far transfer** (measures containing content not closely

Figure 10.1   Examples of four types of figural relations problems. (a) series, (b) classification, (c) topology, (d) matrices.

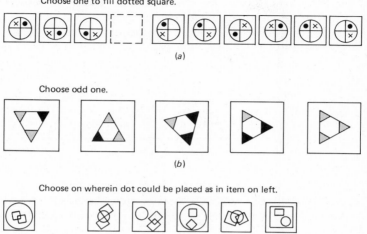

Choose one to fill dotted square.

(a)

Choose odd one.

(b)

Choose on wherein dot could be placed as in item on left.

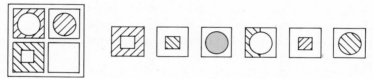

(c)

Choose one to fill empty square at left.

(d)

From *Test of "g": Culture Fair* (Scales II and III), by R. B. Cattell and A. K. S. Cattell, 1957, Champaign, IL: Institute for Personality and Ability Testing. Copyright 1957 by R. B. Cattell. Reprinted by permission.

related to the training measures). Far transfer was further divided into two levels: (1) far fluid transfer to another fluid ability and (2) far non-fluid transfer to perceptual speed and crystallized intelligence abilities.

Willis et al.'s (1981) results revealed no significant differences between the training group and the control group on two fluid measures prior to the training sessions. Following training, however, significant differences between the two groups were obtained (see Figure 10.2); and these effects were maintained over a six-month period. Notice in Figure 10.2 that the differences between the two groups are larger for the three near transfer measures (ADEPT Figural Relations Test, Culture Fair Tests, Raven's matrices) than for the four far transfer measures (ADEPT Induction, Induction Composite, Perceptual Speed, Vocabulary). Willis and associates (1981) argued that this pattern of differential transfer would be expected from fluid-crystallized theory. The

Figure 10.2 Mean standardized scores on seven transfer measures for training and control groups averaged across three posttest occasions.

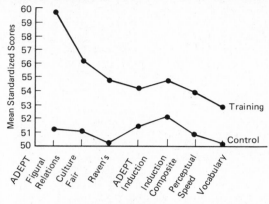

From "Intellectual Training Research in Aging: Modification of Performance on the Fluid Ability of Figural Relations," by S. L. Willis, R. Blieszner, and P. B. Baltes, 1981, *Journal of Educational Psychology, 73*, p. 45. Copyright 1981 by the American Psychological Association. Reprinted by permission.

smaller training effect on the far transfer measures may be due to situational or ability-extraneous factors such as increased testwiseness, response speed improvements, and anxiety reduction. Willis et al.'s data also showed that both the training and control groups evinced significant practice effects across posttest sessions, and these effects did not follow the differential pattern of training transfer. Practice effects noted in training studies with younger and older adults (Hofland et al., 1981; Labouvie-Vief & Gonda, 1976) also provide strong evidence for the plasticity of intellectual functioning because these effects occurred with limited feedback or instruction.

The findings from training studies of children and adults suggest that many cognitive abilities evidence greater plasticity or modifiability than typically acknowledged. Such findings have major implications not only for developmental theory but also for planning educational programs and policy for various age segments of the population. These findings suggest the feasibility of designing special intervention programs to train, enhance, and maintain cognitive development across the life span. We now turn to such large-scale programs.

Practical-Educational Research

In the 1960s many psychologists and educators became quite concerned with the mounting evidence that children from low social class backgrounds perform poorly in school and on standardized intelligence tests. With governmental assistance, professionals began to develop a series of educational intervention programs for children from socially disadvantaged backgrounds. The most visible public program that resulted from these efforts was Project Head Start, although various other special intervention programs existed, some of which preceded Head Start (see Horowitz & Paden, 1973). These programs varied in duration (summer, full year) and approach, but they all shared the beliefs that the early effects of environmental deprivation could be reversed, or at least neutralized, and that providing an enriched environment would enable preschool children to cope better with the demands of school.

The immediate goal of Project Head Start was practical: to help children acquire the requisite cognitive skills for academic work. Another pragmatic goal was to improve the physical health of children by giving them medical and dental examinations one or two years before they normally had health examinations (Horowitz & Paden, 1973). Beyond these practical goals was a theoretical goal involving the relative effects of nurture (environment) and nature (genetics) on childhood development. During the 1960s evidence on the effects of early environmental experience on later development had generated optimism about altering the course of development (B. Bloom, 1964; Hunt, 1961; Skeels, 1966). Moreover, this research suggested that the optimal time for intervention was during the first few years of life. Therefore, designers of Head Start assumed that developmental outcomes are not immutably fixed by genetic background, but have the potential to be changed by programmed environmental experience.

One of the most intense and successful early intervention programs was developed by Rick Heber and colleagues at the University of Wisconsin Infant Education Center (Garber & Heber, 1982; Heber, Garber, Harrington, & Hoffman, 1972). The treatment program, called the Milwaukee Project, involved a group of children chosen from disadvantaged families whose mothers had IQs below 75. All of these children and a comparable control group were considered at high risk for mental retardation. The children in the treatment condition received regular daily visits from a special teacher beginning at ages 3–6 months. Then the children began to spend several hours each day at the center, where they were exposed to a variety of intellectual stimulation experiences under the supervision of a trained adult paraprofessional. During this time, their mothers received rehabilitation training which included job training, home management, and remedial education. After 2 years of age, the children attended the center's classes for the entire day with small groups of adult teachers and different-sized groups of children. The all-day program included learning experiences such as language training, free play, viewing *Sesame Street*, problem-solving sessions, and science and art periods. Later in the program, two additional teachers were introduced to teach reading and mathematics. Children continued in the program until they reached age 6 or entered elementary school.

The results of the Milwaukee Project revealed remarkable differences between children in the treatment group and in the control group. The major finding was a difference of 20 points in Wechsler IQ in favor of the treatment group at the end of the program. In addition, treated children showed a six-month advantage in language skills (speech communication, imitation, comprehension) around 2 years of age, which increased in subsequent years to a full two-year advantage. Garber and Heber (1982) interpreted these findings as evidence that an intensive preschool program specially designed for high-risk children can prevent mental retardation. Moreover, the intellectual advantage of the treated children was maintained across the first four grades of school. The treatment group was significantly superior to the control group in reading and mathematics as measured by a standard achievement test.

As Horowitz and Paden (1973) indicated, these are probably the most impressive data yet on IQ and language gains. However, serious questions have been raised about the validity of the results from the Milwaukee study because its authors did not publish their findings in journals requiring rigorous reviews (Sommer & Sommer, 1983). Therefore, we must exercise caution in interpreting the reported data. Moreover, in the Milwaukee program, as in many of the other projects, slippage occurred once the program was discontinued and sometimes while it was still in operation (see Bronfenbrenner, 1976; Horowitz, 1980). In general, the more intense the programs are and the more involved the parents are, the stronger and more long-lasting are the effects (Horowitz, 1980).

Slippage in scores should not be automatically interpreted as a sign of program failure. Lazar and Darlington (1982) examined over 2000 Head Start children (aged 9–19 years) from 11 different programs. The programs failed to produce a durable effect on IQ scores because program participants' initial gains faded within four years after the programs ceased. Nevertheless, the Head Start children were much less likely than control children to be in special education classes or to have been held back in school. Investigators such as David Weikart and colleagues (see Schweinhart & Weikart, 1980) also have reported such **sleeper effects** for preschool intervention programs. A sleeper effect is not immediately apparent, but appears at a later point in development. Although Schweinhart and Weikart found few differences in cognitive achievement during elementary school for children with and without early enrichment experience in preschool, by junior high school, children with this experience outperformed those without it. While impressive, such sleeper effects would be more convincing if they were replicated and if they were predicted by a developmental theory (Montada & Schmitt, 1982).

The failure to maintain IQ gains over time has been explained in various ways. Early in the Head Start program, Arthur Jensen (1969) concluded that "Compensatory education has been tried and it apparently has failed" (p. 2). Jensen asserted that genetic factors control intellectual development and that environmental factors could have only minimal effect (see Chapter 8). Jensen's opponents countered that he was unrealistic to expect long-term effects solely on the basis of early intervention. This would be like expecting to prevent Vitamin C deficiencies at 10 years of age by having a child drink extra orange juice at age 4 (Horowitz, 1980). Therefore, the latter investigators recommended more intense and longer intervention programs beginning earlier in infancy and continuing well into the school years.

The Head Start experience made psychologists realize that early developmental intervention is much more complex than originally supposed. Because of the haste to initiate social action, intervention programs were undertaken without a sufficient knowledge base and a clear evaluation component. Consequently, one question that remains unanswered is how to judge the short-term and long-term effectiveness of these programs. During the 20-year history of Head Start and related programs, the outcome measure of choice has been the IQ score or magnitude of change in IQ score (Zigler & Trickett, 1978). IQ tests have many desirable properties which made them attractive—wide availability, ease of administration, known reliability, and close relationship to school performance (Zigler & Berman, 1983). However, given the methodological and theoretical problems associated with the use of IQ scores (see Chapter 8), IQ may not have been a particularly good choice as an outcome measure. As an alternative, Zigler and Trickett (1978; see also S. Anderson & Messick, 1974; McClelland, 1973) recommended the development of measures of social competence that include assessments of physical health, cognitive functioning, achievement, and motivational and emotional variables. Such measures may provide a more global and sensitive index of performance gains than IQ. They also may be employed to evaluate the impact of intervention programs on parents' participation in a child's educational experience. Several studies have indicated that parents from lower-class households develop greater feelings of social competence and control by serving as active participants in education intervention projects (see Bronfenbrenner, 1976).

Intervention to prevent the negative effects of early deprivation and to enrich cognitive and emotional development in children has become a major goal in developmental psychology. Although most intervention work now focuses on the early phases of the life cycle (see Box 10.1), broad-scale intervention programs need not be reserved for the young (Birren & Woodruff, 1973). Increasingly, intervention studies are being designed and tested on the adult population, especially in the past 10

Box 10.1   Do We Want Superbabies?

More parents are pushing their children to learn at an earlier and earlier age. This emphasis on intellectual attainment has been spawned, in part, by the expanding knowledge on early infant development, which suggests that infants are more competent than we presumed. Does an emphasis on intense early learning lead to higher intelligence and achievement in later years? The evidence is not clear.

According to some proponents, babies can learn cognitive skills such as simple arithmetic and reading before age 1. In one program developed by Glenn Doman, a 63-year-old physiotherapist and founder of the Better Baby Institute, flashcard educational techniques are used to teach young babies reading, math, and any other subject from foreign languages to zoology. Parents are instructed to present the flashcards for brief periods at least three times a day. In other programs, children as young as age 2 are taught to play concertos on the Suzuki violin and to use computer language skills. In addition, bookstores are flooded with books with achievement-promoting titles such as *Give Your Child a Superior Mind, How to Multiply Your Baby's Intelligence*, and *Growing Wisdom, Growing Wonder*.

Most of these better-babying efforts have drawn sharp criticism from developmental psychologists and other child-care specialists. Psychologists do not dispute that children can learn at an earlier age, but they question the long-range advantage of such attempts. Childhood experts worry that the overemphasis on intellectual skills may impede infants' normal physical, emotional, and creative growth. David Elkind (1981), an internationally known developmental child psychologist, has discussed the dangers of pushing infants and young children toward early intellectual achievement in his book *The Hurried Child: Growing Up Too Fast Too Soon*. Elkind is critical of the "home school" movement, which encourages parents to provide formal instruction in their homes and to think of themselves as teachers. He claims that this emphasis on early learning produces needless anxiety in young children, which can lead to later physical and emotional problems. Parents can and should do many things to encourage intellectual development of their children, but parental efforts need not and probably should not include formal instruction (Elkind, 1981). Taking the time to answer children's questions, reading to them, visiting museums with them, and going on nature hikes with them are some of the things parents can do to encourage learning. As Jerome Kagan of Harvard University has said, "It's not the activity per se but the melody behind the words" (quoted in "Bringing Up Superbaby," 1983, p. 65). In other words, what you teach is less critical than how you demonstrate to the child that learning is important and enjoyable.

years (Sterns & Sanders, 1980). The major thrust of this work is to identify strategies and processes deemed critical to cognitive performance and to develop training activities to improve subjects' usage of such strategies and processes (Willis, 1985).

As Birren and Woodruff (1973) pointed out in their influential essay on life-span education, the likely settings for intervention activities are the educational institutions of society. By their very nature, schools at all levels are geared to intervention, although their programs have traditionally been aimed at children and adolescents. Using educational intervention to promote cognitive growth and psychological well-being throughout the life span may become an important research objective in the future. Before psychologists design life-span educational intervention programs, they should observe the failures of childhood intervention and base their efforts on developmental theory, not simply social need.

GOALS OF INTERVENTION

In setting goals for intervention, developmental psychologists need to consider many criteria. For example, normative data on cognitive development and achievement, such as those provided by Piaget's theory, can and have been used to design early childhood educational programs. Frequently, intervention goals are established in relation to proposed developmental end states or mature stages such as formal operations. Intervention plans are then made, incorporating the specific steps needed to move the individual toward the goal. Intervention goals are also determined by psychologists' beliefs about the antecedents of developmental events. Such beliefs not only allow psychologists to predict the probability of success for any intervention project but also allow them to estimate the project's limitations. For instance, if early childhood interventionists believe school failure is caused by the cognitive and motivational deficits of the child, then they will target interventions to remove these deficits. On the other hand, if they think the causal factor is in the environment, they may direct interventions to upgrade the school curriculum, increase family involvement in the child's learning, and so on. The Head Start program is a good example of an intervention that incorporated both "fix the child" and "fix the environment" points of view.

In planning intervention programs, developmentalists cannot ignore the fact that goal setting is determined by what is considered most desirable in the society, which is a matter of values (Brandstädter & Schneewind, 1977; Reese & Overton, 1980). For example, a developmental scientist may decide that boosting IQ scores is a beneficial intervention goal because high intelligence is a prerequisite for technological, scientific progress. But many other societies and cultures may not share the investigator's notion of intelligence, much less the need to raise IQ scores. Producing happy, well-adjusted people may be seen as more important than creating a society of smart people. Thus, the concept of intervention cannot be understood in isolation. It gains meaning from theories about individual development and behavior as well as from societal values and norms about what is desirable (Baltes & Danish, 1980).

A number of writers have pointed out that the goals of intervention have been too narrow (Baltes, 1973; Birren & Woodruff, 1973). In many instances, the goal is simply to remove or *remediate* a cognitive deficit that already exists rather than to *prevent* such deficits or *enrich* cognitive functioning. A notable exception to this trend is the Head Start program, which attempts not only to alleviate existing deficiencies but also to provide an enrichment experience to prevent future learning problems. To be effective, intervention must aim at all three goals: remediation, prevention, and enrichment.

Remediation

Remediation involves removing or correcting an existing problem behavior. For example, memory problems plague many older adults, and psychologists are interested in correcting these problems through remedial training (Fozard, 1980; Poon, Walsh-Sweeney, & Fozard, 1980). Memory training generally consists of instructing elderly adults in the use of mnemonic aids and imagery techniques (see Chapter 6). Remediation may also involve counseling to reduce anxiety about memory problems, and incentive programs to encourage older people to continue cognitive training (Fozard, 1980). Some cautions are needed in using intervention programs to remediate memory deficits. Psychologists should be certain that the person has a problem remembering. As discussed in Chapter 6, people who complain about memory difficulties do not always show real memory loss (Kahn, Zarit, Hilbert, & Niederehe, 1975). Moreover, it is important to determine the antecedents of any observed memory loss (e.g., brain damge, depression, anxiety, fatigue, information overload). Intervention research will help reveal which memory problems can be ameliorated and which cannot be.

Prevention

Some interventions aim to prevent a problem from occurring or recurring. For example, the goal of early childhood education programs is the **prevention** of subsequent learning difficulties in elementary and junior high school students. Madden, O'Hara, and Levenstein (1984) recently reported the results of a nine-year evaluation of the early intervention Mother-Child Home Program (MCHP), designed to prevent later educational disadvantages in 2–4-year-old children from low-income families. The program focused on developing cognitively stimulating mother-child interactions by having the mother model certain verbal behaviors while she demonstrated the use of educational toys or read a book to her child. The children were selected from four successive cohorts (1973, 1974, 1975, 1976) and randomly assigned to either a home-based intervention training program or to a comparison treatment group. In the home-based program, a college student visited the mother's home on several occasions over a two-year period and demonstrated the use of the toys and ways to engage the child verbally. In the comparison condition, stimulating toys were provided, but the mother received no visits or training.

Madden et al. (1984) reported large effects of the intervention on maternal interaction style during videotaped observations. Mothers in the training condition were more likely to provide labels for their child, to verbalize the child's action, to solicit information, and to encourage the use of many toys. There was also a modest short-term cognitive effect, with children in the home-based program (1976 cohort only) performing better than the comparison children on a cognitive achievement test and the Stanford-Binet IQ test. However, little evidence was found for the long-term effects of the home-based program. Three years after the program ended, children in the home-based and comparison groups did not differ on achievement or IQ measures, nor in teachers' ratings of children's school problems or socioemotional adjustment. In this early intervention program, like so many others, the long-term advantages of prevention intervention are difficult to demonstrate. As indicated, the focus on cognitive and intellectual skills may have obscured the intervention's beneficial effects on the overall quality of life of parents and children (Madden et al., 1984).

Successful prevention of later learning difficulties requires the identification of children who are at risk for these behaviors. Identification might be based on parental characteristics, personality characteristics of the child, intelligence, temperament, motivation, health, or some combination of these. Although infants' and young children's characteristics are not good predictors of later intellectual change patterns, longitudinal research in adult cognitive development has succeeded in identifying variables (e.g., health, educational level, socioeconomic status, environmental variables, intensity of social contact) that predict developmental changes in cognition (Montada & Schmitt, 1982; Schaie, 1979). Individuals at risk do not automatically develop the problem behavior. Genetic background factors, relations with a significant other, and a positive self-concept may mitigate the effects of early negative experience.

Enrichment

The term **enrichment** has often been used as a synonym for intervention (Horowitz & Paden, 1973). By "enrichment" we mean enhancing or optimizing development beyond what it would be under naturally occurring conditions. This approach assumes that the individual has both skills and deficits and participates actively in the intervention (Danish, Smyer, & Nowak, 1980). One example is the Study of Mathematically Precocious Youth, established in 1971 at Johns Hopkins University (Stanley & Benbow, 1983). This program identifies mathematically talented seventh and eighth graders and gives them accelerated mathematical instruction. In many cases the children attend a local high school for advanced mathematics classes, while remaining in junior high school for other subjects and activities.

The results of this enrichment program have been dramatic. As of 1982 over 35,000 mathematically precocious youth had been identified and given special mathematical instruction. Many of these individuals later took college courses while in high school or graduated from high school after two or three years and entered college early.

Nonaccelerated enrichment programs have also been designed for academically talented children. These programs often provide gifted children with special classes in science, art, or social studies or free time to explore subjects of interest. However, many psychologists question whether such enrichment experiences benefit the child or are simply a form of busywork. Little empirical evidence supports the claim that children will automatically profit from unstructured enrichment activities.

An example of an enrichment program for adults is the educational program called "Elderhostel." Elderhostel is a unique educational opportunity for older adults, which began in 1975 at four colleges in New Hampshire and has since been extended to more than 400 campuses in the United States, Canada, and Europe. Through the Elderhostel program, older adults can take college-level courses and combine their academic work with travel to various colleges and universities. Retirement intervention programs aimed at maximizing postemployment skills and activities are another example of an enrichment experience.

From a life-span developmental perspective, the goals of intervention are multidimensional and changing. Depending on the life circumstances, resources, and the developmental status of an individual, the goal may assume one or more of the above forms. Thus, an intervention with an older student may aim to remediate an immediate problem (e.g., poor memory) and at the same time focus on enrichment (e.g., promoting artistic appreciation). Similarly, with children and adolescents, educational intervention can be remedial or preventative as well as enriching.

LEVELS OF INTERVENTION

Once the goals of intervention have been identified, the next step is to determine the *level* of intervention. Interventions can be aimed at individuals, small groups of individuals, or societal organizations and institutions. This is an important decision for the intervenor because differences in the level of intervention may dictate different kinds of intervention strategies or techniques. For example, the intervenor who believes that cognitive problems result from poor social environments or culture may be more likely to employ a large-scale intervention aimed at modifying social conditions than the intervenor who views the problems as a product of the individual's cognitive deficits. The latter intervenor may decide that a small-scale intervention aimed at modifying the individual's cognitive skills is the most appropriate level.

Different kinds of intervention can be used at the same level of intervention, and the same kind of intervention can be used at different levels (Reese & Overton, 1980). For example, the most frequently used intervention procedure at the individual level is behavior modification, but behavioral techniques can—and often are—used to change whole communities or societies.

Individual and Small-Group Level

As mentioned, the most frequently employed intervention procedure at the individual level is behavior modification. The goal of behavior modification is to weaken undesirable behaviors through punishment or extinction and to strengthen desirable behaviors via reinforcement (Risley & Baer, 1973; Risley & Wolf, 1973). Because behavior modifiers wish to instate desirable behaviors, not merely eliminate undesirable ones, behavior modification programs are based primarily upon reinforcement techniques. To illustrate the use of a reinforcement approach to modify cognitive behaviors, consider the following experiment by Clingman and Fowler (1976). They investigated the effects of candy reinforcers on IQ scores among groups of first- and second-grade children. Subjects were first divided into three blocks according to their IQ scores on Form A of the Peabody Picture Vocabulary Test (PPVT), a commonly used vocabulary measure for children. Children in each of the three blocks (low IQ, medium IQ, high IQ) were randomly assigned to one of three experimental conditions: (1) a contingent candy reward for correct responses on the PPVT, (2) noncontingent reward according to the number of candies earned by the first group, and (3) no reward. A month after Form A was administered, all subjects received Form B of the same vocabulary test under one of these three conditions.

The results of this study are displayed in Figure 10.3, which shows that contingent reward raised IQ scores of children from the low-IQ group, but not the scores from the medium- or high-IQ groups. The authors suggest that the provision of candy rewards for correct responses by low-IQ children served to increase their test-taking motivation. Quite likely the medium-IQ and high-IQ children were already functioning at a higher motivational level than children in the low-IQ group. Based on these results and comparable findings, Clingman and Fowler advocate the systematic reinforcement of all children taking standardized tests.

A reinforcement program was used as a long-term intervention to improve cognitive behavior by Wolf, Giles, and Hall (1968). These

Figure 10.3 Mean change in IQ scores for low, medium, and high groups in all reward conditions.

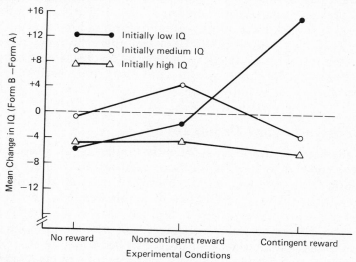

From "The Effects of Primary Reward on the IQ Performance of Grade-School children as a Function of Initial IQ Level" by J. Clingman and R. L. Fowler, 1976, *Journal of Applied Behavior Analysis, 9*, p. 21. Copyright 1976 by the Society for the Experimental Analysis of Behavior, Inc. Reprinted by permission.

investigators employed token reinforcers to improve the reading skills of a group of low-achieving fifth and six graders in an urban school. Token reinforcers are similar to trading stamps; tokens have little inherent value, but can be exchanged for items that are valuable.

In this experiment the treatment group (token plan) received remedial training in reading and arithmetic during a year-and-a-half program at school. For correct completion of an assignment, each child received points from the teacher; these points could be exchanged for reinforcers such as weekly field trips, a snack, money, or items from a token store. By the end of the experiment, children in the treatment group showed a gain of one full year on tests of reading and achievement level. Children in the control group (no-token plan) showed about half of this gain. Moreover, children in the treatment condition improved their grades from D-level to C-level work; the control group evidenced no such gains.

Both of the behavior modification studies discussed above achieved dramatic success. However, the widespread use of behavior modification to modify children's intelligence and achievement has provoked serious objections (Kazdin, 1981). Many parents, teachers, and psychologists contend that using points, chips, or gold stars as reinforcers may foster an overreliance on external rewards and deprive children of the inherent satisfaction of performing an activity (e.g., reading) for its own sake. This reduced satisfaction in engaging in a once rewarding activity is known as the **overjustification effect** (Lepper, 1981; Lepper, Greene, & Nisbett, 1973). By rewarding a child for something he or she already enjoys, one may undermine the child's intrinsic interest in performing the activity in some situations. However, rewards may be indispensable in motivating children to perform an initially unappealing or uninteresting activity such as learning multiplication tables. Also at issue is the manipulative character of behavior modification studies. Will children resent being manipulated and grow to dislike and mistrust teachers and other persons in authority? Will children alter their behavior temporarily to suit the teacher or trainee, but not cooperate once the program has ended? Even though behavior modification is a highly effective technique, we cannot uncritically accept it as a panacea for remediating cognitive deficiencies and enhancing intellectual growth.

Societal Level

Intervention at the societal level is directed at changing organizations, institutions, or large social groups rather than individuals or small groups of individuals (Reese & Overton, 1980). The logic behind this approach is that organizations and institutions are more powerful than individuals, so that the easiest way to change individuals is to change their institutions. From a societal perspective, knowing how an intervention affects a particular behavior or set of behaviors is insufficient. Rather, the need is to develop intervention concepts and approaches that take into account the scope and complexity of real-world ecology (Harshbarger, 1973; Urban, 1978). The use of ecological change strategies (to be discussed later) exemplifies intervention at a societal level.

Typical interventions at the societal level focus on discrete definable environmental units such as a school, office, library, or hospital ward (Harshbarger, 1973). Much of this work considers how the environment can be rearranged to produce a better fit between environmental conditions and user characteristics. For example, intervenors may attempt to increase communication interactions among mental patients by rearranging the furniture on a hospital ward. Or the intervention goal may involve changing from a traditional form of classroom organization to something resembling an open classroom (Harshbarger, 1973). To the extent that the intervenor succeeds in matching the environment with its inhabitants' cognitive and behavioral characteristics, more ecologically adaptive behavior will occur.

Societal interventions can be aimed at identifiable environmental units, but need not be. For example, consider the television program *Sesame Street*, which has been broadcast to millions of children since 1969. The producers hoped that the program would prepare preschool viewers for the academic demands of public school. Not only did the show feature clever skits and a cast of zany characters such as Big Bird, Cookie Monster, and Ernie but it also had a set of concrete educational goals. Subsequent studies reported that children who watched the program showed significant gains in cognitive skills and mental representation.

In a comprehensive evaluation of *Sesame Street*, Ball and Bogatz (1972) measured children's knowledge of letters, numbers, body parts, geometric forms, and matching, sorting, and classification skills before and after a six-month viewing period. The children were 3-, 4-, and 5-year-olds from middle- and lower-class households, who were divided into groups according to how frequently they viewed the program. As Figure 10.4 shows, scores increased with children's increased amount of viewing; 3-year-olds and 4-year-olds who saw the program more than five times a week did better than 5-year-olds who watched it three times a week or less. Furthermore, frequent viewers made substantial gains in performance regardless of whether they came from middle- or lower-class families. Unexpectedly, children's reading scores showed significant improvement, even though reading was not specifically taught on the program. These results indicate that television can be an important intervention tool for effecting intellectual change at a societal level.

Figure 10.4   Pretest and posttest scores of 3-, 4-, and 5-year-olds from lower- and middle-class families. Pretest scores on the cognitive tests sorted almost entirely by age; posttest scores sorted by how often children watched *Sesame Street.* Q1 = children who viewed rarely or never (*N* = 198), Q2 = children who viewed 2–3 times a week (*N* = 197), Q3 = children who viewed 4–5 times a week (*N* = 172), Q4 = children who viewed more than 5 times a week (*N* = 164).

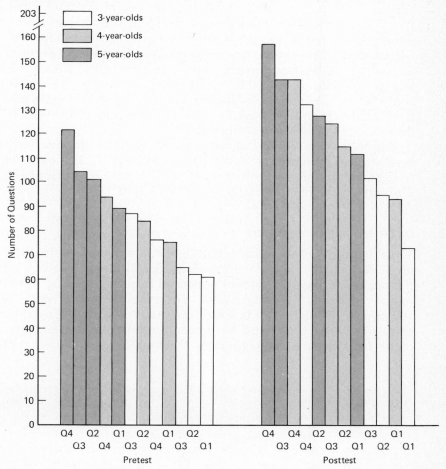

From "Summative Research of *Sesame Street:* Implications for the Study of Preschool Children" by S. Ball and G. A. Bogatz, 1972, in *Minnesota Symposia on Child Psychology* (Vol. 6, p. 13) edited by A. D. Pick, Minneapolis: University of Minnesota Press. Copyright 1972 by University of Minnesota Press. Reprinted by permission.

INTERVENTION STRATEGIES

The term *strategies* refers to concrete modes or techniques of implementation (Baltes & Danish, 1980). In the intervention literature, the term encompasses a wide array of dimensions including the general goals of intervention (e.g., remediation, prevention, enrichment), the "target" behaviors to be modified, the settings for the intervention, the types of intervention mechanisms, and the timing and duration of intervention. Baltes (1973) has presented a taxonomic model of psychological intervention strategies based on an earlier model proposed by A. Jacobs (1974). This taxonomy, shown in Table 10.1, shows the scope and complexity of possible intervention activities. This taxonomy could easily be expanded by adding techniques and strategies borrowed from other disciplines such as genetics (e.g., genetic counseling) or medicine (e.g., preventive surgery).

The following sections concentrate on some of the mechanisms of intervention presented in Table 10.1. In each case, the target behavior considered will be a cognitive function discussed in previous chapters. The settings will be primarily laboratory based.

Social Learning Strategies

Social learning refers to the learning of adaptive behaviors using stimulus cues from the social environment. Social forms of learning follow the same learning principles of nonsocial forms of learning, but involve stimuli provided by other people. For example, much reinforcement and modeling of behavior in learning situations is social. Social learning principles such as modeling have been used successfully to induce people to behave morally (Bandura & McDonald, 1963; Turiel, 1973), to

Table 10.1
A Taxonomy of Psychological Intervention Strategies

Goal	Target Behavior	Setting	Mechanism
Enrichment	Cognition	Laboratory	Training-practice
Prevention	Language	Family	Social learning
Remediation	Intellectual abilities	Classroom	Psychotherapy
	Social interactions	Senior citizen center	Ecological change
	Motivational states	Hospital	Health delivery
	Personality traits	Community	Economic support
	Attitudes	Macroecology	

Note: From "Intervention in Life-Span Development and Aging: Issues and Concepts" by P. B. Baltes and S. J. Danish, 1980, in *Life-Span Developmental Psychology: Intervention* (p. 62) edited by R. R. Turner and H. W. Reese, New York: Academic Press. Copyright 1980 by Academic Press. Reprinted by permission.

overcome debilitating fears (Bandura, Grusec, & Menlove, 1967; Kling-man, Melamed, Cuthbert, & Hermecz, 1984), and to respond altruisti-cally (Hay & Murray, 1982; Midlarsky, Bryan, & Brickman, 1973). Thus, the application of social learning procedures to the realm of cog-nitive behavior is not surprising.

Two of the most frequently targeted behaviors in social learning studies are language and creativity–problem solving. Because imitation was reviewed as a mechanism in language learning (see Chapter 5), lan-guage studies will not be reviewed here. Instead, we will concentrate on modeling effects on creative and problem-solving behaviors. Zim-merman and Dialessi (1973) reported on a modeling study designed to improve children's divergent thinking on an unusual-uses task and a verbal fluency test. (Remember that divergent thinking underlies much creative thought.) The investigators assigned fifth-grade children to one of four experimental groups. The four groups were exposed to an adult male model who was either high or low in fluency (number of words produced) and either high or low in flexibility (number of response cat-egories) on a divergent thinking item. The results showed that high model fluency enhanced subjects' fluency on both divergent thinking measures, particularly for the female subjects. Contrary to what one might expect, high model flexibility depressed the number of divergent thinking responses. Zimmerman and Dialessi (1973) believed that the diversity of the response categories produced by the high-flexibility model introduced an evaluation component into the study by making children aware of the requirement to produce dissimilar responses. The implication is that creativity can be increased by exposing children to fluent models rather than to flexible ones.

Modeling techniques have also been employed to modify problem-solving performance on convergent thinking tasks requiring elimina-tion of solution alternatives. For example, N. Denney and Denney (1974; D. Denney, Denney, & Ziobrowski, 1973) reported that model-ing is a quick and efficient way to modify the question-asking strategies of young children and older adults on the twenty-questions task. As you may remember, in this task the subject is presented with an array of everyday objects and asked to choose the one the experimenter has in mind by asking questions that can be answered either "yes" or "no." Children and older adults typically ask hypothesis-seeking questions, which eliminate only one item at a time from the array, rather than constraint-seeking questions, which eliminate groups of items (N. Den-ney, 1979). However, when exposed to a model who asks constraint-seeking questions, children and adults quickly adopt this strategy as their own. Moreover, they do not merely passively mimic specific ques-tions asked by the model, but use a general constraint-seeking strategy to generate original questions.

The studies reviewed here suggest that children as well as adults can learn to generate novel responses by observing models who demonstrate such use. Apparently, subjects do so, not by imitating or being reinforced for specifically modeled responses, but by abstracting a rule or strategy from the model's performance. According to social learning theory, the *rule* is the fundamental unit of cognitive activity (Zimmerman, 1983). Simpler rules can be used to formulate higher-order plans, and superordinate rules can be used to organize basic rules. An individual's current level of cognitive functioning is a critical variable in determining rule acquisition.

In general, social learning theorists attempt to establish people's current level of cognitive development by first identifying groups of individuals who have not "naturally" attained a particular cognitive level. These individuals are then exposed to a more developmentally advanced model, who demonstrates the rule. If subjects acquire the rule, certain estimations about their degree of cognitive sophistication can be made. For example, Zimmerman (1983) has noted that complex rules such as Piaget's conservation of number depend on the mastery of subordinate rules such as counting and one-to-one-matching. These subordinate rules should be taught first. Once they are acquired, individuals can use them to abstract more complex rules from modeled performances. The main point is that sequences of logically interdependent rules—or *measurement sequences* as Brainerd (1978) calls them—do not require constructs such as Piagetian stages for their explication. In contrast to stage assumptions, rule learning explanations suggest that children and adults can learn cognitively complex material if they are first taught subordinate rules.

Training-Practice Strategies

Earlier in this chapter we reviewed Piagetian training studies with children and fluid intelligence training programs with adults. This section takes a broader look at the whole notion of cognitive training and practice. We will discuss interventions that range all the way from complexly structured training experiences (involving feedback, instructions, and modeling) to simple practice without feedback.

A good example of a training study with complex intervention procedures is Parker, Rieff, and Sperr's (1971) investigation of multiple classification ability. As you read in Chapter 7, multiple classification skill is an important component of concrete operations and typically does not emerge until age 7 or 8. In Parker et al.'s study, children aged 4½, 6, and 7½ years were pretested on a series of multiple classification problems and then assigned to one of two conditions: a 13-step feedback training and instruction program sequenced according to difficulty level or a contact-control condition. The experimental training program involved a series of "remedial loops." When subjects failed to reach a solution on any step, they were branched to a remedial loop consisting of the subordinate skills considered prerequisite to that step. The steps involved skills such as labeling the attributes of the stimuli in the problem (color and shape), sorting the stimuli by these attributes, and placing the correct stimuli in the rows and columns of the classification matrix. In the contact-control condition, children had equal contact with an experimenter playing a game, but no training. From one to four days following the training program or contact-control condition, all subjects were posttested on another series of multiple classification problems. As Figure 10.5 shows, the 7½-year-olds and, to a lesser degree, the 6-year-olds benefited from the experimental training program, but the 4½-year-olds who received training did less well than the control group on the multiple classification tasks. As the authors explain, the youngest children may have lacked the cognitive structures necessary to benefit from training, or the training procedure may have been too complex and attention demanding. The same differential pat-

Figure 10.5   Mean number of correct responses on five multiple classification tasks as a function of age and treatment condition.

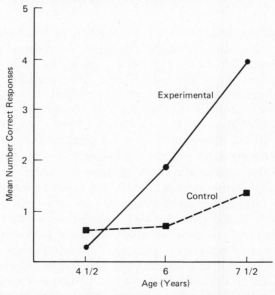

From "Teaching Multiple Classification to Young Children" by R. K. Parker, M. L. Rieff, and S. J. Sperr, 1971, *Child Development, 42,* p. 1785. Copyright 1971 by The Society for Research in Child Development, Inc. Reprinted by permission.

tern of results by age was found on a series of nine multiple classification transfer problems. Again, the oldest children's performance improved on the transfer tasks relative to the youngest children's as a consequence of feedback training.

In a study with older adults, Hornblum and Overton (1976) employed a simple feedback training procedure to train conservation in female nonconservers. The feedback procedure involved informing older women about the correctness or incorrectness of their responses to a series of area conservation problems. Control subjects solved the same problems, but did not receive feedback about their responses. The results showed a significant effect on the posttest, with the feedback group giving more conservation responses than the no-feedback control group. The feedback group also performed better than the control group on a series of near and far transfer measures of conservation.

These two studies indicate that feedback training results in significant improvement in different types of cognitive performance—at least among subjects whose existing cognitive competencies or capacities are developed enough to benefit from it. Feedback *activates* these competencies into performance, but is not effective with individuals (e.g., the 4½-year-olds in Parker et al.'s (1971) study) who lack the requisite cognitive abilities or structures. Such results highlight the need to distinguish between competence and performance not only in describing intellectual development (see Chapter 8) but also in attempting to modify it.

An equally important issue is whether individuals spontaneously improve their performances in the absence of direct training procedures such as feedback. In other words, is practice sufficient to boost cognitive performance, or are more highly structured interventions required? Several studies in the adult developmental literature have included a practice-only control group (e.g., F. Hoyer, Hoyer, Treat, & Baltes, 1978–1979; Labouvie-Vief & Gonda, 1976; Sanders, Sterns, Smith, & Sanders, 1975). The results of these studies provide mixed support for the effectiveness of practice. Labouvie-Vief and Gonda (1976) have reported that unspecific training (practice only) on a fluid intelligence task yielded stronger effects than two other types of training involving modeling and direct instructions in solution rules. But the data were sufficiently mixed that the results must be viewed with caution. In a study designed to improve older subjects' performance on a concept-learning problem, Sanders et al. (1975) included a practice and a control condition as well as two training conditions. In contrast to Labouvie-Vief and Gonda (1976), Sanders and colleagues found that the training conditions yielded better performance on the posttest than either the practice or control condition. In this case practice-only subjects received the solution to a problem if they failed the problem, but were given no other feedback. Control subjects received only the pretest and the posttest. F. Hoyer et al. (1978–1979) included a practice-with-feedback condition in a study of response speed in younger and older women. Both age groups' speed improved with practice and feedback, but the younger women benefited more from a training condition than the older women. The dependent measure in this case was a series of paper-and-pencil tasks.

The studies cited above bear on a general issue that has raised considerable debate in the Piagetian training literature, namely, the relative effectiveness of tutorial versus self-discovery instructional approaches (Brainerd, 1983; Sterns & Sanders, 1980). Tutorial approaches are characterized by *passive reception* of information, in which the experimenter imposes certain strategies on the subject. Some familiar examples of tutorial training procedures are modeling, direct rule instruction, and corrective feedback. In contrast, self-discovery approaches, favored by Piagetians, involve the active manipulation of the cognitive environment (e.g., constructing things, transforming ideas, and removing conflict). Piagetians claim that self-discovery training is superior to tutorial methods. By manipulating the environment to produce cognitive conflict in the learner, one promotes active efforts at cognitive discovery. A similar suggestion regarding the superiority of self-discovery methods has been made by researchers of adult development (Labouvie-Vief & Gonda, 1976).

The experimental evidence does not permit firm conclusions about the relative effectiveness of self-discovery and tutorial methods. In a series of Piagetian training experiments, Inhelder and colleagues (1974) trained children to solve conservation and class inclusion problems. They encouraged children to discover the rule for solving the problems by having them manipulate a variety of experimental apparatuses. For example, on a conservation-of-liquid problem, nonconserving children were encouraged to pour a fixed quantity of liquid from one beaker to another with the expectation that they would discover the principle that the quantity of liquid remains the same, regardless of the size or shape of its container. The results suggested that children can benefit greatly from self-discovery methods. These results were challenged by Brainerd (1983), who cited evidence supporting an opposite conclusion. For example, Cantor, Dunlap, and Rettie (1982) looked at kindergartners' performance on a series of probability tasks and found that tutorial methods led to greater gains on these tasks than self-discovery training. Thus, neither approach seems superior. We definitely need further research to directly compare the efficacy of alternative intervention training strategies (Sterns & Sanders, 1980).

Ecological Change Strategies

As intervention studies become more prevalent, there is a growing need to consider the wider ecological context of intervention. Developmentalists such as Urie Bronfenbrenner (1976) have called for intervention at the ecological (i.e., community, societal) level, which involves a more radical restructuring of the entire environment. Garber and Heber's (1982) study on early childhood intervention (discussed earlier) is a prime example of intervention at an ecological level. Some of the study's major ecological features were that mothers as well as teachers participated in the training; children received training first alone and then in small groups of children and teachers; the training involved perceptual, language, and intellectual abilities; and the project had a long time span.

An ecological perspective on intervention focuses on time trajectories, patterns of intervention treatments and effects, and types of intervention targets (Baltes & Danish, 1980). It emphasizes long time trajectories, multiple treatment and assessment periods, and multiple targets. Intervention efforts directed at one or two behaviors at a given point in development may overlook possible negative side effects produced by the intervention (Urban, 1978; Willems, 1973). For example, many intervention programs focus on a single aspect of the cognitive system—perceptual ability, memory, language, creativity, or intelligence—or a combination of two systems such as language and cognitive abilities. The order and patterning of these programmed interventions may have a significant impact on their outcome. Sigel and Olmsted (as cited in Sigel, 1972) reported the side effects of a training program for lower-class Black kindergarten children which included two training sequences: (1) classification training, which explored object characteristics and categorization skills, and (2) attention training, which emphasized specific dimensions of objects. When attention training preceded classification training, positive gains in categorization skills resulted. However, when attention training followed classification training, initial benefits of training were undone and a negative effect resulted. Thus, the patterning of intervention is an important variable in designing training programs.

The timing of intervention is also a critical variable in cognitive training research. Historically, the accepted view has been that early experience exerts a disproportionate influence upon later development (Clarke & Clarke, 1976; Kagan, 1976; Wachs & Gruen, 1982). Accordingly, early intervention research (e.g., Project Head Start) was believed to produce long-range effects even if the child's ecological context remained unaltered. But interventions that ignore the person's current developmental level of functioning and long-term ecological context are unlikely to be as productive as interventions that take these factors into account (Baltes & Danish, 1980; Sigel, 1972). Box 10.2 discusses a well-planned ecological intervention with elderly persons.

THE EVALUATION OF INTERVENTION RESEARCH

The observation that interventions do not always produce the intended effects underscores the need for evaluation. Evaluation involves collecting information about an intervention program in order to judge its

Box 10.2 An Ecological Intervention with the Institutionalized Aged

The number of aged persons residing in long-term care institutions has increased rapidly over the past two decades. Accompanying this increase has been a growing concern among psychologists about the long-range effects of institutionalization on physical and psychological well-being (Ransen, 1981). Psychologists know that institutionalization is associated with such adverse developmental consequences as dramatically increased mortality rates, physiological declines, loss of perceived control, and feelings of hopelessness. The cognitive consequences of institutionalization may be equally severe. Since residents of institutions are confined to a very restricted living space and a highly redundant daily routine, they may have little new information to process; as a result, their ability to think and remember may deteriorate.

In a series of well-planned studies, Ellen Langer and her associates (E. Langer, Rodin, Beck, Weinman, & Spitzer, 1979) explored the effects of institutional living on the cognitive functioning of different groups of elderly nursing home residents. The researchers hypothesized that increasing the cognitive demands of the environment and the residents' motivation to attend to and remember their environment would improve the residents' mental functioning. In E. Langer et al.'s (1979) first study, 54 middle-class elderly residents of a private nursing home were visited several times over a six-week period by one of five young adult interviewers. The interviewers were instructed to either disclose a lot of information about events in their personal lives (high reciprocal self-disclosure group) or to ask the residents about events in the residents' lives (low reciprocal self-disclosure group). After each

visit, the interviewers also asked the residents to think about topics for discussion during future visits. The results showed that
subjects in the high reciprocal self-disclosure group were more
likely to follow the interviewers' suggestion to think about a discussion topic than subjects in the low reciprocal self-disclosure
group. The former group also achieved higher scores on two recall
memory tasks. The investigators explained these results in terms
of the degree of subjects' involvement in the interviews. Subjects
who heard new information from a self-disclosing interviewer
apparently were more cognitively involved during the interview
(and thus performed better) than subjects who simply were asked
questions about their own lives.

In their second study, E. Langer et al. (1979) employed practical
incentives rather than personal incentives to increase subjects'
cognitive activity; 45 residents of another nursing home participated. Each resident was visited several times over a three-week
period, with various cognitive demands made during each visit.
For example, residents were asked about nursing home activities
and names of other residents and staff members. Residents who
could not remember the answers were asked to try to find the correct information by the next visit. In the contingent condition, residents received a poker chip for each correct response, which could
be redeemed at the end of the experiment for a gift. Subjects in the
noncontingent condition received chips at each visit regardless of
their answers. Subjects in a no-treatment control condition
received no chips, but got a gift at the end of the experiment. Four
days after the last visit all subjects received a test of immediate
memory (word recall) and memory for remote events (e.g., "When
was the Great Depression?"). Subjects in the contingent condition
remembered significantly more meals than subjects in the noncontingent condition, and they took less time to find out information
regarding activities in the nursing home. The contingent group
also outperformed the other two groups on the recall memory
measures.

Both of these studies provide impressive support for the impact
of a relatively brief ecological intervention on cognitive functioning in the aged. The results suggest that interventionists must be
sensitive to the social environmental factors influencing performance in the testing context as well as to the motivation of people
to practice and perform well in general (E. Langer et al., 1979). In
addition, the long-term effects of intervention need to be better
understood. Interventions that produce such impressive initial
gains do not always result in enduring improvements.

effectiveness. There are two principal types of evaluation: (1) **formative evaluation** and (2) **summative evaluation.** Formative evaluation emphasizes monitoring the process, strategy, and targets of intervention. This type of evaluation is designed to provide a solid basis for improving the intervention or abandoning it in favor of a more effective one. In areas where knowledge about the effects of intervention is sparse (e.g., gerontological cognition), formative evaluations should be employed.

Summative evaluations provide information about the overall effectiveness and outcome of the intervention procedure. Less often, they give information about competing modes of intervention. Summative evaluations are complex because they must consider not only the intervention strategies but also such factors as the costs and time required, the meeting of certain target needs, and the relationship of the intervention to the ecological context. Generally, summative evaluations, unlike formative evaluations, are performed by a team of outside evaluators specially trained in the theory and politics of intervention. Because summative evaluations examine the results of efforts to manipulate critical variables in people's lives, they have the potential to add to our knowledge base about human behavior and development.

Effective evaluation of intervention programs begins during the initial proposal and design phases of intervention, not after their completion. As Danish and Conter (1978) have remarked, "Evaluation becomes a part of the intervention program development, not a process applied after its development" (p. 345). In evaluating interventions for children and adults, the life-span researcher must be aware of relevant theoretical issues such as those discussed below.

Developmental Plasticity versus Invariance

A primary theme in the study and evaluation of psychological intervention is the relative degree of developmental plasticity and developmental invariance that exists for different age levels. As discussed in Chapter 8, *plasticity* refers to the possible range of individual variations that can occur in intraindividual development over time (Gollin, 1981, p. 231). *Invariance* refers to the view that abilities are fixed and unchanging over a lifetime; that is, abilities show trait-like properties. These fixed abilities are used to compare one individual with another, usually at one point in development. The research we have cited in this text should make clear that intellectual and cognitive abilities are not fixed, contrary to the assumptions of many early investigators of cognition.

According to N. Denney (1982), individuals of any age possess a certain amount of plasticity, so that the real question is not one of absolute plasticity. There is growing evidence for a large amount of intraindividual plasticity and modifiability in cognitive performance in adults as well as children (Baltes, Reese, & Lipsitt, 1980; Willis & Baltes, 1980). Rather, the important question is the *relative* plasticity of cognition and intelligence across the life span. That is, do certain age groups show more responsiveness to training or other forms of intervention than other age groups? This question is not easily answered because only studies comparing two or more age groups are appropriate. Furthermore, cross-sectional intervention research has the same set of potential methodological problems as purely descriptive age-comparative studies.

The research on this topic suggests increasing plasticity of cognitive development through childhood and adulthood, at least for some abilities, and then decreasing plasticity in later life. For example, in the Parker et al. (1971) study, corrective feedback improved multiple classification performance for school-aged children, but not for 4½-year-olds. Similarly, in the F. Hoyer et al. (1978–1979) study, younger women were more responsive to feedback training than older women on speed-of-response measures. Thus, intervention research undertaken to reduce age differences in performance does not always succeed in eliminating these differences. In some cases, age-related differences may increase as a result of intervention because certain aged individuals show more plasticity than others.

N. Denney (1982) has proposed a theoretical framework that attempts to integrate the current empirical findings on intraindividual development and plasticity. Denney's formulation considers two developmental functions: (1) untrained or **unexercised ability** and (2) optimally trained or **optimally exercised ability.** The first function represents what a normal healthy person would be able to do in a cognitive domain if not given any special training or exercise. It reflects both normal biological potential and normally occurring environmental conditions. The second function is what an individual is capable of doing (i.e., competence or capacity) when given optimal exercise or training in a cognitive skill. This function is assumed to reflect maximum biological potential under normal environmental conditions with optimal exercise and training.

The developmental curves for these two functions are presented in Figure 10.6. As you can see, both unexercised and optimally exercised abilities increase with age up to adolescence or early adulthood and then decline gradually throughout the remainder of the life span. The potential effect of exercise or training on performance (i.e., the degree of plasticity) is represented in Figure 10.6 by the area between the unexercised and optimally exercised ability. Through proper exercise and intervention, individuals can improve their performance appreciably over what it would be under ordinary conditions. Nevertheless, the

Figure 10.6 Developmental functions of unexercised and optimally exercised cognitive abilities.

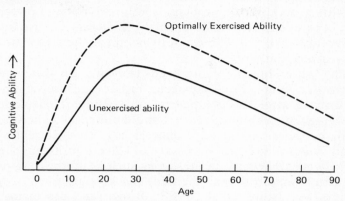

From "Aging and Cognitive Changes" by N. W. Denney, 1982, in *Handbook of Developmental Psychology* (p. 819) edited by B. B. Wolman, Englewood Cliffs, NJ: Prentice-Hall. Copyright 1982 by Prentice-Hall, Inc. Reprinted by permission.

overall trend depicted in Figure 10.6 is downward, reflecting the probable decline in intellectual abilities with age, even among abilities considered most resistant to aging (i.e., verbal abilities). Notice also that the two curves are closer together in childhood and old age than in young or middle adulthood. Thus, exercise and training may benefit young children and older adults less than other age groups, although there is room for improvement at any age level.

N. Denney's (1982) theoretical model provides an integrative conceptual framework for studying intraindividual variation in the effects of training across the life span. The model makes different predictions about the effects of training depending on the degree and timing of the experience and the difficulty level of the ability. For example, on easy tasks, children and older adults may be more responsive to training than young adults, who may already be performing near ceiling levels. On difficult tasks, young adults would be expected to gain more from training than young children or older adults, who may lack the ability to reach optimal performance levels (N. Denney, 1982). Additional research is needed to extend N. Denney's model to interindividual factors such as cohort differences and sex differences.

Maintenance and Generalization

One major limitation of intervention studies is that training often helps individuals learn how to perform well on the trained task, but does not necessarily alter how they approach similar problems. In short, intervention procedures may fail to produce **maintenance,** or durability of the cognitive strategies over time, and **generalization,** or transfer of strategies across tasks (A. Brown et al., 1983). A familiar example of a real-life generalization problem is failure to transfer material learned in school to out-of-school situations. Instructors are usually reluctant to claim that a student who can only compute the problems given in class has learned mathematics.

The successful intervenor needs to plan for maintenance and generalization effects before they occur, rather than simply report their non-occurrence after the completion of a study. This planning involves knowing which skills to teach. Should one teach concrete, task-specific skills or more abstract and general cognitive strategies? The former might involve routines necessary to solve a problem; the latter might include general cognitive strategies such as monitoring one's progress, exhorting oneself to stay focused, and keeping track of solution alternatives (A. Brown et al., 1983). Brown and associates have recommended the teaching of intermediate-level skills, which are more general than specific routines, but more powerful and relevant than the broad sets of skills taught in current educational curricula. A. Brown et al. (1983) have argued that specific skills may be powerful for solving problems, but may not always be accessible when needed. On the other hand, general skills may be appropriate in almost any situation, but do not require close attention to task demands and may be less powerful than more specialized routines.

In a theoretical vein, the failure of maintenance and generalization of training can be attributed to the lack of a conceptual rationale for transfer. To adequately evaluate the degree of learning requires a conceptual framework that defines the target ability for training, the design of the intervention program, and the criteria for training and transfer effects. The ADEPT program, discussed earlier in this chapter, is an example of an intervention approach based on a theoretical model. Using the fluid-crystallized model of intelligence, the investigators targeted fluid abilities for training and selected transfer tasks that were related by theory to the training task (Willis et al., 1981). Their design also examined the maintenance of training and transfer effects across a six-month posttest period. The predicted pattern of transfer occurred at posttest. However, few developmental intervention studies incorporate transfer and delayed training effects into their design. As a result, most studies are not sensitive to the occurrence of long-term side effects or sleeper effects from intervention.

U-Shaped Development

One final problem in evaluating the effects of intervention programs is trying to assess developmental changes that may not be linear. In a recent provocative book, Strauss (1982) has called attention to *U-shaped*

functions in behavioral growth and development. Such functions involve the initial appearance of a behavior, an apparent disappearance of this behavior, and a later reappearance or recovery period (Strauss, 1982). These behavior changes, when plotted on a graph, show a *U*-shaped curve. For example, a common observation, supported by empirical research, is that creative activities and abilities appear to decline with age in early childhood and then increase late in childhood and adolescence (H. Gardner & Winner, 1982; Lowenfeld & Brittain, 1970; Strauss & Stavy, 1982). These declines are typically attributed to the conformity and suppression of individuality produced by the public school system. Strauss (1982), however, has explained the *U*-shaped curves for creativity and other cognitive abilities in terms of the individual's reorganization of representational systems. Taking an organismic developmental perspective, Strauss has claimed that these declines reflect a developmental advance to a higher level of functioning, not a regression. When the child tries to apply rules from one representational system to another representational system, a temporary drop in performance may occur; after the representational systems are reorganized, the child's performance rebounds.

Strauss (1982) has noted several developmental phenomena to which *U*-shaped curves may pertain: language acquisition, metaphor production, number conservation, and facial representation. Thus, the implications of *U*-shaped functions for developmental interventions are far-reaching. These functions may help explain why programs such as Head Start produced immediate cognitive gains, which disappeared within two or three years, and reappeared later in junior high and high school. By junior high school, children who had Head Start experience in preschool were less likely to be enrolled in special education classes and were more likely to view their schools favorably than control children, although these benefits had not been immediately apparent (Lazar & Darlington, 1982). The existence of *U*-shaped curves might also prepare researchers to expect temporary setbacks in performance as individuals attempt to reorganize their representational system to accommodate new learning. Eventually, their performance should return to or exceed earlier levels.

ETHICAL CONCERNS

The use of interventions to alter cognitive development and other aspects of psychological functioning raises thorny ethical questions. Should psychologists intervene, or should they allow development to run its natural course? Is intervention targeted at one individual or group unfair to other individuals or groups not benefiting from the intervention? If interventions are producing a beneficial effect, is terminating them ethical? In this section, we will examine these questions with the aim of developing a more ethically aware stance toward intervention.

Whether to intervene is an age-old philosophical issue. During the Middle Ages, human beings were conceived to be naturally sinful and corrupt; harsh training was thought necessary to eradicate sinful tendencies. Reacting to this view, the eighteenth-century French philosopher Jean-Jacques Rousseau stressed the inherent purity and goodness of human beings. Rousseau believed that children would develop into compassionate and competent human beings if left to their inborn devices.

These early philosophical belief systems still color our views about the necessity of intervention. For example, one of the best-known and widely employed intervention approaches to preschool education for children from "disadvantaged" backgrounds was developed by Bereiter and Engelmann (1966). These intervenors took the position that it is unrealistic to expect children from low-income households and poor social backgrounds to profit from traditional public school experience. The major problem in Bereiter and Engelmann's (1966) view was that low-income children are deficient in their use of the English language. These investigators developed a highly structured training program focusing on rewards and punishments to teach linguistic and conceptual skills. They concluded that a structured curriculum has greater impact on IQ and linguistic achievement than traditional child-centered approaches.

In contrast to Bereiter and Engelmann (1966), A. S. Neill's (1960) school, Summerhill, represented an approach based on child-centered principles. Drawing on Rousseau's philosophy, Neill (1960) argued that the child must be free to be himself: "How can happiness be bestowed? My own answer is: Abolish authority. Let the child be himself. Don't push him around. Don't teach him. Don't lecture him. Don't elevate him. Don't force him to do anything" (p. 297). The currently popular free school and open school movements represent this approach. They do not attempt to change the child's language or behavior so much as to encourage individual differences.

Which approach is "right" and which one is "wrong" is impossible to say. As Horowitz and Paden (1973) emphasized, the general portrayal of lower-class children's deficits has been both right and wrong. On one hand, lower-class children often do not possess the linguistic and cognitive responses needed to negotiate a public school system based on White middle-class standards and values. But on the other hand, they may develop rich language repertoires that are appropriate and meaningful within their own social-cultural context. Perhaps the most ethically enlightened way to deal with this issue is to think about "differences" in functioning, rather than "deficits" in functioning. Once we label people as deficient, disadvantaged, or deprived, we ignore their cultural integrity and value. This problem can also be seen in gerontological research that labels elderly individuals as deficient in cognitive functioning compared to young White upper-middle-class adults. By thinking of older people as cognitively disadvantaged, we are likely to ignore the unique characteristics and features of their thinking (Labouvie-Vief, 1977, 1982).

Another practice that raises serious ethical questions is targeting an intervention at a single individual or group. In the past many interventions were conducted by a trained professional rather than by the primary agents of a person's socialization (i.e., parents, siblings, peers). If it alters the nature of family interactions, this practice may have the unintended side effect of isolating the individual from his or her social group. There is also a problem in giving an intervention that is perceived to be highly beneficial to a treatment group and using an untreated group as a control for experimental purposes. People in the control condition may view this practice as unfair and arbitrary, particularly if they are in need of the treatment. A compromise solution is to design experiments in which people are given different types or levels of intervention, rather than no intervention (Riecken & Boruch, 1974). Another solution is to give intervention to the groups most likely to benefit from it.

A final question concerns the termination of intervention. Most research in psychology, including longitudinal research, is conducted for a limited time. In theory, it would be possible to conduct an experiment in which the treatment group was treated as long as was needed or desirable (Riecken & Boruch, 1974). However, because of practical restrictions, this is seldom done. In research, the intervention is often ended because of financial or political reasons, not because the intervention failed to produce the intended effect. The ethical problem is whether it is ethically defensible to enrich people's lives temporarily and then return them to their original condition (Riecken & Boruch, 1974). Perhaps a little intervention is worse than no intervention if the former raises people's expectations about their ability to achieve cognitively only to destroy such expectations when the intervention is removed. Much more attention should be paid to the duration of intervention as an experimental variable in developmental studies.

In concluding this chapter, we encourage cognitive developmental researchers to avoid narrowly limiting their interventions to IQ and related cognitive behaviors in the here-and-now environment. Rather, interventions should be geared to the whole person functioning within a complexly changing ecology over long time spans (Bronfenbrenner, 1977). As we have said before, cognitive development is best understood not in isolation from, but in relation to, the total psychological functioning of the person.

SUMMARY

1. "Intervention" can be defined as the systematic attempt to alter the course of cognitive change in order to prevent intellectual deficits and to maximize cognitive functioning.

2. Because the area of intervention research is relatively new, not all psychologists accept the need for or understand the objectives of intervention.

3. Intervention research can be categorized into two broad areas. Theoretical-developmental approaches emphasize research on the amount of age-related plasticity or potential in cognitive development; practical-educational approaches stress training of cognitive abilities for academic achievement. These two approaches are not exclusive of each other.

4. The majority of training studies with children focus on the acquisition of Piagetian concepts. Those with adults attempt to modify performance on standardized intelligence measures, especially measures of fluid ability.

5. Project Head Start and similar intervention programs for preschool children were designed to overcome the effects of early environmental deprivation and to equip children with the cognitive skills necessary for academic work. Although these programs often fail to produce durable increases in intelligence, they appear to have some long-term benefits for children.

6. Intervention has three major interrelated goals: (1) remediation, (2) prevention, and (3) enrichment. Remediation involves removing or correcting an existing problem behavior, whereas prevention seeks to prevent the occurrence or recurrence of a problem. Enrichment aims at the enhancement or optimization of psychological development.

7. Intervention can occur at the individual level, small-group level, or societal level. The level of intervention is important in choosing an appropriate intervention strategy.

8. An intervention strategy is the actual mode or technique of intervention used. Three major intervention strategies are social learning, training-practice, and ecological change.

9. The patterning and the timing of intervention are influential vari-

ables in intervention research. Interventions may produce negative side effects if they are introduced in an inappropriate order or at a nonoptimal time in development.

10. The frequent failure of intervention programs to yield intended outcomes underscores the need for evaluation research. The principal types of evaluation are (1) formative evaluation and (2) summative evaluation.

11. Several theoretical issues are critical in evaluating the effectiveness of intervention programs on cognitive development. These include the relative amount of intellectual plasticity at different age levels, the maintenance and generalization of intervention over time and tasks, and the existence of curvilinear patterns or U-shaped functions of development.

12. The increasing use of intervention to modify cognitive functioning raises important ethical issues. Attention to these issues will help developmental psychologists design more effective and more humane intervention programs.

Key Terms

intervention

cognitive conflict

near transfer

far transfer

sleeper effects

remediation

prevention

enrichment

overjustification effect

social learning

formative evaluation

summative evaluation

unexercised ability

optimally exercised ability

maintenance

generalization

U-shaped functions

Suggested Readings

Allen, K. E., & Goetz, E. M. (Eds.). (1982). *Early childhood education: Special problems, special solutions.* Rockville, MD: Aspen Systems Corporation. This book presents an integrated look at the behavior analysis approach to intervention with a focus on developmental problems in young handicapped, normal, and at-risk children. Several chapters deal with intervention to lessen linguistic and cognitive skill deficiencies.

Bronfenbrenner, U. (1979). *The ecology of human development: Experiments by nature and design.* Cambridge, MA: Harvard University Press. Bronfenbrenner proposes an ecological model for the study of development in context. Empirical investigations which satisfy ecological criteria are reviewed, and the implications of the findings for modifying human behavior are discussed.

Feuerstein, R., Rand, Y., Hoffman, M. B., & Miller, R. (1980). *Instrumental enrichment: An intervention program for cognitive modifiability.* Baltimore, MD: University Park Press. This book describes an intervention strategy for modifying cognitive development in retarded adolescents. The success of the strategy challenges prevailing beliefs that interventions must begin in early infancy and continue well into the school years.

Gottfried, A. W. (Ed.). (1984). *Home environment and early cognitive development: Longitudinal research.* New York: Academic Press. This volume is based on seven longitudinal studies investigating the relationship of home environment variables to cognitive development during infancy and the preschool years. The last chapter deals with the implications of the findings for intervention.

Lerner, R. M. (1984). *On the nature of human plasticity.* New York: Cambridge University Press. A major premise of this book is that plasticity exists at many different levels of analysis (biological, cognitive, sociocultural), and intervention aimed at one level may influence functioning at another level. According to Lerner, this reciprocal influence provides a rationale for a multidisciplinary life-span approach to research and intervention.

CHAPTER 11

Epilogue

OVERVIEW

During the past two decades the cognitive revolution in psychology has had a profound influence, affecting the conceptions of investigators who 10 or 20 years ago would have avoided references to terms such as *cognition*. But as Baltes and Schaie (1973) have aptly pointed out in their discussion of the life-span revolution in developmental psychology, "it appears easier to start a revolution than it is to carry it to impressive heights or even victory" (p. 395). Although the current research activity, the multitude of research articles, and the proliferation of models in cognitive psychology suggest that there may be no immediate cause for alarm, the history of science is replete with examples of approaches that outran their scientific value by promising too much and delivering too little. This Epilogue will review the current status of life-span cognitive developmental psychology; we will not present any new empirical research findings. Rather, we wish to point out areas in the field that represent genuine progress and identify emerging areas that may give us a clue about the field's directions in the future. Critical questions about present conceptions and methods which may need revision will also be considered.

THE COGNITIVE REVOLUTION: REVOLUTION OR CONSPIRACY?

The cognitive approach to psychology, though very old (Baldwin, 1906; James, 1890), reemerged during the 1960s and 1970s with renewed vigor. As psychology began to feel the full impact of the cognitive revolution, two major forces became evident: (1) Piaget, with his structural theory of intelligence, and (2) information-processing psychologists, with their model of an input-throughput-output cognitive system. Both of these approaches employ radically different theoretical constructs and methods of study, but they have become so popular as to almost drown out opposing voices. Does this mean that the cognitive revolution is over and victory is won? Not exactly. As Datan (1977) has remarked, "a revolution is incomplete until the counterrevolutionaries have begun to be heard" (p. 55). If this is true, then we must examine not only the positive contributions of each approach but also what the critics are saying.

Challenges to Piaget's Theory

Piaget's death on September 16, 1980, marked the passing of the greatest child psychologist of the twentieth century. His thoughts about children's cognitive and conceptual abilities revolutionized developmental psychology and influenced generations of psychologists. Prior to Piaget, few psychologists were seriously interested in studying the unique features of children's thinking. Researchers generally assumed that children are merely immature (or less bright) versions of adults. But Piaget's ideas dramatically altered our thinking about cognitive development and will continue to have an impact. Questions about qualitative changes in the structures of thought with age, the nature of cognitive operations, and the coherence of thought have received much more attention than in the decades before Piaget's introduction to North American psychologists (Keating, 1984).

Although many investigators will continue to be influenced by the questions Piaget raised, their answers to these questions are likely to be very different (L. Siegel & Brainerd, 1978). For example, Chapter 2 noted the growing dissatisfaction with Piaget's stage account of cognitive development. Cognitive development seems less stage-like than Piaget thought, or at least the stages are somewhat different than he proposed (Broughton, 1984; Flavell & Markman, 1983). Investigators are now proposing more limited sequences of development within circumscribed task domains rather than universal cognitive stages defined by logical-mathematical structures (Feldman, 1980; Fischer, 1980; Gelman & Baillargeon, 1983). In addition, researchers have vigorously criticized the vagueness and emptiness of Piaget's adaptive mechanism of *equilibration* (see Chapter 2). As you may recall, Piaget described equilibration as an interaction of assimilative and accommodative processes which serves to maintain the equilibrium of all self-regulatory systems. He believed that equilibration was a factor of tremendous psychological importance and could characterize self-regulation at the biological, psychological, or social level. However, with the possible exception of the sensorimotor period, Piaget did not formulate the concept of equilibration except in very global, abstract terms. A description of the characteristics of the interaction between organismic structures and environmental and maturational factors is lacking in his theory (A. Siegel, Bisanz, & Bisanz, 1983).

Current cognitive developmental approaches have attempted to provide a more adequate account of stage-to-stage transitions. Pascual-Leone (1970) has proposed that the Piagetian stages of cognitive development are determined by increases in cognitive capacity because of growing central computing space, which he calls *M-space*. Case and colleagues (Case, 1978; Case, Kurland, & Goldberg, 1982) have taken a similar "neo-Piagetian" approach. They suggest that the automaticity of basic processes (e.g., encoding, retrieval) that accompany development frees processing space, resulting in improved cognitive functioning. Both of these approaches incorporate information-processing components into Piagetian theory and thus reflect a beginning synthesis of cognitive structuralist and information-processing formulations.

Researchers have also begun to question the usefulness of Piaget's assessment tasks. Tasks that are limited to physics and mathematical reasoning may not tell us much about children's or adults' cognitive potential in real life. When researchers modify task materials and procedures in order to make them more true to life, some surprising discoveries about childhood and adulthood cognition often occur. For example, under certain task conditions young children seem to have remarkably well-developed knowledge of classification, number, and social cognition (Flavell & Markman, 1983). Similarly, many adults may perform better when the assessment tasks are more contextually valid, a possibility Piaget (1972) also acknowledged.

In the adolescent and adult portions of the life span, there have been major reconceptualizations of Piaget's theory. In Piaget's account, formal operations culminate in adolescence and represent the final and most developmentally mature stage of thinking. But life-span researchers are now arguing that the contextual variability of adult thinking demands a new interpretation of postadolescent thought. For example, Labouvie-Vief (1980, 1982, 1985) claims that adulthood is characterized by a major reorganization of the structures of self-regulation. Rather than view logic as the organizing principle of adult cognition, Labouvie-Vief sees the integration of adult thinking with the practical and real-life constraints of the culture as most significant. Cognitive abilities of adults should not be interpreted as regression, but as a growth of more highly differentiated skills marked by autonomy, social orientation, and a dialectical mode of reasoning (Labouvie-Vief, 1982). Life-span cognitive developmental research is likely to be heavily influenced by these theoretical notions in the future.

Challenges to Information-Processing Theories

In a recent review chapter, Siegler (1983) has claimed that at present the information-processing approach "is arguably *the* leading strategy for the study of cognitive development" (p. 129). Based on the spiraling number of references to information-processing research, Siegler may be correct. Although it is not intrinsically a developmental framework, information processing has considerably enriched our understanding of the way children and adults think. The approach offers developmental psychologists a distinctive way to conceptualize the organism and also influences the kinds of questions they must ask to understand the organism (Kail & Bisanz, 1982). In particular, it has focused attention on the similarities in children's and adults' thought processes and the transitional mechanisms that may explain continued developmental change across the life span.

The two processes that have received the most developmental speculation are increases in attentional capacity and knowledge base modifications. The bulk of the research evidence on the capacity of working memory suggests invariance across the life span, but this claim remains equivocal (Salthouse, 1985; Siegler, 1983). The main problem appears to be whether increases occur in absolute capacity (size), or whether less processing space must be devoted to executing basic operations because of increased use and automatization of memory strategies. Actually, both explanations could be partly correct in the sense that the underlying capacity of working memory may remain unchanged, but increased automaticity may increase memory's "effective" capacity. More empirical work will undoubtedly examine the question of capacity differences in the future.

Much less attention has been focused on changes in knowledge of a specific content area as an explanation of developmental changes, perhaps because increases in the knowledge base with age have always been assumed. However, as research by Chi (1978) has shown, changes in the knowledge base may overshadow all other age-related differences and, on occasion, developmental differences may be reversed. Given that changes in knowledge are omnipresent yet poorly understood, they seem to be likely targets for future study. Some questions for further research are the following: How do modifications in knowledge influence memory and other cognitive processes at different ages? How can the knowledge base be used to compensate for a failing memory system? Do structural or qualitative transformations in the knowledge base occur in later adulthood?

The potential for modifications in the knowledge base highlights the role of learning in information-processing analyses of cognitive development. For many years, psychology emphasized the core concept of learning (W. Hoyer, 1980; Sigel, 1981). Psychologists constructed global theories of learning based on basic learning principles such as the so-called law of effect. The law of effect refers to the strengthening or weakening of a stimulus-response association as a result of its consequences. However, until recently information-processing theorists resembled Piaget in not making learning an issue in spite of its central importance to development. This omission is especially surprising in view of the necessity of learning for acquiring, organizing, and responding to incoming information. Part of the reason for this neglect is that an understanding of learning requires knowledge about stimulus inputs, problems of representation, and response outputs (D. A. Norman, 1981). As information-processing psychologists began to better understand these processes, they began to pay increased attention to the problem of learning and development (A. Brown, 1982; Siegler & Klahr, 1982).

Like Piagetian studies, information-processing studies often employ laboratory tasks that have little connection to everyday-life cognitive activities. However, whereas Piagetian structural theorists are concerned with identifying abstract intellectual structures that can be applied across a wide range of tasks, information-processing theorists are concerned with identifying precise cognitive skills or sets of skills for specific tasks. The task specificity of information-processing analyses limits their generalizability to other problem situations. Moreover, it raises the issue of whether the cognitive processes are isomorphic with the tasks in which they have been "discovered" (Keating, 1984; Newell, 1973). The real danger is that the cognitive skills may be so constrained by the nature of the task that the researcher is unable to form a more general theory of cognition.

Information-processing theories have not proven especially fruitful in studying the "hotter" side of cognition—that is, emotional, social, and personality characteristics. Like Piaget's theory, they seem better suited to the "cold" cognition of logical problem solving and mathematical reasoning. One problem has been an inability to capture the complexities of human emotion and personality in computer-programming language. Attempts are now being made to develop information-processing models of emotion that integrate cognition and emotion (e.g., Zajonc, 1980, 1984). Moreover, psychologists are describing models of knowing that involve abilities to access one's own feelings and perceive the feelings of others, to visually analyze the world, and to learn music and faces (H. Gardner, 1983).

NEW DIRECTIONS IN COGNITIVE DEVELOPMENT

The mounting challenges to Piagetian and information-processing approaches to cognitive development signal a major shift in the direction of the cognitive revolution. At this juncture it may be useful to consider issues that will be at the forefront of the field in the future.

Context and Cognition

Most approaches to the study of cognitive development have considered internal aspects of the person (e.g., strategies, representations) as primary and as relatively stable across settings and tasks. Until recently, understanding of the properties of the context has been considered secondary. The role of context in development has been most often discussed as a problem of generalizing from performance in laboratory situations to the real world of ordinary individuals and real-life tasks. The significance of context is highlighted in Bronfenbrenner's (1977) complaint that developmental psychology is "the science of the strange behavior of children in strange situations with strange adults for the briefest possible periods of time" (p. 513).

A consideration of context is critical for developmental researchers who need valid assessments of individual competencies and behaviors at different ages in order to describe, explain, and predict cognitive changes across the life span (Hultsch & Hickey, 1978; Rogoff, 1982). For example, as noted in Chapter 5, on language development, young children as well as the elderly often have difficulty in laboratory-based social communication tasks, yet they seem to be able to communicate well in everyday life. This observation has led psycholinguists to try to identify pragmatic rules that govern the use of language in various communication contexts. Similarly, children who are often unable to recall objects on laboratory memory tasks demonstrate impressive skills in searching for objects hidden in their homes by their parents (Wellman, 1985). In these examples, individuals who do not appear to have competencies in the laboratory show them in the real world.

When discrepant findings arise, the typical recommendation is to abandon laboratory research in favor of more contextually valid naturalistic studies. But such a recommendation misses the point: naturalistic studies are not necessarily valid because they are conducted in a real-life setting or with more meaningful tasks, nor are laboratory experiments invalid because they use settings and tests that do not represent real-life conditions. Many laboratory findings do generalize to behaviors in daily life.

The objective should be to find suitable experimental methods that include context as an integral variable. Two possible methods for accomplishing this objective are (1) *protocol analysis* and (2) *ethnographic analysis.* In protocol analysis, the researcher provides a rich description of the structure and process of cognitive events observed in context. Anzai and Simon (1979) used a detailed protocol analysis to study changes in problem-solving strategies of one person on the tower of Hanoi problem. J. Meyer and Rebok (1985) have applied this same type of analysis to planning protocols in their study of life-span differences in problem solving (see Chapter 7). Ethnographic analysis of cognition involves detailed descriptive analysis and interpretation of a few cases. Ethnographers use their knowledge of behavioral and cultural norms as well as analyses of data in the form of verbal transcripts and videotapes. Cognitive researchers often use ethnographic methods to analyze communication interactions in parent-child dyads or to study transmission of cognitive skills as adults assist children in problem solving (Rogoff, 1982). Both protocol analysis and ethnographic analysis are methodologically rigorous ways of carrying out contextually oriented experimental studies of cognitive development.

Intellectual Plasticity and Constraints

One of the long-standing debates in life-span developmental psychology concerns the amount of age-related plasticity in intellectual functioning. Baltes, Schaie, and other life-span researchers have emphasized the high degree of intellectual plasticity or intraindividual variability in intellectual functioning in the later years of the life span (Willis & Baltes, 1980; Schaie, 1983). Using results from cohort-sequential studies of intelligence and intervention training studies, they argue for the possibility of genuine improvements in intellectual abilities and performance with age. In contrast, Horn and Donaldson (1976) have suggested that cognitive development and aging are marked by limitations in an organism's intellectual plasticity because of biological and neurological losses.

To conclude that either side has won the battle over plasticity would be premature. However, the controversy has served to focus attention on the need to differentiate aging effects from other forms of developmental variance. Thus, researchers have turned to studies showing the effects of cohort variables (e.g., education, occupation, health) and specific life events (e.g., marriage, illness, retirement) as factors in age-related cognitive changes. In addition, life-span investigators have employed the concept of "testing the limits" to obtain information on the range of variability or modifiability of intellectual performance. The testing-the-limits approach involves the assessment of performance under varying levels of support and difficulty and reveals what a person can do under maximally supportive (or maximally unsupportive) biological and environmental conditions. In other words, the strategy defines the boundaries of plasticity.

The debate about plasticity also poses a challenge to the assumption that intellectual change is characterized by universal, biologically based declines in the adult years. Recent evidence on the plasticity of the aging brain (G. Lynch, 1983) suggests that biology may not invariably constrain or limit further intellectual and cognitive growth. This is not to say that we can ignore the constraints imposed by biological capacities of individuals at different points in their life span. Biomedical evidence indicates that loss of vital capacity and resistance to disease and death are inevitable facts of later life (Finch & Schneider, 1985).

Arguing from a very different perspective, Keil (1981) has claimed that psychologists need to consider developmental constraints on natural concepts such as number concepts, natural language syntax, knowledge of basic categories, and deductive reasoning. According to Keil, *constrained* knowledge is acquired effortlessly and rapidly in early life without much formal instruction (e.g., certain spatial and orienting skills, esthetics, linguistic skills). For example, some type of constraint must enable young children to discover the complex structure of language or to show a propensity to use numbers. Thus, although it may show a great deal of developmental plasticity, knowledge also appears to obey a set of constraints. Identifying these constraints will be a major advance in cognitive developmental theory.

Interindividual Differences in Cognitive Change

Closely related to the notion of plasticity in cognition is the issue of interindividual differences. As noted at the beginning of this book, wide interindividual differences appear in cognitive change patterns, especially during adulthood and old age. The existence of such large interindividual variability has led many life-span researchers to question the search for universal and normative patterns in cognitive developmental change (Baltes, Dittmann-Kohli, & Dixon, 1984; Willis, 1985). This view differs markedly from some models of child development (such as Piaget's organismic developmental approach) in which universality and homogeneity of change across individuals is assumed.

Identifying the pattern and sources of interindividual differences in intraindividual cognitive change has been and will continue to be a major research objective for many life-span developmental investigators. For example, work by Schaie (1983) on individual differences in several primary mental abilities indicates that interindividual differences remain high for certain abilities (e.g., verbal meaning) into people's 80s, whereas for other abilities (e.g., space, number, reasoning) variability declines. Schaie has suggested that such differences may stem from an increased incidence of cardiovascular disease, differential exposure to favorable environmental conditions, and flexibility in personality style earlier in life. Because some of these variables are under environmental control, they may be subjected to various types of cognitive intervention programs. For example, advances in treating cardiovascular diseases, improved health practices, and stimulating educational programs may help prevent declines in intellectual functioning earlier as well as later in life.

As they become more aware of interindividual differences in performance, investigators will pay greater attention to whether or not differences in health, ability, education, background, or gender confound aging effects on cognitive measures (I. Krauss, Poon, Gilewski, & Schaie, 1982). As noted, controlling for educational differences between age groups often reduces or eliminates age-related cognitive differences. Great care will be needed when selecting subject samples to ensure that developmental effects are not accounted for by differences in these individual difference variables, rather than in chronological age.

Applications of Cognitive Developmental Research

One of the biggest advances in the years ahead will come as cognitive developmental researchers spell out the applications of their work. We are likely to see increasing numbers of cognitive developmentalists turn to applied problems in education, social policy, and mental health. Such efforts will sharpen the definition of key concepts, test the results of laboratory research in real-life settings, and highlight the limitations of the available data base (Flavell & Markman, 1983). But applied research also has its dangers, especially if researchers oversimplify their findings or make immodest claims about the extent of their knowledge. Therefore, cognitive developmental researchers will have to serve as interpreters as well as producers of scientific knowledge.

Cognitive developmental psychologists will be faced with stiff methodological problems as they investigate applied problems in complex interactive situations. Life-span developmentalists have been particularly sensitive to the need for research methods that involve multiple sources of causation and multiple dependent variables. Increasingly, we see the use of more powerful data analytic techniques such as structural equations models to explain life-span developmental differences and changes (Baltes, Reese, & Nesselroade, 1977; Schaie & Hertzog, 1985). Structural equations models are used to test well-articulated hypotheses about causal relationships among variables in cross-sectional and longitudinal data sets. Given the current limitations of investigating short-term and long-term developmental changes with experimental manipulative methods, structural equations models open up vast new possibilities for life-span developmental investigations (for technical discussions of this technique, see Jöreskog & Sörbom, 1979; Rogosa, 1979). One likely outcome is a greater emphasis on longitudinal research and other repeated measures strategies. Many investigators feel that longitudinal designs are the only truly developmental designs because they focus on intraindividual change, rather than on static age differences. Finally, developmental multivariate research strategies, in which several dependent variables are studied at a time, are being employed more frequently (especially in longitudinal work) and promise to provide a more comprehensive account of life-span behavioral change.

CONCLUSION

We talk about progress in cognitive developmental psychology, about paradigmatic shifts and rapid advances in theoretical knowledge. If progress is judged by the number of new theories or new research methods, then we can conclude that the field has advanced a great deal over the past two decades. But if we want to know more—if we want to know how the organism thinks, feels, and acts in real time and real life—then a great deal is yet to be done. This will be the challenging enterprise for cognitive developmental psychology in coming decades.

Let us conclude by reemphasizing three points originally presented in Chapter 1. These points provide challenges to current thinking about life-span cognition and offer an agenda for future research. They can be summarized as follows:

1. Cognitive developmental change occurs continually across the life span and is not limited to one particular age or period of time.
2. Cognitive development occurs as a complex result of changing person-environment interactions; it cannot be studied apart from the biological, psychological, and sociological context in which the person thinks and behaves.
3. Cognitive development shows both progressive and regressive features across the life span, and its course is influenced by multiple determinants.

By challenging long-held assumptions about the nature and direction of cognitive development, the life-span approach offers us new insights into human intellectual potential and a basis for developing a more integrative conception of child and adult cognition.

References

Abrahams, J. P. (1976). Health status as a variable in aging research. *Experimental Aging Research, 2,* 63–71.

Abravanel, E. (1968). The development of intersensory patterning with regard to selected spatial dimensions. *Monographs of the Society for Research in Child Development, 3* (2, Serial No. 118).

Achenbach, T. M. (1978). *Research in developmental psychology: Concepts, strategies, methods.* New York: Free Press.

Acredolo, L. P. (1976). Frames of reference used by children for orientation in unfamiliar spaces. In G. T. Moore & R. G. Golledge (Eds.), *Environmental knowing* (pp. 165–172). Stroudsburg, PA: Dowden, Hutchinson, & Ross.

Acredolo, L. P. (1981). Small- and large-scale spatial concepts in infancy and childhood. In L. S. Liben, A. H. Patterson, & N. Newcombe (Eds.), *Spatial representation and behavior across the life span* (pp. 63–81). New York: Academic Press.

Acredolo, L. P., & Hake, J. L. (1982). Infant perception. In B. B. Wolman (Ed.), *Handbook of developmental psychology* (pp. 244–283). Englewood Cliffs, NJ: Prentice-Hall.

Acredolo, L., Pick, H. L., Jr., & Olsen, M. G. (1975). Environmental differentiation and familiarity as determinants of children's memory for spatial location. *Developmental Psychology, 11,* 495–501.

Allen, G. L., Kirasic, K. C., Siegel, A. W., & Herman, J. F. (1979). Developmental issues in cognitive mapping: The selection and utilization of environmental landmarks. *Child Development, 50,* 1062–1070.

Alpaugh, P. K., & Birren, J. E. (1977). Variables affecting creative contributions across the adult life span. *Human Development, 20,* 240–248.

Altemeyer, R., Fulton, D., & Berney, K. (1969). Long-term memory improvement: Confirmation of a finding by Piaget. *Child Development, 40,* 845–857.

American Psychiatric Association (1980). *Diagnostic and statistical manual of mental disorders* (3rd ed.). Washington, DC.

Anastasi, A. (1958). Heredity, environment, and the question "How?" *Psychological Review, 65,* 197–208.

Anderson, J. E. (1939). The limitations of infant and preschool tests in the measurement of intelligence. *Journal of Psychology, 8,* 351–379.

Anderson, J. R. (1983). *The architecture of cognition.* Cambridge, MA: Harvard University Press.

Anderson, J. R. (1985). *Cognitive psychology and its implications* (2nd ed.). San Francisco: Freeman.

Anderson, S., & Messick, S. (1974). Social competency in young children. *Developmental Psychology, 10,* 282–293.

Anzai, Y., & Simon, H. A. (1979). The theory of learning by doing. *Psychological Review, 86,* 124–140.

Arenberg, D. (1968). Concept problem solving in young and old adults. *Journal of Gerontology, 23,* 279–282.

Arenberg, D. (1974). A longitudinal study of problem solving in adults. *Journal of Gerontology, 29,* 650–658.

Arenberg, D. (1976). The effects of input condition on free recall in young and old adults. *Journal of Gerontology, 31,* 551–555.

Arenberg, D. (1982). Changes with age in problem solving. In F. I. M. Craik & S. Trehub (Eds.), *Advances in the study of communication and affect: Vol. 8. Aging and cognitive processes* (pp. 221–235). New York: Plenum Press.

Arlin, P. K. (1975). Cognitive development: A fifth stage? *Developmental Psychology, 11,* 602–606.

Arlin, P. K. (1984). Adolescent and adult thought: A structural interpretation. In M. L. Commons, F. A. Richards, & C. Armon (Eds.), *Beyond formal operations: Late adolescent and adult cognitive development* (pp. 258–271). New York: Praeger.

Aronfreed, J. (1968). *Conduct and conscience.* New York: Academic Press.

Aronson, E., & Rosenbloom, S. (1971). Space perception within a common auditory-visual space. *Science, 172,* 1161–1163.

Ashton, P. T. (1975). Cross-cultural Piagetian research: An experimental perspective. *Harvard Educational Review, 45,* 475–506.

Aslin, R. N., Pisoni, D. B., & Jusczyk, P. W. (1983). Auditory development and speech perception in infancy. In M. M. Haith & J. J. Campos (Eds.), *Handbook of child psychology: Vol. 2. Infancy and developmental psychobiology* (pp. 573–687). New York: Wiley.

Atkinson, R. C., & Shiffrin, R. M. (1968). Human memory: A proposed system and its control processes. In K. W. Spence & J. T. Spence (Eds.), *The psychology of learning and motivation: Advances in research and theory* (Vol. 2, pp. 89–195). New York: Academic Press.

Baddeley, A. D. (1978). The trouble with levels: A reexamination of Craik and Lockhart's framework for memory research. *Psychological Review, 85,* 139–152.

Baddeley, A. D. (1981). Cognitive psychology of everyday life. *British Journal of Psychology, 72,* 257-269.

Baddeley, A. D., & Hitch, G. (1974). Working memory. In G. H. Bower (Ed.), *The psychology of learning and motivation: Advances in research and theory* (Vol. 8, pp. 47–89). New York: Academic Press.

Bahrick, H. P., Bahrick, P. O., & Wittlinger, R. P. (1975). Fifty years of memory for names and faces: A cross-sectional approach. *Journal of Experimental Psychology: General, 104,* 54–75.

Baldwin, J. M. (1906). *Mental development in the child and the race: Methods and processes* (3rd ed.). New York: Macmillan.

Ball, S., & Bogatz, G. A. (1972). Summative research of *Sesame Street:* Implications for the study of preschool children. In A. D. Pick (Ed.), *Minnesota Symposia on Child Psychology* (Vol. 6, pp. 3–17). Minneapolis: University of Minnesota Press.

Baltes, P. B. (Ed.). (1973). Strategies for psychological intervention in old age: A symposium. *Gerontologist, 13,* 4–38.

Baltes, P. B. (Ed.). (1978). *Life-span development and behavior* (Vol. 1). New York: Academic Press.

Baltes, P. B. (1979). Life-span developmental psychology: Some converging observations on history and theory. In P. B. Baltes & O. G. Brim, Jr. (Eds.), *Life-span development and behavior* (Vol. 2, pp. 255–279). New York: Academic Press.

Baltes, P. B., & Danish, S. J. (1980). Intervention in life-span development and aging: Issues and concepts. In R. R. Turner & H. W. Reese (Eds.), *Life-span developmental psychology: Intervention* (pp. 49–78). New York: Academic Press.

Baltes, P. B., Dittmann-Kohli, F., & Dixon, R. (1984). New perspectives on the development of intelligence in adulthood: Toward a dual-process conception and a model of selective optimization with compensation. In P. B. Baltes & O. G. Brim, Jr. (Eds.), *Life-span development and behavior* (Vol. 6, pp. 33–76). New York: Academic Press.

Baltes, P. B., & Goulet, L. R. (1971). Exploration of developmental variables by manipulation and simulation of age differences in behavior. *Human Development, 14,* 149–170.

Baltes, P. B., & Nesselroade, J. R. (Eds.). (1979). *Longitudinal research in the study of behavior and development.* New York: Academic Press.

Baltes, P. B., Reese, H. W., & Lipsitt, L. P. (1980). Life-span developmental psychology. *Annual Review of Psychology, 31,* 65–110.

Baltes, P. B., Reese, H. W., & Nesselroade, J. R. (1977). *Life-span developmental psychology: Introduction to research methods.* Monterey, CA: Brooks-Cole.

Baltes, P. B., & Schaie, K. W. (Eds.). (1973). *Life-span developmental psychology: Personality and socialization.* New York: Academic Press,.

Baltes, P. B., & Willis, S. L. (1977). Toward psychological theories of aging and development. In J. E. Birren & K. W. Schaie (Eds.), *Handbook of the psychology of aging* (pp. 128–154). New York: Van Nostrand Reinhold.

A ban on IQ tests. (1976, March 22). *Newsweek,* p. 49.

Bandura, A. (1977). *Social learning theory.* Englewood Cliffs, NJ: Prentice-Hall.

Bandura, A., Grusec, J. E., & Menlove, F. L. (1967). Vicarious extinction of avoidance behavior. *Journal of Personality and Social Psychology, 5,* 16–23.

Bandura, A., & McDonald, F. J. (1963). Influence of social reinforcement and the behavior of models in shaping children's moral judgments. *Journal of Abnormal and Social Psychology, 67,* 274–281.

Bandura, A., & Schunk, D. H. (1981). Cultivating competence, self-efficacy, and intrinsic interest through proximal self-motivation. *Journal of Personality and Social Psychology, 42,* 586–598.

Banks, M. S. (1980). The development of visual accommodation during early infancy. *Child Development, 51,* 646–666.

Barenboim, C. (1981). The development of person perception in childhood and adolescence: From behavioral comparisons to psychological constructs to psychological comparisons. *Child Development, 52,* 129–144.

Barron, F. (1969). *Creative person and creative process.* New York: Holt, Rinehart and Winston.

Barron, F., & Harrington, D. M. (1981). Creativity, intelligence, and personality. *Annual Review of Psychology, 32,* 439–476.

Bartlett, F. C. (1932). *Remembering.* New York: Cambridge University Press.

Bates, E. (1979). *The emergence of symbols: Cognition and communication in infancy.* New York: Academic Press.

Bates, E., Benigni, L., Bretherton, I., Camaioni, L., & Volterra, V. (1979). Cognition and communication from nine to thirteen months: Correlational findings. In E. Bates (Ed.), *The emergence of symbols: Cognition and communication in infancy* (pp. 69–140). New York: Academic Press.

Bates, E., Camaioni, L., & Volterra, V. (1975). The acquisition of performatives prior to speech. *Merrill-Palmer Quarterly, 21,* 205–226.

Bayley, N. (1943). Mental growth during the first three years. In R. G. Barker, J. S. Kounin, & H. F. Wright (Eds.), *Child behavior and development* (pp. 87–105). New York: McGraw-Hill.

Bayley, N. (1968). Behavioral correlates of mental growth: Birth to thirty-six years. *American Psychologist, 23,* 1–17.

Bayley, N. (1969). *Bayley Scales of Infant Development.* New York: Psychological Corporation.

Bayley, N., & Oden, M. H. (1955). The maintenance of intellectual ability in gifted adults. *Journal of Gerontology, 10,* 91–107.

Beal, C. R., & Flavell, J. H. (1983). Young speakers' evaluations of their listeners' comprehension in a referential communication task. *Child Development, 54,* 148–153.

Bearison, D. J. (1974). The construct of regression: A Piagetian approach. *Merrill-Palmer Quarterly, 20,* 21–30.

Bearison, D. J. (1982). New directions in studies of social interaction and cognitive growth. In F. C. Serafica (Ed.), *Social-cognitive development in context* (pp. 199–221). New York: Guilford Press.

Beilin, H. (1965). Learning and operational convergence in logical thought development. *Journal of Experimental Child Psychology, 2,* 317–339.

Beilin, H. (1980). Piaget's theory: Refinement, revision, or rejection? In R. H. Kluwe & H. Spada (Eds.), *Developmental models of thinking* (pp. 245–261). New York: Academic Press.

Benedict, H. (1975, April). *The role of repetition in early language comprehension.* Paper presented at the meeting of the Society for Research in Child Development, Denver, CO.

Benedict, H. (1979). Early lexical development: Comprehension and production. *Journal of Child Language, 6,* 183–200.

Bereiter, C., & Engelmann, S. (1966). *Teaching disadvantaged children in the preschool.* Englewood Cliffs, NJ: Prentice-Hall.

Berg, C., Hertzog, C., & Hunt, E. (1982). Age differences in the speed of mental rotation. *Developmental Psychology, 18,* 95–107.

Berg, C. A., & Sternberg, R. J. (1985). A triarchic theory of intellectual development during adulthood. *Developmental Review, 5,* 334–370.

Berg-Cross, L. G. (1975). Intentionality, degree of damage, and moral judgments. *Child Development, 46,* 970–974.

Berko, J. (1958). The child's learning of English morphology. *Word, 14,* 50–177.

Berry, J. W. (1966). Temne and Eskimo perceptual skills. *International Journal of Psychology, 1,* 207–229.

Berry, J. W., & Dasen, P. R. (Eds.). (1974). *Culture and cognition: Readings in cross-cultural psychology.* New York: Methuen.

Bielby, D. D., & Papalia, D. E. (1975). Moral development and egocentrism: Their development and interrelationship across the life-span. *International Journal of Aging and Human Development, 6,* 293–308.

Birren, J. E. (1973). A summary: Prospects and problems of research on the longitudinal development of man's intellectual capacities throughout life. In L. F. Jarvik, C. Eisdorfer, & J. E. Blum (Eds.), *Intellectual functioning in adults: Psychological and biological influences* (pp. 149–154). New York: Springer.

Birren, J. E., Kinney, D. K., Schaie, K. W., & Woodruff, D. S. (1981). *Developmental psychology: A life-span approach.* Boston: Houghton Mifflin.

Birren, J. E., & Morrison, D. F. (1961). Analysis of the WAIS subtests in relation to age and education. *Journal of Gerontology, 16,* 363–369.

Birren, J. E., & Woodruff, D. S. (1973). Human development over the life span through education. In P. B. Baltes & K. W. Schaie (Eds.), *Life-span developmental psychology: Personality and socialization* (pp. 305–337). New York: Academic Press.

Bjork, E. L., & Cummings, E. M. (1984). Infant search errors: Stage of concept development or stage of memory development. *Memory and Cognition, 12,* 1–19.

Black, J. B., & Wilensky, R. (1979). An evaluation of story grammars. *Cognitive Science, 3,* 213–230.

Blasi, A. (1980). Bridging moral cognition and moral action: A critical review of the literature. *Psychological Bulletin, 88,* 1–45.

Blieszner, R., Willis, S. L., & Baltes, P. B. (1981). Training research on induction ability in aging: A short-term longitudinal study. *Journal of Applied Developmental Psychology, 2,* 247–265.

Bloom, B. S. (1964). *Stability and change in human characteristics.* New York: Wiley.

Bloom, L. (1970). *Language development: Form and function in emerging grammars.* Cambridge, MA: MIT Press.

Bloom, L. (1973). *One word at a time: The use of single word utterances before syntax.* The Hague: Mouton.

Bloomfield, L. (1933). *Language.* New York: Holt.

Boles, D. B. (1980). X-linkage of spatial ability: A critical review. *Child Development, 51,* 625–635.

Boring, E. G. (1923, June 6). Intelligence as the tests test it. *New Republic,* pp. 35–37.

Boring, E. G. (1950). *A history of experimental psychology.* Englewood Cliffs, NJ: Prentice-Hall.

Borke, H. (1971). Interpersonal perception of young children: Egocentrism or empathy? *Developmental Psychology, 7,* 107–109.

Borke, H. (1975). Piaget's mountains revisited: Changes in the egocentric landscape. *Developmental Psychology, 11,* 240–243.

Boswell, S. L. (1974). *The development of verbal and spatial organization for materials presented tachistoscopically.* Unpublished doctoral dissertation, University of Colorado.

Botwinick, J. (1977). Intellectual abilities. In J. E. Birren & K. W. Schaie (Eds.), *Handbook of the psychology of aging* (pp. 580–605). New York: Van Nostrand Reinhold.

Botwinick, J. (1979). Methodological issues in the study of aging. JSAS *Catalog of Selected Documents in Psychology, 9,* 26 (Ms. No. 1836).

Botwinick, J. (1984). *Aging and behavior* (3rd ed.). New York: Springer.

Botwinick, J., & Storandt, M. (1974a). *Memory, related functions, and age.* Springfield, IL: Charles C Thomas.

Botwinick, J., & Storandt, M. (1974b). Vocabulary ability in later life. *Journal of Genetic Psychology, 125,* 303–308.

Bower, T. G. R. (1966, December). The visual world of infants. *Scientific American,* pp. 80–92.

Bower, T. G. R. (1975). Infant perception of the third dimension and object concept development. In L. B. Cohen & P. Salapatek (Eds.), *Infant perception: From sensation to cognition: Vol. 2. Perception of space, speech, and sound* (pp. 33–50). New York: Academic Press.

Bower, T. G. R. (1974). *Development in infancy.* San Francisco: Freeman.

Bower, T. G. R. (1982). *Development in infancy* (2nd ed.). San Francisco: Freeman.

Bower, T. G. R., Broughton, J. M., & Moore, M. K. (1970). The coordination of vision and tactual input in infancy. *Perception and Psychophysics, 8,* 51–53.

Bowerman, M. (1978). Semantic and syntactic development. In R. L. Schiefelbusch (Ed.), *The bases of language intervention* (pp. 97–189). Baltimore: University Park Press.

Boylin, W., Gordon, S. K., & Nehrke, M. F. (1976). Reminiscing and ego integrity in institutionalized elderly males. *Gerontologist, 16,* 118–124.

Braddick, O., Atkinson, J., French, J., & Howland, H. C. (1979). A photorefractive study of infant accommodation. *Vision Research, 19,* 1319–1330.

Braine, M. D. S. (1963). The ontogeny of English phrase structure: The first phase. *Language, 39,* 1–14.

Brainerd, C. J. (1974). Training and transfer of transitivity, conservation, and class inclusion of length. *Child Development, 45,* 324–334.

Brainerd, C. J. (1978). Learning research and Piagetian theory. In L. S. Siegel & C. J. Brainerd (Eds.), *Alternatives to Piaget: Critical essays on the theory* (pp. 69–109). New York: Academic Press.

Brainerd, C. J. (1981). Working memory and the developmental analysis of probability judgments. *Psychological Review, 88,* 463–502.

Brainerd, C. J. (1983). Modifiability of cognitive development. In S. Meadows (Ed.), *Developing thinking: Approaches to children's cognitive development* (pp. 26–66). New York: Methuen.

Brainerd, C. J., & Allen, T. W. (1971). Experimental inductions of the conservation of "first order" quantitative invariants. *Psychological Bulletin, 75,* 128–144.

Brandstädter, J., & Schneewind, K. A. (1977). Optimal human development: Some implications for psychology. *Human Development, 20,* 48–64.

Breslow, L. (1981). Reevaluation of the literature on the development of transitive inferences. *Psychological Bulletin, 89,* 325–351.

Bringing up superbaby. (1983, March 28). *Newsweek,* pp. 62–68.

Broadbent, D. E. (1958). *Perception and communication.* New York: Pergamon.

Broadbent, D. E. (1971). *Decision and stress.* New York: Academic Press.

Bromley, D. B. (1958). Some effects of age on short-term learning and memory. *Journal of Gerontology, 13,* 398–406.

Bronfenbrenner, U. (1976). Is early intervention effective? Facts and principles of early intervention: A summary. In A. M. Clarke & A. D. B. Clarke (Eds.), *Early experience: Myth and evidence* (pp. 247–256). New York: Free Press.

Bronfenbrenner, U. (1977). Toward an experimental ecology of human development. *American Psychologist, 32,* 513–531.

Brooks, J., & Lewis, M. (1976). Infant's response to strangers: Midget, adult, and child. *Child Development, 47,* 323–332.

Brooks-Gunn, J., & Weinraub, M. (1983). Origins of infant intelligence testing. In M. Lewis (Ed.), *Origins of intelligence: Infancy and early childhood* (2nd ed., pp. 25–66). New York: Plenum Press.

Broughton, J. M. (1984). Not beyond formal operations but beyond Piaget. In M. L. Commons, F. A. Richards, & C. Armon (Eds.), *Beyond formal operations: Late adolescent and adult cognitive development* (pp. 395–411). New York: Praeger.

Broverman, D. M., Klaiber, E. L., Kobayashi, Y., & Vogel, W. (1968). Roles of activation and inhibition in sex differences in cognitive abilities. *Psychological Review, 75,* 23–50.

Brown, A. L. (1975). The development of memory: Knowing, knowing about knowing, and knowing how to know. In H. W. Reese (Ed.), *Advances in child development and behavior* (Vol. 10, pp. 103–152). New York: Academic Press.

Brown, A. L. (1982). Learning and development: The problem of compatibility, access, and induction. *Human Development, 25,* 89–115.

Brown, A. L., Bransford, J. D., Ferrara, R. A., & Campione, J. C. (1983). Learning, remembering, and understanding. In J. H. Flavell & E. M. Markman (Eds.), *Handbook of child psychology: Vol. 3. Cognitive development* (pp. 77–166). New York: Wiley.

Brown, A. L., & French, L. A. (1979). The zone of potential development: Implications for intelligence testing in the year 2000. *Intelligence, 3,* 255–277.

Brown, A. L., & Scott, M. S. (1971). Recognition memory for pictures in preschool children. *Journal of Experimental Child Psychology, 11,* 401–412.

Brown, R. (1973). *A first language: The early stages.* Cambridge, MA: Harvard University Press.

Bruce, P. R., Coyne, A. C., & Botwinick, J. (1982). Adult age differences in metamemory. *Journal of Gerontology, 37,* 354–357.

Brückner, R. (1967). Longitudinal research on the eye. *Gerontologia Clinica, 9,* 87–95.

Bruner, J. S. (1973). *Beyond the information given: Studies in the psychology of knowing.* New York: Norton.

Bruner, J. S. (1983). *Child's talk: Learning to use language.* New York: Norton.

Bruner, J. S., Goodnow, J. J., & Austin, G. A. (1956). *A study of thinking.* New York: Wiley.

Bruner, J. S., Olver, R. R., & Greenfield, P. M. (1966). *Studies in cognitive growth.* New York: Wiley.

Bryant, P. E., Jones, P., Claxton, V., & Perkins, J. (1972). Recognition of shapes across modalities by infants. *Nature, 240,* 303–304.

Bryant, P. E., & Trabasso, T. (1971). Transitive inferences and memory in young children. *Nature, 232,* 456–458.

Burke, D. M., & Light, L. L. (1981). Memory and aging: The role of retrieval processes. *Psychological Bulletin, 90,* 513–546.

Butler, R. N. (1963). The life review: An interpretation of reminiscence in the aged. *Psychiatry, 26,* 65–76.

Cairns, R. B. (1979). *Social development: The origins and plasticity of interchanges.* San Francisco: Freeman.

Campos, J. J., Hiatt, S., Ramsay, D., Henderson, C., & Svejda, M. (1978). The emergence of fear on the visual cliff. In M. Lewis & L. A. Rosenblum (Eds.), *The development of affect* (Vol. 1, pp. 149–182). New York: Plenum Press.

Cantor, G. N., Dunlap, L. L., & Rettie, C. S. (1982). Effects of reception and discovery instruction on kindergartners' performance on probability tasks. *American Educational Research Journal, 19,* 453–463.

Caporael, L. R. (1981). The paralanguage of caregiving: Baby talk to the institutionalized aged. *Journal of Personality and Social Psychology, 40,* 876–884.

Carey, S. (1978). The child as word learner. In M. Halle, J. Bresnan, & G. A. Miller (Eds.), *Linguistic theory and psychological reality* (pp. 264–293). Cambridge, MA: MIT Press.

Carlson, J. S., & Wiedl, K. H. (1978). Use of testing-the-limits procedure in the assessment of intellectual capabilities in children with learning difficulties. *American Journal of Mental Deficiency, 82,* 559–564.

Carroll, J. B. (1976). Psychometric tests as cognitive tasks: A new "structure of intellect." In L. B. Resnick (Ed.), *The nature of intelligence* (pp. 27–56). Hillsdale, NJ: Erlbaum.

Case, R. (1978). Intellectual development from birth to adulthood: A neo-Piagetian interpretation. In R. S. Siegler (Ed.), *Children's thinking: What develops?* (pp. 37–71). Hillsdale, NJ: Erlbaum.

Case, R., Kurland, D. M., & Goldberg, J. (1982). Operational efficiency and the growth of short-term memory span. *Journal of Experimental Child Psychology, 33,* 386–404.

Cattell, R. B. (1963). Theory of fluid and crystallized intelligence: A critical experiment. *Journal of Educational Psychology, 54,* 1–22.

Cattell, R. B. (1971). *Abilities: Their structure, growth, and action.* Boston: Houghton Mifflin.

Cavanaugh, J. C., & Perlmutter, M. (1982). Metamemory: A critical evaluation. *Child Development, 53,* 11–28.

Chandler, M. J. (1976). Social cognition and life-span approaches to the study of child development. In H. W. Reese (Ed.), *Advances in child development and behavior* (Vol. 11, pp. 225–239). New York: Academic Press.

Chandler, M. J. (1977). Social cognition: A selective review of current research. In W. F. Overton & J. M. Gallagher (Eds.), *Knowledge and development: Vol. 1. Advances in theory and research* (pp. 93–147). New York: Plenum Press.

Charness, N. (1979). Components of skill in bridge. *Canadian Journal of Psychology, 33,* 1–16.

Charness, N. (1981). Aging and skilled problem solving. *Journal of Experimental Psychology: General, 110,* 21–38.

Chase, W. G., & Ericsson, K. A. (1981). Skilled memory. In J. R. Anderson (Ed.), *Cognitive skills and their acquisition* (pp. 141–189). Hillsdale, NJ: Erlbaum.

Chase, W. G., & Simon, H. A. (1973). Perception in chess. *Cognitive Psychology, 4,* 55–81.

Cherry, E. C. (1953). Some experiments on the recognition of speech, with one and with two ears. *Journal of the Acoustical Society of America, 25,* 975–979.

Chi, M. T. H. (1976). Short-term memory limitations in children: Capacity or processing deficits? *Memory and Cognition, 4,* 559–572.

Chi, M. T. H. (1978). Knowledge structures and memory development. In R. S. Siegler (Ed.), *Children's thinking: What develops?* (pp. 73–96). Hillsdale, NJ: Erlbaum.

Chi, M. T. H., & Koeske, R. D. (1983). Network representation of a child's dinosaur knowledge. *Developmental Psychology, 19,* 29–39.

Chomsky, C. (1969). *The acquisition of syntax in children from 5 to 10.* Cambridge, MA: MIT Press.

Chomsky, N. (1957). *Syntactic structures.* The Hague: Mouton.

Chomsky, N. (1965). *Aspects of the theory of syntax.* Cambridge, MA: MIT Press.

Cicirelli, V. G. (1976). Categorization behavior in aging subjects. *Journal of Gerontology, 36,* 676–680.

Clark, E. V. (1973). What's in a word? On the child's acquisition of semantics in his first language. In T. E. Moore (Ed.), *Cognitive development and the acquisition of language* (pp. 65–110). New York: Academic Press.

Clark, E. V. (1979). Building a vocabulary: Words for objects, actions, and relations. In P. Fletcher & M. Garman (Eds.), *Language acquisition* (pp. 149–160). New York: Cambridge University Press.

Clark, E. V. (1983). Meanings and concepts. In J. H. Flavell & E. M. Markman (Eds.), *Handbook of child psychology: Vol. 3. Cognitive development* (pp. 787–840). New York: Wiley.

Clarke, A. M., & Clarke, A. D. B. (Eds.). (1976). *Early experience: Myth and evidence.* New York: Free Press.

Clayton, V. (1975). Erikson's theory of human development as it applies to the aged: Wisdom as contradictive cognition. *Human Development, 18,* 119–128.

Clayton, V. (1982). Wisdom and intelligence: The nature and function of knowledge in the later years. *International Journal of Aging and Human Development, 15,* 315–323.

Clayton, V., & Birren, J. E. (1980). The development of wisdom across the life span: A reexamination of an ancient topic. In P. B. Baltes & O. G. Brim, Jr. (Eds.), *Life-span development and behavior* (Vol. 3, pp. 103–135). New York: Academic Press.

Clingman, J., & Fowler, R. L. (1976). The effects of primary reward on the IQ performance of grade-school children as a function of initial IQ level. *Journal of Applied Behavior Analysis, 9,* 19–23.

Coates, S. (1974). Sex differences in field dependence–independence between the ages of 3 and 6. *Perceptual Motor Skills, 39,* 1307–1310.

Coates, S. (1978). Sex differences in field independence among preschool children. In R. C. Friedman, R. M. Richart, & R. L. Vande Wiele (Eds.), *Sex differences in behavior* (pp. 259–274). Huntington, New York: Krieger.

Cohen, D., & Wilkie, F. (1979). Sex-related differences in cognition among the elderly. In M. A. Wittig & A. C. Petersen (Eds.), *Sex-related differences in cognitive functioning: Developmental issues* (pp. 145–159). New York: Academic Press.

Cohen, D., & Wu, S. (1980). Language and cognition during aging. *Annual Review of Gerontology and Geriatrics, 1,* 71–96.

Cohen, G. (1979). Language comprehension in old age. *Cognitive Psychology, 11,* 412–429.

Cohen, L., & Salapatek, P. (Eds.). (1975). *Infant perception.* New York: Academic Press.

Cohen, L. B., DeLoache, J. S., & Strauss, M. S. (1979). Infant visual perception. In J. Osofsky (Ed.), *Handbook of infant development* (pp. 393–438). New York: Wiley.

Coie, J. D., Costanzo, P. R., & Farnill, D. (1973). Specific transitions in the development of spatial perspective-taking ability. *Developmental Psychology, 9,* 167–177.

Coie, J. D., & Dorval, B. (1973). Sex differences in the intellectual structure of social interaction skills. *Developmental Psychology, 8,* 261–267.

Cole, M., Gay, J., Glick, J. A., & Sharp, D. W. (1971). *The cultural context of learning and thinking.* New York: Basic Books.

Cole, M., & Scribner, S. (1977). Cross-cultural studies of memory and cognition. In R. V. Kail, Jr., & J. W. Hagen (Eds.), *Perspectives on the development of memory and cognition* (pp. 239–271). Hillsdale, NJ: Erlbaum.

Cole, S. (1979). Age and scientific performance. *American Journal of Sociology, 84,* 958–977.

Collins, A. M., & Loftus, E. F. (1975). A spreading-activation theory of semantic memory. *Psychological Review, 82,* 407–428.

Comalli, P. E. (1965). Cognitive functioning in a group of 80–90-year-old men. *Journal of Gerontology, 20,* 14–17.

Commons, M. L., Richards, F., & Kuhn, D. (1982). Metasystematic reasoning: A case for a level of systematic reasoning beyond Piaget's stage of formal operations. *Child Development, 53*, 1058–1069.

Coren, S., & Porac, C. A. (1978). A new analysis of life-span age trends in visual illusion. *Developmental Psychology, 14*, 193–194.

Corrigan, R. (1978). Language development as related to Stage 6 object permanence development. *Journal of Child Language, 5*, 173–189.

Cowart, B. J. (1981). Development of taste perception in humans: Sensitivity and preference throughout the life span. *Psychological Bulletin, 90*, 43–73.

Cox, M. V. (Ed.). (1980). *Are young children egocentric?* New York: St. Martin's Press.

Coyne, A. C., Whitbourne, S. K., & Glenwick, D. S. (1978). Adult age differences in reflection-impulsivity. *Journal of Gerontology, 33*, 402–407.

Craik, F. I. M. (1971). Age differences in recognition memory. *Quarterly Journal of Experimental Psychology, 23*, 316–323.

Craik, F. I. M. (1977). Age differences in human memory. In J. E. Birren & K. W. Schaie (Eds.), *Handbook of the psychology of aging* (pp. 384–420). New York: Van Nostrand Reinhold.

Craik, F. I. M., & Lockart, R. S. (1972). Levels of processing: A framework for memory research. *Journal of Verbal Learning and Verbal Behavior, 11*, 671–684.

Craik, F. I. M., & Tulving, E. (1975). Depth of processing and the retention of words in episodic memory. *Journal of Experimental Psychology: General, 104*, 268–294.

Cromer, R. F. (1981). Reconceptualizing language acquisition and cognitive development. In R. L. Schiefelbusch & D. Bricker (Eds.), *Early language: Acquisition and intervention* (pp. 51–137). Baltimore, University Park Press.

Crowder, R. G. (1980). Echoic memory and the study of aging memory systems. In L. W. Poon, J. L. Fozard, L. S. Cermak, D. Arenberg, & L. W. Thompson (Eds.), *New directions in memory and aging: Proceedings of the George A. Talland Memorial Conference* (pp. 181–204). Hillsdale, NJ: Erlbaum.

Cultice, J. C., Somerville, S. C., & Wellman, H. M. (1983). Preschoolers' memory monitoring: Feeling of knowing judgments. *Child Development, 54*, 1480–1486.

Cunningham, W. R. (1981). Ability factor structure differences in adulthood and old age. *Multivariate Behavioral Research, 16*, 3–22.

Cunningham, W. R., & Owens, W. A., Jr. (1983). The Iowa State study of the adult development of intellectual abilities. In K. W. Schaie (Ed.), *Longitudinal studies of adult psychological development* (pp. 20–39). New York: Guilford Press.

Curtis, L. E., Siegel, A. W., & Furlong, N. E. (1981). Developmental differences in cognitive mapping: Configurational knowledge of familiar large-scale environments. *Journal of Experimental Child Psychology, 31*, 456–469.

Curtiss, S. (1977). *Genie: A psychoanalytic study of a modern day "wild child."* New York: Academic Press.

Cutrona, C. E., & Feshbach, S. (1979). Cognitive and behavioral correlates of children's differential use of social information. *Child Development, 50*, 1036–1042.

Dale, P. S. (1976). *Language development: Structure and function* (2nd ed.). New York: Holt, Rinehart and Winston.

Damon, W. (1979). Why study social-cognitive development? *Human Development, 22*, 206–211.

Damon, W., & Hart, D. (1982). The development of self-understanding from infancy through adolescence. *Child Development, 53*, 841–864.

Danish, S. J., & Conter, K. R. (1978). Intervention and evaluation: Two sides of the same community coin. In L. Goldman (Ed.), *Research methods for counselors* (pp. 343–359). New York: Wiley.

Danish, S. J., Smyer, M. A., & Nowak, C. A. (1980). Developmental intervention: Enhancing life-event processes. In P. B. Baltes & O. G. Brim, Jr. (Eds.), *Life-span development and behavior* (Vol. 3, pp. 339–366). New York: Academic Press.

Darwin, C. J., Turvey, M. T., & Crowder, R. G. (1972). An auditory analogue of the Sperling partial-report procedure: Evidence for brief auditory storage. *Cognitive Psychology, 3,* 255–267.

Dasen, P. R. (1972). Cross-cultural Piagetian research: A summary. *Journal of Cross-Cultural Psychology, 3,* 23–29.

Datan, N. (1977). After the apple: Post-Newtonian metatheory for jaded psychologists. In N. Datan & H. W. Reese (Eds.), *Life-span developmental psychology: Dialectical perspectives on experimental research* (pp. 47–57). New York: Academic Press.

Datan, N., & Ginsberg, L. H. (Eds.). (1975). *Life-span developmental psychology: Normative life crises.* New York: Academic Press.

Datan, N., & Reese, H. W. (Eds.). (1977). *Life-span developmental psychology: Dialectical perspectives on experimental research.* New York: Academic Press.

Day, R. H., & McKenzie, B. E. (1977). Constancies in the perceptual world of the infant. In W. Epstein (Ed.), *Stability and constancy in visual perception: Mechanisms and processes* (pp. 285–320). New York: Wiley.

DeCasper, A. J., & Fifer, W. P. (1980). Of human bonding: Newborns prefer their mothers' voices. *Science, 208,* 1174–1176.

de Lemos, M. M. (1969). The development of conservation in Aboriginal children. *International Journal of Psychology, 4,* 255–269.

Demming, J. A., & Pressey, S. L. (1957). Tests indigenous to the adult and older years. *Journal of Counseling Psychology, 4,* 144–148.

Denney, D. R. (1972). Modeling effects upon conceptual style and cognitive tempo. *Child Development, 43,* 105–119.

Denney, D. R., Denney, N. W., & Ziobrowski, M. (1973). Alterations in the information-processing strategies of young children following observation of adult models. *Developmental Psychology, 8,* 202–208.

Denney, N. W. (1979). Problem solving in later adulthood: Intervention research. In P. B. Baltes & O. G. Brim, Jr. (Eds.), *Life-span development and behavior* (Vol. 2, pp. 37–66). New York: Academic Press.

Denney, N. W. (1982). Aging and cognitive changes. In B. B. Wolman (Ed.), *Handbook of developmental psychology* (pp. 807–827). Englewood Cliffs, NJ: Prentice-Hall.

Denney, N. W., & Cornelius, S. W. (1975). Class inclusion and multiple classification in middle and old age. *Developmental Psychology, 11,* 521–522.

Denney, N. W., & Denney, D. R. (1974). Modeling effects on the questioning strategies of the elderly. *Developmental Psychology, 10,* 458.

Denney, N. W., & List, J. A. (1979). Adult age differences in performance on the Matching Familiar Figures Test. *Human Development, 22,* 137–144.

Denney, N. W., & Palmer, A. M. (1981). Adult age differences on traditional and practical problem-solving measures. *Journal of Gerontology, 36,* 323–328.

Denney, N. W., & Wright, J. C. (1976). Cognitive changes during the adult years: Implications for developmental theory and research. In H. W. Reese (Ed.), *Advances in child development and behavior* (Vol. 11, pp. 213–224). New York: Academic Press.

Dennis, W. (1966). Creative productivity between the ages of 20 and 80 years. *Journal of Gerontology, 21,* 1–8.

Derwing, B. L. (1977). Is the child really a "little linguist"? In J. Macnamara (Ed.), *Language learning and thought* (pp. 79–84). New York: Academic Press.

Deutsch, J. A., & Deutsch, D. (1963). Attention: Some theoretical considerations. *Psychological Review, 70,* 80–90.

deVilliers, J. G., & deVilliers, P. A. (1974). Competence and performance in child language: Are children really competent to judge? *Journal of Child Language, 1,* 11–22.

Dirks, J., & Neisser, U. (1977). Memory for objects in real scenes: The development of recognition and recall. *Journal of Experimental Child Psychology, 23,* 315–328.

Dittmann-Kohli, F., & Baltes, P. B. (in press). Towards a neofunctionalist conception of adult intellectual development: Wisdom as a prototypical case of intellectual growth. In C. N. Alexander & E. Langer (Eds.), *Beyond formal operations: Alternative endpoints to human development.* New York: Oxford University Press.

Dixon, R. A., Simon, E. W., Nowak, C. A., & Hultsch, D. F. (1982). Text recall in adulthood as a function of level of information, input modality, and delay interval. *Journal of Gerontology, 37,* 358–364.

Dove, A. (1968, July 15). The Chitling Test. *Newsweek,* pp. 51–52.

Downing, J., & Leong, C. K. (1982). *Psychology of reading.* New York: Macmillan.

Doyle, A. B. (1973). Listening to distraction: A developmental study of selective attention. *Journal of Experimental Child Psychology, 15,* 100–115.

Dubin, R., & Dubin, E. R. (1965). Children's social perceptions: A review of research. *Child Development, 36,* 809–838.

Dudek, S. Z. (1974). Creativity in young children: Attitude or ability? *Journal of Creative Behavior, 8,* 282–292.

Dulit, E. (1972). Adolescent thinking à la Piaget: The formal stage. *Journal of Youth and Adolescence, 1,* 281–301.

Duncker, K. (1945). On problem solving. *Psychological Monographs, 58* (5, Whole No. 270).

Dusek, J. B., & Flaherty, J. F. (1981). The development of the self-concept during the adolescent years. *Monographs of the Society for Research in Child Development, 46*(4, Serial No. 191).

Easterbrook, J. A. (1959). The effect of emotion on cue utilization and organization of behavior. *Psychological Review, 66,* 183–201.

Eilers, R. E., Wilson, W. R., & Moore, J. M. (1977). Developmental changes in speech discrimination in three-, six-, and twelve-month-old infants. *Journal of Speech and Hearing Research, 20,* 766–780.

Eimas, P. D. (1969). A developmental study of hypothesis behavior and focusing. *Journal of Experimental Child Psychology, 8,* 160–172.

Eimas, P. D. (1970). Information processing in problem solving as a function of developmental level and stimulus saliency. *Developmental Psychology, 2,* 224–229.

Eimas, P. D. (1975). Speech perception in early infancy. In L. B. Cohen & P. Salapatek (Eds.), *Infant perception: From sensation to cognition: Vol. 2. Perception of space, speech, and sound* (pp. 193–231). New York: Academic Press.

Eimas, P., Siqueland, E., Jusczyk, P., & Vigorito, J. (1971). Speech perception in infants. *Science, 171,* 303–306.

Eisenberg, R. B. (1976). *Auditory competence in early life.* Baltimore: University Park Press.

Eisner, D. A., & Schaie, K. W. (1971). Age changes in response to visual illusions from middle to old age. *Journal of Gerontology, 26,* 146–150.

Elias, M. F., & Streeten, D. H. P. (Eds.). (1980). *Hypertension and cognitive processes.* Mount Desert, ME: Beech Hill.

Elkind, D. (1967). Egocentrism in adolescence. *Child Development, 38,* 1025–1034.

Elkind, D. (1977). Perceptual development in children. In I. Janis (Ed.), *Current trends in psychology* (pp. 121–129). Los Altos, CA: Kaufmann.

Elkind, D. (1980). Strategic interactions in early adolescence. In J. Adelson (Ed.), *Handbook of adolescent psychology* (pp. 432–444). New York: Wiley.

Elkind, D. (1981). *Children and adolescents: Interpretative essays on Jean Piaget* (3rd ed.). New York: Oxford University Press.

Engle, R. W., Fidler, D. S., & Reynolds, L. H. (1981). Does echoic memory develop? *Journal of Experimental Child Psychology, 32,* 459–473.

Epstein, H. T. (1974). Phrenoblysis: Special brain and neural growth periods: II. Human mental development. *Developmental Psychobiology, 7,* 217–224.

Erber, J. T. (1974). Age differences in recognition memory. *Journal of Gerontology, 29*, 171–181.

Eriksen, C. W., & Collins, J. F. (1967). Some temporal characteristics of visual pattern perception. *Journal of Experimental Psychology, 74*, 476–484.

Erikson, E. H. (1963). *Childhood and society* (2nd ed.). New York: Norton.

Erikson, E. H. (1968). *Identity: Youth and crisis.* New York: Norton.

Ervin, S. (1961). Changes with age in the verbal determinants of word association. *American Journal of Psychology, 74*, 361–372.

Evans, G. W., Brennan, P. L., Skorpanich, M. A., & Held, D. (1984). Cognitive mapping and elderly adults: Verbal and location memory for urban landmarks. *Journal of Gerontology, 39*, 452–457.

Eysenck, M. W. (1974). Age differences in incidental learning. *Developmental Psychology, 10*, 936–941.

Eysenck, M. W., & Eysenck, M. C. (1979). Processing depth, elaboration of encoding, memory stores, and expended processing capacity. *Journal of Experimental Psychology: Human Learning and Memory, 5*, 472–484.

Fagan, J. F., III. (1982). Infant memory. In T. M. Field, A. Huston, H. C. Quay, L. Troll, & G. E. Finley (Eds.), *Review of human development* (pp. 79–92). New York: Wiley.

Fakouri, M. (1976). Cognitive development in adulthood: A fifth stage? *Developmental Psychology, 12*, 472.

Fantz, R. L. (1966). Pattern discrimination and selective attention as determinants of perceptual development from birth. In A. H. Kidd & J. L. Rivoire (Eds.), *Perceptual development in children* (pp. 143–173). New York: International Universities Press.

Fantz, R. L., Fagan, J. F., III, & Miranda, S. B. (1975). Early visual selectivity. In L. B. Cohen & P. Salapatek (Eds.), *Infant perception: From sensation to cognition: Vol. 1. Basic visual processes* (pp. 249–345). New York: Academic Press.

Feffer, M., & Gourevitch, V. (1960). Cognitive aspects of role taking in children. *Journal of Personality, 28*, 383–396.

Feldman, D. H. (1980). *Beyond universals in cognitive development.* Norwood, NJ: Ablex.

Ferguson, C. A. (1977). Baby talk as a simplified register. In C. E. Snow & C. A. Ferguson (Eds.), *Talking to children: Language input and acquisition* (pp. 209–235). New York: Cambridge University Press.

Feshbach, N. D. (1978). Studies of empathic behavior in children. In B. A. Maher (Ed.), *Progress in experimental personality research* (Vol. 8, pp. 1–47). New York: Academic Press.

Field, D. (1981). Can preschool children really learn to conserve? *Child Development, 52*, 326–334.

Field, T. M. (1982). Social perception and responsivity in early infancy. In T. M. Field, A. Huston, H. C. Quay, L. Troll, & G. E. Finley (Eds.), *Review of human development* (pp. 20–31). New York: Wiley.

Fillmore, C. J., Kempler, D., & Wang, W. S-Y. (1979). *Individual differences in language ability and language behavior.* New York: Academic Press.

Finch, C. E., & Schneider, E. L. (Eds.). (1985). *Handbook of the biology of aging* (2nd ed.). New York: Van Nostrand Reinhold.

Fischer, K. W. (1980). Theory of cognitive development: The control and construction of hierarchies of skills. *Psychological Review, 87*, 477–531.

Fisher, R. P., & Craik, F. I. M. (1977). The interaction between encoding and retrieval operations in cued recall. *Journal of Experimental Psychology: Human Learning and Memory, 3*, 701–711.

Fitzgerald, J. M. (1978). Actual and perceived sex and generational differences in interpersonal style: Structural and quantitative issues. *Journal of Gerontology, 33*, 394–401.

Fitzgerald, J. M. (1981). Research methods and research questions for the study of person-perception in adult development. *Human Development, 24*, 138–144.

Flapan, D. (1968). *Children's understanding of social interaction.* New York: Teachers College Press.

Flavell, J. H. (1963). *The developmental psychology of Jean Piaget.* New York: Van Nostrand Reinhold.

Flavell, J. H. (1970). Developmental studies of meditated memory. In H. W. Reese & L. P. Lipsitt (Eds.), *Advances in child development and behavior* (Vol. 5, pp. 181–211). New York: Academic Press.

Flavell, J. H. (1971a). Stage-related properties of cognitive development. *Cognitive Psychology, 2,* 421–453.

Flavell, J. H. (1971b). What is memory development the development of? *Human Development, 14,* 272–275.

Flavell, J. H. (1977). *Cognitive development.* Englewood Cliffs, NJ: Prentice-Hall.

Flavell, J. H. (1985). *Cognitive development* (2nd ed.). Englewood Cliffs, NJ: Prentice-Hall.

Flavell, J. H., Beach, D. H., & Chinsky, J. M. (1966). Spontaneous verbal rehearsal in a memory task as a function of age. *Child Development, 37,* 283–299.

Flavell, J. H., Botkin, P. T., Fry, C. L., Jr., Wright, J. W., & Jarvis, P. E. (1968). *The development of role-taking and communication skills in children.* New York: Wiley.

Flavell, J. H., Friedrichs, A. G., & Hoyt, J. D. (1970). Developmental changes in memorization processes. *Cognitive Psychology, 1,* 324–340.

Flavell, J. H., & Markman, E. M. (1983). Preface to Volume III. In J. H. Flavell & E. M. Markman (Eds.), *Handbook of child psychology: Vol. 3. Cognitive development* (pp. viii–x). New York: Wiley.

Flavell, J. H., & Ross, L. (Eds.). (1981). *Social and cognitive development.* New York: Cambridge University Press.

Flavell, J. H., & Wellman, H. M. (1977). Metamemory. In R. V. Kail & J. W. Hagen (Eds.), *Perspectives on the development of memory and cognition* (pp. 3–33). Hillsdale, NJ: Erlbaum.

Ford, M. (1979). The construct validity of egocentrism. *Psychological Bulletin, 86,* 1169–1188.

Ford, M. E. (1985). Two perspectives on the validation of developmental constructs: Psychometric and theoretical limitations in research on egocentrism. *Psychological Bulletin, 97,* 497–501.

Forman, G. E. (1975). On the components of spatial representation. In J. Eliot & N. J. Salkind (Eds.), *Children's spatial development* (pp. 111–155). Springfield, IL: Charles C Thomas.

Forman, G. E., & Sigel, I. E. (1979). *Cognitive development: A life-span view.* Monterey, CA: Brooks-Cole.

Fouts, R. S., & Fouts, H. (1985, May). *Signs of conversations in chimpanzees.* Paper presented at the meeting of the American Association for the Advancement of Science, Los Angeles.

Fowler, W., & Swenson & A. (1979). The influence of early language stimulation on development: Four studies. *Genetic Psychology Monographs, 100,* 73–109.

Fozard, J. L. (1980). The time for remembering. In L. W. Poon (Ed.), *Aging in the 1980s: Psychological issues* (pp. 273–287). Washington, DC: American Psychological Association.

Fozard, J. L., & Nuttall, R. L. (1971). General Aptitude Test Battery scores by age and socioeconomic status. *Journal of Applied Psychology, 55,* 372–379.

Fozard, J. L., & Popkin, S. J. (1978). Optimizing adult development: Ends and means of an applied psychology of aging. *American Psychologist, 33,* 975–989.

Fozard, J. L., Wolf, E., Bell, B., McFarland, R. A., & Podolsky, S. (1977). Visual perception and communication. In J. E. Birren & K. W. Schaie (Eds.), *Handbook of the psychology of aging* (pp. 497–534). New York: Van Nostrand Reinhold.

Freud, S. (1930). *Civilization and its discontents.* London: Hogarth Press.

Fromkin, V. A., Krashen, S., Curtiss, S., Rigler, D., & Rigler, M. (1974). The development of language in Genie: A case of language acquisition beyond the "critical period." *Brain and Language, 1,* 81–107.

Furth, H. G. (1966). *Thinking without language: Psychological implications of deafness.* New York: Free Press.

Furth, H. G. (1971). Linguistic deficiency and thinking: Research with deaf subjects, 1964–1969. *Psychological Bulletin, 75,* 58–72.

Gagné, R. M. (1977). *The conditions of learning* (3rd ed.). New York: Holt, Rinehart and Winston.

Galton, F. (1883). *Inquiries into human faculty and its development.* London: Macmillan.

Garber, H., & Heber, R. (1982). Modification of predicted cognitive development in high-risk children through early intervention. In D. K. Detterman & R. J. Sternberg (Eds.), *How and how much can intelligence be increased?* (pp. 121–137). Norwood, NJ: Ablex.

Gardner, H. (1978). *Developmental psychology.* Boston: Little, Brown.

Gardner, H. (1982). *Developmental psychology* (2nd ed.). Boston: Little, Brown.

Gardner, H. (1983). *Frames of mind: The theory of multiple intelligences.* New York: Basic Books.

Gardner, H., & Winner, E. (1982). First intimations of artistry. In S. Strauss (Ed.), *U-shaped behavioral growth* (pp. 147–168). New York: Academic Press.

Gardner, R. A., & Gardner, B. T. (1978). Comparative psychology and language acquisition. *Annals of the New York Academy of Sciences, 309,* 37–76.

Garrett, H. E. (1946). A developmental theory of intelligence. *American Psychologist, 1,* 372–378.

Gaylord, S. A., & Marsh, G. R. (1975). Age differences in the speed of a spatial cognitive process. *Journal of Gerontology, 30,* 674–678.

Gelman, R. (1969). Conservation acquisition: A problem of learning to attend to relevant attributes. *Journal of Experimental Child Psychology, 7,* 167–187.

Gelman, R. (1972). The nature and development of early number concepts. In H. W. Reese (Ed.), *Advances in child development and behavior* (Vol. 7, pp. 115–167). New York: Academic Press.

Gelman, R. (1979). Preschool thought. *American Psychologist, 34,* 900–906.

Gelman, R., & Baillargeon, R. (1983). A review of some Piagetian concepts. In J. H. Flavell & E. M. Markman (Eds.), *Handbook of child psychology: Vol. 3. Cognitive development* (pp. 167–230). New York: Wiley.

Gelman, R., & Gallistel, C. R. (1978). *The child's understanding of number.* Cambridge, MA: Harvard University Press.

Gesell, A., & Thompson, H. (1934). *Infant behavior.* New York: McGraw-Hill.

Getzels, J. W., & Jackson, P. W. (1962). *Creativity and intelligence.* New York: Wiley.

Gholson, B., & Schuepfer, T. (1979). Commentary on Kendler's paper: An alternative perspective. In H. W. Reese & L. P. Lipsitt (Eds.), *Advances in child development and behavior* (Vol. 13, pp. 137–144). New York: Academic Press.

Giambra, L. M., & Arenberg, D. (1980). Problem solving, concept learning, and aging. In L. W. Poon (Ed.), *Aging in the 1980s: Psychological issues* (pp. 253–259). Washington, DC: American Psychological Association.

Gibbs, J. C. (1979). Kohlberg's moral stage theory: A Piagetian revision. *Human Development, 22,* 89–112.

Gibson, E. J. (1969). *Principles of perceptual learning and development.* New York: Appleton-Century-Crofts.

Gibson, E. J. (1982). The concept of affordances in development: The renascence of functionalism. In W. A. Collins (Ed.), *Minnesota Symposia on Child Psychology: Vol. 15. The concept of development* (pp. 55–81). Hillsdale, NJ: Erlbaum.

Gibson, E. J., & Spelke, E. S. (1983). The development of perception. In J. H. Flavell &

E. M. Markman (Eds.), *Handbook of child psychology: Vol. 3. Cognitive development* (pp. 1–76). New York: Wiley.

Gibson, E. J., & Walk, R. D. (1960, April). The "visual cliff." *Scientific American*, pp. 64–71.

Gibson, J. J. (1966). *The senses considered as perceptual systems.* Boston: Houghton Mifflin.

Gibson, J. J. (1979). *The ecological approach to visual perception.* Boston: Houghton Mifflin.

Gibson, J. J., & Gibson, E. J. (1955). Perceptual learning: Differentiation or enrichment? *Psychological Review, 62,* 32–41.

Gilligan, C. F. (1977). In a different voice: Women's conceptions of self and morality. *Harvard Educational Review, 47,* 481–517.

Gilligan, C. (1982). *In a different voice: Psychological theory and women's development.* Cambridge, MA: Harvard University Press.

Gilligan, C., & Murphy, J. M. (1979). Development from adolescence to adulthood: The philosopher and the dilemma of the fact. In D. Kuhn (Ed.), *Intellectual development beyond childhood* (pp. 85–99). San Francisco: Jossey-Bass.

Gleitman, L. R., Newport, E. L., & Gleitman, H. (1984). The current status of the motherese hypothesis. *Journal of Child Language, 11,* 43–79.

Golden, M., & Birns, B. (1976). Social class and infant intelligence. In M. Lewis (Ed.), *Origins of intelligence: Infancy and early childhood* (pp. 299–351). New York: Plenum Press.

Goldin-Meadow, S., Seligman, M., & Gelman, R. (1976). Language in the two-year-old. *Cognition, 4,* 189–202.

Gollin, E. S. (Ed.). (1981). *Developmental plasticity.* New York: Academic Press.

Gordon, F. R., & Yonas, A. (1976). Sensitivity to binocular depth information in infants. *Journal of Experimental Child Psychology, 22,* 413–422.

Gordon, W. J. (1961). *Synectics: The development of creative capacity.* New York: Harper & Row.

Goulet, L. R., & Baltes, P. B. (Eds.). (1970). *Life-span developmental psychology: Research and theory.* New York: Academic Press.

Granick, S., & Friedman, A. D. (1967). The effect of education on the decline of psychometric test performance with age. *Journal of Gerontology, 22,* 191–195.

Granick, S., Kleban, M. H., & Weiss, A. D. (1976). Relationships between hearing loss and cognition in normally hearing aged persons. *Journal of Gerontology, 31,* 434–440.

Gratch, G. (1975). Recent studies based on Piaget's view of object concept development. In L. B. Cohen & P. Salapatek (Eds.), *Infant perception: From sensation to cognition: Vol. 2. Perception of space, speed, and sound* (pp. 51–99). New York: Academic Press.

Greenfield, P. M. (1972). Oral or written language: The consequences for cognitive development. *Language and Speech, 15,* 169–178.

Greenfield, P. M. (1976). Cross-cultural research and Piagetian theory: Paradox and progress. In K. F. Riegel & J. A. Meacham (Eds.), *The developing individual in a changing world. Historical and cultural issues* (Vol. 1, pp. 322–345). Chicago: Aldine.

Greenfield, P. M., & Smith, J. H. (1976). *The structure of communication in early language development.* New York: Academic Press.

Greeno, J. G. (1976). Indefinite goals in well-structured problems. *Psychological Review, 83,* 479–491.

Greeno, J. G. (1980). Trends in the theory of knowledge for problem solving. In D. T. Tuma & F. Reif (Eds.), *Problem solving and education: Issues in teaching and learning* (pp. 9–23). Hillsdale, NJ: Erlbaum.

Guilford, J. P. (1959). Three faces of intellect. *American Psychologist, 14,* 469–479.

Guilford, J. P. (1979). *Cognitive psychology with a frame of reference.* San Diego, CA: Edits.

Guilford, J. P. (1980). Fluid and crystallized intelligence: Two fanciful concepts. *Psychological Bulletin, 88,* 408–412.

Guilford, J. P. (1982). Cognitive psychology's ambiguities: Some suggested remedies. *Psychological Review, 89,* 48–59.

Haan, N., Smith, M. B., & Block, J. (1968). Moral reasoning of young adults: Political-social behavior, family background, and personality correlates. *Journal of Personality and Social Psychology, 10,* 183–201.

Hagen, J. W., & Hale, G. H. (1973). The development of attention in children. In A. D. Pick (Ed.), *Minnesota Symposia on Child Psychology* (Vol. 7, pp. 117–140). Minneapolis: University of Minnesota Press.

Haith, M. M. (1971). Developmental changes in visual information processing and short-term visual memory. *Human Development, 14,* 249–261.

Haith, M. M. (1980). *Rules that babies look by: The organization of newborn visual activity.* Hillsdale, NJ: Erlbaum.

Hall, V. C., & Kaye, D. B. (1980). Early patterns of cognitive development. *Monographs of the Society for Research in Child Development, 45*(2, Serial No. 184).

Harding, C., & Golinkoff, R. (1979). The origins of intentional vocalization in prelinguistic infants. *Child Development, 50,* 33–40.

Hardwick, D. A., McIntyre, C. W., & Pick, H. L. (1976). The content and manipulation of cognitive maps in children and adults. *Monographs of the Society for Research in Child Development, 41*(3, Serial No. 166).

Harker, J. O., Hartley, J. T., & Walsh, D. A. (1982). Understanding discourse: A life-span approach. *Advances in Reading/Language Research, 1,* 155–202.

Harper, L. V., & Sanders, K. M. (1975). Preschool children's use of space: Sex differences in outdoor play. *Developmental Psychology, 11,* 119.

Harris, J. E. (1984). Remembering to do things: A forgotten topic. In J. E. Harris & P. E. Morris (Eds.), *Everyday memory, actions and absent-mindedness* (pp. 71–92). New York: Academic Press.

Harris, L. J. (1978). Sex differences in spatial ability: Possible environmental, genetic, and neurological factors. In M. Kinsbourne (Ed.), *Asymmetrical function of the brain* (pp. 405–522). New York: Cambridge University Press.

Harris, L. J. (1981). Sex-related variations in spatial skill. In L. S. Liben, A. H. Patterson, & N. Newcombe (Eds.), *Spatial representation and behavior across the life span* (pp. 83–125). New York: Academic Press.

Harris, P. L. (1975). Development of search and object permanence during infancy. *Psychological Bulletin, 81,* 332–334.

Harris, P. L. (1983). Infant cognition. In M. M. Haith & J. J. Campos (Eds.), *Handbook of child psychology: Vol. 2. Infancy and developmental psychobiology* (pp. 689–782). New York: Wiley.

Harshbarger, D. (1973). Some ecological implications for the organization of human intervention throughout the life span. In P. B. Baltes & K. W. Schaie (Eds.), *Life-span developmental psychology: Personality and socialization* (pp. 339–364). New York: Academic Press.

Hart, J. T. (1965). Memory and the feeling-of-knowing experience. *Journal of Educational Psychology, 56,* 208–216.

Hart, J. T. (1967). Memory and the memory-monitoring process. *Journal of Verbal Learning and Verbal Behavior, 6,* 685–691.

Hartley, A. A., & Anderson, J. W. (1983). Task complexity and problem-solving performance in younger and older adults. *Journal of Gerontology, 38,* 72–77.

Hasher, L., & Zacks, R. T. (1979). Automatic and effortful processes in memory. *Journal of Experimental Psychology: General, 108,* 356–388.

Hay, D. F., & Murray, P. (1982). Giving and requesting: Social facilitation of infants' offers to adults. *Infant Behavior and Development, 5,* 301–310.

Hayes, K. J., & Hayes, C. (1951). Intellectual development of a home-raised chimpanzee. *Proceedings of the American Philosophical Society, 95*, 105–109.

Haynes, H., White, B. L., & Held, R. (1965). Visual accommodation in human infants. *Science, 148*, 528–530.

Heber, R., Garber, H., Harrington, S., & Hoffman, C. (1972). *Rehabilitation of families at risk for mental retardation.* Madison: University of Wisconsin, Rehabilitation Research and Training Center in Mental Retardation.

Heglin, H. J. (1956). Problem solving set in different age groups. *Journal of Gerontology, 11*, 310–317.

Heider, F. (1958). *The psychology of interpersonal relations.* New York: Wiley.

Herman, J. F., Kail, R. V., & Siegel, A. W. (1979). Cognitive maps of a college campus: A new look at freshman orientation. *Bulletin of the Psychonomic Society, 13*, 183–186.

Herman, J. F., & Siegel, A. W. (1978). The development of cognitive mapping of the large-scale environment. *Journal of Experimental Child Psychology, 26*, 389–406.

Hess, E. H. (1973). *Imprinting.* New York: Van Nostrand Reinhold.

Hildyard, A., & Olson, D. R. (1982). On the structure and meaning of prose text. In W. Otto & S. White (Eds.), *Reading expository material* (pp. 155–184). New York: Academic Press.

Hoffman, C. D., & Dick, S. A. (1976). A developmental investigation of recognition memory. *Child Development, 47*, 794–799.

Hoffman, M. L. (1977a). Moral internalization: Current theory and research. In L. Berkowitz (Ed.), *Advances in experimental social psychology* (Vol. 10, pp. 85–133). New York: Academic Press.

Hoffman, M. L. (1977b). Empathy, its development and prosocial implications. In C. B. Keasey (Ed.), *Nebraska Symposium on Motivation* (Vol. 25, pp. 169–217). Lincoln: University of Nebraska Press.

Hoffman, M. L. (1979). Development of moral thought, feeling, and behavior. *American Psychologist, 34*, 958–966.

Hoffman, M. L. (1981). Perspectives on the difference between understanding people and understanding things: The role of affect. In J. H. Flavell & L. Ross (Eds.), *Social cognitive development: Frontiers and possible futures* (pp. 67–81). New York: Cambridge University Press.

Hoffman, M. L. (1983). Empathy, guilt, and social cognition. In W. F. Overton (Ed.), *The relationship between social and cognitive development* (pp. 1–51). Hillsdale, NJ: Erlbaum.

Hoffman, R. F. (1978). Developmental changes in human infant visual-evoked potentials to patterned stimuli recorded at different scalp locations. *Child Development, 49*, 110–118.

Hofland, B. F., Willis, S. L., & Baltes, P. B. (1981). Fluid intelligence performance in the elderly: Retesting and conditions of assessment. *Journal of Educational Psychology, 73*, 573–586.

Hogan, R. (1973). Moral conduct and moral character: A psychological perspective. *Psychological Bulletin, 79*, 217–232.

Hogan, R. (1975). Moral development and the structure of personality. In D. J. DePalma & J. M. Foley (Eds.), *Moral development: Current theory and research* (pp. 153–168). Hillsdale, NJ: Erlbaum.

Hogan, R., & Emler, N. P. (1978). Moral development. In M. E. Lamb (Ed.), *Social and personality development* (pp. 200–223). New York: Holt, Rinehart and Winston.

Holstein, C. (1976). Irreversible, stepwise sequence in the development of moral judgment: A longitudinal study of males and females. *Child Development, 47*, 51–61.

Honzik, M. P. (1976). Value and limitations of infant tests: An overview. In M. Lewis (Ed.), *Origins of intelligence: Infancy and early childhood* (pp. 59–95). New York: Plenum Press.

Honzik, M. P., & Macfarlane, J. W. (1973). Personality development and intellectual functioning from 21 months to 40 years. In L. F. Jarvik, C. Eisdorfer, & J. E. Blum (Eds.), *Intellectual functioning in adults: Psychological and biological influences* (pp. 45–58). New York: Springer.

Honzik, M. P., Macfarlane, J., & Allen, L. (1948). The stability of mental test performance between 2 and 18 years. *Journal of Experimental Education, 4*, 309–324.

Horn, J. L. (1970). Organization of data on life-span development of human abilities. In L. R. Goulet & P. B. Baltes (Eds.), *Life-span developmental psychology: Research and theory* (pp. 423–466). New York: Academic Press.

Horn, J. L. (1972). The structure of intellect: Primary abilities. In R. M. Dreger (Ed.), *Multivariate personality research* (pp. 451–511). Baton Rouge, LA: Claitor.

Horn, J. L. (1978). Human ability systems. In P. B. Baltes (Ed.), *Life-span development and behavior* (Vol. 1, pp. 211–256). New York: Academic Press.

Horn, J. L. (1982). The aging of human abilities. In B. B. Wolman (Ed.), *Handbook of developmental psychology* (pp. 847–870). Englewood Cliffs, NJ: Prentice-Hall.

Horn, J. L., & Cattell, R. B. (1967). Age differences in fluid and crystallized intelligence. *Acta Psychologia, 26*, 107–129.

Horn, J. L., & Donaldson, G. (1976). On the myth of intellectual decline in adulthood. *American Psychologist, 31*, 701–719.

Hornblum, J. N., & Overton, W. F. (1976). Area and volume conservation among the elderly: Assessment and training. *Developmental Psychology, 12*, 68–74.

Horowitz, F. D. (1980). Intervention and its effects on early development: What model of development is appropriate? In R. R. Turner & H. W. Reese (Eds.), *Life-span developmental psychology: Intervention* (pp. 235–248). New York: Academic Press.

Horowitz, F. D., & Paden, L. Y. (1973). The effectiveness of environmental intervention programs. In B. M. Caldwell & H. N. Ricciuti (Eds.), *Review of child development research* (Vol. 3, pp. 331–402). Chicago: University of Chicago Press.

Horton, D. L., & Turnage, T. W. (1976). *Human learning.* Englewood Cliffs, NJ: Prentice-Hall.

Houston, S. H. (1970). A re-examination of some assumptions about the language of the disadvantaged child. *Child Development, 41*, 947–963.

Howe, G. F. (1931). The teaching of directions in space. *Journal of Geography, 30*, 298–304.

Hoyer, F. W., Hoyer, W. J., Treat, N. J., & Baltes, P. B. (1978–1979). Training response speed in young and elderly women. *International Journal of Aging and Human Development, 9*, 247–253.

Hoyer, W. J. (1980). Information processing, knowledge acquisition, and learning: Developmental perspectives. *Human Development, 23*, 389–399.

Hoyer, W. J. (1985). Aging and the development of expert cognition. In T. M. Shlechter & M. P. Toglia (Eds.), *New directions in cognitive science* (pp. 69–87). Norwood, NJ: Ablex.

Hoyer, W. J., Raskind, C. L., & Abrahams, J. P. (1984). Research practices in the psychology of aging: A survey of research published in the *Journal of Gerontology,* 1975–1982. *Journal of Gerontology, 39*, 44–48.

Hoyer, W. J., Rebok, G. W., & Sved, S. M. (1979). Effects of varying irrelevant information on adult age differences in problem solving. *Journal of Gerontology, 34*, 553–560.

Hughes, C. P. (1978). The differential diagnosis of dementia in the senium. In K. Nandy (Ed.), *Senile dementia: A biomedical approach.* New York: Elsevier.

Hulicka, I. M. (1967). Age differences in retention as a function of interference. *Journal of Gerontology, 22*, 180–184.

Hulicka, I. M., & Grossman, J. L. (1967). Age group comparisons for the use of mediators in paired-associate learning. *Journal of Gerontology, 22*, 46–51.

Hultsch, D. F. (1969). Adult age differences in the organization of free recall. *Developmental Psychology, 1,* 673–678.

Hultsch, D. F. (1971). Adult age differences in free classification and free recall. *Developmental Psychology, 4,* 338–342.

Hultsch, D. F., & Dixon, R. A. (1984). Memory for text materials in adulthood. In P. B. Baltes & O. G. Brim, Jr. (Eds.), *Life-span development and behavior* (Vol. 6, pp. 77–108). New York: Academic Press.

Hultsch, D. F., & Hickey, T. (1978). External validity in the study of human development: Theoretical and methodological issues. *Human Development, 21,* 76–91.

Hultsch, D. F., & Pentz, C. A. (1980). Encoding, storage, and retrieval in adult memory: The role of model assumptions. In L. W. Poon, J. L. Fozard, L. S. Cermak, D. Arenberg, & L. W. Thompson (Eds.), *New directions in memory and aging: Proceedings of the George A. Talland Memorial Conference* (pp. 73–94). Hillsdale, NJ: Erlbaum.

Hunt, J. McV. (1961). *Intelligence and experience.* New York: Ronald Press.

Huston-Stein, A., & Baltes, P. B. (1976). Theory and method in life-span developmental psychology: Implications for child development. In H. W. Reese (Ed.), *Advances in child development and behavior* (Vol. 11, pp. 169–188). New York: Academic Press.

Huttenlocher, J. (1974). The origins of language comprehension. In R. Solso (Ed.), *Theories of cognitive psychology* (pp. 331–368). Hillsdale, NJ: Erlbaum.

Huttenlocher, J., & Burke, D. (1976). Why does memory span increase with age? *Cognitive Psychology, 8,* 1–31.

Huyck, M. H. (1982). From gregariousness to intimacy: Marriage and friendship over the adult years. In T. M. Field, A. Huston, H. C. Quay, L. Troll, & G. E. Finley (Eds.), *Review of human development* (pp. 471–484). New York: Wiley.

Inhelder, B., & Piaget, J. (1958). *The growth of logical thinking from childhood to adolescence.* New York: Basic Books.

Inhelder, B., & Piaget, J. (1964). *The early growth of logic in the child.* New York: Harper & Row.

Inhelder, B., Sinclair, H., & Bovet, M. (1974). *Thinking and the development of cognition.* Cambridge, MA: Harvard University Press.

Irwin, M. H., & McLaughlin, D. H. (1970). Ability and preference in category sorting by Mano schoolchildren and adults. *Journal of Social Psychology, 82,* 15–24.

Irwin, M., Schafer, G., & Frieden, C. (1974). Emic and unfamiliar category sorting of Mano farmers and U.S. undergraduates. *Journal of Cross-Cultural Psychology, 5,* 407–423.

Istomina, Z. M. (1975). The development of voluntary memory in preschool-age children. *Soviet Psychology, 13,* 5–64.

Izard, C. E. (1977). *Human emotions.* New York: Plenum Press.

Izard, C. E. (1978). On the ontogenesis of emotions and emotion-cognition relationships in infancy. In M. Lewis & L. A. Rosenblum (Eds.), *The development of affect* (pp. 389–413). New York: Plenum Press.

Jacewicz, M. M., & Hartley, A. A. (1979). Rotation of mental images by young and old college students: The effects of familiarity. *Journal of Gerontology, 34,* 396–403.

Jackson, P. W., & Messick, S. (1965). The person, the product, and the response: Conceptual problems in the assessment of creativity. *Journal of Personality, 33,* 309–329.

Jacobs, A. (1974). Strategies of social intervention: Past and future. In A. Jacobs & W. Spradlin (Eds.), *The group as agent of change* (pp. 18–37). New York: Behavioral Publications.

Jacobs, P. I., & Vandeventer, M. (1971). The learning and transfer of double classification skills by first graders. *Child Development, 42,* 149–159.

James, W. (1890). *The principles of psychology.* New York: Holt.

Jenkins, J. J. (1974). Remember that old theory of memory? Well, forget it! *American Psychologist, 29*, 785–795.

Jensen, A. R. (1969). How much can we boost IQ and scholastic achievement? *Harvard Educational Review, 39*, 1–123.

Jensen, A. R. (1971). Hebb's confusion about heritability. *American Psychologist, 26*, 394–395.

Jerome, E. A. (1962). Decay of heuristic processes in the aged. In C. Tibbitts & W. Donahue (Eds.), *Social and psychological aspects of aging* (pp. 802–823). New York: Columbia University Press.

Johnson-Laird, P., Hermann, D., & Chaffin, R. (1984). Only connections: A critique of semantic networks. *Psychological Bulletin, 96*, 292–315.

Johnston, W. A., & Heinz, S. P. (1978). Flexibility and capacity demands of attention. *Journal of Experimental Psychology: General, 107*, 420–435.

Jones, E. E., & Davis, K. E. (1965). From acts to dispositions: The attribution process in person perception. In L. Berkowitz (Ed.), *Advances in experimental social psychology* (Vol. 2, pp. 219–266). New York: Academic Press.

Jones, H. E., & Conrad, H. S. (1933). The growth and decline of intelligence: A study of a homogeneous group between the ages of ten and sixty. *Genetic Psychology Monographs, 13*, 223–294.

Jones, W. R. (1960). A critical study of bilingualism and non-verbal intelligence. *British Journal of Educational Psychology, 30*, 71–77.

Jöreskog, K. G., & Sörbom, D. (1979). *Advances in factor analysis and structural equations models.* Cambridge, MA: Abt Associates.

Jusczyk, P. W. (1981). Infant speech perception: A critical appraisal. In P. D. Eimas & J. L. Miller (Eds.), *Perspectives on the study of speech* (pp. 113–164). Hillsdale, NJ: Erlbaum.

Kagan, J. (1971). *Change and continuity in infancy.* New York: Wiley.

Kagan, J. (1972, March). Do infants think? *Scientific American*, pp. 74–82.

Kagan, J. (1976). Resilience and continuity in psychological development. In A. M. Clarke & A. D. B. Clarke (Eds.), *Early experience: Myth and evidence* (pp. 97–121). New York: Free Press.

Kagan, J. (1978). *The growth of the child.* New York: Norton.

Kagan, J., Kearsley, P., & Zelazo, P. (1978). *Infancy: Its place in human development.* Cambridge, MA: Harvard University Press.

Kagan, J., Rosman, B. L., Day, D., Albert, J., & Phillips, W. (1964). Information processing in the child: Significance of analytic and reflective attitudes. *Psychological Monographs, 78*(1, Whole No. 578).

Kahn, R. L., Zarit, S. H., Hilbert, N. M., & Niederehe, M. A. (1975). Memory complaint and impairment in the aged: The effect of depression and altered brain function. *Archives of General Psychiatry, 32*, 1569–1573.

Kahneman, D. (1973). *Attention and effort.* Englewood Cliffs, NJ: Prentice-Hall.

Kail, R. (1984). *The development of memory in children* (2nd ed.). San Francisco: Freeman.

Kail, R., & Bisanz, J. (1982). Information processing and cognitive development. In H. W. Reese (Ed.), *Advances in child development and behavior* (Vol. 17, pp. 45–81). New York: Academic Press.

Kail, R., Carter, P., & Pellegrino, J. (1979). The locus of sex differences in spatial ability. *Perception & Psychophysics, 26*, 102–116.

Kail, R., & Hagen, J. W. (1982). Memory in childhood. In B. B. Wolman (Ed.), *Handbook of developmental psychology* (pp. 350–366). Englewood Cliffs, NJ: Prentice-Hall.

Kail, R., & Pellegrino, J. W. (1985). *Human intelligence: Perspectives and prospects.* San Francisco: Freeman.

Kail, R., Pellegrino, J., & Carter, P. (1980). Developmental changes in mental rotation. *Journal of Experimental Child Psychology, 29*, 102–116.

Kallio, K. D. (1982). Developmental change on a five-term transitive inference. *Journal of Experimental Child Psychology, 33*, 142–164.

Kamin, L. J. (1974). *The science and politics of IQ.* Hillsdale, NJ: Erlbaum.

Kamin, L. (1981a). Separated identical twins. In H. J. Eysenck & L. Kamin, *The intelligence controversy* (pp. 106–113). New York: Wiley.

Kamin, L. (1981b). Studies of adopted children. In H. J. Eysenck & L. Kamin, *The intelligence controversy* (pp. 114–125). New York: Wiley.

Karmel, B. Z., & Maisel, E. B. (1975). A neuronal activity model for infant visual attention. In. L. B. Cohen & P. Salapatek (Eds.), *Infant perception: From sensation to cognition: Vol. 1. Basic visual processes* (pp. 77–131). New York: Academic Press.

Karmiloff-Smith, A. (1979). Language development after five. In P. Fletcher & M. Garman (Eds.), *Language acquisition* (pp. 307–323). New York: Cambridge University Press.

Karplus, R., & Karplus, E. F. (1972, November). Intellectual development beyond elementary school: Ratio, a longitudinal study. *School Science and Mathematics*, pp. 735–742.

Kastenbaum, R. (1968). Perspectives on the development and modification of behavior in the aged: A developmental-field perspective. *Gerontologist, 8*, 280–283.

Kausler, D. H. (1970). Retention-forgetting as a nomological network for developmental research. In L. R. Goulet & P. B. Baltes (Eds.), *Life-span developmental psychology: Research and theory* (pp. 305–353). New York: Academic Press.

Kausler, D. H. (1974). *Psychology of verbal learning and memory.* New York: Academic Press.

Kausler, D. H. (1982). *Experimental psychology and human aging.* New York: Wiley.

Kausler, D. H., & Hakami, M. K. (1982). Frequency judgments by young and elderly adults for relevant stimuli with simultaneously present irrelevant stimuli. *Journal of Gerontology, 37*, 438–442.

Kausler, D. H., & Puckett, J. M. (1980). Frequency judgments and correlated cognitive abilities in young and elderly adults. *Journal of Gerontology, 35*, 376–382.

Kazdin, A. E. (1981). Uses and abuses of behavior modification in education: A rejoinder. *Developmental Review, 1*, 61–62.

Keating, D. P. (1978). A search for social intelligence. *Journal of Educational Psychology, 70*, 218–223.

Keating, D. P. (1984). The emperor's new clothes: The "new look" in intelligence research. In R. J. Sternberg (Ed.), *Advances in the psychology of human intelligence* (Vol. 2, pp. 1 –45). Hillsdale, NJ: Erlbaum.

Keil, F. C. (1981). Constraints on knowledge and cognitive development. *Psychological Review, 88*, 197–227.

Kelley, H. H. (1973). The processes of causal attribution. *American Psychologist, 28*, 107–128.

Kendler, H. H., & Kendler, T. S. (1962). Vertical and horizontal processes in problem solving. *Psychological Review, 69*, 1–16.

Kendler, H. H., & Kendler, T. S. (1975). From discrimination learning to cognitive development: A neobehavioristic odyssey. In W. K. Estes (Ed.), *Handbook of learning and cognitive processes* (Vol. 1, pp. 191–247). Hillsdale, NJ: Erlbaum.

Kendler, T. S. (1979). The development of discrimination learning: A levels-of-functioning explanation. In H. W. Reese & L. P. Lipsitt (Eds.), *Advances in child development and behavior* (Vol. 13, pp. 83–117). New York: Academic Press.

Kendler, T. S., & Kendler, H. H. (1959). Reversal and nonreversal shifts in kindergarten children. *Journal of Experimental Psychology, 58*, 56–60.

Kennedy, W. A. (1969). A follow-up normative study of Negro intelligence and achievement. *Monographs of the Society for Research in Child Development, 34*(6, Serial No. 90).

Kerr, N. H., Corbitt, R., & Jurkovic, G. J. (1980). Mental rotation: Is it stage related? *Journal of Mental Imagery, 4,* 49–56.

Kessel, F. S. (1970). The role of syntax in children's comprehension from ages six to twelve. *Monographs of the Society for Research in Child Development, 35*(6, Serial No. 139).

Kingsley, R. C., & Hall, V. C. (1967). Training conservation through the use of learning sets. *Child Development, 38,* 1111–1126.

Kintsch, W., & van Dijk, T. A. (1978). Toward a model of text comprehension and production. *Psychological Review, 85,* 363–394.

Kirasic, K. C. (1985). A roadmap to research for spatial cognition in the elderly adult. In R. Cohen (Ed.), *The development of spatial cognition* (pp. 185–198). Hillsdale, NJ: Erlbaum.

Kirasic, K. C., Allen, G. L., & Siegel, A. W. (1984). Expression of configurational knowledge of large-scale environments: Students' performance of cognitive tasks. *Environment and Behavior, 16,* 687–712.

Klahr, D. (1978). Goal formation, planning, and learning by pre-school problem solvers or: "My socks are in the dryer." In R. S. Siegler (Ed.), *Children's thinking: What develops?* (pp. 181–212). Hillsdale, NJ: Erlbaum.

Klahr, D. (1984). Transition processes in quantitative development. In R. J. Sternberg (Ed.), *Mechanisms of cognitive development* (pp. 101–139). San Francisco: Freeman.

Klahr, D., & Robinson, M. (1981). Formal assessment of problem solving and planning processes in preschool children. *Cognitive Psychology, 13,* 113–148.

Klahr, D., & Wallace, J. G. (1976). *Cognitive development: An information-processing view.* Hillsdale, NJ: Erlbaum.

Klann-Delius, G. (1981). Sex and language acquisition: Is there any influence? *Journal of Pragmatics, 5,* 1–25.

Klatzky, R. L. (1984). *Memory and awareness: An information-processing perspective.* San Francisco: Freeman.

Kleemeier, R. W. (1962). Intellectual change in the senium. *Proceedings of the Social Statistics Section of the American Statistical Association, 1,* 290–295.

Kline, D. W., Culler, M. P., & Susec, J. (1977). Differences in inconspicuous word identification as a function of age and reversible-figure training. *Experimental Aging Research, 3,* 203–213.

Kline, D. W., & Orme-Rogers, C. (1978). Examination of stimulus persistence as the basis for superior visual identification performance among older adults. *Journal of Gerontology, 33,* 76–81.

Kline, D. W., & Schieber, F. (1981). What are the age differences in visual sensory memory? *Journal of Gerontology, 36,* 86–89.

Kline, D. W., & Schieber, F. (1985). Vision and aging. In J. E. Birren & K. W. Schaie (Eds.), *Handbook of the psychology of aging* (2nd ed., pp. 296–331). New York: Van Nostrand Reinhold.

Klingman, A., Melamed, B. G., Cuthbert, M. I., & Hermecz, D. A. (1984). Effects of participant modeling on information acquisition and skill utilization. *Journal of Consulting and Clinical Psychology, 52,* 414–422.

Klodin, V. M. (1976). The relationship of scoring treatment and age in perceptual integrative performance. *Experimental Aging Research, 2,* 303–313.

Kogan, N. (1973). Creativity and cognitive style: A life-span perspective. In P. B. Baltes & K. W. Schaie (Eds.), *Life-span developmental psychology: Personality and socialization* (pp. 145–178). New York: Academic Press.

Kogan, N. (1974). Categorizing and conceptualizing styles in younger and older adults. *Human Development, 17,* 218–230.

Kogan, N. (1982). Cognitive styles in older adults. In T. M. Field, A. Huston, H. C. Quay, L. Troll, & G. E. Finley (Eds.), *Review of human development* (pp. 586–601). New York: Wiley.

Kogan, N. (1983). Stylistic variation in childhood and adolescence: Creativity, metaphor, and cognitive styles. In J. H. Flavell & E. M. Markman (Eds.), *Handbook of child psychology: Vol. 3. Cognitive development* (pp. 630–706). New York: Wiley.

Kogan, N., & Wallach, M. A. (1961). Age changes in values and attitudes. *Journal of Gerontology, 16,* 272–280.

Kohen-Raz, R. (1974). Physiological maturation and mental growth at preadolescence and puberty. *Journal of Child Psychology and Psychiatry and Allied Disciplines, 15,* 199–213.

Kohlberg, L. (1963). Development of children's orientation towards a moral order. 1. Sequence in the development of moral thought. *Vita Humana, 6,* 11–36.

Kohlberg, L. (1969). Stage and sequence: The cognitive developmental approach to socialization. In D. A. Goslin (Ed.), *Handbook of socialization theory and research* (pp. 347–480). Skokie, IL: Rand McNally.

Kohlberg, L. (1973). Continuities in childhood and adult moral development revisited. In P. B. Baltes & K. W. Schaie (Eds.), *Life-span developmental psychology: Personality and socialization* (pp. 179–204). New York: Academic Press.

Kohlberg, L. (1976). Moral stages and moralization: The cognitive-developmental approach. In T. Lickona (Ed.), *Moral development and behavior: Theory, research, and social issues* (pp. 31–53). New York: Holt, Rinehart and Winston.

Kohlberg, L. (1978). Revisions in the theory and practice of moral development. *New Directions for Child Development, 2,* 83–88.

Kohlberg, L., Colby, A., Gibbs, J., & Speicher-Dubin, B. (1978). *Standard form scoring manual.* Cambridge, MA: Harvard Graduate School of Education, Center for Moral Education.

Kohlberg, L., & Kramer, R. B. (1969). Continuities and discontinuities in childhood and adult moral development. *Human Development, 12,* 93–120.

Köhler, W. (1927). *The mentality of apes.* New York: Harcourt.

Korchin, S. J., & Basowitz, H. (1956). The judgment of ambiguous stimuli as an index of cognitive functioning in the aged. *Journal of Personality, 25,* 81–95.

Koslowski, B. (1980). Quantitative and qualitative changes in the development of seriation. *Merrill-Palmer Quarterly, 26,* 391–405.

Kosslyn, S. M. (1983). *Ghosts in the mind's machine: Creating and using images in the brain.* New York: Norton.

Kosslyn, S. M., Pick, H. L., Jr., & Fariello, G. R. (1974). Cognitive maps in children and men. *Child Development, 45,* 707–716.

Kosslyn, S. M., & Pomerantz, J. R. (1977). Imagery, propositions, and the form of the internal representations. *Cognitive Psychology, 9,* 52–76.

Kramer, D. A. (1983). Post-formal operations? A need for further conceptualization. *Human Development, 26,* 91–105.

Krauss, I., Poon, L. W., Gilewski, M., & Schaie, K. W. (1982, November). *Effects of biased sampling on cognitive performance.* Paper presented at the meeting of the Gerontological Society of America, Boston.

Krauss, R. M., & Glucksberg, S. (1969). The development of communication as a function of age. *Child Development, 40,* 255–266.

Krauss, R. M., & Glucksberg, S. (1977, February). Social and nonsocial speech. *Scientific American,* pp. 100–105.

Kuczaj, S., II (Ed.). (1982). *Language development: Vol. 1. Syntax and semantics.* Hillsdale, NJ: Erlbaum.

Kuhn, D. (1974). Inducing development experimentally: Comments on a research paradigm. *Developmental Psychology, 10,* 590–600.

Kuhn, D. (1978). Mechanisms of cognitive and social development: One psychology or two? *Human Development, 21*, 92–118.

Kuhn, D., & Angelev, J. (1976). An experimental study of the development of formal operational thought. *Child Development, 47*, 697–706.

Kuhn, D., & Brannock, J. (1977). Development of the isolation of variables scheme in experimental and "natural experiment" contexts. *Developmental Psychology, 13*, 9–14.

Kuhn, T. (1970). *The structure of scientific revolutions* (2nd ed.). Chicago: University of Chicago Press.

Kurdek, L. R. (1977). Structural components and intellectual correlates of cognitive perspective taking in first- through fourth-grade children. *Child Development, 48*, 1503–1511.

Kurtines, W., & Grief, E. (1974). The development of moral thought: Review and evaluation of Kohlberg's approach. *Psychological Bulletin, 81*, 453–470.

LaBerge, D., & Samuels, S. J. (1974). Toward a theory of automatic information processing in reading. *Cognitive Psychology, 6*, 293–323.

Labouvie, E. W. (1980). Identity versus equivalence of psychological measures and constructs. In L. W. Poon (Ed.), *Aging in the 1980s: Psychological issues* (pp. 493–502). Washington, DC: American Psychological Association.

Labouvie-Vief, G. (1977). Adult cognitive development: In search of alternative interpretations. *Merrill-Palmer Quarterly, 23*, 227–263.

Labouvie-Vief, G. (1980). Beyond formal operations: Use and limits of pure logic in life-span development. *Human Development, 23*, 141–161.

Labouvie-Vief, G. (1982). Dynamic development and mature autonomy: A theoretical prologue. *Human Development, 25*, 161–191.

Labouvie-Vief, G. (1985). Intelligence and cognition. In J. E. Birren & K. W. Schaie (Eds.), *Handbook of the psychology of aging* (2nd ed., pp. 500–530). New York: Van Nostrand Reinhold.

Labouvie-Vief, G., & Chandler, M. J. (1978). Cognitive development and life-span developmental theory: Idealistic versus contextual perspectives. In P. B. Baltes (Ed.), *Life-span development and behavior* (Vol. 1, pp. 181–210). New York: Academic Press.

Labouvie-Vief, G., & Gonda, J. N. (1976). Cognitive strategy training and intellectual performance in the elderly. *Journal of Gerontology, 31*, 327–332.

Labov, W. (1970). The logic of nonstandard English. In F. Williams (Ed.), *Language and poverty* (pp. 153–189). Chicago: Markham.

Labov, W. (1972). The study of language in its social context. In W. Labov (Ed.), *Sociolinguistic patterns* (pp. 183–259). Philadelphia: University of Pennsylvania Press.

Lachman, J. L., Lachman, R., & Thronesbery, C. (1979). Metamemory through the adult life-span. *Developmental Psychology, 15*, 543–551.

Lachman, M. E. (1983). Perceptions of intellectual aging: Antecedent or consequence of intellectual functioning? *Developmental Psychology, 19*, 482–498.

Lachman, R., Lachman, J. L., & Butterfield, E. C. (1979). *Cognitive psychology and information processing: An introduction.* Hillsdale, NJ: Erlbaum.

Lakatos, I. (1978). *The methodology of scientific research programs.* New York: Cambridge University Press.

Langer, E. J. (1978). Rethinking the role of thought in social interaction. In J. H. Harvey, W. J. Ickes, & R. F. Kidd (Eds.), *New directions in attribution research* (Vol. 2, pp. 35–58). Hillsdale, NJ: Erlbaum.

Langer, E. J., Rodin, J., Beck, P., Weinman, C., & Spitzer, L. (1979). Environmental determinants of memory improvement in late adulthood. *Journal of Personality and Social Psychology, 37*, 2003–2013.

Langer, J. (1970). Werner's comparative organismic theory. In P. H. Mussen (Ed.), *Carmichael's manual of child psychology* (Vol. 1, 3rd ed., pp. 733–771). New York: Wiley.

Laurendeau, M., & Pinard, A. (1970). *The development of the concept of space in the child.* New York: International Universities Press.

Lawton, M. P. (1970). Ecology and aging. In L. A. Pastalan & D. H. Carson (Eds.), *Spatial behavior of older people* (pp. 40–67). Ann Arbor: University of Michigan Press.

Lazar, I., & Darlington, R. (1982). Lasting effects of early education: A report from the Consortium for Longitudinal Studies. *Monographs of the Society for Research in Child Development, 47*(2–3, Serial No. 195).

Lee, J. A., & Pollack, R. H. (1978). The effects of age on perceptual problem-solving strategies. *Experimental Aging Research, 4,* 37–54.

Lee, J. A., & Pollack, R. H. (1980). The effects of age on perceptual field dependence. *Bulletin of the Psychonomic Society, 15,* 239–241.

Lehman, H. C. (1953). *Age and achievement.* Princeton, NJ: Princeton University Press.

Lehman, H. C. (1956). Reply to Dennis' critique of *Age and Achievement. Journal of Gerontology, 11,* 333–337.

Leibowitz, H. W., & Gwozdecki, J. (1967). The magnitude of the Poggendorf illusion as a function of age. *Child Development, 38,* 573–580.

Leibowitz, H., & Judisch, J. M. (1967). The relation between age and magnitude of the Ponzo illusion. *American Journal of Psychology, 80,* 105–109.

Lenneberg, E. H. (1967). *Biological foundations of language.* New York: Wiley.

Lepper, M. R. (1981). Intrinsic and extrinsic motivation in children: Detrimental effects of superfluous social controls. In W. H. Collins (Ed.), *Minnesota Symposia on Child Psychology* (Vol. 14, pp. 155–214). Hillsdale, NJ: Erlbaum.

Lepper, M. R., Greene, D., & Nisbett, R. E. (1973). Undermining children's intrinsic interest with extrinsic reward: A test of the overjustification hypothesis. *Journal of Personality and Social Psychology, 28,* 129–137.

Lerner, R. M. (Chair). (1982). Child development: Life-span perspectives. *Human Development, 25,* 38–88.

Lerner, R. M. (1986). *Concepts and theories of human development* (2nd ed.). New York: Random House.

Lerner, R. M., & Busch-Rossnagel, N. A. (Eds.). (1981). *Individuals as producers of their development: A life-span perspective.* New York: Academic Press.

Levelt, W. J. M. (1975). *What became of LAD?* The Hague: Peter de Ridder.

Leventhal, A. S., & Lipsitt, L. P. (1964). Adaptation, pitch discrimination, and sound localization in the neonate. *Child Development, 35,* 756–767.

Levin, J. R., McCabe, R. E., & Bender, B. G. (1975). A note on imagery-inducing motor activity in young children. *Child Development, 46,* 263–266.

Levine, M. (1963). Mediating processes in humans at the outset of discrimination learning. *Psychological Review, 70,* 254–276.

Levine, M. (1975). *A cognitive theory of learning: Research on hypothesis-testing.* Hillsdale, NJ: Erlbaum.

Lewis, M. (1983). On the nature of intelligence: Science or bias? In M. Lewis (Ed.), *Origins of intelligence: Infancy and early childhood* (2nd ed., pp. 1–24). New York: Plenum Press.

Lewis, M., & Brooks, J. (1975). Infants' social perception: A constructivist view. In L. B. Cohen & P. Salapatek (Eds.), *Infant perception: From sensation to cognition: Vol. 2. Perception of space, speech, and sound* (pp. 101–148). New York: Academic Press.

Lewis, M., & Freedle, R. O. (1973). Mother-infant dyad: The cradle of meaning. In P. Pliner, L. Krames, & T. Alloway (Eds.), *Communication and affect: Language and thought* (pp. 127–155). New York: Academic Press.

Lewis, T. L., Mauer, D., & Kay, D. (1978). Newborns' central vision: Whole or hole? *Journal of Experimental Child Psychology, 26,* 193–203.

Liben, L. S. (1975a). Evidence for developmental differences in spontaneous seriation and its implication for past research on long-term memory improvement. *Developmental Psychology, 11,* 121–125.

Liben, L. S. (1975b). Long-term memory for pictures related to seriation, horizontality, and verticality concepts. *Developmental Psychology, 11,* 795–806.

Liben, L. S. (1981). Spatial representation and behavior: Multiple perspectives. In L. S. Liben, A. H. Patterson, & N. Newcombe (Eds.), *Spatial representation and behavior across the life-span* (pp. 3–36). New York: Academic Press.

Lickona, T. (Ed.). (1976). *Moral development and behavior: Theory, research, and social issues.* New York: Holt, Rinehart and Winston.

Lieberman, D. A. (1979). Behaviorism and the mind: A (limited) call for a return to introspection. *American Psychologist, 34,* 319–333.

Lieven, E. V. M. (1978). Conversations between mothers and young children: Individual differences and their possible implications for the study of language learning. In N. Waterson & C. Snow (Eds.), *The development of communication* (pp. 173–187). New York: Wiley.

Light, P. (1983). Social interaction and cognitive development: A review of post-Piagetian research. In S. Meadows (Ed.), *Developing thinking: Approaches to children's cognitive development* (pp. 67–88). New York: Methuen.

Lindsay, P. H., & Norman, D. A. (1977). *Human information processing: An introduction to psychology* (2nd ed.). New York: Academic Press.

Lipsitt, L. P., Engen, T., & Kaye, H. (1963). Developmental changes in the olfactory threshold of the neonate. *Child Development, 34,* 371–376.

Livesley, W. J., & Bromley, D. B. (1973). *Person perception in childhood and adolescence.* New York: Wiley.

Loehlin, J. C., Lindzey, G., & Spuhler, J. N. (1975). *Race differences in intelligence.* San Francisco: Freeman.

Looft, W. R. (1972). Egocentrism and social interaction across the life-span. *Psychological Bulletin, 78,* 75–92.

Looft, W. R., & Charles, D. C. (1971). Egocentrism and social interaction in young and old adults. *Aging and Human Development, 2,* 21–28.

Lovaas, O. I. (1977). *The autistic child: Language development through behavior modification.* New York: Irvington.

Lowenfeld, V., & Brittain, W. L. (1970). *Creative and mental growth* (5th ed.). New York: Macmillan.

Luchins, A. S. (1942). Mechanization in problem solving. *Psychological Monographs, 54*(6, Whole No. 248).

Lynch, G. S. (1983, August). *Aging and brain plasticity.* Paper presented at the meeting of the American Psychological Association, Anaheim, CA.

Lynch, K. (1960). *The image of the city.* Cambridge, MA: MIT Press.

Macauley, R. K. S. (1978). The myth of female superiority in language. *Journal of Child Language, 5,* 353–374.

Maccoby, E. E., & Jacklin, C. N. (1974). *The psychology of sex differences.* Stanford, CA: Stanford University Press.

Maccoby, E. E., & Konrad, K. W. (1966). Age trends in selective listening. *Journal of Experimental Child Psychology, 3,* 113–122.

Maccoby, E. E., & Konrad, K. W. (1967). Effect of preparatory set on selective listening: Developmental trends. *Monographs of the Society for Research in Child Development, 32*(4, Serial No. 112).

Macfarlane, J. A. (1975). Olfaction in the development of social preferences in the human neonate. In M. A. Hofer (Ed.), *Parent-infant interaction* (pp. 103–117). New York: Elsevier.

MacKinnon, D. W. (1962). The nature and nurture of creative talent. *American Psychologist, 17,* 484–495.

Macnamara, J. (1972). Cognitive basis of language learning in infants. *Psychological Review, 79*, 1–13.

MacWhinney, B. (1978). The acquisition of morphophonology. *Monographs of the Society for Research in Child Development, 43*(1–2, Serial No. 174).

Madden, J., O'Hara, J., & Levenstein, P. (1984). Home again: Effects of the Mother-Child Home Program on mother and child. *Child Development, 55*, 636–647.

Malatesta, C. Z. (1981). Affective development over the lifespan: Involution or growth? *Merrill-Palmer Quarterly, 27*, 145–173.

Mandler, J. M. (1978). A code in the node: The use of story schema in retrieval. *Discourse Processes, 1*, 14–35.

Mandler, J. M., & DeForest, M. (1979). Is there more than one way to recall a story? *Child Development, 50*, 886–889.

Mandler, J. M., & Johnson, N. S. (1977). Remembrance of things parsed: Story structure and recall. *Cognitive Psychology, 9*, 111–151.

Mandler, J. M., & Robinson, C. A. (1978). Developmental changes in picture recognition. *Journal of Experimental Child Psychology, 26*, 122–136.

Mandler, J. M., & Stein, N. L. (1974). Recall and recognition of pictures by children as a function of organization and distractor similarity. *Journal of Experimental Psychology, 102*, 657–669.

Mans, L., Cicchetti, D., & Sroufe, L. A. (1978). Mirror reactions of Down's syndrome infants and toddlers: Cognitive underpinnings of self-recognition. *Child Development, 49*, 1247–1250.

Marks, L., & Miller, G. A. (1964). The role of semantic and syntactic constraints in the memorization of English sentences. *Journal of Verbal Learning and Verbal Behavior, 3*, 1–5.

Marmor, G. (1975). Development of kinetic images: When does the child first represent movement in mental images? *Cognitive Psychology, 7*, 548–559.

Marmor, G. (1977). Mental rotation and number conservation: Are they related? *Developmental Psychology, 13*, 320–325.

Marsh, D. T., Serafica, F. C., & Barenboim, C. (1980). Effect of perspective-taking training on interpersonal problem solving. *Child Development, 51*, 140–145.

Mason, S. E. (1979). Effects of orienting tasks on the recall and recognition performance of subjects differing in age. *Developmental Psychology, 15*, 467–469.

Matarazzo, J. D. (1972). *Wechsler's measurement and appraisal of adult intelligence* (5th ed.). Baltimore: Williams & Wilkins.

Matlin, M. (1983). *Cognition.* New York: Holt, Rinehart and Winston.

Matlin, M. W. (1985). Current issues in psycholinguistics. In T. M. Shlechter & M. P. Toglia (Eds.), *New directions in cognitive science* (pp. 217–241). Norwood, NJ: Ablex.

Maurer, D., & Salapatek, P. (1976). Developmental changes in the scanning of faces by young infants. *Child Development, 47*, 523–527.

Maurer, D., Siegel, L. S., Lewis, T. L., Kristofferson, M. W., Barnes. R. A., & Levy, B. A. (1979). Long-term memory improvement. *Child Development, 50*, 106–118.

Mayer, R. E. (1983). *Thinking, problem solving, cognition.* San Francisco: Freeman.

McCall, R. B. (1981). Nature-nurture and the two realms of development: A proposed integration with respect to mental development. *Child Development, 52*, 1–12.

McCall, R. B., Applebaum, M., & Hogarty, P. S. (1973). Developmental changes in mental performance. *Monographs of the Society for Research in Child Development, 38*(3, Serial No. 150).

McClelland, D. C. (1973). Testing for competence rather than for "intelligence." *American Psychologist, 28*, 1–14.

McCluskey, K. A., & Reese, H. W. (Eds.). (1986). *Life-span developmental psychology: Historical and generational effects.* New York: Academic Press.

McGee, M. G. (1979). Human spatial abilities: Psychometric studies and environmental, genetic, hormonal, and neurological influences. *Psychological Bulletin, 86,* 889–918.

McKenzie, B. E., Tootell, H. E., & Day, R. H. (1980). Development of visual size constancy during the 1st year of human infancy. *Developmental Psychology, 16,* 163–174.

McLaughlin, B. (1977). Second-language learning in children. *Psychological Bulletin, 84,* 438–459.

McNeill, D. (1970). The development of language. In P. H. Mussen (Ed.), *Carmichael's manual of child psychology* (Vol. 1, 3rd ed., pp. 1061–1161). New York: Wiley.

McNemar, Q. (1964). Lost: Our intelligence? Why? *American Psychologist, 19,* 871–882.

Meacham, J. A. (1972). The development of memory abilities in the individual and society. *Human Development, 42,* 205–228.

Meacham, J. A. (1977). A transactional model of remembering. In N. Datan & H. W. Reese (Eds.), *Life-span developmental psychology: Dialectical perspectives on experimental research* (pp. 261–283). New York: Academic Press.

Meicler, M., & Gratch, G. (1980). Do 5-month-olds show object conception in Piaget's sense? *Infant Behavior and Development, 3,* 265–282.

Mendelson, M. J., & Haith, M. M. (1976). The relation between audition and vision in the human newborn. *Monographs of the Society for Research in Child Development, 41*(4, Serial No. 167).

Mercer, J. R. (1971). Sociocultural factors in labeling mental retardates. *Peabody Journal of Education, 48,* 188–203.

Mergler, N. L., Dusek, J. B., & Hoyer, W. J. (1977). Central/incidental recall and selective attention in young and elderly adults. *Experimental Aging Research, 3,* 49–60.

Mergler, N. L., & Goldstein, M. D. (1983). Why are there old people? Senescence as biological and cultural preparedness for the transmission of information. *Human Development, 26,* 72–90.

Meyer, B. J. F. (1975). *The organization of prose and its effect on memory.* New York: Elsevier.

Meyer, B. J. F., & Rice, G. E. (1981). Information recalled from prose by young, middle, and old adult readers. *Experimental Aging Research, 7,* 253–268.

Meyer, J. S. (1983, April). *A cognitive developmental theory of creativity.* Paper presented at the meeting of the Eastern Psychological Association, Philadelphia.

Meyer, J. S., & Rebok, G. W. (1985). Planning-in-action across the life span. In T. M. Shlecter & M. P. Toglia (Eds.), *New directions in cognitive science* (pp. 47–68). Norwood, NJ: Ablex.

Midlarsky, E., Bryan, J. H., & Brickman, P. (1973). Aversive approval: Interactive effects of modeling and reinforcement on altruistic behavior. *Child Development, 44,* 321–328.

Miller, E. (1981). The nature of the cognitive deficit in dementia. In N. E. Miller & G. D. Cohen (Eds.), *Clinical aspects of Alzheimer's disease and senile dementia* (pp. 103–120). New York: Raven Press.

Miller, G. A. (1956). The magical number seven, plus or minus two: Some limits on our capacity for processing information. *Psychological Review. 63,* 81–97.

Miller, P. H. (1983). *Theories of developmental psychology.* San Francisco: Freeman.

Miller, P. H., & Weiss, M. G. (1981). Children's attention allocation, understanding of attention, and performance on the incidental learning task. *Child Development, 52,* 1183–1190.

Minton, H. L., & Schneider, F. W. (1980). *Differential psychology.* Monterey, CA: Brooks-Cole.

Mischel, W. (1968). *Personality and assessment.* New York: Wiley.

Moates, D. R., & Schumacher, G. M. (1980). *An introduction to cognitive psychology.* Belmont, CA: Wadsworth.

Molfese, D. L., Molfese, V. J., & Carrell, P. L. (1982). Early language development. In B. B. Wolman (Ed.), *Handbook of developmental psychology* (pp. 301–322). Englewood Cliffs, NJ: Prentice-Hall.

Monge, R. H. (1973). Developmental trends in factors of adolescent self-concept. *Developmental Psychology, 8,* 382–393.

Monge, R. H., & Gardner, E. F. (1976). Education as an aid to adaptation in the adult years. In K. F. Riegel & J. A. Meacham (Eds.), *The developing individual in a changing world: Vol. 2. Social environmental issues* (pp. 611–620). Chicago: Aldine.

Montada, L., & Schmitt, M. (1982). Issues in applied developmental psychology: A lifespan perspective. In P. B. Baltes & O. G. Brim, Jr. (Eds.), *Life-span development and behavior* (Vol. 4, pp. 1–32). New York: Academic Press.

Montemayor, R., & Eisen, M. (1977). The development of self-conceptions from childhood to adolescence. *Developmental Psychology, 13,* 314–319.

Moore, G. T. (1976). Theory and research on the development of environmental knowing. In G. T. Moore & R. G. Golledge (Eds.), *Environmental knowing* (pp. 138–164). Stroudsburg, PA: Dowden, Hutchinson & Ross.

Morris, C. D., Bransford, J. D., & Franks, J. J. (1977). Levels of processing versus transfer appropriate processing. *Journal of Verbal Learning and Verbal Behavior, 16,* 519–533.

Morrison, F. J., Holmes, D. L., & Haith, M. M. (1974). A developmental study of the effects of familiarity on short-term visual memory. *Journal of Experimental Child Psychology, 18,* 412–425.

Morsbach, G., & Steel, P. M. (1976). 'John is easy to see' re-investigated. *Journal of Child Language, 3,* 443–447.

Morse, P. A., & Cowan, N. (1982). Infant auditory and speech perception. In T. M. Field, A. Huston, H. C. Quay, L. Troll, & G. E. Finley (Eds.), *Review of human development* (pp. 32–61). New York: Wiley.

Mortimer, J. T., Finch, M. D., & Kumka, D. (1982). Persistence and change in development: The multidimensional self-concept. In P. B. Baltes & O. G. Brim, Jr. (Eds.), *Life-span development and behavior* (Vol. 4, pp. 263–313). New York: Academic Press.

Mosher, F. A., & Hornsby, J. R. (1966). On asking questions. In J. S. Bruner, R. R. Olver, & P. M. Greenfield (Eds.), *Studies in cognitive growth* (pp. 86–102). New York: Wiley.

Murphy, J. M., & Gilligan, C. (1980). Moral development in late adolescence and adulthood: A critique and reconstruction of Kohlberg's theory. *Human Development, 23,* 77–104.

Murphy, M. D., & Brown, A. L. (1975). Incidental learning in preschool children as a function of level of cognitive analysis. *Journal of Experimental Child Psychology, 19,* 509–523.

Murphy, M. D., Sanders, R. E., Gabriesheski, A. S., & Schmitt, F. A. (1981). Metamemory in the aged. *Journal of Gerontology, 36,* 185–193.

Murray, F. B. (1978). Teaching strategies and conservation training. In A. M. Lesgold, J. W. Pellegrino, S. D. Fokkema, & R. Glaser (Eds.), *Cognitive psychology and instruction* (pp. 419–428). New York: Plenum Press.

Muson, H. (1979, February). Moral thinking: Can it be taught? *Psychology Today,* pp. 48–58, 92.

Myers, N. A., & Perlmutter, M. (1978). Memory in the years from two to five. In P. A. Ornstein (Ed.), *Memory development in children* (pp. 191–218). Hillsdale, NJ: Erlbaum.

Nardi, A. H. (1973). Person-perception research and the perception of life-span development. In P. B. Baltes & K. W. Schaie (Eds.), *Life-span developmental psychology: Personality and socialization* (pp. 285–301). New York: Academic Press.

Nehrke, M. F., Hulicka, I. M., & Morganti, J. B. (1980). Age differences in life satisfaction, locus of control, and self-concept. *International Journal of Aging and Human Development, 11,* 25–33.

Neill, A. S. (1960). *Summerhill: A radical approach to child rearing.* New York: Hart.

Neimark, E. D. (1975a). Intellectual development during adolescence. In F. D. Horowitz (Ed.), *Review of child development research* (Vol. 4, pp. 541–594). Chicago: University of Chicago Press.

Neimark, E. D. (1975b). Longitudinal development of formal operations thought. *Genetic Psychology Monographs, 91,* 171–225.

Neimark, E. D. (1982). Adolescent thought: Transition to formal operations. In B. B. Wolman (Ed.), *Handbook of developmental psychology* (pp. 486–502). Englewood Cliffs, NJ: Prentice-Hall.

Neimark, E., Slotnick, N. S., & Ulrich, T. (1971). Development of memorization strategies. *Developmental Psychology, 5,* 427–432.

Neisser, U. (1967). *Cognitive psychology.* New York: Appleton-Century-Crofts.

Neisser, U. (1976). *Cognition and reality: Principles and implications of cognitive psychology.* San Francisco: Freeman.

Neisser, U. (1979). The concept of intelligence. In R. J. Sternberg & D. K. Detterman (Eds.), *Human intelligence: Perspectives on its theory and measurement* (pp. 179–189). Norwood, NJ: Ablex.

Neisser, U., & Becklen, R. (1975). Selective looking: Attending to visually-specified events. *Cognitive Psychology, 7,* 480–494.

Neisser, U., Hirst, W., & Spelke, E. S. (1981). Limited capacity theories and the notion of automaticity: Reply to Lucas and Bub. *Journal of Experimental Psychology: General, 110,* 499–500.

Nelson, K. (1973a). Structure and strategy in learning to talk. *Monographs of the Society for Research in Child Development, 38*(1–2, Serial No. 149).

Nelson, K. (1973b). Some evidence for the cognitive primacy of categorization and its functional basis. *Merrill-Palmer Quarterly, 19,* 21–40.

Nelson, K. (1974). Concept, word, and sentence: Interrelations in acquisition and development. *Psychological Review, 81,* 267–285.

Nelson, K. (1981). Individual differences in language development: Implications for development and language. *Developmental Psychology, 17,* 170–187.

Nelson, K., & Brown, A. L. (1978). The semantic-episodic distinction in memory development. In P. A. Ornstein (Ed.), *Memory development in children* (pp. 233–241). Hillsdale, NJ: Erlbaum.

Nelson, S. A. (1980). Factors influencing young children's use of motives and outcomes as moral criteria. *Child Development, 51,* 823–829.

Nesselroade, J. R., & Baltes, P. B. (Eds.). (1979). *Longitudinal research in the study of behavior and development.* New York: Academic Press.

Newell, A. (1973). You can't play 20 questions with nature and win: Projective comments on the papers of this symposium. In W. G. Chase (Ed.), *Visual information processing* (pp. 283–308). New York: Academic Press.

Newell, A., & Simon, H. A. (1972). *Human problem solving.* Englewood Cliffs, NJ: Prentice-Hall.

Newport, E. L. (1976). Motherese: The speech of mothers to young children. In N. J. Castellan, Jr., D. B. Pisoni, & G. R. Potts (Eds.), *Cognitive theory* (Vol. 2, pp. 177–217). Hillsdale, NJ: Erlbaum.

Ninio, A., & Bruner, J. S. (1978). The achievement and antecedents of labeling. *Journal of Child Language, 5,* 1–15.

Nisbett, R. E., Borgida, E., Crandall, R., & Reed, H. (1976). Popular induction: Information is not necessarily informative. In J. S. Carroll & J. W. Payne (Eds.), *Cognition and social behavior* (pp. 113–133). Hillsdale, NJ: Erlbaum.

Norman, D. A. (1968). Toward a theory of memory and attention. *Psychological Review, 75,* 522–536.

Norman, D. A. (1976). *Memory and attention* (2nd ed.). New York: Wiley.

Norman, D. A. (1981). Twelve issues for cognitive science. In D. A. Norman (Ed.), *Perspectives on cognitive science* (pp. 265–295). Norwood, NJ: Ablex.

Norman, D. K. A. (1980). A comparison of children's spatial reasoning: Rural Appalachia, suburban, and urban New England. *Child Development, 51,* 288–291.

Oden, M. H. (1968). The fulfillment of promise: 40-year follow-up of the Terman gifted group. *Genetic Psychology Monographs, 77,* 3–93.

Odom, R. D. (1972). Effects of perceptual salience on the recall of relevant and incidental dimensional values. *Journal of Experimental Psychology, 92,* 285–291.

Odom, R. D. (1978). A perceptual salience account of décalage relations and developmental change. In L. S. Siegel & C. J. Brainerd (Eds.), *Alternatives to Piaget: Critical essays on the theory* (pp. 111–130). New York: Academic Press.

Odom, R. D., Cunningham, J. G., & Astor-Stetson, E. C. (1977). The role of perceptual salience and type of instruction in children's recall of relevant and incidental dimensional values. *Bulletin of the Psychonomic Society, 9,* 77–80.

Ohta, R. J., Walsh, D. A., & Krauss, I. K. (1981). Spatial perspective-taking ability in young and elderly adults. *Experimental Aging Research, 7,* 45–63.

Olson, D. R. (1966). On conceptual strategies. In J. S. Bruner, R. R. Olver, & P. M. Greenfield (Eds.), *Studies in cognitive growth* (pp. 135–153). New York: Wiley.

Olson, D. R., & Torrance, N. G. (1983). Literacy and cognitive development: A conceptual transformation in the early school years. In S. Meadows (Ed.), *Developing thinking: Approaches to children's cognitive development* (pp. 142–160). New York: Methuen.

Ornstein, P. A., & Naus, M. J. (1978). Rehearsal processes in children's memory. In P. A. Ornstein (Ed.), *Memory development in children* (pp. 69–99). Hillsdale, NJ: Erlbaum.

Osborn, A. (1957). *Applied imagination.* New York: Scribner's.

Oster, H. (1978). Facial expression and affect development. In M. Lewis & L. Rosenblum (Eds.), *The development of affect* (pp. 43–75). New York: Plenum Press.

Overton, W. F. (1973). On the assumptive base of the nature-nurture controversy: Additive versus interactive conceptions. *Human Development, 16,* 74–89.

Overton, W. F. (Ed.). (1983). *The relationship between social and cognitive development.* Hillsdale, NJ: Erlbaum.

Overton, W. F. (1984). World views and their influence on psychological theory and research: Kuhn-Lakatos-Laudan. In H. W. Reese (Ed.), *Advances in child development and behavior* (Vol. 18, pp. 191–226). New York: Academic Press.

Overton, W., & Reese, H. (1973). Models of development: Methodological implications. In J. R. Nesselroade & H. W. Reese (Eds.), *Life-span developmental psychology: Methodological issues* (pp. 65–86). New York: Academic Press.

Owens, W. A. (1953). Age and mental abilities: A longitudinal study. *Genetic Psychology Monographs, 48,* 3–54.

Owens, W. A. (1959). Is age kinder to the initially more able? *Journal of Gerontology, 14,* 334–337.

Paivio, A. (1969). Mental imagery in associative learning and memory. *Psychological Review, 76,* 241–263.

Palermo, D. S., & Molfese, D. L. (1972). Language acquisition from age five onward. *Psychological Bulletin, 78,* 409–428.

Palmore, E., & Cleveland, W. (1976). Aging, terminal decline, and terminal drop. *Journal of Gerontology, 31,* 76–81.

Panek, P. E. (1985). Age differences in field-dependence/independence. *Experimental Aging Research, 11,* 97–99.

Papalia, D. E. (1972). The status of several conservation abilities across the life-span. *Human Development, 15,* 229–243.

Papalia, D. E., Kennedy, E., & Sheehan, N. (1973). Conservation of space in noninstitutionalized old people. *Journal of Psychology, 84,* 75–79.

Papalia, D. E., Salverson, S. M., & True, M. (1973). An evaluation of quantity conservation performance during old age. *Aging and Human Development, 4,* 103–110.

Parikh, B. (1980). Moral judgment development and its relation to family factors in Indian and American families. *Child Development, 51,* 1030–1039.

Paris, S. G. (1978). Coordination of means and goals in the development of mnemonic skills. In P. A. Ornstein (Ed.), *Memory development in children* (pp. 259–273). Hillsdale, NJ: Erlbaum.

Paris, S. G., & Lindauer, B. K. (1982). The development of cognitive skills during childhood. In B. B. Wolman (Ed.), *Handbook of developmental psychology* (pp. 333–349). Englewood Cliffs, NJ: Prentice-Hall.

Park, D. C., Puglisi, J. T., & Lutz, R. (1982). Spatial memory in older adults: Effects of intentionality. *Journal of Gerontology, 37,* 330–335.

Parker, R. K., Rieff, M. L., & Sperr, S. J. (1971). Teaching multiple classification to young children. *Child Development, 42,* 1779–1789.

Parkinson, S. R., Lindholm, J. M., & Urell, T. (1980). Aging, dichotic memory, and digit span. *Journal of Gerontology, 35,* 87–95.

Parkinson, S. R., & Perey, A. (1980). Aging, digit span, and the stimulus suffix effect. *Journal of Gerontology, 35,* 736–742.

Pascual-Leone, J. (1970). A mathematical model for the transition rule in Piaget's developmental stages. *Acta Psychologia, 32,* 301–345.

Pastalan, L. A., Mautz, R. K., & Merrill, J. (1973). The simulation of age-related sensory losses: A new approach to the study of environmental barriers. In W. F. E. Preiser (Ed.), *Environmental design research* (Vol. 1, pp. 383–391). Stroudsburg, PA: Dowden, Hutchinson & Ross.

Peevers, B., & Secord, P. (1973). Developmental changes in attribution of descriptive concepts to persons. *Journal of Personality and Social Psychology, 27,* 120–128.

Pepper, S. (1942). *World hypotheses.* Berkeley: University of California Press.

Perky, C. W. (1910). An experimental study of imagination. *American Journal of Psychology, 21,* 422–452.

Perlmutter, M. (1978). What is memory aging the aging of? *Developmental Psychology, 14,* 330–345.

Perlmutter, M. (1979). Age differences in adults' free recall, cued recall, and recognition. *Journal of Gerontology, 34,* 533–539.

Perlmutter, M., & Myers, N. A. (1974). Recognition memory development in two- to four-year olds. *Developmental Psychology, 10,* 447–450.

Perry, W. I. (1970). *Forms of intellectual and ethical development in the college years.* New York: Holt, Rinehart and Winston.

Petersen, A. C. (1976). Physical androgyny and cognitive functioning in adolescence. *Developmental Psychology, 12,* 524–533.

Piaget, J. (1926). *The language and thought of the child.* New York: Harcourt.

Piaget, J. (1932). *The moral judgment of the child.* New York: Harcourt.

Piaget, J. (1951). *Play, dreams, and imitation in childhood.* London: Heinemann.

Piaget, J. (1952). *The child's conception of number.* New York: Norton.

Piaget, J. (1954). *The construction of reality in the child.* New York: Basic Books.

Piaget, J. (1963). *The psychology of intelligence.* New York: International Universities Press.

Piaget, J. (1967). *The language and thought of the child.* London: Routledge.

Piaget, J. (1970). Piaget's theory. In P. H. Mussen (Ed.), *Carmichael's manual of child psychology* (Vol. 1, 3rd ed., pp. 703–732). New York: Wiley.

Piaget, J. (1971). *Biology and knowledge.* Chicago: University of Chicago Press.

Piaget, J. (1972). Intellectual evolution from adolescence to adulthood. *Human Development, 15,* 1–12.

Piaget, J. (1978). What is psychology? *American Psychologist, 33,* 648–652.

Piaget, J., & Inhelder, B. (1967). *The child's conception of space.* New York: Norton.

Piaget, J., & Inhelder, B. (1969). *The psychology of the child.* New York: Basic Books.

Piaget, J., & Inhelder, B. (1971). *Mental imagery in the child.* New York: Basic Books.

Piaget, J., & Inhelder, B. (1973). *Memory and intelligence.* London: Routledge.

Piaget, J., Inhelder, B., & Szeminska, A. (1960). *A child's conception of geometry.* New York: Basic Books.

Pick, A. D., Frankel, D. G., & Hess, V. L. (1975). Children's attention: The development of selectivity. In E. M. Hetherington (Ed.), *Review of child development research* (Vol. 5, pp. 325–383). Chicago: University of Chicago Press.

Pick, H. L., Jr., & Lockman, J. J. (1981). From frames of reference to spatial representations. In L. S. Liben, A. H. Patterson, & N. Newcombe (Eds.), *Spatial representation and behavior across the life span* (pp. 39–61). New York: Academic Press.

Platt, J. J., & Spivack, G. (1973, Summer). Studies in problem-solving thinking of psychiatric patients: Patient-control differences and factorial structure of problem-solving thinking. *Proceedings of the 81st Annual Convention of the American Psychological Association, 8,* 461–462.

Platt, J. J., Spivack, G., Altman, N., Altman, D., & Peizer, S. B. (1974). Adolescent problem-solving thinking. *Journal of Consulting and Clinical Psychology, 42,* 787–793.

Plomin, R. (1983). Developmental behavioral genetics. *Child Development, 54,* 253–259.

Plude, D. J., & Hoyer, W. J. (1981). Adult age differences in visual search as a function of stimulus mapping and processing load. *Journal of Gerontology, 36,* 598–604.

Pollack, R. H., & Atkeson, B. M. (1978). A life-span approach to perceptual development. In P. B. Baltes (Ed.), *Life-span development and behavior* (Vol. 1, pp. 85–109). New York: Academic Press.

Poon, L. W. (1985). Differences in human memory with aging: Nature, causes, and clinical implications. In J. E. Birren & K. W. Schaie (Eds.), *Handbook of the psychology of aging* (2nd ed., pp. 427–462). New York: Van Nostrand Reinhold.

Poon, L. W., Fozard, J. L., Paulshock, D. R., & Thomas, J. C. (1979). A questionnaire assessment of age differences in retention of recent and remote events. *Experimental Aging Research, 5,* 401–411.

Poon, L. W., Walsh-Sweeney, L., & Fozard, J. L. (1980). Memory skill training for the elderly: Salient issues on the use of imagery mnemonics. In L. W. Poon, J. L. Fozard, L. S. Cermak, D. Arenberg, & L. W. Thompson (Eds.), *New directions in memory and aging: Proceedings of the George A. Talland Memorial Conference* (pp. 461–484). Hillsdale, NJ: Erlbaum.

Postman, L., & Underwood, B. J. (1973). Critical issues in interference theory. *Memory and Cognition, 1,* 19–40.

Pratt, M. W., & Bates, K. R. (1982). Young editors: Preschoolers' evaluations and production of ambiguous messages. *Developmental Psychology, 18,* 30–42.

Premack, D. (1976). Language and intelligence in ape and man. *American Scientist, 64,* 674–683.

Pressey, S. L., & Kuhlen, R. G. (1957). *Psychological development through the life span.* New York: Harper & Row.

Pribram, K. H. (1986). The cognitive revolution and mind/brain issues. *American Psychologist, 41,* 507–520.

Pylyshyn, Z. W. (1973). What the mind's eye tells the mind's brain: A critique of mental imagery. *Psychological Bulletin, 80,* 1–24.

Pylyshyn, Z. W. (1981). The imagery debate: Analogue media versus tacit knowledge. *Psychological Review, 88,* 16–45.

Rabbitt, P. M. A. (1965). An age decrement in the ability to ignore irrelevant information. *Journal of Gerontology, 20,* 233–238.

Rader, N., Bausano, M., & Richards, J. E. (1980). On the nature of the visual-cliff avoidance response in human infants. *Child Development, 51,* 61–68.

Rankin, J. L., & Kausler, D. H. (1979). Adult age differences in false recognitions. *Journal of Gerontology, 34,* 58–65.

Ransen, D. L. (1981). Long-term effects of two interventions with the aged: An ecological analysis. *Journal of Applied Developmental Psychology, 2*, 13–27.

Rebok, G. W. (1981). Age effects in problem solving in relation to irrelevant information, dimensional preferences, and feedback. *Experimental Aging Research, 7*, 393–403.

Reese, H. W. (1972). Imagery and multiple paired-associate learning in young children. *Journal of Experimental Child Psychology, 13*, 310–323.

Reese, H. W. (1973a). Life-span models of memory. *Gerontologist, 13*, 472–478.

Reese, H. W. (1973b). Models of memory and models of development. *Human Development, 16*, 398–416.

Reese, H. W. (1976). Models of memory development. *Human Development, 19*, 291–303.

Reese, H. W., & Overton, W. F. (1970). Models of development and theories of development. In L. R. Goulet & P. B. Baltes (Eds.), *Life-span developmental psychology: Research and theory* (pp. 115–145). New York: Academic Press.

Reese, H. W., & Overton, W. F. (1980). Models, methods, and ethics of intervention. In R. R. Turner & H. W. Reese (Eds.), *Life-span developmental psychology: Intervention* (pp. 29–47). New York: Academic Press.

Reinert, G. (1970). Comparative factor analytic studies of intelligence throughout the human life span. In L. R. Goulet & P. B. Baltes (Eds.), *Life-span developmental psychology: Research and theory* (pp. 467–484). New York: Academic Press.

Reitman, W. R. (1965). *Computers and thought: An information-processing approach.* New York: Wiley.

Reno, R. (1979). Attribution of success and failure as a function of perceived age. *Journal of Gerontology, 34*, 709–715.

Rest, J. R. (1983). Morality. In J. H. Flavell & E. M. Markman (Eds.), *Handbook of child psychology: Vol. 3. Cognitive development* (pp. 556–629). New York: Wiley.

Rest, J., Turiel, E., & Kohlberg, L. (1969). Levels of moral development as a determinant of preference and comprehension of moral judgments made by others. *Journal of Personality, 37*, 225–252.

Rheingold, H. L., & Cook, K. V. (1975). The content of boys' and girls' rooms as an index of parents' behavior. *Child Development, 46*, 459–463.

Rice, B. (1979, September). Brave new world of intelligence testing. *Psychology Today*, pp. 26–41.

Rice, M. L. (1982). Child language: What children know and how. In T. M. Field, A. Huston, H. C. Quay, L. Troll, & G. E. Finley (Eds.), *Review of human development* (pp. 253–268). New York: Wiley.

Richards, J. E., & Rader, N. (1981). Crawling-onset age predicts visual cliff avoidance in infants. *Journal of Experimental Psychology: Human Perception and Performance, 7*, 382–387.

Riecken, H. W., & Boruch, R. F. (Eds.). (1974). *Social experimentation: A method for planning and evaluating social intervention.* New York: Academic Press.

Riegel, K. F. (1973a). Dialectic operations: The final period of cognitive development. *Human Development, 16*, 346–370.

Riegel, K. F. (1973b). Language and cognition: Some life-span developmental issues. *Gerontologist, 13*, 478–482.

Riegel, K. F., & Riegel, R. M. (1964). Changes in associative behavior during later years of life: A cross-sectional analysis. *Vita Humana, 7*, 1–32.

Riegel, K. F., & Riegel, R. M. (1972). Development, drop, and death. *Developmental Psychology, 6*, 306–319.

Risley, T. R., & Baer, D. M. (1973). Operant behavior modification: The deliberate development of behavior. In B. M. Caldwell & N. Ricciuti (Eds.), *Review of child development research* (Vol. 3, pp. 283–329). Chicago: University of Chicago Press.

Risley, T. R., & Wolf, M. M. (1973). Strategies for analyzing behavioral change over time.

In J. R. Nesselroade & H. W. Reese (Eds.), *Life-span developmental psychology: Methodological issues* (pp. 175–183). New York: Academic Press.

Robinson, A. R. (1912). *Memory and the executive mind.* Chicago: Donahue.

Rogoff, B. (1982). Integrating context and cognitive development. In M. E. Lamb & A. L. Brown (Eds.), *Advances in developmental psychology* (Vol. 2, pp. 125–170). Hillsdale, NJ: Erlbaum.

Rogosa, D. (1979). Causal models in longitudinal research: Rationale, formulation, and interpretation. In J. R. Nesselroade & P. B. Baltes (Eds.), *Longitudinal research in the study of behavior and development* (pp. 263–302). New York: Academic Press.

Rohwer, W. D., Jr. (1973). Elaboration and learning in childhood and adolescence. In H. W. Reese (Ed.), *Advances in child development and behavior* (Vol. 8, pp. 1–57). New York: Academic Press.

Romaniuk, J. G., & Romaniuk, M. (1981). Creativity across the life span: A measurement perspective. *Human Development, 24,* 366–381.

Roodin, P. A., Rybash, J. M., & Hoyer, W. J. (1984). Affect in adult cognition: A constructivist view of moral thought and action. In C. Malatesta & C. Izard (Eds.), *Emotion in adult development* (pp. 297–316). Beverly Hills, CA: Sage.

Rosch, E. (1973). On the internal structure of perceptual and semantic categories. In T. E. Moore (Ed.), *Cognitive development and the acquisition of language* (pp. 111–144). New York: Academic Press.

Rosch, E. H., & Mervis, C. B. (1975). Family resemblances: Studies in the internal structure of categories. *Cognitive Psychology, 7,* 573–605.

Rose, S. A., Gottfried, A. W., & Bridger, W. H. (1981). Cross-modal transfer and information-processing by the sense of touch in infancy. *Developmental Psychology, 17,* 90–98.

Rosenberg, S., & Sedlak, A. (1972). Structural representations of implicit personality theory. In L. Berkowitz (Ed.), *Advances in experimental social psychology* (Vol. 6, pp. 173–220). New York: Academic Press.

Ross, D. M., & Ross, S. A. (1976). *Hyperactivity: Research, theory, and action.* New York: Wiley.

Ross, L. (1977). The intuitive psychologist and his shortcomings: Distortions in the attribution process. In L. Berkowitz (Ed.), *Advances in experimental social psychology* (Vol. 10, pp. 173–220). New York: Academic Press.

Rotenberg, K. J. (1980). Children's use of intentionality in judgments of character and disposition. *Child Development, 51,* 282–284.

Rotenberg, K. J. (1982). Development of character constancy in self and other. *Child Development, 53,* 505–515.

Rothenberg, B. (1970). Children's social sensitivity and the relationship to interpersonal competence, intrapersonal comfort, and intellectual level. *Developmental Psychology, 2,* 335–350.

Rovee, C. K., Cohen, R. Y., & Shlapack, W. (1975). Life-span stability in olfactory sensitivity. *Developmental Psychology, 11,* 311–318.

Rubin, K. H. (1974). The relationship between spatial and communicative egocentrism in children and young and old adults. *Journal of Genetic Psychology, 125,* 295–301.

Rubin, K. H. (1976). Extinction of conservation: A life-span investigation. *Developmental Psychology, 12,* 51–56.

Rubin, K. H. (1978). Role taking in childhood: Some methodological considerations. *Child Development, 49,* 428–433.

Rubin, K., Attewell, P., Tierney, M., & Tumolo, P. (1973). The development of spatial egocentrism and conservation across the life span. *Developmental Psychology, 9,* 432.

Rubin, R., & Balow, B. (1979). Measures of infant development and socioeconomic status as predictors of later intelligence and school achievement. *Developmental Psychology, 15,* 225–227.

Ruff, H. A., & Halton, A. (1978). Is there directed reaching in the human neonate? *Developmental Psychology, 14,* 425–426.

Rybash, J. M., Roodin, P. A., & Hoyer, W. J. (1983). Expressions of moral thought in later adulthood. *Gerontologist, 23,* 254–260.

Salapatek, P., & Kessen, W. (1966). Visual scanning of triangles by the human newborn. *Journal of Experimental Child Psychology, 3,* 155–167.

Salkind, N. J. (1978). The development of norms for the Matching Familiar Figures Test. *JSAS Catalog of Selected Documents in Psychology, 8,* p. 61. (Ms. No. 1718).

Salkind, N. J. (1981). *Theories of human development.* New York: Van Nostrand Reinhold.

Salkind, N. J., & Nelson, C. F. (1980). A note on the developmental nature of reflection-impulsivity. *Developmental Psychology, 16,* 237–238.

Salthouse, T. A. (1976). Age and tachistoscopic perception. *Experimental Aging Research, 2,* 91–103.

Salthouse, T. (1982). *Adult cognition: An experimental psychology of human aging.* New York: Springer.

Salthouse, T. A. (1985). Speed of behavior and its implications for cognition. In J. E. Birren & K. W. Schaie (Eds.), *Handbook of the psychology of aging* (2nd ed., pp. 400–426). New York: Van Nostrand Reinhold.

Salthouse, T. A., & Kail, R. (1983). Memory development throughout the life span: The role of processing rate. In P. B. Baltes & O. G. Brim, Jr. (Eds.), *Life-span development and behavior* (Vol. 5, pp. 89–116). New York: Academic Press.

Sameroff, A. (1975). Transactional models in early social relations. *Human Development, 18,* 65–79.

Sampson, E. E. (1981). Cognitive psychology as ideology. *American Psychologist, 36,* 730–743.

Samuel, A. G. (1978). Organizational vs. retrieval factors in the development of digit span. *Journal of Experimental Child Psychology, 26,* 308–319.

Sanders, J. C., Sterns, H. L., Smith, M., & Sanders, R. E. (1975). Modification of concept identification performance in older adults. *Developmental Psychology, 11,* 824–829.

Sapir, E. (1921). *Language: An introduction to the study of speech.* New York: Harcourt.

Scarr, S. (1983). An evolutionary perspective on infant intelligence: Species patterns and individual variations. In M. Lewis (Ed.), *Origins of intelligence: Infancy and early childhood* (2nd ed., pp. 191–223). New York: Plenum Press.

Scarr, S., & Weinberg, R. A. (1976). IQ test performance of Black children adopted by White families. *American Psychologist, 31,* 726–739.

Scarr, S., & Weinberg, R. A. (1977). Intellectual similarities within families of both adopted and biological children. *Intelligence, 32,* 170–191.

Scarr, S., & Weinberg, R. A. (1983). The Minnesota adoption studies: Genetic differences and malleability. *Child Development, 54,* 260–267.

Scarr-Salapatek, S. (1975). Genetics and the development of intelligence. In F. D. Horowitz (Ed.), *Review of child development research* (Vol. 4, pp. 1–57). Chicago: University of Chicago Press.

Schaie, K. W. (1958). Rigidity-flexibility and intelligence: A cross-sectional study of the adult life span from 20 to 70 years. *Psychological Monographs, 72*(9, Whole No. 462).

Schaie, K. W. (1965). A general model for the study of developmental problems. *Psychological Bulletin, 64,* 92–107.

Schaie, K. W. (1967). Age changes and age differences. *Gerontologist, 7,* 128–132.

Schaie, K. W. (1977–1978). Toward a stage theory of adult cognitive development. *International Journal of Aging and Human Development, 8,* 129–138.

Schaie, K. W. (1978). External validity in the assessment of intellectual development in adulthood. *Journal of Gerontology, 33,* 695–701.

Schaie, K. W. (1979). The primary mental abilities in adulthood: An exploration in the development of psychometric intelligence. In P. B. Baltes & O. G. Brim, Jr. (Eds.), *Life-span development and behavior* (Vol. 2, pp. 67–115). New York: Academic Press.

Schaie, K. W. (1983). The Seattle Longitudinal Study: A 21-year exploration of psychometric intelligence in adulthood. In K. W. Schaie (Ed.), *Longitudinal studies of adult psychological development* (pp. 64–135). New York: Guilford Press.

Schaie, K. W., & Baltes, P. B. (1975). On sequential strategies and developmental research. *Human Development, 18,* 384–390.

Schaie, K. W., & Hertzog, C. (1985). Measurement in the psychology of adulthood and aging. In J. E. Birren & K. W. Schaie (Eds.), *Handbook of the psychology of aging* (2nd ed., pp. 61–92). New York: Van Nostrand Reinhold.

Schaie, K. W., & Labouvie-Vief, G. V. (1974). Generational versus ontogenetic components of change in adult cognitive behavior: A fourteen-year cross-sequential study. *Developmental Psychology, 10,* 305–320.

Schaie, K. W., & Willis, S. L. (1978). Life-span development: Implications for education. *Review of Educational Research, 6,* 120–156.

Scheidt, R. J., & Schaie, K. W. (1978). A taxonomy of situations for an elderly population: Generating situational criteria. *Journal of Gerontology, 33,* 848–857.

Schneider, W., & Shiffrin, R. M. (1977). Controlled and automatic human information processing: I. Detection, search, and attention. *Psychological Review, 84,* 1–66.

Schonfield, D., & Robertson, E. H. (1966). Memory storage and aging. *Canadian Journal of Psychology, 20,* 228–236.

Schultz, N. R., Jr., Elias, M. F., Robbins, M. A., Streeten, D. H. P., & Blakeman, N. (1986). A longitudinal comparison of hypertensives and normotensives on the Wechsler Adult Intelligence Scale: Initial findings. *Journal of Gerontology, 41,* 169–175.

Schultz, N. R., Jr. & Hoyer, W. J. (1976). Feedback effects on spatial egocentrism in old age. *Journal of Gerontology, 31,* 72–75.

Schwartz, A., Campos, J., & Baisel, E. (1973). The visual cliff: Cardiac and behavioral responses on the deep and shallow sides at five and nine months of age. *Journal of Experimental Child Psychology, 15,* 86–99.

Schweinhart, L. J., & Weikart, D. P. (1980). Young children grow up: The effects of the Perry Preschool Program on youths through age 15. *Monographs of the High/Scope Educational Research Foundation* (No. 7). Ypsilanti, MI: High/Scope Press.

Sears, R. R. (1977). Sources of life satisfaction of Terman gifted men. *American Psychologist, 32,* 119–128.

Selman, R. L. (1976). Toward a structural analysis of developing interpersonal relations concepts: Research with normal and disturbed preadolescent boys. In A. D. Pick (Ed.), *Minnesota Symposia on Child Psychology* (Vol. 10, pp. 156–200). Minneapolis: University of Minnesota Press.

Selman, R. L. (1981). The child as a friendship philosopher. In S. R. Asher & J. M. Gottman (Eds.), *The development of children's friendships* (pp. 242–272). New York: Cambridge University Press.

Selman, R. L., & Byrne, D. F. (1974). A structural-developmental analysis of levels of role-taking in middle childhood. *Child Development, 45,* 803–806.

Selman, R. L., & Jaquette, D. (1978). Stability and oscillation in interpersonal awareness: A clinical-developmental analysis. In C. B. Keasey (Ed.), *Nebraska Symposium on Motivation* (Vol. 25, pp. 261–304). Lincoln: University of Nebraska Press.

Selzer, S. C., & Denney, N. W. (1980). Conservation abilities in middle-aged and elderly adults. *International Journal of Aging and Human Development, 11,* 135–146.

Sexton, M. A., & Geffen, G. (1979). Development of three strategies of attention in dichotic monitoring. *Developmental Psychology, 15,* 299–310.

Shaklee, H. (1979). Bounded rationality and cognitive development: Upper limits on growth? *Cognitive Psychology, 11,* 327–345.

Shantz, C. U. (1975). The development of social cognition. In E. M. Hetherington (Ed.), *Review of child development research* (Vol. 5, pp. 257–323). Chicago: University of Chicago Press.

Shantz, C. U. (1983). Social cognition. In J. H. Flavell & E. M. Markman (Eds.), *Handbook of child psychology: Vol. 3. Cognitive development* (pp. 495–555). New York: Wiley.

Shatz, M. (1983). Communication. In J. H. Flavell & E. M. Markman (Eds.), *Handbook of child psychology: Vol. 3. Cognitive development* (pp. 841–889). New York: Wiley.

Shatz, M., & Gelman, R. (1973). The development of communication skills: Modifications in the speech of young children as a function of listener. *Monographs of the Society for Research in Child Development, 38*(5, Serial No. 152).

Shaw, R., & Bransford, J. D. (1977). *Perceiving, acting, and knowing: Toward an ecological psychology.* Hillsdale, NJ: Erlbaum.

Sheingold, K. (1973). Developmental differences in intake and storage of visual information. *Journal of Experimental Child Psychology, 16,* 1–11.

Shepard, R. N. (1978). The mental image. *American Psychologist, 33,* 125–137.

Shepard, R. N., & Feng, C. (1972). A chronometric study of mental paper folding. *Cognitive Psychology, 3,* 228–243.

Shepard, R. N., & Metzler, J. (1971). Mental rotation of three-dimensional objects. *Science, 171,* 701–703.

Shiffrin, R. M., & Schneider, W. (1977). Controlled and automatic information processing: II. Perceptual learning, automatic attending, and a general theory. *Psychological Review, 84,* 127–190.

Shure, M. B. (1982). Interpersonal problem solving: A cog in the wheel of social cognition. In F. C. Serafica (Ed.), *Social-cognitive development in context* (pp. 133–166). New York: Guilford Press.

Shure, M. B., & Spivack, G. (1978). *Problem solving techniques in childrearing.* San Francisco: Jossey-Bass.

Shwartz, S. P., & Kosslyn, S. M. (1982). A computer simulation approach to studying mental imagery. In J. Mehler, E. C. T. Walker, & M. Garrett (Eds.), *Perspectives on mental representation* (pp. 69–85). Hillsdale, NJ: Erlbaum.

Siegel, A. W. (1981). The externalization of cognitive maps by children and adults: In search of ways to ask better questions. In L. S. Liben, A. H. Patterson, & N. Newcombe (Eds.), *Spatial representation and behavior across the life span* (pp. 167–194). New York: Academic Press.

Siegel, A. W., & Allik, J. P. (1973). A developmental study of visual and auditory short-term memory. *Journal of Verbal Learning and Verbal Behavior, 12,* 409–418.

Siegel, A. W., Bisanz, J., & Bisanz, G. L. (1983). Developmental analysis: A strategy for the study of psychological change. In D. Kuhn & J. A. Meacham (Eds.), *On the development of developmental psychology: Vol. 8. Contributions to human development* (pp. 53–80). Basel, Switzerland: Karger.

Siegel, A. W., & Schadler, M. (1977). Young children's cognitive maps of their classroom. *Child Development, 48,* 388–394.

Siegel, A. W., & White, S. H. (1975). The development of spatial representations of large-scale environments. In H. W. Reese (Ed.), *Advances in child development and behavior* (Vol. 10, pp. 9–55). New York: Academic Press.

Siegel, L. S. (1981). Infant tests as predictors of cognitive and language development at two years. *Child Development, 52,* 545–557.

Siegel, L. S., & Brainerd, C. J. (Eds.). (1978). *Alternatives to Piaget: Critical essays on the theory.* New York: Academic Press.

Siegler, R. S. (Ed.). (1978). *Children's thinking: What develops?* Hillsdale, NJ: Erlbaum.

Siegler, R. S. (1981). Developmental sequences within and between concepts. *Monographs of the Society for Research in Child Development, 46*(2, Serial No. 189).

Siegler, R. S. (1983). Information-processing approaches to development. In W. Kessen (Ed.), *Handbook of child psychology: Vol. 1. History, theory, and methods* (pp. 129–211). New York: Wiley.

Siegler, R. S., & Klahr, D. (1982). When do children learn: The relationship between existing knowledge and the ability to acquire new knowledge. In R. Glaser (Ed.), *Advances in instructional psychology* (pp. 121–212). Hillsdale, NJ: Erlbaum.

Siegler, R. S., & Richards, D. D. (1982). The development of intelligence. In R. J. Sternberg (Ed.), *Handbook of human intelligence* (pp. 897–971). New York: Cambridge University Press.

Siegler, R. S., & Richards, D. D. (1983). The development of two concepts. In C. J. Brainerd (Ed.), *Recent advances in cognitive developmental theory: Progress in cognitive development research* (pp. 51–121). New York: Springer.

Sigel, I. E. (1972). Developmental theory: Its place and relevance in early intervention programs. *Young Children, 37,* 364–372.

Sigel, I. E. (1981). Child development research in learning and cognition in the 1980s: Continuities and discontinuities from the 1970s. *Merrill-Palmer Quarterly, 27,* 347–371.

Sigel, I., & Hooper, F. (1968). *Logical thinking in children.* New York: Holt, Rinehart and Winston.

Silverman, I., & Reimanis, G. (1966). A test of two interpretations of age deficit in the ability to reverse an ambiguous figure. *Journal of Gerontology, 21,* 89–92.

Simon, H. A. (1975). The functional equivalence of problem solving skills. *Cognitive Psychology, 7,* 268–288.

Simon, H. (1979). Information-processing models of cognition. *Annual Review of Psychology, 30,* 363–396.

Simonton, D. K. (1975). Age and literary creativity: A cross-cultural and transhistorical survey. *Journal of Cross-Cultural Psychology, 6,* 259–277.

Simonton, D. K. (1977). Creative productivity, age, and stress: A biographical time-series analysis. *Journal of Personality and Social Psychology, 35,* 791–804.

Sinclair-de Zwart, H. (1969). Developmental psycholinguistics. In D. Elkind & J. H. Flavell (Eds.), *Studies in cognitive development* (pp. 315–336). New York: Oxford University Press.

Sinnott, J. D. (1981). The theory of relativity: A metatheory for development? *Human Development, 24,* 293–311.

Sinnott, J. D. (1984). Postformal reasoning: The relativistic stage. In M. L. Commons, F. A. Richards, & C. Armor (Eds.), *Beyond formal operations: Late adolescent and adult cognitive development* (pp. 298–325). New York: Praeger.

Skeels, H. M. (1966). Adult status of children with contrasting early experiences. *Monographs of the Society for Research in Child Development, 31*(3, Serial No. 105).

Skinner, B. F. (1957). *Verbal behavior.* New York: Appleton-Century-Crofts.

Slobin, D. I. (1979). *Psycholinguistics* (2nd ed.). Glenview, IL: Scott, Foresman.

Smedslund, J. (1961a). The acquisition of conservation of substance and weight in children. I: Introduction. *Scandinavian Journal of Psychology, 2,* 11–20.

Smedslund, J. (1961b). The acquisition of conservation of substance and weight in children. II: External reinforcement of conservation of weight and of the operations of addition and subtraction. *Scandinavian Journal of Psychology, 2,* 71–84.

Smedslund, J. (1961c). The acquisition of conservation of substance and weight in children. III: Extinction of conservation of weight acquired "normally" and by means of empirical controls on a balance scale. *Scandinavian Journal of Psychology, 2,* 85–87.

Smith, A. D. (1977). Adult age differences in cued recall. *Developmental Psychology, 13,* 326–331.

Smith, A. D. (1980). Age differences in encoding, storage, and retrieval. In L. W. Poon, J. L. Fozard, L. S. Cermak, D. Arenberg, & L. W. Thompson (Eds.), *New directions in memory and aging: Proceedings of the George A. Talland Memorial Conference* (pp. 23–45). Hillsdale, NJ: Erlbaum.

Smith, E. E., Shoben, E. J., & Rips, L. J. (1974). Structure and process in semantic memory: A featural model for semantic decision. *Psychological Review, 81*, 214–241.

Smith, J., Heckhausen, J., Kliegl, R., & Baltes, P. B. (1984, November). *Cognitive reserve capacity, expertise, and aging: Plasticity of digit span performance.* Paper presented at the meeting of the Gerontological Society of America, San Antonio.

Smith, M. E. (1926). An investigation of the development of the sentence and the extent of vocabulary in young children. *University of Iowa Studies in Child Welfare, 3*(No. 5).

Smith, S. W., Rebok, G. W., Smith, W. R., Hall, S. E., & Alvin, M. (1983). Adult age differences in the use of story structure in delayed free recall. *Experimental Aging Research, 9*, 191–195.

Smothergill, D. W. (1973). Accuracy and variability in the localization of spatial targets at three age levels. *Developmental Psychology, 8*, 62–66.

Smothergill, D. W., Hughes, F. P., Timmons, S. A., & Hutko, P. (1975). Spatial visualizing in children. *Developmental Psychology, 11*, 4–13.

Snow, C. E. (1972). Mothers' speech to children learning language. *Child Development, 43*, 549–565.

Snow, C. E. (1978). The conversational context of language acquisition. In R. N. Campbell & P. T. Smith (Eds.), *Recent advances in the psychology of language: Vol. 4a. Language development and mother-child interaction* (pp. 253–269). New York: Plenum Press.

Snow, C. E., & Hoefnagel-Höhle, M. (1978). The critical period for language acquisition: Evidence from second language learning. *Child Development, 49*, 1114–1128.

Solso, R. L. (1979). *Cognitive psychology.* New York: Harcourt.

Sommer, R., & Sommer, B. A. (1983). Mystery in Milwaukee: Early intervention, IQ, and psychology textbooks. *American Psychologist, 38*, 982–985.

Spelke, E. S. (1979a). Exploring audible and visible events in infancy. In A. D. Pick (Ed.), *Perception and its development: A tribute to Eleanor J. Gibson* (pp. 221–235). Hillsdale, NJ: Erlbaum.

Spelke, E. S. (1979b). Perceiving bimodally specified events in infancy. *Developmental Psychology, 15*, 626–636.

Spelke, E., Hirst, W., & Neisser, U. (1976). Skills of divided attention. *Cognition, 4*, 215–230.

Sperling, G. (1960). The information available in brief visual presentations. *Psychological Monographs, 74*(11, Whole No. 498).

Spilich, G. J. (1983). Life-span components of text processing: Structural and procedural changes. *Journal of Verbal Learning and Verbal Behavior, 22*, 231–244.

Spivack, G., & Shure, M. B. (1974). *Social adjustment of young children: A cognitive approach to solving real-life problems.* San Francisco: Jossey-Bass.

Spoehr, K. T., & Lehmkuhle, S. W. (1982). *Visual information processing.* San Francisco: Freeman.

Stanley, J. C., & Benbow, C. P. (1983). SMPY's first decade: Ten years of posing problems and solving them. *Journal of Special Education, 17*, 11–25.

Stein, M. I. (1974). *Stimulating creativity: Vol. 1. Individual procedures.* New York: Academic Press.

Stein, N. L., & Glenn, C. G. (1979). An analysis of story comprehension in elementary school children. In R. O. Freedle (Ed.), *New directions in discourse processing* (Vol. 2, pp. 53–120). Hillsdale, NJ: Erlbaum.

Sternberg, R. J. (1977). *Intelligence, information processing, and analogical reasoning: The componential analysis of human abilities.* Hillsdale, NJ: Erlbaum.

Sternberg, R. J. (Ed.). (1984). *Mechanisms of cognitive development.* San Francisco: Freeman.

Sternberg, R. J. (1985). *Beyond IQ: A triarchic theory of human intelligence.* New York: Cambridge University Press.

Sternberg, R. J., Conway, B. E., Ketron, J. L., & Bernstein, M. (1981). People's conceptions of intelligence. *Journal of Personality and Social Psychology, 41,* 37–55.

Sternberg, R. J., & Powell, J. S. (1983). The development of intelligence. In J. H. Flavell & E. M. Markman (Eds.), *Handbook of child psychology: Vol. 3. Cognitive development* (pp. 341–419). New York: Wiley.

Sterns, H. L., & Sanders, R. E. (1980). Training and education of the elderly. In R. R. Turner & H. W. Reese (Eds.), *Life-span developmental psychology: Intervention* (pp. 307–330). New York: Academic Press.

Stewart, N. (1947). A.G.C.T. scores of army personnel grouped by occupation. *Occupation, 26,* 5–41.

Storck, P. A., Looft, W. R., & Hooper, F. H. (1972). Interrelationships among Piagetian tasks and traditional measures of cognitive abilities in mature and aged adults. *Journal of Gerontology, 27,* 461–465.

Strauss, S. (Ed.). (1982). *U-shaped behavioral growth.* New York: Academic Press.

Strauss, S., & Stavy, R. (1982). U-shaped behavioral growth: Implications for theories of development. In W. W. Hartup (Ed.), *Review of child development research* (Vol. 6, pp. 547–599). Chicago: University of Chicago Press.

Sugarman-Bell, S. (1978). Some organizational aspects of pre-verbal communication. In I. Markova (Ed.), *The social context of language* (pp. 49–66). New York: Wiley.

Szafran, J., & Birren, J. E. (1969). Perception. In J. E. Birren (Ed.), *Contemporary gerontology: Concepts and issues* (pp. 1–26). Los Angeles: University of Southern California, Gerontology Center.

Tamir, L. M. (1979). *Communication and the aging process: Interaction throughout the life cycle.* New York: Pergamon.

Tapley, S. M., & Bryden, M. P. (1977). An investigation of sex differences in spatial ability: Mental rotation of three-dimensional objects. *Canadian Journal of Psychology, 31,* 122–130.

Taylor, S. E., & Fiske, S. T. (1978). Salience, attention, and attribution: Top of the head phenomena. In L. Berkowitz (Ed.), *Advances in experimental social psychology* (Vol. 11, pp. 249–288). New York: Academic Press.

Templin, M. C. (1957). Certain language skills in children: Their development and interrelationships. *University of Minnesota Institute of Child Welfare Monograph* (No. 26).

Terman, L. M. (Ed.). (1959). *Genetic studies of genius* (Vols. 1–5). Stanford, CA: Stanford University Press.

Terrace, H. S. (1979). *Nim: A chimpanzee who learned to talk.* New York: Knopf.

Tesch, S. A. (1983). Review of friendship development across the life span. *Human Development, 26,* 266–276.

Thomas, R. M. (1985). *Comparing theories of child development* (2nd ed.). Belmont, CA: Wadsworth.

Thompson, L. W., & Marsh, G. R. (1973). Psychophysiological studies of aging. In C. Eisdorfer & M. P. Lawton (Eds.), *The psychology of adult development and aging* (pp. 112–148). Washington, DC: American Psychological Association.

Thomson, G. H. (1939). *The factorial analysis of human ability.* London: University of London Press.

Thurstone, L. L. (1938). *Primary mental abilities.* Chicago: University of Chicago Press.

Thurstone, T. G. (1958). *Manual for the SRA Primary Mental Abilities.* Chicago: Science Research Associates.

Till, R. E., & Jenkins, J. J. (1973). The effects of cued orienting tasks on the free recall of words. *Journal of Verbal Learning and Verbal Behavior, 12,* 489–498.

Tomlinson-Keasey, C. (1972). Formal operations in females from eleven to fifty-four years of age. *Developmental Psychology, 6,* 364.

Torrance, E. P. (1966). *Torrance Tests of Creative Thinking: Verbal Form A and B.* Princeton, NJ: Personnel Press.

Trabasso, T. (1975). Representation, memory, and reasoning: How do we make transitive inferences? In A. D. Pick (Ed.), *Minnesota Symposia on Child Psychology* (Vol. 9, pp. 135–172). Minneapolis: University of Minnesota Press.

Trabasso, T. (1977). The role of memory as a system in making transitive inferences. In R. V. Kail & J. W. Hagen (Eds.), *Perspectives on the development of memory and cognition* (pp. 333–366). Hillsdale, NJ: Erlbaum.

Treat, N. J., & Reese, H. W. (1976). Age, pacing, and imagery in paired-associate learning. *Developmental Psychology, 12,* 119–124.

Treffinger, D. J., Runzulli, J. S., & Feldhusen, J. F. (1971). Problems in the assessment of creative thinking. *Journal of Creative Behavior, 5,* 104–112.

Treisman, A. M. (1964). Monitoring and storage of irrelevant messages and selective attention. *Journal of Verbal Learning and Verbal Behavior, 3,* 449–459.

Trowbridge, C. C. (1913). Fundamental methods of orientation and imaginary maps. *Science, 38,* 888–897.

Tuckman, J., & Lorge, I. (1953). Attitudes toward old people. *Journal of Social Psychology, 37,* 249–260.

Tulving, E. (1972). Episodic and semantic memory. In E. Tulving & W. Donaldson (Eds.), *Organization of memory* (pp. 381–403). New York: Academic Press.

Tulving, E. (1983). *Elements of episodic memory.* New York: Oxford University Press.

Tulving, E., & Thomson, D. M. (1973). Encoding specificity and retrieval processes in episodic memory. *Psychological Review, 80,* 352–373.

Tumblin, A., & Gholson, B. (1981). Hypothesis theory and the development of conceptual learning. *Psychological Bulletin, 90,* 102–124.

Turiel, E. (1973). Stage transition in moral development. In R. Travers (Ed.), *Second handbook of research on teaching* (pp. 732–758). Skokie, IL: Rand McNally.

Turiel, E. (1974). Conflict and transition in adolescent moral development. *Child Development, 45,* 14–29.

Urban, H. B. (1978). The concept of development from a systems perspective. In P. B. Baltes (Ed.), *Life-span development and behavior* (Vol. 11, pp. 45–83). New York: Academic Press.

U.S. National Health Survey. (1968). Monocular-binocular visual acuity of adults (Public Health Service Publication No. 100, Series 11, No. 30, 1960–1962). Washington, DC: U.S. Government Printing Office.

Uzgiris, I. C., & Hunt, J. Mc V. (1975). *Assessment in infancy: Ordinal scales of psychological development.* Champaign: University of Illinois Press.

Versey, J. (1980). Longitudinal studies and Piaget's theory of cognitive development. In S. Modgil & C. Modgil (Eds.), *Toward a theory of psychological development* (pp. 501–539). Windsor, England: National Foundation for Educational Research.

Vygotsky, L. S. (1962). *Thought and language.* Cambridge, MA: MIT Press.

Vygotsky, L. S. (1978). *Mind in society: The development of higher psychological processes* (M. Cole, V. John-Steiner, S. Scribner, & E. Souberman, Eds.). Cambridge, MA: Harvard University Press.

Wachs, T. D., & Gruen, C. E. (1982). *Early experiences and human development.* New York: Plenum Press.

Waddington, C. H. (1957). *The strategy of the genes.* London: Allen & Unwin.

Wagner, D. A. (1978). Memories of Morocco: The influence of age, schooling, and environment on memory. *Cognitive Psychology, 10,* 1–28.

Wagner, D. A. (1981). Culture and memory development. In H. C. Triandis & A. Heron (Eds.), *Handbook of cross-cultural psychology* (Vol. 4, pp. 187–232). Boston: Allyn & Bacon.

Wagner, D. A., & Paris, S. G. (1981). Problems and prospects in comparative studies of memory. *Human Development, 24,* 412–424.

Walk, R. D. (1981). *Perceptual development.* Monterey, CA: Brooks-Cole.

Walk, R. D., & Gibson, E. J. (1961). A comparative and analytical study of visual depth perception. *Psychological Monographs, 75*(15, Whole No. 519).

Wallach, M. (1970). Creativity. In P. Mussen (Ed.), *Carmichael's manual of child psychology* (Vol. 1, 3rd ed., pp. 1211–1272). New York: Wiley.

Wallach, M. A., & Kogan, N. (1965). *Modes of thinking in young children.* New York: Holt, Rinehart and Winston.

Walsh, D. A., & Jenkins, J. J. (1973). Effects of orienting tasks on free recall in incidental learning: "Difficulty," "effort," and "process" explanations. *Journal of Verbal Learning and Verbal Behavior, 12,* 481–488.

Walsh, D. A., Krauss, I. K., & Regnier, V. A. (1981). Spatial ability, environmental knowledge, and environmental use: The elderly. In L. S. Liben, A. H. Patterson, & N. Newcombe (Eds.), *Spatial representation and behavior across the life span* (pp. 321–357). New York: Academic Press.

Walsh, D. A., & Prasse, M. J. (1980). Iconic memory and attentional processes in the aged. In L. W. Poon, J. L. Fozard, L. S. Cermak, D. Arenberg, & L. W. Thompson (Eds.), *New directions in memory and aging: Proceedings of the George A. Talland Memorial Conference* (pp. 153–180). Hillsdale, NJ: Erlbaum.

Wapner, S., Werner, H., & Comalli, P. E. (1960). Perception of part-whole relationships in middle and old age. *Journal of Gerontology, 15,* 412–416.

Warren, R. M. (1961). Illusory changes in repeated words: Differences between young adults and the aged. *American Journal of Psychology, 74,* 506–516.

Waugh, N. C., & Norman, D. A. (1965). Primary memory. *Psychological Review, 72,* 89–104.

Weale, R. A. (1963). *The aging eye.* New York: Harper & Row.

Wechsler, D. (1939). *Measurement of adult intelligence.* Baltimore: Williams & Wilkins.

Wechsler, D. (1955). *Manual for the Wechsler Adult Intelligence Scale.* New York: Psychological Corporation.

Wechsler, D. (1958). *The measurement and appraisal of adult intelligence.* Baltimore: Williams & Wilkins.

Wechsler, D. (1974). *Wechsler Intelligence Scale for Children.* New York: Psychological Corporation.

Weir, M. W. (1964). Developmental changes in problem-solving strategies. *Psychological Review, 71,* 473–490.

Weisberg, R. W., & Alba, J. W. (1981). An examination of the alleged role of "fixation" in the solution of several "insight" problems. *Journal of Experimental Psychology: General, 110,* 169–192.

Weisberg, R., & Suls, J. (1973). An information-processing analysis of Duncker's candle problem. *Cognitive Psychology, 4,* 255–276.

Weiss, G., & Hechtman, L. (1979). The hyperactive child syndrome. *Science, 205,* 1348–1354.

Weiss, S. L., Robinson, G., & Hastie, R. (1977). The relationship of depth of processing to free recall in second and fourth graders. *Developmental Psychology, 13,* 525–526.

Wellman, H. M. (1977). Tip of the tongue and feeling of knowing experiences: A developmental study of memory monitoring. *Child Development, 48,* 13–21.

Wellman, H. M. (Ed.). (1985). *Children's searching: The development of search skills and spatial representation.* Hillsdale, NJ: Erlbaum.

Wellman, H. M., & Lempers, J. D. (1977). The naturalistic communicative abilities of two-year-olds. *Child Development, 48,* 1052–1057.

Werner, H. (1948). *Comparative psychology of mental development.* New York: International Universities Press.

Werner, H. (1957). The concept of development from a comparative and organismic point of view. In D. Harris (Ed.), *The concept of development: An issue in the study of human behavior* (pp. 125–148). Minneapolis: University of Minnesota Press.

West, R. L., Odom, R. D., & Aschkenasy, J. R. (1978). Perceptual sensitivity and conceptual coordination in children and younger and older adults. *Human Development, 21,* 334–345.

Whitehurst, G. J. (1982). Language development. In B. B. Wolman (Ed.), *Handbook of developmental psychology.* Englewood Cliffs, NJ: Prentice-Hall.

Whorf, B. (1956). *Language, thought, and reality.* Cambridge, MA: MIT Press.

Wilkie, F., & Eisdorfer, C. (1971). Intelligence and blood pressure in the aged. *Science, 172,* 959–962.

Wilkinson, A. (1976). Counting strategies and semantic analyses as applied to class inclusion. *Cognitive Psychology, 8,* 64–85.

Willems, E. P. (1973). Behavioral ecology and experimental analysis: Courtship is not enough. In J. R. Nesselroade & H. W. Reese (Eds.), *Life-span developmental psychology: Methodological issues* (pp. 195–217). New York: Academic Press.

Willis, S. L. (1985). Towards an educational psychology of the older adult learner: Intellectual and cognitive bases. In J. E. Birren & K. W. Schaie (Eds.), *Handbook of the psychology of aging* (2nd ed., pp. 818–847). New York: Van Nostrand Reinhold.

Willis, S. L., & Baltes, P. B. (1980). Intelligence in adulthood and aging: Contemporary issues. In L. W. Poon (Ed.), *Aging in the 1980s: Psychological issues* (pp. 260–272). Washington, DC: American Psychological Association.

Willis, S. L., Blieszner, R., & Baltes, P. B. (1981). Intellectual training research in aging: Modification of performance on the fluid ability of figural relations. *Journal of Educational Psychology, 73,* 41–50.

Wilson, J. R., DeFries, J. C., McClearn, G. E., Vandenberg, S. G., Johnson, R. C., & Rashed, M. N. (1975). Cognitive abilities: Use of family data as a control to assess sex differences in two ethnic groups. *International Journal of Aging and Human Development, 6,* 261–276.

Wimer, R. E. (1960). Age differences in incidental and intentional learning. *Journal of Gerontology, 15,* 79–82.

Winer, G. A. (1980). Class-inclusion reasoning in children: A review of the empirical literature. *Child Development 51,* 309–328.

Witkin, H. A., Dyk, R. B., Faterson, G. E., Goodenough, D. R., & Karp, S. A. (1962). *Psychological differentiation.* New York: Wiley.

Witkin, H. A., & Goodenough, D. R. (1981). *Cognitive style: Essence and origins.* New York: International Universities Press.

Witkin, H. A., Lewis, H. B., Hertzman, M., Machover, K., Meissner, P. B., & Wapner, S. (1954). *Personality through perception.* New York: Harper.

Wolf, M. M., Giles, D. K., & Hall, R. V. (1968). Experiments with token reinforcement in a remedial classroom. *Behavioral Research and Therapy, 6,* 51–64.

Wolman, B. B. (1973). *Dictionary of behavioral science.* New York: Van Nostrand Reinhold.

Wood, D. J., Bruner, J. S., & Ross, G. (1976). The role of tutoring in problem solving. *Journal of Child Psychology and Psychiatry, 17,* 89–100.

Yerkes, R. M., & Dodson, J. D. (1908). The relation of strengths of stimulus to rapidity of habit-formation. *Journal of Comparative Neurological Psychology, 18,* 459–482.

Yonas, A., Oberg, C., & Norcia, A. (1978). Development of sensitivity to binocular information for the approach of an object. *Developmental Psychology, 14,* 147–152.

Yonas, A., & Pick, H. L., Jr. (1975). An approach to the study of infant space perception. In L. B. Cohen & P. Salapatek (Eds.), *Infant perception: From sensation to cognition: Vol. 2. Perception of space, speech, and sound* (pp. 3–31). New York: Academic Press.

Young, M. L. (1966). Problem-solving performance in two age groups. *Journal of Gerontology, 21,* 505–510.

Youniss, J. (1975). Another perspective on social cognition. In A. D. Pick (Ed.), *Minnesota Symposia on Child Psychology* (Vol. 9, pp. 173–193). Minneapolis: University of Minnesota Press.

Yussen, S. R., & Levy, V. M., Jr. (1975). Developmental changes in predicting one's own span of short-term memory. *Journal of Experimental Child Psychology, 19,* 502–508.

Zachry, W. (1978). Ordinality and interdependence of representation and language development in infancy. *Child Development, 49,* 681–687.

Zajonc, R. B. (1980). Feeling and thinking: Preferences need no inferences. *American Psychologist, 35,* 151–175.

Zajonc, R. B. (1984). On the primacy of affect. *American Psychologist, 39,* 117–123.

Zaporozhets, A. V. (1965). The development of perception in the preschool child. *Monographs of the Society for Research in Child Development, 30*(2, Serial No. 100).

Zarit, S. H., Cole, K. D., & Guider, R. L. (1981). Memory training strategies and subjective complaints of memory in the aged. *Gerontologist, 21,* 158–164.

Zelniker, T., & Jeffrey, W. E. (1976). Reflective and impulsive children: Strategies of information processing underlying differences in problem solving. *Monographs of the Society for Research in Child Development, 41*(5, Serial No. 168).

Zentall, S. (1975). Optimal stimulation as theoretical basis of hyperactivity. *American Journal of Orthopsychiatry, 45,* 549–563.

Zigler, E., & Berman, W. (1983). Discerning the future of early childhood intervention. *American Psychologist, 38,* 894–906.

Zigler, E., & Trickett, P. K. (1978). IQ, social competence, and evaluation of early childhood intervention programs. *American Psychologist, 33,* 789–798.

Zimmerman, B. J. (1983). Social learning theory: A contextualist account of cognitive functioning. In C. J. Brainerd (Ed.), *Recent advances in cognitive developmental theory: Progress in cognitive development research* (pp. 1–50). New York: Springer.

Zimmerman, B. J., & Dialessi, F. (1973). Modeling influences on children's creative behavior. *Journal of Educational Psychology, 65,* 127–134.

Glossary

Absolute space the view that space exists independently of any objects contained within it and remains unchanged even if those objects are removed.

Accommodation adapting to the environment by modifying one's internal organization or mental structures to fit external conditions.

Adaptation the process of adjusting to the demands of one's environment.

Age differentiation hypothesis the hypothesis that abstract intelligence changes in organization with age from a general ability factor to a more loosely organized group of special abilities or factors.

Algorithms problem-solving strategies or methods that are guaranteed, sooner or later, to generate a solution to a problem.

Allocentric a type of spatial reference system in which spatial locations are defined by positions external to the person.

Analogical relating to a form of mental representation or imagery which closely corresponds to the actual physical object being represented.

Anticipatory schemata the mental structures or plans that direct perceptual exploration.

Aphasia a condition characterized by a variety of language dysfunctions including an inability to talk, to understand language, or both.

Arousal a general level of alertness that serves to keep the attentional system activated to receive perceptual inputs.

Assimilation adapting to the environment by fitting external conditions to one's internal cognitive structures or organization.

Associative learning according to Jensen, a type of learning involving abilities such as short-term memory, attention, and simple associative thinking.

Attenuation model a model of attention proposed by Treisman that involves multiple channels of processing; the greater the number of channels that operate, the weaker or more attenuated the incoming signals become.

Attribution the inferences people draw about the cause for others', as well as their own, behavior.

Automatic detection on perceptual search tasks, detection that does not require attentional control from subjects.

Automatic processing a rapid, parallel process that requires little attentional effort and demands little direct subject control.

Behaviorism a school of thought founded by John B. Watson that favors stimulus-response learning as the explanation of development.

Black English a distinctive dialect used mainly by inner-city Black children that has its own complex language structure and logical rules.

Blank-trials procedure a procedure that provides subjects with feedback or no feedback over a series of learning trials and that can be used to predict what hypotheses or rules they are using.

Canalization Waddington's concept that genes channel development along a predetermined path or track.

Cataracts a condition occurring primarily in later adulthood in which the lens of the eye becomes opaque.

Categorical perception the perception of sounds as discontinuous or distinctive even though they lie along a speech continuum.

Central learning a type of learning frequently measured in studies of attentional development which reflects the amount of attention devoted to the relevant (or central) features of a task.

Class inclusion the ability to classify objects hierarchically in terms of a superordinate class and two or more subclasses while simultaneously maintaining the identity of the subclasses.

Clinical method a type of interview procedure in which a child's unexpected answers to a series of loosely structured questions are followed up with additional questions.

Cognition in the most general sense, any process which allows an organism to know and be aware.

Cognitive conflict a procedure used by Piagetian researchers to induce contradictions in children's reasoning in order to study their cognitive development.

Cognitive learning according to Jensen, a type of learning involving abstract reasoning, symbolic thinking, and problem-solving skills.

Cognitive map the internal representation of a small-scale or large-scale spatial environment.

Cognitive styles an individual's distinctive ways of organizing, attending, processing, remembering, and thinking about perceptual and cognitive tasks.

Cohort a group of persons born during approximately the same period of historical time or experiencing the same historical events.

Complementary groupings categorization of objects according to their complementarity in functions.

Concept formation a type of concept learning problem in which the subject must identify the dimensions and values in the problem as well as learn the relevant concept.

Concept identification a type of concept learning problem in which all the dimensions and values of the problem are described in advance and the subject must identify the rule or concept.

Configuration well-organized spatial knowledge that represents an integration of landmark and route information.

Conscious the aspect of people's mental life about which they are fully aware.

Constraint-seeking on the twenty-questions task, a question that eliminates several items from the stimulus array and that constrains the number of remaining possibilities.

Constructivist view in philosophy, the view that organisms construct their experience and knowledge through their interactions with the world.

Content the raw data of intelligence that can be measured by a standardized intelligence test.

Contextual validity the extent to which developmental changes that have been observed or manipulated under laboratory conditions can be generalized to those occurring in the real world.

Contrast the principle that any pairs of words in a language have contrasting meanings.

Controlled processing a slow, serial process that requires a good deal of mental effort and allows the subject a large degree of control.

Controlled search   a serial search procedure in which subjects compare each member of a perceptual set.

Conventional   in Kohlberg's theory, the level of moral thinking at which the individual is concerned with maintaining social conventions and the expectations of social groups for their own sake.

Conventionality   the principle that contrasts in word meanings depend on the conventional meanings assigned by the language community.

Convergent thinking   the ability to converge upon or generate the appropriate or correct answer to a problem.

Creod   the path along which all members of a species tend to develop unless their environment is atypical.

Cross-sectional method   a research design in which different age groups are compared on a particular behavior at approximately the same time.

Crystallized intelligence   in Horn and Cattell's theory, a type of intelligence that depends on systematic schooling and acculturation experiences and that steadily increases over most of the life span.

Dedifferentiation   the return of the organization of specialized intellectual abilities in adulthood to the general, global structure characteristic of childhood intelligence.

Deep structure   the abstract structures and relations between words in a sentence as well as the intended meaning of a sentence.

Depth perception   the capacity to perceive a third dimension projecting outward from a flat, two-dimensional surface.

Developmental psycholinguistics   a field of study involving the developmental investigation of language acquisition.

Deviation IQs   intelligence quotients computed on the basis of an individual's performance on an intelligence test relative to the performance of others within the same age group.

Differentiation   the ability to detect perceptual features that distinguish one class of objects or events from others.

Discrepancy principle   Kagan's principle that infants prefer to look at moderately novel stimuli and that this preference is most optimal for eliciting attentional development.

Distinctive features   in Eleanor Gibson's theory of perception, the dimensions of difference between two or more objects.

Divergent thinking   the ability to generate many novel associations to a stimulus; a measure of creativity.

Divided attention   an individual's capacity to pay attention to more than one task at a time.

Echoic   a type of sensory memory involving the auditory modality.

Egocentric   a type of spatial reference system in which spatial positions are defined in relation to the person's body.

Egocentric speech   speech occurring in social circumstances, but not intended for communicative purposes.

Egocentrism   a general inability or failure to differentiate between the views of one's self and those of others.

Elementarism   in the mechanistic model of development, the assumption that all behaviors are reducible to their simplest parts or elements.

Empathy   the ability to be consciously aware of other people's inner feelings and respond affectively to their situation.

Empiricism   the philosophical position that all knowledge comes by way of the senses and grows through experience.

Enrichment an intervention designed to enhance or optimize development beyond what it would be under naturally occurring conditions.

Episodic memory in contrast to semantic memory, memory that primarily involves recall of personal experiences and their temporal relations.

Epistemology a branch of philosophy dealing with the processes of knowing and the nature of knowledge.

Equilibration in Piagetian theory, the successive shifts in an organism's balance with the environment to increasingly higher adaptive levels.

Euclidean a three-dimensional model of space which includes the dimensions of height, width, and distance.

Factor analysis a correlational technique for observing the clustering of relationships among a large number of items or responses on a test.

Far transfer measures which contain content not closely related to training measures and which are used to assess the generalizability or transfer of training.

Field dependence a cognitive style characterized by dependence on the surrounding perceptual field for contextual cues.

Field independence a cognitive style characterized by an ability to function independently of the surrounding perceptual field and to ignore misleading contextual cues.

Figurative knowledge in Piaget's theory, knowledge that is based on static perception of the properties of objects or events in the world.

Filtering model a type of attentional model in which only one informational input gets processed at a single time.

Fluid intelligence in Horn and Cattell's theory, a type of intelligence that is relatively independent of any systematic educational or acculturation experiences and that increases through adolescence and then declines in middle and later adulthood.

Formative evaluation a type of evaluation that focuses on monitoring the process, strategy, and targets of intervention.

Function referring to inborn intellectual operations or functioning.

Functional core hypothesis Katherine Nelson's hypothesis that the child initially names objects or events in terms of their functional relation to the child's actions.

Functional fixedness the tendency to view an object in terms of its characteristic function rather than envisioning novel uses.

Functionality the degree to which children wish to express an intention in their speech.

Generalizability when results of a study can be applied to individuals or cultures other than those studied.

Generalization the transfer of cognitive strategies over tasks or situations.

Generative the ability to generate a practically infinite variety of novel sentences from a finite set of rules.

Gerontology the scientific study of the aging process and the factors that influence it.

Gestalt psychology a school of psychology which emphasizes the role of organized wholes in perception, problem solving, and other psychological processes.

Heuristic search a problem-solving strategy that is limited to the portion of the problem space most likely to produce a solution.

Holophrase the single-word utterances that children use to stand for whole phrases or sentences.

Horizontal décalages lags or gaps occurring in the cognitive developmental sequence when the attainment of the mental structure to solve one problem precedes the attainment of structures to solve another problem.

Hypothesis-scanning on the twenty-questions task, a type of question that eliminates only one item at a time from a stimulus array.

Hypothetical constructs concepts invented to describe and explain relationships among events, objects, properties, or variables.

Iconic a type of sensory memory involving the visual modality.

Illocutionary a stage in the development of intentional communication when infants begin to use signals to make nonverbal requests and to initiate social interactions.

Illusion a perceptual phenomenon that occurs when the perceived properties of objects differ from their actual properties.

Imaginary audience a self-conscious feeling of always being "on stage" which results from adolescents' belief that the concerns of others are the same as theirs.

Immanent justice the child's belief that any violation of rules results in strict and swift punishment inflicted by nature or God.

Impulsivity a cognitive style characterized by rapid responses to a problem without consideration of all solution alternatives.

Incidental learning a type of learning frequently measured in studies of attentional development which reflects the amount of attention devoted to the irrelevant (or incidental) features of a task.

Information processing a term borrowed from communications theory referring to the acquisition, coding, processing, storage, and transformation of information.

Inner speech in Vygotsky's theory, speech that is internalized, highly abbreviated, and consists mostly of predicates rather than subjects.

INRC group a higher-order system of transformational rules, comprising identity, negation, reciprocity, and correlation, which are used to manipulate mental operations.

Insight the experience of suddenly grasping or seeing how the elements of a problem fit together to form a solution.

Intelligence quotient the ratio of a person's mental age to his or her chronological age multiplied by 100.

Intervention the systematic attempt to modify the course of cognitive development and aging for purposes of preventing cognitive deficits and enhancing cognitive functioning and psychological well-being.

Introspection a technique by which subjects are taught to observe and report on the content of their thoughts and feelings.

Invariants objects that have the same perceptual features across individual members despite variations in other features.

Kinetic imagery the ability to mentally represent the transformation of an object in motion from an initial state to a final state.

Landmarks the salient locations, objects, and points in the environment around which people organize their spatial ability.

Language acquisition device an inborn propensity or predisposition for acquiring and understanding language.

Levels-of-processing model a model in which memory is characterized as a continuum of processing ranging from shallow, less permanent encoding of sensory features of stimuli to deeper, more permanent encoding of semantic features.

Lexical contrast theory a recently proposed theory of the acquisition of word meaning based on the principles of contrast and conventionality.

Linear syllogism a special type of transitive inference problem in which subjects are presented with two premises, each describing a relation between two terms, and are asked to order the terms in the premises in a linear sequence.

Linguistic determinism Whorf's hypothesis that the structure of one's language determines all other forms of one's perception and thinking.

Linguistic relativity Whorf's hypothesis that thinking is relative to the forms of language characteristic of one's particular culture; a corollary to the linguistic determinism hypothesis.

Linguistics the formal study of the structure of language.

Locutionary a stage in the development of intentional communication when infants begin to use speech sounds together with nonverbal signals to convey requests and to interact socially.

Longitudinal method a research design in which behavior changes in a single age group are studied over two or more points in time.

Long-term store in information-processing models, a permanent storage structure that can hold a virtually limitless amount of information and that contains very old as well as more recent memories.

Maintenance the durability of the effects of cognitive training or intervention procedures over time.

Means-ends analysis a problem-solving strategy involving a comparison of differences between the initial state and the goal state of a problem and an identification of the operators and subgoals that will reduce those differences.

Mediation deficiencies conditions that occur when a memory strategy is produced either spontaneously or after training but does not benefit recall performance.

Memory decay the weakening of the memory trace in the storage structures of the information-processing system.

Mental age a measure of mental ability based on the number of items a person gets correct on an intelligence test relative to the number of items the average person of the same chronological age gets correct.

Mental imagery the mental representation of objects or events in either verbal or nonverbal form.

Mental rotation the ability to turn a mental image clockwise or counterclockwise in your mind so that it matches a standard.

Metacognition knowledge of one's own cognitive processes and the factors that influence them.

Metalinguistic knowledge a person's knowledge or awareness of the rules of language.

Metamemory knowledge or awareness of one's own memory processes and how they operate.

Minimum distance principle the principle that the noun or pronoun phrase immediately preceding an infinitive in a sentence is the subject of the verb.

Morphemes the smallest units of sound that convey meaning in a language.

Morphology the study of the basic units of meaning in a language.

Motherese a simplified form of speech characterized by pauses between sentences, repetition of key phrases, and simple syntax; also known as baby talk.

Multiple classification the capacity to reason simultaneously about two separate classes and to identify the dimensions common to both as the multiple class.

Nativism the philosophical position that infants are innately equipped to organize rudimentary knowledge about time and space.

Nature referring to inner biological or genetic causes of behavior.

Near transfer measures which contain content similar to training measures and which are used to evaluate the generalizability or transfer of training.

Non-Euclidean a model of space, such as in Einstein's theory, that allows for the possibility of more than three dimensions.

Nonreversal shift a type of shift occurring on an optional-shift problem that involves switching to a completely different dimension to solve the problem.

Nurture referring to environmental or experiential causes of behavior.

Object concept the knowledge that objects that have disappeared from one's immediate view still continue to exist.

Operative knowledge in Piaget's theory, knowledge which derives from the ability to think about and envision transformations from one state of a problem to another.

Operators in problem solving, the actions or sequences of steps taken to reach a goal.

Optimally exercised ability a developmental function which is determined by what an individual is capable of doing when given optimal exercise or training in a cognitive domain.

Organization the tendency of all organisms to organize and systematize their psychological functioning into integrated wholes.

Orthogenetic principle in Werner's theory, the principle that development proceeds from a global, undifferentiated state to a state of differentiation and hierarchic integration.

Overextension the phenomenon in which children employ a single word to cover much more than the conventional meaning of the word.

Overjustification effect the reduced satisfaction in engaging in a once rewarding activity that occurs when a person receives an external reward for something he or she enjoys doing for its own sake.

Overregularization a phenomenon occurring when children first acquire the rules for regular plural and past tense endings and overextend these rules to irregular forms.

Paired-associate learning a learning task involving memorization of paired stimulus-response items and recall of the response items when the stimulus items are presented alone.

Paradigmatic associations word associations that are the same part of speech as the stimulus word.

Paradigmatic shifts in science, a change that occurs when an accumulation of unexpected discoveries leads to a new way of thinking about scientific phenomena.

Perception the process by which organisms organize and extract meaning from the sensory information in their environment.

Perceptual cycle Neisser's model of perception depicting the perceptual process as a continuous and cyclic activity.

Perceptual salience the relative sensitivity of the perceptual system to dimensions, relations, and categories in the stimulus environment.

Perlocutionary the earliest stage in the development of intentional communication when an infant's communicative acts such as babbling or smiling have an effect on the listener but the infant is unaware of the effect.

Person perception the way in which people view the internal and external attributes of others.

Personal fable a story an adolescent constructs which idealizes his or her unique feelings and experiences.

Perspectivism the capacity to differentiate between one's own point of view and the views of others.

Philosophical wisdom wisdom or judgment that involves the relationship of the self to human life and the world at large.

Phonemes the most basic units of sound used to distinguish one utterance from another by producing a change in meaning.

Phonemic contraction a process that begins at the end of the first year of life when the number of phonemes produced decreases as a result of linguistic shaping by the child's particular culture.

Phonemic expansion a process occurring during the first year of life when the number of phonemes increases dramatically.

Pivot–open grammar a grammatical system used to characterize children's early multiword utterances, especially those combining adjectival words and nouns.

Postconventional in Kohlberg's theory, the highest level of moral thinking where an effort is made to define moral values and principles that have universal and logical validity apart from a group or society.

Practical space the capacity to move in space or to manipulate spatial objects.

Practical wisdom wisdom or judgment that relates to one's personal life and life span.

Pragmatics term referring to the appropriate use of language in its physical and social context.

Preconventional in Kohlberg's theory, the first level of moral thinking in which the individual interprets right or wrong according to physical needs and rewarding or punishing consequences.

Presbyopia the inability of the eye to focus on near objects; also called farsightedness.

Prevention an intervention aimed at preventing a problem behavior from occurring or recurring.

Primacy effect an effect indicating that initial items have been recalled better than items in the middle of a series; depends on long-term store processes.

Primary memory a system for maintaining information in conscious awareness in short-term store.

Proactive interference a phenomenon that occurs when previously learned material interferes with the memorization of new material.

Problem-finding stage a postformal stage of cognitive development, characterized by an ability to think creatively, to find new problems, and to raise general questions about ill-defined problems.

Problem-solving set a habitual way of solving a problem based on familiar or routine solutions which creates difficulty in envisioning alternative problem solutions.

Problem space a problem solver's mental representation of the initial and final states of a problem as well as the various intermediate states.

Production deficiencies conditions that exist when individuals, for reasons other than ability or skill, do not spontaneously generate mnemonic activities that would benefit their memory recall.

Production inefficiency an inability to carry out a memory strategy skillfully and effectively.

Production system a set of condition-action rules for changing one problem state into another.

Projective spatial concepts involving the idea that certain linear properties of objects remain invariant with different changes in perspective.

Propositional the representation of objects or events in verbal or conceptual form rather than pictorial form.

Prosocial behaviors behaviors such as cooperation or altruism that are intended to benefit another person without the expectation of a personal reward.

Prospective memory memory for future actions or events.

Psycholinguistics a field of study focusing on the psychological aspects of language.

Psychometric models models of intelligence that are concerned with practical issues such as the construction of tests and the prediction of future performance as well as the theoretical nature of intelligence.

Pupillary reflex the automatic contraction of the iris and the pupil in response to bright light.

Random search the random application of operators or permissible moves in a problem until the correct solution is generated.

Recall a memory task involving retrieval of information from storage in the absence of any stimulus information.

Recast a sentence with the same core meaning as the original but with a simplified, limited structural change such as the addition of articles or auxiliary verbs.

Recency effect superior recall for the last three or four items on a list, assumed to come from short-term memory store.

Reception method in concept learning studies, a method in which the experimenter chooses the stimulus items and the subject decides if each item is a positive or negative instance of the concept.

Recognition a memory task requiring subjects to match information in storage with the presence of certain stimulus information.

Recruitment a shortening of the loudness scale which leads to the perception of a change in stimulus intensity of an auditory signal as much greater than it actually is.

Reflectivity a cognitive style characterized by a careful approach to problems and consideration of all solution alternatives.

Relative space the view that space does not exist independently of the objects within it and is transformed by changes in the relative position of objects and observer.

Remediation an intervention designed to remove or correct an existing problem behavior.

Reminiscence the act or process of calling to mind a past life experience or event.

Representational space the capacity to mentally represent spatial objects and their relationships.

Retroactive interference a phenomenon that occurs when recently learned material interferes with memory for previously learned information.

Retrospective memory memory for past experiences and events.

Reversal shift a type of shift occurring on an optional-shift problem when the same dimension continues to be reinforced but the subject "reverses" on that dimension by selecting the alternate value.

Reversibility   the ability to mentally reverse an action or operation by returning an object to its original state.

Role taking   the ability to adopt the roles and perspectives of other people.

Routes   patterns of action that guide a person's travel between spatial landmarks.

Scaffold   a support device used to extend the linguistic skills of children and to simplify their task in the learning process.

Schema   an abstract representation of a story or an event that guides subsequent recall.

Secondary memory   a permanent long-term storage system for information processing that has a practically limitless storage capacity.

Selection method   in concept learning studies, a method in which the subject selects the stimulus items and identifies each as a positive or negative instance of the concept.

Selective survival   a process involving differential survivorship of particular individuals or subgroups in the population which may bias results of longitudinal studies.

Self-concept   the sum total of ideas and perceptions an individual has about himself or herself.

Semantic differential scale   a self-rating scale that is used to assess self-concept and that consists of several bipolar adjectives describing different personality dimensions.

Semantic feature hypothesis   Eve Clark's hypothesis that the meaning of a word depends on the semantic components or features attached to the word.

Semantic memory   memory that consists of organized knowledge about meanings of words and other verbal symbols, about relations among them, and about rules for the manipulation of these words and symbols.

Semantics   the ways in which words and sentences are combined together to form meaning.

Semiotic function   term referring to the symbolic functioning that marks the beginning of the preoperational stage of thought.

Senile miosis   a gradual decrease in the size of the pupil from late adolescence onward which affects brightness discrimination.

Sensation   the initial activation of the sense organ receptors by sensory stimuli in the environment.

Sensorimotor scheme   an infant's organized pattern of activity or series of actions for dealing with environmental demands.

Sensory register   in information-processing models, the storage structure that briefly registers sensory information before it is transferred to short-term storage.

Sequential methods   complex research designs which involve combinations of cross-sectional and longitudinal designs.

Serial position curve   a curve that plots recall scores as a function of when an item appeared in a series of items recalled.

Seriation   the ability to order objects in a series along some abstract dimension such as number or height.

Shadowing   an experimental technique in which subjects listen to two spoken messages simultaneously and are asked to pay attention to one message and ignore the other.

Short-term store   in information-processing models, a temporary storage structure that can hold only a limited number of items in conscious awareness for a brief period of time.

Similarity groupings categorization of objects according to similarity in function or category.

Situationist the view that personality characteristics depend upon particular situations and may vary from one situation to another.

Size constancy the capacity to perceive that the size of an object remains constant despite changes in the retinal image resulting from a change in viewing position.

Sleeper effects effects which may not be immediately apparent in an intervention program but which become manifest at a later point in development.

Social cognition knowledge about the self, social roles, and relations between individuals or groups.

Social learning the learning of adaptive behaviors using stimulus cues from the social environment.

Sociolinguistics the study of language focusing on the social and cultural context of language use.

Span of immediate memory the upper limit on the number of items that can be reported from sensory memory.

Spatial reference system a point or set of points with respect to which spatial position is defined.

Stereopsis the process by which visual images from each of our eyes are combined to produce one image with depth.

Structure in the most general sense, an organism's level of mental organization or ability.

Structure-of-intellect model Guilford's multidimensional model of intelligence consisting of the dimensions of operations, content, and product.

Summative evaluation a type of evaluation designed to provide information about the overall effectiveness and outcome of an intervention procedure.

Surface structure the phonological features of words and their order in a sentence.

Surroundingness the concept that large-scale space surrounds individuals, forcing them to construct and explore their spatial environment.

Syntagmatic word associations that are a different part of speech than the stimulus word.

Syntax the rules by which morphemes and words are combined to produce more complex clauses, phrases, and sentences.

Telegraphic speech a type of abbreviated speech that lacks less informative or communicatively nonessential words such as conjunctions and prepositions.

Terminal drop the rapid and precipitous drop in mental abilities a few months or years prior to physical death.

Theories sets of concepts and ideas designed to provide specific explanations for scientific phenomena.

Topological spatial concepts in which spatial relationships are defined by very general principles such as proximity, order, enclosure, and continuity.

Totalism a conception of self characterized by arbitrary, rigid, and absolute boundaries.

Trait a characteristic aspect of one's personality that manifests itself regardless of particular situations or circumstances.

Transformational grammar a grammatical system proposed by Noam Chomsky consisting of a set of transformational rules for converting the deep structure of sentences into surface structures.

Transitive inference a type of inference involving logical reasoning about the comparative relations among a seriated set of objects.

Transitivity   the ability to note that a relation between one object and a second object, and between a second object and a third object, implies something about the relation between the first object and the third object.

Type I illusions   illusions resulting from physiological changes in the sensory receptors.

Type II illusions   illusions which are based on the functioning of intellectual mechanisms.

Type I processing   a type of maintenance rehearsal characterized by rote repetition of material in working memory.

Type II processing   a type of elaborative rehearsal involving the generation of images of items and semantic associations between these images.

Unconscious   the part of people's mental life about which they are unaware.

Underextension   the phenomenon in which children use a single word to refer to less than is conventionally conveyed by the word.

Unexercised ability   a developmental function representing what a normal healthy person would be able to do in a cognitive domain if not given any special training or exercise.

U-shaped functions   nonlinear developmental changes involving the initial appearance of a behavior, an apparent disappearance of this behavior, and a later reappearance or recovery period.

Verbal transformation effect   an auditory illusion that occurs when a sound or word presented repeatedly is perceived as having changed.

Virtual object   a visible, but not tangible, object produced by stereoscopic glasses that is used in studies of infant depth perception.

Visual accommodation   the ability of the lens of the eye to adjust its shape to bring a distant object into sharp focus.

Visual acuity   a term referring to how clearly the visual system can discern fine detail.

Visual cliff   an apparatus frequently used in studies of infant perception to test infants' ability to perceive depth.

Working memory   the amount of processing or mental work that can be carried out in short-term memory.

Zeitgeist   the prevailing ideology and outlook characteristic of a particular time.

Name Index

Subject Index

Formal operational period (*cont.*)
  and self-concept, 398–399
  structured wholes, 380–381
Freud's theory, 8, 24

Generalizability, 10, 68, 72, 482–483
Generalization, 35, 469–470
Genetic epistemology, 28
Gerontology, 14
Gestalt psychology, 8–9, 86–88
  figure-ground reversals, 87–88
  perceptual principles of, 86–87, 161
  theory of problem solving, 286–288

Habituation techniques, 193
Hemispheric differences, 170–171, 214–215
Hormonal differences, 170–171
Hyperactivity *See* Attention deficit disorder
Hypothesis testing, 37, 309–313
Hypothetical constructs, 24

Imitation, 26, 35–36
  deferred, 188–189
  and language learning, 209–210
Individual differences in cognition, 18, 62–63, 119–124, 145, 167–171, 221–225, 357, 360, 362, 366–376, 485–486
Inference abilities, 55, 208, 271, 303–305, 395, 398, 412
Information processing, 10, 25, 40–48, 448
  adaptive production system, 46
  advantages of, 44–45
  and affective behavior, 431, 482
  balance-scale apparatus, 45–48, 380–381
  changes with age, 44
  chronometric methods, 44
  computer simulation, 10, 43, 46
  contextualistic influences on, 53
  descriptions of change, 56–59
  input-throughput-output, 41
  limitations of, 53, 480–482
  and memory, 232–233, 236–238, 264
  and problem solving, 288–294
  production system, 46
  protocol analysis, 44–45, 483–484
  tree diagram, 46
INRC group, 380

Intellectual development
  in adulthood, 363–366
  in childhood and adolescence, 356–363
  cross-sectional vs. longitudinal findings, 364–366
  in infancy, 354–356
  prediction of, 354–358, 373
Intelligence
  adoption studies of, 363
  Alzheimer's disease, 369–371
  and blood pressure, 369
  and brain damage, 337, 349
  content of, 30–31
  definitions of, 29–30, 334–335
  divergent vs. convergent thinking, 324, 328, 346, 382, 459
  and education, 371
  exceptionality in, 337, 342–343
  factor analytic approaches, 344–347, 350–351
  fluid vs. crystallized, 346–350, 442–444, 470
  function of, 30–32
  G factor, 344, 350
  and health status, 368–371
  hereditary factors in, 361–363, 445
  and language ability, 355
  multiple intelligences, 336–339
  and occupation, 372–373
  parenting effects on, 361
  performance intelligence, 17–18, 152, 344
  and personality, 371–372
  psychometric models, 338–351
  racial and ethnic differences in, 360–363
  S factors, 344, 350
  social class differences in, 360–363, 372–373
  structure of, 30, 32–33
  structure-of-intellect model, 324, 345–346
  traits of, 335–336
  triarchic theory, 351–353
  verbal intelligence, 17–18, 152, 205, 344
Intelligence test, 13, 28, 31, 71, 359–360
  age-fair, 375
  biases in, 358–360
  Binet-Simon test, 341–342, 363
  culture-fair, 358–359
  development of the, 339–342
  deviation IQs, 341